SUPPLEMENTARY FILMSTRIPS

Continued on back end sheet

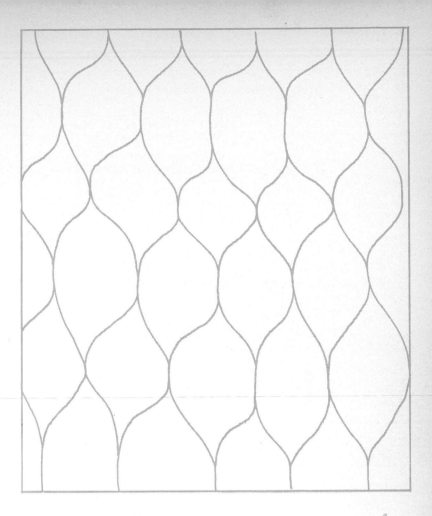

HISTOLOGY

second edition

THOMAS S. LEESON, M.D.

Professor and Chairman, Department of
Anatomy, University of Alberta, Faculty
of Medicine, Edmonton, Alberta, Canada

AND

C. ROLAND LEESON, M.D.

Professor and Chairman, Department of
Anatomy, The University of Missouri
School of Medicine, Columbia, Missouri

W. B. SAUNDERS COMPANY
Philadelphia   London   Toronto

W. B. Saunders Company: West Washington Square
Philadelphia, Pa. 19105

12 Dyott Street
London, WC1A 1DB

1835 Yonge Street
Toronto 7, Ontario

Listed here is the latest translated edition of this book together with the language of the translation and the publisher.

Spanish (1st Edition) — Editorial Interamericana, Mexico

HISTOLOGY   SBN 0-7216-5711-7

Print No.:   9   8   7   6   5   4

PREFACE

The first edition of *Histology* was an attempt to offer a textbook that was sufficiently detailed to satisfy the requirements of professional students and senior science undergraduates, but which eliminated all unnecessary detail and material that is not usually considered a legitimate part of a course in histology. Its acceptance by both students and faculty was extremely gratifying. Since the first edition was published in the summer of 1966, the trend toward more basic and abbreviated courses in the basic sciences has continued and the justification for a "short" textbook has perhaps increased.

In preparing the second edition, the greatest problem undoubtedly has been to prevent an unreasonable growth in size of the book. Knowledge of the subject has increased and continues to increase. We are aware that standard textbooks of histology show a tendency to wax progressively in content and weight with succeeding editions. We consider this unfortunate and in this edition we have attempted to include reviews of recent advances without augmenting substantially the length of the text. All chapters have undergone critical review and revision. A conscious effort has been made to increase both the quality and number of the illustrations. In great part, it is the increase in illustrative material which accounts for the modest increase in the number of pages. Among the most significant additions are light photomicrographs of Epon-embedded sections. We feel that a study of such material, representing as it does an application of refined electron microscopic techniques to light microscopy, will assist the student in his attempts to integrate knowledge gained from his perusal of traditional light microscopic preparations and from electron photomicrographs.

Another innovation in illustration is the availability of two 35 mm. supplementary filmstrips carrying a total of 100 color photomicrographs. The instructor may project these transparencies, and the individual student may, if he wishes, study them privately with an inexpensive desk-top viewer.* The color pictures are keyed to the text and the text to them. These filmstrips are not intended to include a comprehensive selection of all histological material. Many illustrations gain little by color presentation. However, an attempt has been made to select tissues

---

*Two such viewers we recommend are Viewlex Jr., and the Standard; they can be ordered directly through the W. B. Saunders Company.

which are more effectively shown in color than in black and white, with a spectrum of different staining techniques.

We have retained the previous order of presentation of subject matter and the basic division of the text into two parts. The student is urged to acquire a firm understanding of the appearance and functions of the cell and of the primary tissues and their specializations, as presented in Part I, before proceeding to a study of the organ systems (Part II).

In the preparation of this edition we have been guided in no small part by the comments of reviewers and of the many colleagues and students who have criticized constructively both text and illustrations. It is a real pleasure to acknowledge the assistance of colleagues in permitting us to use their illustrations. We particularly wish to express our gratitude to Dr. Fritz Jacoby and Dr. Richard Ellis, who provided us with comprehensive evaluations of the first edition. Many improvements in this edition are the direct result of their thoughtful suggestions. We also wish to thank Mrs. M. Wylie and Mrs. Mildred Lind for secretarial assistance and our publishers for their encouragement, courtesy, and patience.

C. ROLAND LEESON

THOMAS S. LEESON

CONTENTS

Part Two HISTOLOGY OF THE ORGAN SYSTEMS

Chapter 11

THE CIRCULATORY SYSTEM

Chapter 12

Chapter 13

Chapter 14

Part I—The Oral Cavity

Part II—The Tubular Digestive Tract

PART ONE

GENERAL PRINCIPLES AND PRIMARY TISSUES

CHAPTER 1

INTRODUCTION

Histology is a term derived from the Greek *histos*, meaning tissue, and *logia*, meaning "the study of" or knowledge. Literally, then, it refers to the knowledge, or science, of tissues, both plant and animal. This textbook is restricted, in the main, to a consideration of human histology.

What does the term "histology" encompass today? Anatomy can be subdivided into that which is visible to the naked eye, gross anatomy, and that which can be seen only with the aid of a microscope, microscopic anatomy. The latter can be further subdivided into organology (the study of organs), histology (tissues), and cytology (cells). Today the term "histology" is used loosely to include all subdivisions of microscopic anatomy, and it is in this sense that the term is used here.

Histology involves, therefore, the study not only of tissues but of individual cells and organ systems. And since histology refers to the study of cells, tissues, and organs, it embraces a study of function as well as of structure. Thus a study of histology not only complements the study of gross anatomy, but provides a structural basis for the study of physiology. The correlation between structure and function perhaps provides the reason why histology is such an intriguing and readily understandable subject. The student will find that if he ex- amines a structure he can deduce much about its function; conversely, if he knows the function of an organ or tissue, he can forecast much of its microscopic structure.

A knowledge of the normal is a necessary prelude to the study of the abnormal (pathology), which deals with the alterations in structure and function of the body and of its organs, tissues, and cells caused by disease. Hence the study of histology is fundamental within the medical and dental curriculum. For biology students not proceeding to professional degrees, it provides a reservoir of valuable knowledge. Too often in many special fields of biological science the student becomes involved in problems of a functional nature without sufficient consideration of the underlying microscopic structure.

In our study of histology, there are two important considerations with regard to methodology: the kind of microscope used and the preparation of the tissue or organ in a manner suitable for viewing with the microscope. In general, the development of histological techniques has lagged behind the technical achievements made in connection with various types of microscopes. Perhaps the best example of this applies to the electron microscope. Although the electron microscope was developed in the early

1930's, it was not utilized to any extent in biological work until the late 1940's and early 1950's when methods of thin sectioning were developed.

Microscopy dates from the seventeenth century when Robert Hooke and Marcello Malpighi employed simple lenses in the study of various structural features. Between 1673 and 1716, Leeuwenhoek developed compound lenses and published a series of observations upon protozoa, bacteria, muscle, nerve, and many other structures. Microscopic anatomy developed slowly during the eighteenth century, and by the early nineteenth century the compound microscope had become highly developed. Robert Brown (1831) discovered the nucleus, and Schleiden (1838) and Schwann (1839) enunciated the "cell theory." In 1841 Henle published the first comprehensive (for that time) account of human histology. Virchow (1863) described the human body as a "cell state" and listed specialized categories of cells. In the latter part of the nineteenth century, microtomes were developed commercially, and hand in hand with their appearance came the development of fixing, embedding, and staining techniques. The latter are still in the process of development, particularly with regard to their application to the newer forms of microscopy.

In the study of histology, the student will be introduced to the results obtained from various forms of microscopy and of histological technique. How these results were obtained should always be borne in mind since it will influence their interpretation. Thus it is important for the student to understand the applications and limitations of the various types of microscopes in use today and the basic principles underlying the different methods of preparation of tissues.

MICROSCOPY

Several types of microscopes are available for the study of biological material. Basically they can be classified by the type of light source used. In most general use, of course, is the optical microscope using visible light. There are certain modifications of this, namely the polarization, phase contrast, interference, and dark-field microscopes. Microscopes which utilize invisible radiation, the ultraviolet, x-ray, and electron microscopes, are more recent developments.

The usefulness of any type of microscope depends not only upon its ability to magnify but, more important, upon its ability to resolve detail. Beyond certain limits, magnification adds no new details. The useful magnification of an ordinary light microscope is about 1500×. The resolving power is a measure of the capacity of the microscope to separate clearly two points close together. Beyond the resolving power of any microscope, two points will appear as one. The resolution with lens systems is limited by the wave length of light and by the numerical aperture, or light gathering capacity, of the objective lens. The resolving power of a well-constructed light microscope is about 0.2 μ.

The Light (or Optical) Microscope

Basically the light microscope acts as a two stage magnifying device. An objective lens provides the initial magnification, and an ocular lens is placed so as to magnify the primary image a second time. An additional condensing lens is normally employed beneath the stage of the microscope to concentrate the light from its source into a very bright beam illuminating the object, thus providing sufficient light for the inspection of the magnified image.

The Polarizing Microscope

This instrument was developed by mineralogists who employ it in their studies of crystalline materials. Many natural objects, including crystals and fibers, exhibit an optical property known as double refraction, or birefringence. In histological material, birefringence is caused by the orientation of particles too small to be resolved even by the best lenses. Thus an examination of birefringence permits deductions to be made concerning the organization of structure not demonstrable by regular methods of microscopy.

In its simplest form, the polarizing microscope is a conventional microscope in which a Nicol prism (or Polaroid sheet) is interposed in the light path below the condenser. This "polarizer" converts all light passing through the instrument into plane polarized light, or light which vibrates in one optical plane only. A similar, second prism, termed the "analyzer," is placed within the barrel of the microscope above the objective lens. When the analyzer is orientated so that its polarizing direction is parallel to that of the polarizer below, one sees the regular image. However, if the analyzer is rotated until its axis is perpendicular to that of the polarizer, no light can pass through the ocular lens and the field is black. The field will remain black if an *isotropic*, or singly refractive, object is placed on the stage. A birefringent object, however, will appear light upon a dark background when examined in this manner. Birefringence, or *anisotropy*, is exhibited by many biological structures, for example, muscle fibers, certain connective tissue fibers, lipid droplets within the adrenal cortex, and the rods and cones of the retina.

The Phase Contrast Microscope

Lack of contrast has always been a problem in biological work because the refractive indices of cytoplasm and of its inclusions are similar. In normal microscopy, one overcomes this problem by staining differentially, but this is subject to numerous limitations.

Phase microscopy provides a method whereby contrast is created by purely optical means.

The refractive index is a measure of the optical density of an object, or the speed with which it is traversed by a light wave. Air, for instance, has a refractive index of approximately 1.0, water about 1.3, and glass about 1.5. In other words, light travels fastest in air, more slowly in water, and slower still in glass. Light waves traversing equal distances through air, water, and glass will not emerge at the same time; they will emerge out of phase with each other. The phase contrast apparatus consists of optical plates placed within the condenser and objective lenses which convert the phase differences into amplitude differences. Briefly, therefore, differences in refractive index are rendered directly visible. Objects ordinarily transparent become visible through contrast differences. The phase contrast microscope is of no particular assistance in the study of fixed and stained preparations in which transparency differences are not important. The instrument finds its application chiefly in the study of living cells and of unstained tissues.

The Interference Microscope

The interference microscope, like the phase contrast microscope, depends upon the ability of an object to retard light. Unlike the phase microscope, which depends upon the specimen diffracting light, the interference microscope sends through the specimen two separate beams of light which then are combined in the image plane. After recombination, difference in retardation of the light results in interference which can be used to measure the thickness or refractive index of the object under investigation.

The Dark-Field Microscope

This microscope utilizes a strong, oblique light that does not enter the objective lens. A special dark-field condenser, in which no light passes through the center of the lens, is employed. Light thus reaches the object to be viewed at an angle so oblique that none of it can enter the objective lens. The field is therefore dark. Small particles present in the field will reflect some light into the objective lens and appear as glistening spots. Thus it is possible to visualize particles far below the limits of bright light resolution. The effect is similar to the phenomenon of dust particles "seen" in a beam of sunlight entering a darkened room. Dark-field examination is also of use in the examination of small transparent objects such as chylomicrons, which are invisible in the glare of bright field illumination, and of microincineration specimens.

The microscopes just discussed all utilize visible light. However, images can be formed by rays other than visible light and in this instance, since the images cannot be viewed directly, they are made visible by means of a suitably sensitized photographic film. In general the rays used in these special microscopes all have a shorter wave length than that of visible light and thus permit higher resolution.

The Ultraviolet Microscope

Since ordinary optical lenses are nearly opaque to ultraviolet light, quartz lenses are used throughout the lens system. In principle, this system allows an improvement in resolution about twice that of the ordinary microscope (0.1μ).

Ultraviolet light is also employed in *fluorescence microscopy*. Many substances have the property of emitting visible light when irradiated by invisible rays. Ultraviolet light is focused upon the specimen which glows and can be observed by its emitted fluorescence. Fluorescence may be naturally occurring in the specimen or may result from the introduction of fluorescent dyes bound to certain specific components of the specimen.

The X-Ray Microscope

X-rays have a shorter wave length than visible or ultraviolet light and therefore a greater penetration and theoretically a higher resolving power. By using preparation techniques similar to those used in light microscopy, the specimen can be placed upon a photographic emulsion and exposed to soft x-irradiation. The small x-ray picture obtained is subsequently magnified optically. This process is known as contact microradiography. In *projection x-ray microscopy*, a point source of x-rays casts an enlarged image of a nearby object upon a distant fluorescent screen or photographic plate. It is the contrast obtained as a result of differences in x-ray absorption that is utilized in these procedures. Resolution in either case is not particularly high and with the instruments available is still far from the theoretical limits.

The Electron Microscope

The electron microscope utilizes a system which in principle is analogous to that of the light microscope. In the electron microscope, the illuminating source is a beam of high velocity electrons accelerated in a vacuum. The beam is passed through the specimen and is focused upon a fluorescent screen or photographic plate by a series of electromagnetic or electrostatic fields. The wave length of the electrons depends upon the acceleration voltage used. At the voltages used routinely, the wave lengths of the electrons are of the order of 0.05 Å.* The electric or magnetic fields used as lenses are imperfect and do not have the numerical aperture of

---

* Å, an angstrom unit $= 1 \times 10^{-4} \mu$, or 1×10^{-7} mm.

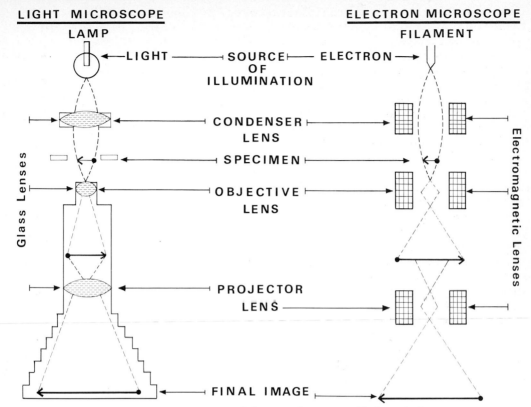

LIGHT MICROSCOPE   **ELECTRON MICROSCOPE**

LAMP   FILAMENT

←——LIGHT——— | SOURCE | ——ELECTRON——→
OF
ILLUMINATION

CONDENSER
LENS

SPECIMEN

OBJECTIVE
LENS

PROJECTOR
LENS

FINAL IMAGE

Glass Lenses

Electromagnetic Lenses

Figure 1-1. Diagrammatic comparison of the optical systems of light and electron microscopes. For ease of comparison the system of the light microscope has been inverted and a camera attachment added.

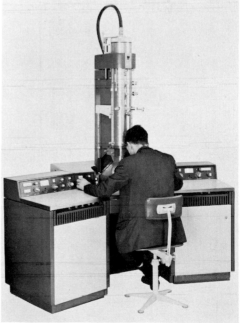

Figure 1-2. A modern electron microscope. (Courtesy of Philips Electronic Instruments.)

optical lenses. Thus the practical limit of resolution of the electron microscope is about 2 Å, and the usual limit for biological preparations about 3.5 Å.

The electron microscope permits the observation of cell and tissue structure beyond that seen with the light microscope. Structures smaller than individual macromolecules can now be visualized. To describe this particular level of structure requires the use of some special term. The one most commonly used is *fine structure*, which refers to those elements of structure which can be visualized only with the electron microscope. The term *ultrastructure*, which is used by some workers in this field, is better avoided since literally it means *beyond structure*.

Just as with light microscopy, electron microscopy requires special techniques for preparing specimens for examination. These will be discussed in the following section.

THE PREPARATION OF TISSUES

It will be obvious to the student that cells, tissues, and organs cannot be studied to advantage unless they are suitably prepared for microscopic examination. The methods of preparation fall logically into two groups: methods involving the direct observation of living cells and methods employed with dead cells (fixed or preserved). In his or her personal study of histology, the student will employ, in the main, fixed and stained preparations of tissues and organs which are permanent. Living tissues are usually more difficult to handle and are valuable for a short period only. Nevertheless, it is important that the student become aware of the methods by which living cells may be observed and understand the ways in which they differ from fixed cells. In the living cell, structure and function may be studied simultaneously. Living

cells may be seen to move, to ingest foreign material, occasionally to divide, and to carry on other functions.

Observation of Living Tissue

Unicellular organisms and, occasionally, free cells from a complex organism may be studied directly under the microscope while they still are alive. Free cells are colorless and structures within them lack contrast. This difficulty may be overcome by using a phase contrast microscope. Human blood cells are easy to obtain and can be studied in thin films while surrounded by their natural environment, plasma. In this way ameboid and phagocytic activity may be recognized within white blood cells.

Membranes may be thin enough to be viewed directly under the microscope: for instance, the web of the frog foot, the wing of the bat, and the buccal pouch of the hamster. Thin sections of relatively thick organs such as liver and kidney may be viewed by *transillumination* with quartz rods, which produce a cold light and avoid coagulation of protoplasm. *Glass windows* may be inserted into ears or backs of animals and so permit extended study of processes such as tissue regeneration or vascular activities. Small pieces of tissue for microscopic examination may be excised, placed in some relatively harmless liquid such as serum or an 0.85 per cent aqueous solution of sodium chloride, and teased apart gently with needles of fine steel or glass.

Prolonged preservation of living cells outside the body can be achieved by a technique known as *tissue culture*. Fragments of tissue are removed aseptically, transferred to a physiological medium, and kept at a temperature normal for the animal from which the tissue was taken. The cultures are placed in thin glass vessels or in hanging drops on a coverglass mounted over a hollow slide. In this way they

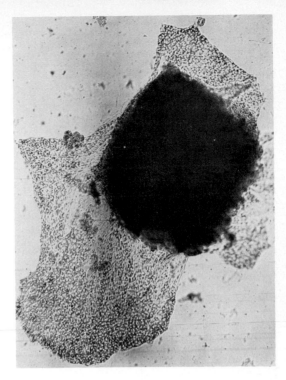

Figure 1-3. Light microphotograph of a tissue culture preparation. A guinea pig kidney explant (dark mass) is surrounded by sheets of epithelial cells which have grown out from the explant into the surrounding nutrient medium. × 50. (Courtesy of F. Jacoby.)

are available for observation under the microscope. In such cultures, growth, multiplication, and in some cases, differentiation of cells into other cell types can be observed directly. Tissue culture is a valuable method for the study of cancer and of many viruses.

Microdissection involves the use of an instrument which moves very fine glass needles with precision under the microscope. In this way small portions of a cell such as a nucleus can be removed and the effect observed.

Two staining methods have been applied successfully to living animals or surviving cells. In *vital staining*, dyes are injected into the living animal. The activity of certain cells will result in the selective absorption of the coloring material by these cells. An example of this procedure is the staining by trypan blue of macrophages on the basis of their ability to phagocytose foreign particles. *Supravital staining* involves the addition of a dyestuff to a medium of cells already removed from the organism. Examples

of this technique are the staining of mitochondria in living cells by Janus green, of lysosomes by neutral red, and of nerve fibers and cells by methylene blue.

Finally, motion picture records aid in the understanding of cellular activities. Lapsed time films made of individual living cells or of tissue cultures help to analyze processes such as mitosis, phagocytosis, and ameboid movement. Slow-motion films of such rapid processes as the beating of cilia permit analysis of the action.

Preparation of Dead Tissue

Light Microscopy. The most convenient way to study histology is to use *sections*, each of which is a more or less permanent preparation. A section is prepared by cutting a thin slice from a small piece of fixed tissue, which is then stained, mounted in a medium of suitable refractive index upon a slide, and finally covered with a coverslip. The various ways in which sections can be prepared constitute *histological technique*, about which many books have been written. Detailed information of this kind is not required by the student of histology, but he should be aware of the general principles involved so that he may use the material intelligently. The production of a histological section involves the following steps:

REMOVAL OF THE SPECIMEN. For cytological purposes, and for the best histological preparations, the material should be removed from an anesthetized animal or immediately after death of the animal. In the case of human material this is scarcely ever possible. Surgical material represents the best source of human material since frequently some normal tissue is removed together with the abnormal or diseased tissue.

FIXATION. The primary objective of fixation is to preserve protoplasm with the least alteration from the living state. Fixing fluids act as preservatives, inhibiting autolytic changes and bacterial growth. They coagulate protoplasm, thus rendering it insoluble, and harden the tissue so that sectioning is facilitated. They may or may not preserve carbohydrates and lipids. Many fixatives also increase the affinity of protoplasm for certain stains.

The reagents that are employed most commonly as fixing agents are formalin, alcohol, mercuric bichloride, potassium bichromate, and certain acids (picric, acetic, osmic). No single fixative possesses all the desirable qualities, and many reagents are used in mixtures such as Bouin's fluid, Zenker's fluid, and Susa's fluid. The choice of a fixative is usually determined by the particular tissue or component that is to be studied and by the staining method to be used.

EMBEDDING. Prior to embedding, the fixed tissue is washed to remove excess fixative and then dehydrated by passing it through increasing strengths of alcohol or some other dehydrating agent. The tissue is then *"cleared."* This process involves the removal of the dehydrating agent and its replacement by some fluid which is miscible both with the dehydrating agent and with the embedding medium. *Clearing agents* include xylol, chloroform, benzene, and cedarwood oil. After clearing, the tissue is infiltrated with the embedding agent, usually paraffin or celloidin. After infiltration, the embedding agent is made to solidify so that a firm homogeneous mass containing the embedded tissue is obtained.

For special studies, tissue can be embedded in paraffin without subjecting it to preliminary treatment with fixatives, dehydrating solutions, or clearing agents. This is known as the *freeze-drying* method in which the fresh tissue is frozen rapidly and dehydrated, while still frozen, in vacuum at a low temperature. The dried tissue is then embedded. In the *freeze-substitution* modification of this method, the ice within the frozen tissue is replaced by alcohol at a very low temperature prior to embedding.

SECTIONING. Tissue embedded in paraffin may be sliced very thin. For the majority of microscopic work, the sections are between 3 and 10 microns thick. To cut such sections, a *microtome* is used. Each section is transferred to a clean glass microscope slide on which a little egg albumen has been smeared. Water is run under the section and the slide placed on a warming stage. The water evaporates and the section settles down onto the glass surface, to which it becomes attached. The mounted section is now ready for staining.

STAINING. The purpose of staining is to enhance natural contrast and to make more evident various cell and tissue components and extrinsic material. Most stains are employed in aqueous solution, and thus to stain a paraffin section it is necessary to remove the paraffin by placing the section in a paraffin solvent or *decerating agent*, usually xylol or toluol. This step is omitted in the case of a section which has been embedded in celloidin. The section is then passed through descending strengths of alcohol prior to staining.

MOUNTING. After staining, excess dye is removed by washing with water or alcohol, depending upon the solvent of the dye, and the section is dehydrated through ascending grades of alcohol. Following absolute alcohol, the section is transferred to a solution of a clearing agent. After removal from the clearing agent, a drop of mounting medium, for instance Canada balsam, which has a similar refractive index to that of glass, is placed on the section. The preparation is covered with a coverslip and allowed to dry.

Electron Microscopy. In general, the method of preparation of sections for electron microscopy is similar to that employed for light microscopy. There are some important points of difference. Much smaller pieces of tissue are used since preservation and fixation of cell fine structure is more critical and requires rapid interaction with the fixative. Blocks are commonly about 1 cu. mm. or less in size. Tissue must be obtained fresh since postmortem changes are more obvious at the higher resolution of the electron microscope. The procedures of fixation, dehydration, and embedding, though similar to those employed in light microscopy, are effected rapidly because of the small pieces of tissue involved. Since paraffin is not suitable for very thin sectioning, it is replaced as an embedding medium by some agent, usually a plastic material such as Epon or Araldite, which produces a firm block. The sections, cut upon a special, precision-built microtome with glass or diamond knives, are minute, about 0.25 mm. square and about 300 to 500 Å thick. They are mounted on perforated copper grids for viewing in the electron microscope. Thick sections, about 0.2 to 1.0 micron thick, of such plastic embedded material can be mounted on a glass slide, stained, and examined by light microscopy. Several photomicrographs of this type of preparation are to be found in this textbook.

Freeze-etching is another method of preparation of material for electron microscopy. This method involves a purely physical preparation which may allow examination of specimens virtually free of artifacts. The specimen is frozen, cut into small pieces, briefly warmed to etch the cut surface by vacuum-sublimation, and a replica of the surface made by heavy metal shadowing. The frozen specimen is thawed and the replica can then be placed on a specimen grid and viewed in a conventional electron microscope or in a *scanning electron microscope (Stereoscan microscope)*, which provides three-dimensional images. The method helps to distinguish natural from artificial structures and allows examination of the surface of single cells or of such structures as cytoplasmic membrane systems.

Autoradiography. Autoradiography is a special technique which employs the microscope, either light or electron, only as a visual aid. The technique is coming into increasing prominence in histology as a method of chemical localization. Tracer isotopes introduced in the organism either by feeding or by injection follow the same metabolic pathways as do the naturally occurring elements. Their presence in an organ or tissue can be detected by autoradiography. After administration of a tracer isotope, the organ or tissue under investigation is removed and processed for light or electron microscopy in the normal manner. The section is placed in close contact with a photographic emulsion and allowed to remain in the dark for a certain period of time. After subsequent photographic development of the sensitive emulsion, the radioactive tracer elements will appear as dark areas lying over the cells or components of cells in which the radioactivity is located. Some excellent results have been achieved by this method: for instance, the localization of radioiodine in the thyroid gland and of phosphorus (using radio-strontium as a substitute) in bone.

THE EXAMINATION AND INTERPRETATION OF SECTIONS

The ability to interpret histological sections is a skill which the student has to develop. In gross anatomy, structure is studied in three dimensions. Histology must be learned from a study of sections which, for all practical purposes, have no depth. *It is important to reconstruct a three dimensional mental picture of cells, tissues, and organs from the two dimensional sections.* In this respect, the plane of sectioning must be borne in mind. A single section of an organ may give a false impression of its architecture. Thus it is important to use several sections taken in different planes in order to make an interpretation of structure of complex organs.

Nor is the mere identification and notation of structures sufficient. One must strive to interpret the functional significance of what one observes. Dead structures are examined for the purpose of throwing light upon their condition in life. Conditions which are dynamic in life have been converted to a static form in the permanent histological section.

It must be appreciated also that not all sections are perfect. Owing to the techniques used in preparation, sections may not be accurate representations. These alterations are termed *artifacts*, and they should be recognized as such by the student. They may be due to different chemicals used in the histological technique, resulting in shrinkage, or due to sectioning, leading to folding or wrinkling of the section, or to defects caused by an imperfect knife.

During the study of a collection of microscopic slides, the student often is confused by the varying appearance of different constituents of cells and tissues due to the use of a number of different staining techniques. With any microscopic preparation, interpretation involves also an appreciation of the staining techniques used. Although it is not necessary for the student to be conversant with details of the various staining techniques used, he should understand the general principles, uses, and results of the common staining procedures.

STAINS

In general the dyes used are complex organic chemicals which often show some variability in performance. They may be classified in numerous ways, but the simplest approach is to base the classification upon use, with regard to tissue and cell components. Dyes may be of general use, staining either the nucleus or the cytoplasm, or they may be more specific with regard to particular components. It must be emphasized that many dyes require special methods of fixation and preparation of the tissue, and the reader is referred to a textbook of histological and histochemical techniques for the details.

Stains in general use are considered to be either acids or bases, but in fact they are neutral salts having both acidic and basic radicals. When the coloring property of the dye is in the basic radical of the neutral salt, the stain is referred to as a basic dye and structures which stain with it are termed *basophil*. In most instances, the basophil substances which attract the basic dyes are themselves acids, for instance, the nucleic acids of the nucleus and the acidic components of the cytoplasm such as ribonucleic acid (RNA). Similarly, when the staining property is in the acidic radical of the neutral salt, the stain is spoken of as an acid dye and the structures stained (for instance, the general cytoplasm) as *acidophil*.

The nuclear stain in most common use is hematoxylin, the staining property of which depends upon the presence in solution of its oxidation product, hematein. (Thus, a freshly prepared solution of hematoxylin must be allowed to "ripen" or "age" for oxidation to occur prior to use.) When stained with such a dye, nuclei appear blue. Iron hematoxylin, which stains nuclei dark blue or black, has a wide application. In most methods employing iron hematoxylin, one overstains with the dye and regressively differentiates in a weak acid or in a ferric salt solution. By careful *differentiation*, which may be viewed directly under the microscope, such organelles as chromosomes, mitochondria, Golgi apparatus, and the contractile elements of muscle may be visualized. Carmine, a red to purple nuclear stain, formerly was very popular but is little used today. The basic aniline dyes are a group of stains used extensively. This group includes azure A, toluidine blue, and methylene blue, stains which are employed also in the identification of mucopolysaccharides which stain *metachromatically* (*meta*, beyond; *chroma*, color). This means that mucopolysaccharides, when stained with one of these dyes, will take on a color different from that of the dye employed. It is thought that substances which demonstrate metachromasia do so because they are capable of concentrating the dye or of altering its molecular state. Mucin, matrix of cartilage, and the granules of mast cells are demonstrated readily by their metachromatic staining. Other basic aniline dyes in common use are brilliant cresyl blue, neutral red, and Janus green, all of which are nontoxic and may be used also as vital or supravital stains.

Acidic dyes, commonly employed to stain the general cytoplasm, include eosin, picric acid, acid azo dyes such as chromotrope, and the acid diazo dyes, trypan blue and trypan red. The latter two are used also as vital stains. Most histological sections are stained with both a basic stain and an acidic stain. The commonest combination is *hematoxylin and eosin* (H and E), in which nuclear structures are stained dark purple or blue, and practically all cytoplasmic structures and intercellular substances are stained pink. Mallory's connective tissue stain and the Mallory-Azan method are good general stains. They stain certain connective tissue fibers bright blue, nuclei red or orange, and various cell constituents blue, red, orange, or purple. Masson's staining procedure is another trichrome method of general use in which connective tissue fibers are stained green, nuclei blue or purple, and cytoplasmic structures red. Although there is no truly specific stain for collagen, it is best shown by the acid aniline dyes in a trichrome method. Elastic fibers are brilliantly acidophil and can be stained selectively with orcein or with resorcin fuchsin. Reticulin can be demonstrated specifically by precipitation of silver from an alkaline solution. Hence these fibers are termed *argyrophil*. It must be realized that special methods of staining are necessary to demonstrate certain constituents of cells and formed extracellular fibers, and that a single staining method does not suffice to demonstrate everything present within a section.

HISTOCHEMISTRY

The fact that deposition of specific stains in certain regions is a result of chemical or physical properties inherent in the tissue forms the basis of histochemistry. This is a field of research which is expanding rapidly and has as its goal the localization within specific areas or cell components of the chemical compounds known already by biochemical analysis to be present. Histochemical methods are now available for many inorganic and organic substances. An example of the former is the adaptation of the Prussian blue reaction for the detection of ferric iron. In sections treated with potassium ferrocyanide, deposits are colored blue.

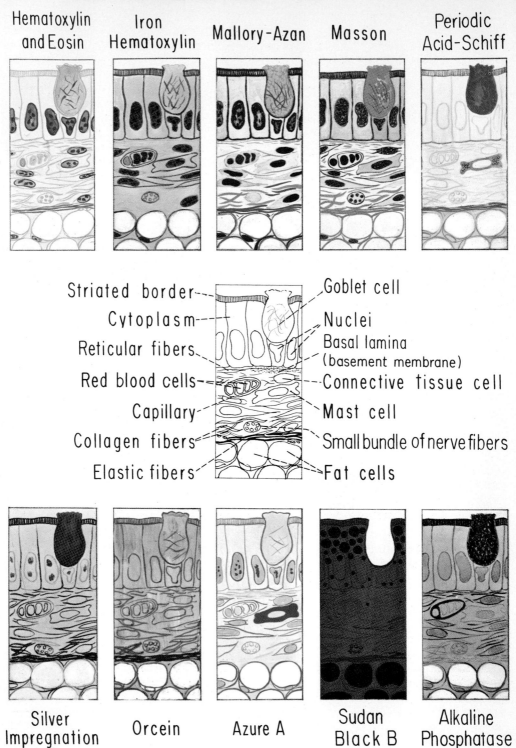

Hematoxylin and Eosin Iron Hematoxylin Mallory-Azan Masson Periodic Acid-Schiff

Striated border Goblet cell
Cytoplasm Nuclei
Reticular fibers Basal lamina (basement membrane)
Red blood cells Connective tissue cell
Capillary Mast cell
Collagen fibers Small bundle of nerve fibers
Elastic fibers Fat cells

Silver Impregnation Orcein Azure A Sudan Black B Alkaline Phosphatase

Figure 1-4. Diagrammatic representation of a section (partly hypothetical) of a portion of the wall of the intestine as it would appear after different staining procedures. Hematoxylin and eosin stains nuclei dark blue and both cytoplasm and connective tissue fibers pink-red. Iron hematoxylin

(Legend continues on opposite page)

The *Feulgen reaction* for the identification of deoxyribonucleic acid (DNA) is an example of a histochemical test which requires preliminary treatment of the section so that the substance under investigation either is liberated or produces a substance for which a specific test exists. Basic fuchsin is a magenta colored dye which can be bleached by treatment with hydrochloric acid and sodium bisulfite. Reaction with the aldehydes produces, in the bleached dye, a new, colored compound, also magenta. Mild hydrolysis of a section with hydrochloric acid will produce aldehydes from DNA. If the section is then immersed in the colorless form of basic fuchsin, the aldehydes formed from DNA will react with the dye and exhibit the magenta color. Since both deoxyribonucleic acid (DNA) and ribonucleic acid (RNA) are basophil, the Feulgen reaction allows a distinction to be made as to which basophil material is DNA. A method which employs a similar histochemical technique is the *periodic acid–Schiff reaction* (PAS reaction). Periodic acid is an oxidizing agent which will produce from certain polysaccharides aldehydes that are insoluble. These then react with the Schiff reagent, which is the colorless form of basic fuchsin.

Not all reactions in histochemistry rely upon chemical affinities. Fat can be detected in sections which have not been exposed to fat solvents by stains such as Sudan III, Sudan IV, and Sudan black B. These stains have a physical affinity for lipid and are adsorbed by the fat. Use of such dyes forms the basis for the term *sudanophilia*, the ability to stain substances with this group of dyes.

Enzymes may be detected by histochemical methods which in principle attempt to localize the site of a specific enzyme by a chemical process similar to that performed by the enzyme *in vivo*. The section under examination is incubated at body temperature in the presence of a suitable substrate, and the product of the resultant chemical reaction with the enzyme is converted into a chemical substance of a definite color. For example, to demonstrate the enzyme alkaline phosphatase, glycerophosphate is used as the substrate in an alkaline medium and the phosphate liberated by the action of the enzyme is deposited in the presence of calcium ions as calcium phosphate. The deposit of calcium phosphate is converted to an easily visualized black precipitate of cobalt sulfide (or metallic silver) by immersing the section in cobalt acetate (or silver acetate) and then rinsing in ammonium sulfide. Methods are available now for a wide variety of enzymes including phosphatases, lipases, oxidases, and esterases.

Glycogen is stained by Best's carmine stain or by the periodic acid–

---

stains nuclei a dark purple-black. It also stains red blood cells. With less differentiation after staining (see text) it would make visible also such cellular components as mitochondria. Mallory-Azan and Masson are examples of trichrome methods of staining which are useful in differentiating between cytoplasm and connective tissue fibers. In the former method, collagen fibers are stained bright blue; in the latter, green. Periodic acid—Schiff stains the brush border, mucus within the goblet cell, the basal lamina, and cytoplasmic granules of the mast cell positively. All other structures on the section are negative with this stain. Silver impregnation and orcein are examples of stains used to differentiate between the various types of connective tissue fibers. Impregnation with silver outlines reticular fibers; hence, commonly, they are termed *argyrophil*. Elastic fibers are stained selectively with orcein (and with resorcin fuchsin). Azure A is one of the group of basic aniline dyes which stains nuclei blue and also is employed in the identification of mucopolysaccharides which stain metachromatically as do the granules of the mast cell here (see text). Sudan black B is a dye which is absorbed by fat and thus stains it selectively. It requires a method of preparation of tissue which avoids the use of fat solvents. Alkaline phosphatase is an enzyme which can be localized by a histochemical method (see text). Here there is a positive reaction in the brush border and, as often happens, in the cytoplasm of endothelium lining blood vessels. (After Garvin.) See filmstrip I, frame 1.

Schiff reagent. In either case, glycogen can be differentiated from other polysaccharides by the fact that the staining property of the latter substances is resistant to digestion by salivary amylase.

Immunocytochemistry is one branch of histochemistry that has received considerable attention recently. At the light microscopic level, the fluorescent antibody technique is a sensitive method for the localization of specific polysaccharides or proteins. The basis of this technique is the fact that the body reacts to foreign protein substances, the *antigens*, by elaborating specific substances, the *antibodies*, which combine with and inactivate the antigens. Fluorescent dye molecules are chemically linked to antibody molecules and the sites of their reaction with antigens can be visualized in the ultraviolet microscope. The method has been used to identify the cells of origin of protein hormones, the intracellular localization of various enzymes, and the sites of proteins such as myosin. The method has been adapted for use with the electron microscope by conjugating an antibody with a metalloprotein such as *ferritin*, which naturally possesses a distinct appearance in the electron microscope. This method enables the investigator to localize precisely the site of the antibody-antigen reaction.

REFERENCES

Baker, J. R.: Cytological Technique: The Principles Underlying Routine Methods, ed. 4. Longon, Methuen & Co., Ltd; New York, John Wiley and Sons, Inc., 1960.

Clark, G. L. (editor): The Encyclopedia of Microscopy. New York, Reinhold Publishing Corp., 1961.

Coons, A. H.: Fluorescent antibody methods. *In* General Cytochemical Methods, edited by J. F. Danielli. New York, Academic Press, 1958, p. 400.

Ficq, A.: Autoradiography. *In* The Cell: Biochemistry, Physiology, Morphology, edited by J. Brachet and A. E. Mirsky. New York, Academic Press, 1959, Vol. 1, p. 67.

Gersh, I.: Fixation and staining. *In* The Cell: Biochemistry, Physiology, Morphology, edited by J. Brachet and A. E. Mirsky. New York, Academic Press, 1959, Vol. 1, p. 21.

Gomori, G.: Microscopic Histochemistry, Principles and Practice. Chicago, University of Chicago Press, 1952.

Hall, C. A.: How to Use the Microscope, ed. 4. New York, Macmillan Co., 1955.

Humason, G. L.: Animal Tissue Techniques. San Francisco, Freeman and Co., 1962.

Journal of the Royal Microscopical Society. Issue in celebration of the Tercentenary of "The Microscope in Living Biology," *83*: 1-229, 1964.

Kay, D. (editor): Techniques for Electron Microscopy, ed. 2. Oxford, Blackwell Scientific Publications, 1965.

Lewis, W. H., and Lewis, M. R.: Behavior of cells in tissue cultures. *In* General Cytology, edited by E. V. Cowdry, Chicago, University of Chicago Press, p. 385.

McManus, J. F. A., and Mowry, R. W.: Staining Methods: Histologic and Histochemical. New York, Paul B. Hoeber, Inc., 1960.

Oster, G., and Pollister, A. W. (editors): Physical Techniques in Biological Research. New York, Academic Press, 1955-1957, Vols. 1-3.

Parker, R. C.: Methods of Tissue Culture, ed. 3. New York, Paul B. Hoeber, Inc., 1961.

Pearse, A. G. E.: Histochemistry: Theoretical and Applied, ed. 3, Vol. I. Boston, Little, Brown and Co., 1968.

Pease, D. C.: Histological Techniques for Electron Microscopy, ed. 2. New York, Academic Press, 1964.

Sjöstrand, F. S.: Electron Microscopy of Cells and Tissues. Vol. 1, Instrumentation and Techniques. New York, Academic Press, 1967.

Sternberger, L. A.: Electron microscopic immunocytochemistry: a review. J. Histochem. Cytochem., *15*:139, 1967.

Wyckoff, R. W. G.: Optical methods in cytology. *In* The Cell: Biochemistry, Physiology, Morphology, edited by J. Brachet and A. E. Mirsky. New York, Academic Press, 1959, Vol. 1, p. 1.

CHAPTER **2**

THE CELL

COMPONENTS OF THE BODY

The body is composed of three different elements: cells, intercellular substance, and the body fluids. The body fluids include blood, confined to the cavities and channels of the vascular system, tissue (intercellular) fluid situated between the cells and in which there is a free exchange of materials on the one side with blood and on the other with the intracellular fluid, and lymph, draining tissue fluid from the tissues of the body at the periphery into a closed system of fine tubes which eventually drains back into the venous system. These fluid components of the body are not seen in a normal histological section because they are lost during preparation, but they must not be forgotten.

The obvious feature of most tissue sections is the presence of cells, although their entire outlines may not be discernible. Each cell is formed by the nucleus and cytoplasm, but in some cases the latter may not be visible. The nucleus, which occasionally is multiple, usually is regularly oval or spherical and darkly staining, while the surrounding cytoplasm is more lightly staining. There is great variation in the appearance, size, and shape of cells and such variation reflects the different functions of different cell types.

Intercellular substance, as the name suggests, is that material which lies between and supports the cells. It is responsible in great degree for the

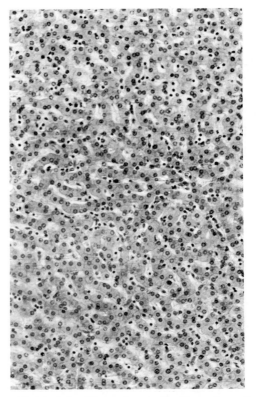

Figure 2-1. Photomicrograph of a section of the rat liver showing irregular cords of cells, each with a spherical nucleus. Cell boundaries are not distinct at this magnification. × 125.

17

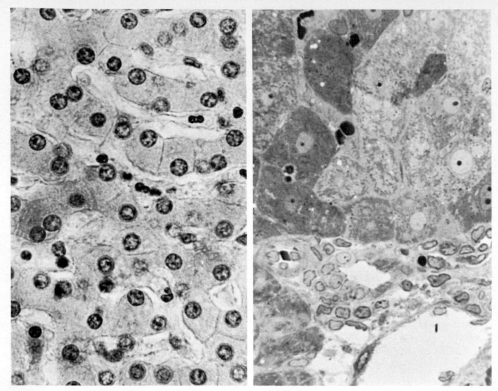

Figure 2-2. Left: a higher magnification of Figure 2-1. Individual cell outlines are recognizable. In the nuclei, chromatin masses and nucleoli are visible. Several cells contain two nuclei. × 750. Right: an Epon section of liver. Cytoplasmic and nuclear detail are more obvious. The discrete dots within some nuclei are nucleoli. × 1200.   See filmstrip I, frame 2.

firmness of tissues, and in histology we recognize two main types, formed and amorphous. The formed type includes the material called collagen (the white, fibrous tissue, for example, that is found in meat and is tough to chew) and elastin, which is largely responsible for the elasticity of tissues. Amorphous intercellular material, or ground substance, is composed of a group of substances termed protein-polysaccharides, long chain polymers of protein-sugar complexes. These intercellular substances are described in detail in the following chapter.

PROTOPLASM

Protoplasm, the material of which cells are composed, has been de-scribed as the physical basis for life. The terms protoplasm and cytoplasm often are used synonymously, but in fact the nucleus also contains protoplasm, termed nucleoplasm or karyoplasm. Hence, each cell is a living, dynamic entity. Approximately 75 per cent of protoplasm is water, partly free and thus available for metabolic processes, and partly bound to protein as a structural component of protoplasm. Salts, particularly potassium and magnesium as cations and phosphate and bicarbonate as anions, account for about 1 per cent of the materials of the body. Other components are the three basic food materials of the body: proteins (10 to 20 per cent), lipids (2 to 3 per cent), and carbohydrates (1 per cent). All percentages are approximate and vary not only from cell type to cell type, but also within any one cell during its metabolic cycle.

Proteins, which are responsible for the characteristic structure of cells, are molecules of high molecular weight composed of amino acids, of which there are some 20 kinds. Lipids function in cells both as food reserves and as components of structures, and all are soluble in fat solvents. During preparation of routine microscopic slides, fat solvents are used, and thus special fixatives or preparative techniques have to be used to preserve lipids. Carbohydrates are present in protoplasm as monosaccharides, disaccharides, polysaccharides, and protein-polysaccharides. Other important components of protoplasm include vitamins, required in very small amounts for the growth and normal metabolism of cells.

Both the vital, living protoplasm of cells and the nonliving materials between cells (intercellular substance) exist in the colloidal state. It is difficult to define a colloid exactly, but the basic feature of a colloidal solution is that its particles are of such a size that they cannot be filtered through natural membranes, the membrane acting as a sieve and holding back the particles. Crystalloids, e.g., glucose, can pass through such membranes. Proteins show all the characteristics of the colloidal state, and some can exist either as a sol or as a gel. Fluid solutions of colloids are sols, but are viscous to some degree, e.g., egg albumen (egg "white"). If, however, the egg albumen is heated or subjected to a change in hydrogen ion concentration, it becomes solid; i.e., it has been transformed into the gel state. In the protoplasm of cells, such sol-gel transformations can occur and often are reversible as is the case, for example, in the "setting" and "melting" of a solution of gelatin.

Substances which mainly are responsible for the form and organization of the protoplasm are the *macromolecules*. These are substances which are constructed from smaller organic building blocks, the *monomers*, linked together repetitively by covalent bonds. Proteins, for instance, are composed of amino acids linked by bonds. Polysaccharides are composed of sugar monomers. The degree of polymerization refers to the number of monomer units linked in a single macromolecule. Within animal cells, macromolecules fall into three principal classes, polysaccharides, proteins, and nucleic acids.

Polysaccharides. Polysaccharides of biological importance include glycogen and protein-polysaccharides. Glycogen, a highly branched polymer of *d*-glucose, constitutes a storage depot from which glucose, needed for many chemical activities within the cell, may be released readily upon demand. Protein-polysaccharides commonly encountered in histological material include hyaluronic acid, often found in association with the connective tissue protein collagen, and chondroitin sulfates, present in large quantities within the ground substance of cartilage.

Proteins. Proteins are large molecules composed of a variety of amino acid monomers linked by peptide bonds in a definite sequence. They occur either as structural proteins or as enzymes. Structural proteins include collagen, the keratins of hair and nail, and the muscle proteins. Enzymes constitute an important group of proteins which function as catalysts in many chemical processes, whether synthetic or degradative. Many hormones, for example, insulin and gonadotrophin, also are proteins.

Nucleic Acids. Nucleic acids are the most restricted geographically of the macromolecules and are concerned with protein synthesis. There are two main classes, known as DNA (deoxyribonucleic acid) and RNA (ribonucleic acid). Each is composed of an alternating sequence of two units, a phosphate group and a sugar group. Attached to each sugar group is a base, either a purine or a pyrimidine. In DNA, the sugar is deoxyribose and the bases are of only four kinds, adenine, thymine, guanine, and cytosine, which follow each other in an irregular order. In RNA, the sugar is ribose, and the bases also are four in number and identical to those of DNA with the exception that uracil replaces thymine. In metazoan cells, DNA is found principally in the nucleus where it constitutes the genetic material. RNA is found both within the nucleus and in the cytoplasm.

In addition to the macromolecules, protoplasm contains lipids, which are smaller molecules and are important since they often interact with proteins to constitute a structural basis of biological membrane formation. Lipids are composed of long aliphatic chains capable of orientating themselves at water interfaces into monomolecular layers. The complex of lipid-protein-water is found in membrane systems of nerve myelin sheaths, mitochondria, Golgi apparatus, and endoplasmic reticulum. The combination of two such complexes back to back constitutes a unit membrane.

Unit Membrane

Unit membrane is a term used to describe the basic trilaminar structure found in all cell membranes. Each membrane is approximately 80 Å thick; at high magnification with the electron microscope it is further resolved into two dense layers about 25 Å thick separated by an intermediate light layer of 30 Å. Although there is some variation in thickness, all cell membranes show this basic trilaminar structure. Chemically the cell membrane probably consists of a bimolecular layer of lipid covered on each surface by a layer of proteins. Although this theory is accepted generally, the evidence is not completely conclusive. It has been suggested that this bimolecular leaflet structure may represent the nonenergized state for the membrane. Alternate theories suggest that the lipid of the unit membrane may form globular micelles between the layers of protein or that there is in all membranes a basic unit of structure resembling a dumbbell with a base and a spherical body connected by a stalk. Regardless of which theory is correct, it must be remembered that all membranes are living dynamic structures and that different membranes differ in chemical composition, metabolism, enzymatic composition, and function. However, the trilaminar structure of the unit membrane seen by electron microscopy is a useful concept.

Metabolism

Metabolism can be defined as the chemical processes of the cell by which nutrition is effected. Metabolism may involve the breakdown of cell protoplasm itself or of the materials brought to the cell as a food supply. In this case it is termed *catabolic*, energy being released. Alternatively, energy may be utilized by the cell to produce materials, which may remain in the cell or be released. This type of metabolism is *anabolic*.

Cell Function

Protoplasm has a variety of physiological properties which indicate the functions of cells. The functions of any particular type of cell are a direct expression of one or more of these properties of its protoplasm, and they include the following:

Irritability. Irritability is the capacity of protoplasm to respond to a stimulus, the response of the cell being detected by one of the other properties of protoplasm. Irritability is an expression of life itself and disappears with cell death.

Conductivity. Conductivity indicates that protoplasm can transmit a wave of excitation (an electrical impulse) throughout the cell from the point of stimulus. This property is highly developed in the cell membrane of nerve and, to a lesser extent, in muscle cells.

Contractility. Contractility is the property of change of shape, usually in the sense of shortening, and is highly developed in muscle cells.

Respiration. Respiration is the process whereby food substances and oxygen within the cell interact chemically to produce energy, carbon dioxide, and water. This process, of course, is essential for life.

Absorption. Absorption involves the imbibition of certain dissolved substances which later may be assimilated by the cell, the cell utilizing such material for metabolism. Fluids may diffuse directly into the cell through the plasma membrane or may be engulfed in bulk, a droplet of fluid passing into the cytoplasm limited by a pinched-off portion of the plasma membrane to form a vacuole. This latter process is called *pinocytosis.* Cells also have the ability to take up particulate matter, this process being called *phagocytosis.*

Secretion and Excretion. Secretion and excretion are the processes by which a cell can extrude material. If the material passed out from the cell is a useful product, e.g., a digestive enzyme or a hormone, then the process is called secretion, but if waste materials are extruded, then the term excretion is applied to the process.

Growth and Reproduction. Although some cells can increase in size as a result of an increase in the amount of cytoplasm, this process is limited by the ratio of nuclear volume to cytoplasmic volume and by a relative loss of surface area in proportion to volume, and many of the metabolic processes are dependent upon a large surface area. Thus, growth of a tissue usually occurs not by an increase in the size of individual cells, although this does occur in some instances (particularly in highly specialized cells), but by an increase in the number of cells. This involves cell division, which will be discussed later.

COMPONENTS OF THE CELL

It is important to appreciate that there are many different kinds of cells in the body—different in size, shape, and function—but that each cell is composed of nucleus and cytoplasm. In the ordinary histological slide, these two components of a cell will be differentially stained; i.e., the cytoplasm will appear to be a different color from that of the nucleus (see page 12). As mentioned previously, the cytoplasm may be small in amount, or very lightly stained, and therefore difficult to see.

CYTOPLASM

In many preparations, cytoplasm has an even, homogeneous appearance, but it does in fact contain many small bodies of varying type and function. Variations in function of cell types, e.g., an enzyme-secreting cell and a nerve cell, are reflected by different appearances of the cytoplasm, in turn consequent upon variations in the number and type of these small cytoplasmic bodies. The cytoplasmic bodies are of two main types: *organelles,* which are living structural components of the cell, and *inclusions,* which are best considered as nonliving accumulations of metabolites or cell products.

Cytoplasmic organelles include the cell (plasma) membrane, the endoplasmic reticulum (ergastoplasm), the Golgi apparatus (Golgi complex), the centrioles (cytocentrum), mitochondria, annulate lamellae, fibrils and filamentous structures, lysosomes, and microtubules.

Cell (Plasma) Membrane

As explained previously, each cell is surrounded by, and separated from its neighbors by, a membrane which not only "isolates" the cell from its en-

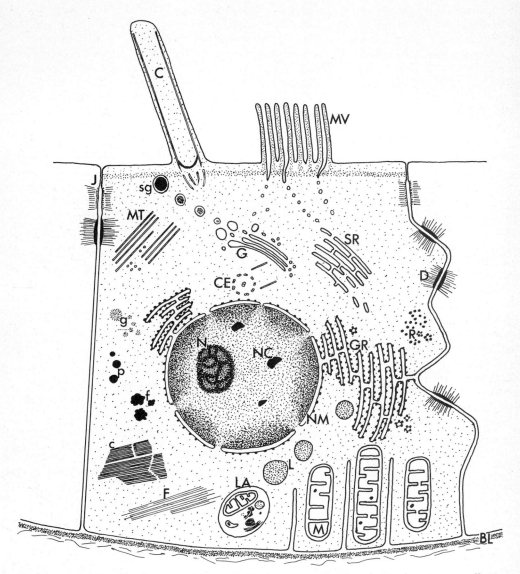

Figure 2-3.   Schematic diagram of the cell. Nuclear components and cytoplasmic organelles are indicated with capital letters, inclusions with small letters, and BL indicates the basal lamina, supported by reticular fibers beneath. C = cilium, CE = centrosome, D = desmosome (macula adherens). F = filaments, G = Golgi apparatus, GR = granular endoplasmic reticulum, J = junctional complex, L = lysosome, LA = autolysosome (secondary lysosome), M = mitochondrion, MT = microtubules, MV = microvillus, N = nucleolus, NC = nuclear chromatin, NM = nuclear envelope, R = ribosomes, and SR = smooth (agranular) endoplasmic reticulum; c = crystal, f = fat, g = glycogen, p = pigment, and sg = secretion granule.

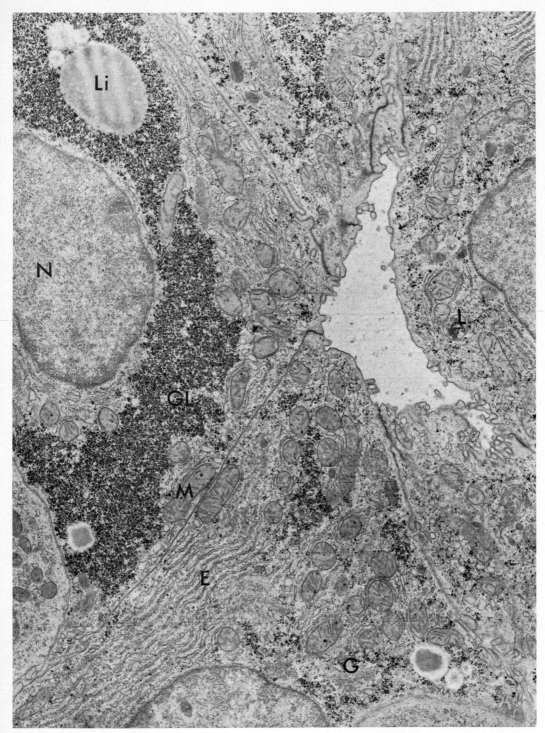

Figure 2-4.   Electron micrograph of rat liver cells illustrating the appearance of several organelles: N = nucleus, M = mitochondrion, G = Golgi apparatus, E = granular endoplasmic reticulum, L = lysosome, GL = glycogen, LI = lipid. The clear space in the center is a bile canaliculus. × 13,000. (Courtesy of J. Steiner.)

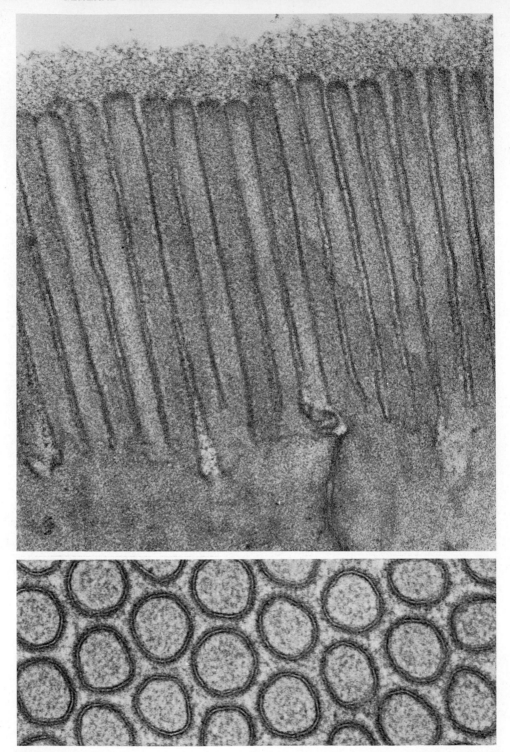

Figure 2-5. Electron micrographs of microvilli from intestinal absorptive epithelial cells of the human ileum. Top, longitudinal section showing an interface between two cells; bottom, cross section. Note the trilaminar unit membranes and the electron dense "fuzz" around microvilli. Top, × 65,000. Bottom, × 145,000. (Courtesy of S. Ito.)

vironment but also creates and maintains the interior cellular environment by active transport of ions and nutrients.

Often by light microscopy the cell membrane or *plasmalemma* is not visible. The membrane is about 0.18 μ thick and thus is beyond the limit of resolution of the light microscope. It is a complex, as shown at the higher magnification of the electron microscope, and can be shown to include material lying outside the cell. For general purposes, it may be defined as the thinnest layer resolved at the cell surface by light microscopy. The term "plasma membrane," now commonly used, indicates that the membrane limits the cell cytoplasm and is a part of the cell.

As viewed with the electron microscope, the plasma membrane is only 80 Å thick and shows the trilaminar structure of the unit membrane (see page 20). In many cells, its outer surface is covered by a surface coat largely composed of protein-polysaccharide. This surface probably is important in

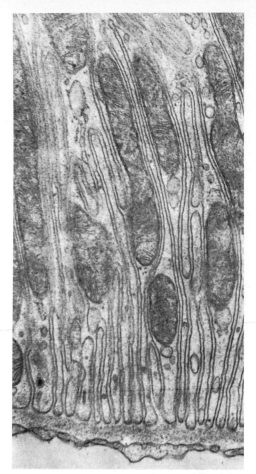

Figure 2-7. Electron micrograph of basal infoldings of the plasma membrane in an epithelial cell of the distal convoluted tubule of the kidney. The line of amorphous material beneath the epithelial cell is the basal lamina. × 26,000.

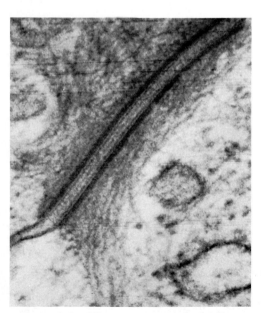

Figure 2-6. Electron micrograph of a desmosome on a cellular interface from corneal epithelium. At the desmosome, opposing plasma membranes are thickened, with an accumulation of fibrillar material in the adjacent cytoplasm. × 90,000.

the selective uptake of material by cells.

In many cell types, the plasma membrane shows modifications associated with function, the majority of these modifications being visible only with the electron microscope. In cells specialized for absorption, there often are at the luminal (apical) border of the cell many small, cylindrical, finger-like processes or microvilli, which collectively form a "brush" or "striated" border of the cell and are visible by light microscopy. These greatly increase the surface area of the cell since each is covered by an extension of the plasma membrane. Laterally, between cells, the adjacent plasma membranes usually are separated by a gap of 100 to 200 Å and may not be straight and parallel, but often show complex "jigsaw" or "zipper" interlocking. This has been considered a factor in cell adhesion. Toward the apices of cells, the lateral cell interfaces may show further complications in the form of dense bodies called *desmosomes*, which are discussed later in relation to epithelial cells. At the base of some epithelial cells, the plasma membrane is infolded into the cytoplasm, another mechanism for increasing surface area. Transport of material in the cell may occur by pinocytosis or phagocytosis, each small mass of fluid or material being surrounded by a pinched-off part of the plasma membrane to form a small vesicle or membrane-bounded inclusion body.

Finally, the relation of the plasma membrane to other membranous parts of the cell may be as indicated in Figure 2-3. It is probable that at some time there is continuity between the plasma membrane and the endoplasmic reticulum, and thus indirectly with the nuclear membrane, with the Golgi apparatus, and perhaps with the mitochondria. However, there is some variation in thickness of these membranes, the plasma membrane being 10 to 15 per cent thicker than the membranes of the other organelles. In each a triple-layered pattern has been demonstrated, and indeed, local variations in thickness of the plasma membrane do occur. For example, it is 75 Å thick at the base and about 100 Å thick at the tip of a microvillus.

Endoplasmic Reticulum

This cytoplasmic organelle, also called cytoplasmic RNA or ergastoplasm, is, as the name suggests, a network of membranes, vesicles, and tubules. Originally it was thought to be confined to the central portion of the cytoplasm ("endo"-plasm), but it is now known to extend throughout the

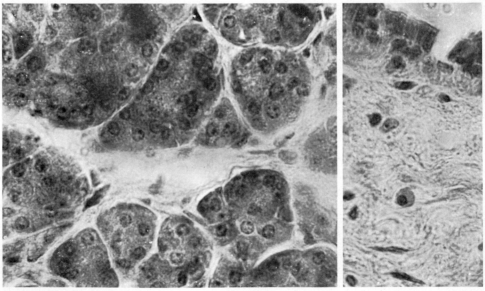

Figure 2-8. Photomicrographs to illustrate cytoplasmic basophilia. The zymogenic cells of the rat pancreas (left) are arranged in groups or acini, and the cytoplasm of each stains intensely basophil owing to the presence of numerous ribosomes associated with the endoplasmic reticulum. The single isolated cell in the center (right) is a plasma cell located near a lactiferous duct in the mammary gland. The cytoplasm is basophil also. × 600.

cell cytoplasm. It consists of a three-dimensional network of cisternae or tubules bounded by a membrane about 80 Å in thickness. The shape of individual elements varies from circular vesicles in perpendicular section to membrane-limited tubules or flattened profiles in longitudinal section. The elements of the endoplasmic reticulum may be single or numerous and packed tightly in parallel or near parallel array with intercommunicating cross channels. This system of fine intracytoplasmic membranes may on the one hand connect intermittently with the plasma membrane and on the other with the outer nuclear membrane. These membranes surround tubules and vesicles of such dimensions as to be visible only with the electron microscope. Two types of endoplas-

mic reticulum are recognized, smooth and rough.

Agranular or Smooth Reticulum. This is characterized by being un-associated with small osmiophilic bodies called RNA particles or *ribosomes* composed of ribonucleic acid. This type of reticulum is present in bulk in certain cell types, e.g., in parietal (acid-secreting) cells of the gastric mucosa where it is thought to be associated with hydrochloric acid secretion, in the interstitial cells of the testis and in cells of the corpus luteum, where it may be concerned with steroid hormone synthesis, in skeletal muscle where it is thought to play some part in the binding of calcium ions, and in liver cells where probably it is associated with glycogen formation and storage and with detoxi-

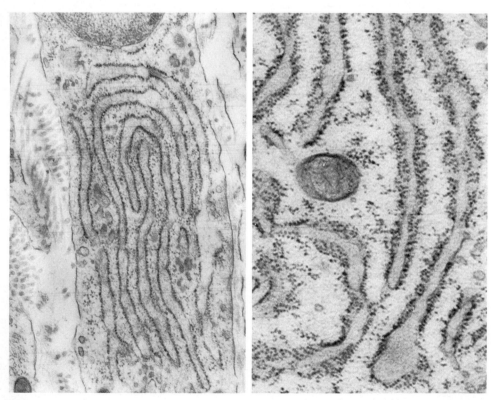

Figure 2-9. Electron micrographs of granular endoplasmic reticulum: Left, in a fibroblast of developing rat ureter. Right, a mesenchymal cell from rat umbilical cord. Note that in each micrograph the cisternae of the endoplasmic reticulum contain some dense (protein) material and that the membranes are studded on their external surfaces with ribosomes. The ribosomes on the right tend to be arranged in chains or groups as polysomes. Left, × 16,000. Right, × 37,000.

cation and cholesterol synthesis. This type of organelle must be distinguished from the membranous elements of the Golgi apparatus, from the small, smooth-walled vesicles previously described in association with pinocytosis, and from the microtubules described later.

Granular or Rough Reticulum. This is studded with the granules mentioned previously, small bodies (ribosomes) lying in rows in contact with the outer surface of the membranes of the endoplasmic reticulum. Small elements of the granular reticulum are present in most cells but are highly developed as series of parallel lamellae in protein-secreting cells, e.g., pancreatic acinar cells. In such cells, as seen by light microscopy, these areas stain with basic dyes. This deeply staining material is known as the *chromidial substance* or the *ergastoplasm*. The areas contain a high content of ribonucleoprotein which is Feulgen negative (whereas all nucleic acids stain with basic dyes, only deoxyribonucleic acid stains with the Feulgen technique). The basophilic staining is not localized directly in the membranous elements of the reticulum but in the ribosomes associated with them.

Ribosomes are small electron-dense granules 120 to 150 Å in diameter. Ribosomes can be isolated and broken down into two dissimilar subunits. Each subunit consists of a single strand of RNA and associated protein, the smaller subunit being about 40 Å in diameter, the larger subunit about 50 Å in diameter. Ribosomes may be found lying free within the cytoplasm in small groups or clumps, an arrangement common in embryonic and tumor cells, or they may be associated with membranes of the granular endoplasmic reticulum. There is some evidence to suggest that the former arrangement is indicative of a capacity for protein formation in cell growth and division and that the latter arrangement is associated with protein formation in cell secretion. This is discussed further on

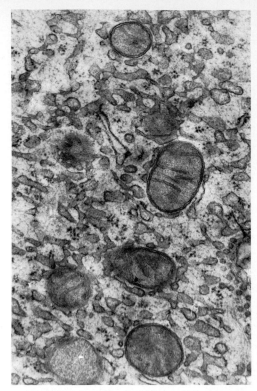

Figure 2-10. Electron micrograph of a portion of an interstitial (Leydig) cell of the human testis. The cytoplasm largely is occupied by smooth or agranular endoplasmic reticulum with a few mitochondria. × 32,000.

page 55. Ribosomes may be grouped in clusters to form *polyribosomes* or *polysomes*, the ribosomes of such a group being held together by a slender filament only about 15 Å in diameter. This filament is messenger RNA (see page 57).

Golgi Apparatus

This organelle, also called the Golgi complex, may be visible with the light microscope as either a "positive" or a "negative" image. After special fixing and staining techniques, e.g., prolonged immersion in osmium tetroxide or chrome-silver impregnation, the Golgi apparatus is visible as a dark net or irregular granular mass, usually situated near the nucleus and sometimes multiple. In most secretory cells, its location is between the nucleus and the apical surface of the cell through which expulsion of the secretory material occurs. In ordinary hematoxylin and eosin (H and E) preparations, this organelle may be visible as a pale area in the characteristic location, particularly in cells in which the cytoplasm stains a deep blue with the basophil dye hematoxylin, e.g., osteoblasts. This is a "negative" Golgi image, the unstained or pale area in deeply staining cytoplasm, as distinct from the specifically stained area ("positive" image) of the special preparations.

Electron microscopy reveals that the Golgi apparatus contains three components: lamellae (plates) of smooth-surfaced membranes bounding flattened sacs piled one upon the other; small microvesicles about 400 Å in diameter, often appearing as strings or necklaces tailing off from the ends of lamellae and presumably derived from them; and large vacuoles probably formed by dilatation of lamellae and often containing electron-dense

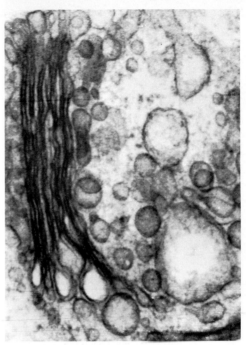

Figure 2-12. Electron micrograph of the Golgi apparatus from an interstitial cell of the human testis. The Golgi membranes or lamellae appear to dilate into vesicles at their ends. × 60,000.

material. The association of the Golgi apparatus with endoplasmic reticulum and cell secretion is discussed on page 57. Radioautographic studies have shown clearly that the Golgi complex is capable of sulfation and strongly suggest that it is involved in glycoprotein and acid mucopolysaccharide synthesis and in intracellular transport or secretion. Recent studies indicate that complex carbohydrate is synthesized in the Golgi vacuoles (saccules) and combined with immigrant protein to form the complex glycoprotein of mucus.

Cell-Center: Centriole

The cell center (centrosome) is located near the nucleus or, often, in an indentation in the nucleus when the latter is of irregular outline. Quite commonly the cell center is surrounded partially by the Golgi appara-

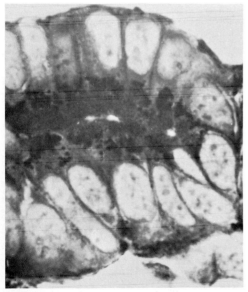

Figure 2-11. Pancreatic acinar cells stained to show the Golgi apparatus (black). Nuclei appear pale. Golgi silver stain. × 600.

tus. Contained in the cell center is a pair of centrioles, small granules or short rods, which for light microscopy can be stained with iron hematoxylin or can be seen by phase microscopy in fresh material. By electron microscopy, each centriole appears as a hollow cylinder about 1500 Å in diameter and 3000 to 5000 Å long. As seen in transverse section, the wall is composed of nine sets of tubular elements, each comprising three tubules fused together (a triplet) and orientated tangentially to the circle. As indicated, centrioles occur usually in pairs and with their long axes at a right angle to each other. They are capable of forming daughter centrioles and their association with, and morphological resemblance to, cilia is very interest-

ing. They are prominent in mitosis, in which they move apart to opposite poles of the nucleus and organize microtubules to form the mitotic spindle and asters (see page 51).

Cilia

Cilia are motile processes protruding from the apices of certain cells. They usually are multiple on some epithelial cells but do occur singly. Cilia are 5 to 10 μ in length and 0.2 μ in diameter, each with a dense granule, the *basal body,* at its base. In living cells they show a rapid beat in one direction with a slower recovery stroke. By their movement they can propel material lying on the cell sur-

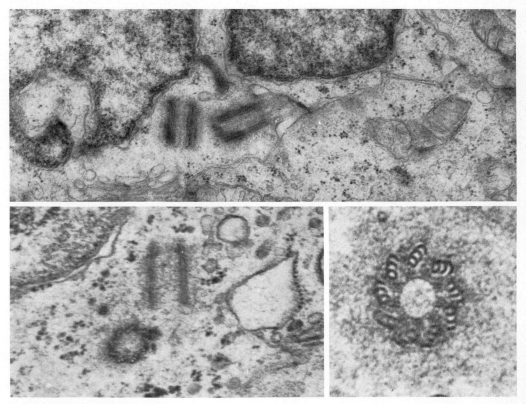

Figure 2-13.   Electron micrographs to demonstrate the appearance of centrioles. Top: a pair of centrioles near the nucleus (top left) of a supporting (Sertoli) cell of the testis. Both are cut longitudinally, but orientated approximately at right angles to each other. × 35,000. Bottom left: a similar pair, but one centriole is cut in cross section and shows nine subunits in its wall. × 42,000. Bottom right: a centriole in cross section to show that each of the nine subunits is composed of triple tubular elements. × 110,000.

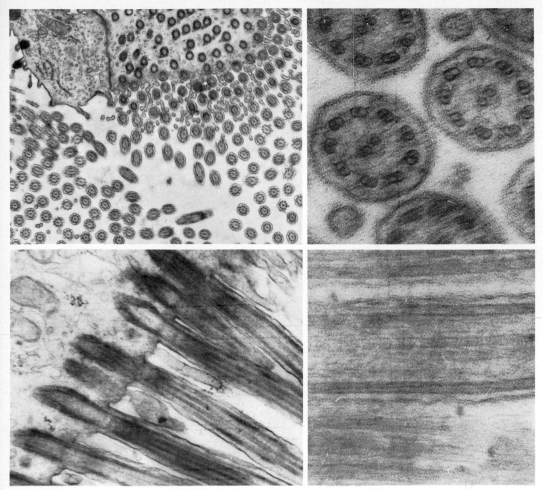

Figure 2-14. Electron micrographs of cilia of bronchiole epithelial cells. Top left: cilia in cross section lying in the lumen and their basal bodies in apical cytoplasm. × 18,000. Top right: cilia in cross section. × 110,000. Bottom left: cilia in longitudinal section. × 35,000. Bottom right: shaft of cilium in longitudinal section showing peripheral and central microtubules. × 110,000.

face. The structure of the basal body is identical to that of a centriole but the shaft of a cilium, covered by a protrusion of the plasma membrane, contains two single, central tubules surrounded by nine peripheral pairs (or doublets) of tubules. At the basal body, the central, single tubules terminate but the peripheral nine doublets are continuous with the inner two tubules of the triplets of the basal body. Flagella show an identical structure. Cilia are formed from centrioles, some of which arise directly from centrioles in the cell center, and some of which

develop from fibrogranular material which accumulates near the Golgi region. This material produces centrioles which progress to form cilia.

Mitochondria

Mitochondria or chondriosomes are present in all animal cells. Although not visible in ordinary H and E preparations, they can be demonstrated, for example, by iron hematoxylin and after supravital staining with Janus green B and other nontoxic dyes. In fresh preparations they are visible by

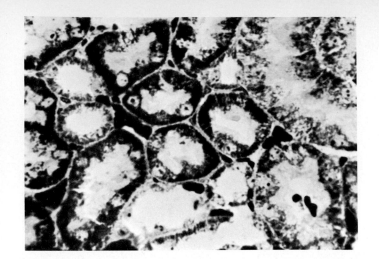

Figure 2-15. Photomicrograph to show mitochondria which appear as dark striations beneath and around nuclei. Kidney tubules, iron hematoxylin stain. × 350. See filmstrip I, frame 3.

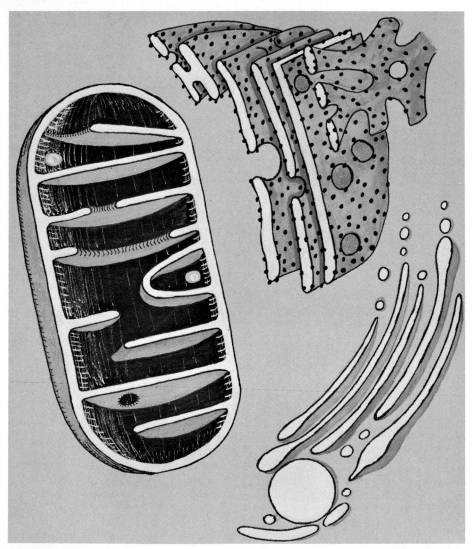

Figure 2-16. Diagram to illustrate the electron microscopic appearance of a mitochondrion (left), elements of the granular endoplasmic reticulum (top right), and the Golgi apparatus (bottom right).

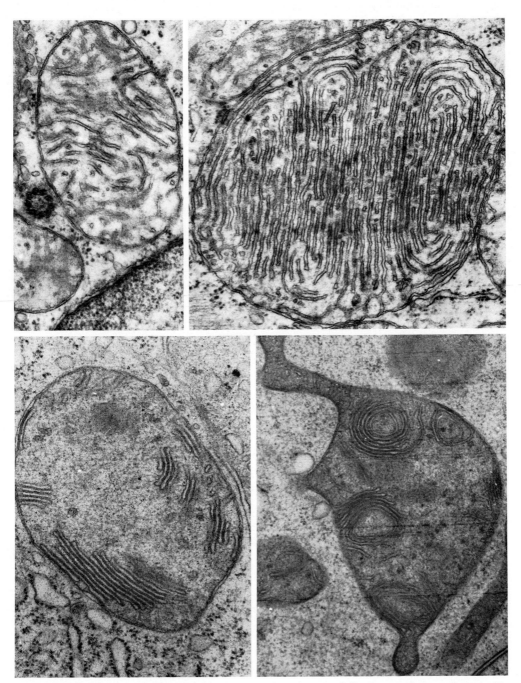

Figure 2-17.   Electron micrographs of mitochondria showing different morphological types. Top left: from striated muscle (note also the presence of a centriole in cross section). Top right: from cardiac muscle. Bottom left and right: from interstitial cells of the human testis. All × 40,000.

phase microscopy. Mitochondria vary in shape and size from small ovoids or spheres less than 0.1 micron in diameter to long, slender threads 10 microns or more in length and 0.5 micron in width. In numbers they range from a few to several thousand in each cell, there being 2000 to 3000 in each parenchymal liver cell, for example. In living cells mitochondria can move within the cytoplasm and change their shape, and often they appear to fuse temporarily and then separate.

By electron microscopy, they have a characteristic basic form. All are bounded by a double membrane structure with the inner membrane being infolded into the center of the organelle, usually as a series of flat membranous plates termed *cristae mitochondriales*. The cristae may show circular fenestrations and they vary in form and extent. Some are relatively short and others appear to extend completely across the mitochondrion. Although in most mitochondria cristae are orientated transversely, in a few they run longitudinally and in others are tubular or villiform in shape, or even appear as prismatic tubules. The outer membrane is about 60 Å thick

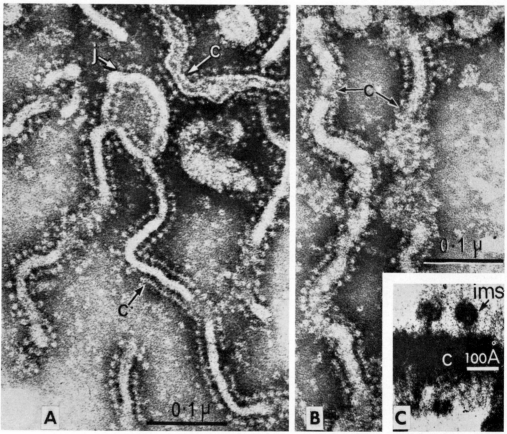

Figure 2-18. Electron micrograph of the subunit (elementary particle) associated with the inner mitochondrial membranes or cristae of mouse liver: *A*, A few cristae (c), consisting of long filaments which sometimes branch (j). The surfaces of the cristae are covered with projecting subunits. × 192,000. *B*, Similar cristae with subunits. × 192,000. *C*, Higher magnification showing a few subunits (ims) with spherical heads having a diameter of approximately 90 Å and stems 30 to 35 Å wide and 45 to 50 Å long. The center to center spacing is 100 Å. Reversed print, × 770,000. (Preparation courtesy of Dr. D. F. Parsons and reproduced by permission from Science, *140*:985, 1963.)

and separated by an intramembranous space of 80 Å from the inner membrane, also 60 Å thick. Because cristae are infoldings of the inner membrane, the intramembranous space extends into the cores of the cristae. The matrix of the mitochondrion is the space bounded by the inner membrane. The matrix usually is homogeneous but may contain small dense granules and also fine filaments which probably are composed of DNA (deoxyribonucleic acid). The matrix is semisolid. The inner surface of the inner membrane is studded with small particles (the *elementary particles*, which can be demonstrated only by special techniques). These are illustrated in Figure 2-18.

Functionally, mitochondria contain most of the enzymes necessary for the citric acid cycle. This process is concerned with the final breakdown of food material (carbohydrate, fatty acids, and many amino acids), and also involves the release of energy. By the electron transport chain, through oxidative phosphorylation, ATP (adenosine triphosphate) is produced from ADP (adenosine diphosphate). ATP then is utilized as an energy source by the cell. Mitochondria, the source of energy-rich ATP, often are located in regions of the cell where energy is utilized to produce metabolic work, e.g., in relation to the contractile elements of muscle cells to produce contraction or in relation to the contractile sperm tail to produce motility. Current knowledge indicates that enzymes for oxidative phosphorylation and electron transport are located on the mitochondrial membranes, and those for the citric acid cycle and biosynthesis in the matrix. In addition, mitochondria are semiautonomous and self-replicating, carrying out some of the biosynthesis necessary for their own replication.

Annulate Lamellae

This term describes an organelle visible only with the electron microscope. Annulate lamellae are usually located near the nucleus and consist of parallel double membranes with numerous pores or annuli. The membranes are about 70 to 90 Å thick enclosing a space of 300 to 500 Å; the pores are 400 to 500 Å in diameter. Generally the pores are spaced regularly at intervals of 1000 to 2000 Å. Thus, annulate lamellae are bilaminar membrane structures with circular pores formed by the union of both membranes. In true transverse section, the pores appear to be closed by a membrane of greater density than those forming the lamellae. This resemblance to the structure of the nuclear envelope gave rise to the hypothesis that the lamellae arose from the nuclear envelope, and recent work has demonstrated stages in the formation of, firstly, blebs of the outer membrane of the nuclear envelope, with subsequent fusion and transformation into lamellae. Similar structures occasionally are seen in an intranuclear position. Functionally, it may be that cytoplasmic annulate lamellae carry information from the nucleus to the cytoplasm, although there is no strong evidence for this hypothesis. Additionally, and again there is no evidence, the process of formation suggests that annulate lamellae may simply be transitory and later break down to form cytoplasmic vesicles. Annulate lamellae to date have been demonstrated in developing stages of male and female germ cells, in embryonic and tumor cells, and in various epithelial cell types.

Fibrils and Filamentous Structures

It is essential to distinguish between a fibril lying within cell cytoplasm—an organelle—and a fibril which lies outside the cell. The latter will be discussed as part of connective tissue. Specific intracellular fibrils are characteristic of various cell types, e.g., muscle cells. In this instance the student must avoid confusion in terminology, for the muscle cell is so elongated and

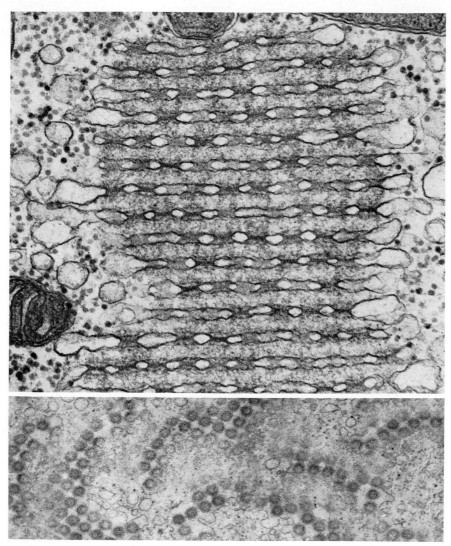

Figure 2-19.   Electron micrographs of annulate lamellae from a frog oocyte, sectioned in different planes. Top × 50,000, bottom × 25,500. (Courtesy of Dr. R. G. Kessel.)

threadlike that often it is referred to as a muscle fiber. Other specific fibrils are present in nerve cells, in certain types of epithelial cells, and in all cells undergoing mitosis. These various types of fibrils will be discussed in detail in the appropriate chapters, but a note on terminology should be included at this time. We have already distinguished between intracellular and extracellular fibrils, but there may be confusion also about fiber size. Generally speaking, a microfibril or filament can be seen only with the electron microscope; microfibrils often are grouped together to form a bundle which is visible with the high power of the light microscope and which usually is termed a fibril; in turn, a bundle of fibrils, visible as a distinct entity with low power, is usually called a fiber.

In many cells cytoplasmic microfibrils are present, probably consisting of elongated protein molecules. They are believed to form a diffuse cytoskeleton providing strength and resiliency. In some epithelial cells, these microfibrils are associated commonly with junctional complexes and desmosomes forming the so-called *terminal web*. Other types of fibrils are seen in specific cell types, for example, keratin in epidermis.

Lysosomes

Lysosomes only recently have been recognized as cytoplasmic organelles and their functions understood. Basically, a lysosome is a membrane-bounded body filled with a droplet of acid hydrolases which functions in many ways as the digestive system of the cell. These enzymes are capable of breaking down all the main constituents of living matter, i.e., proteins, carbohydrates, fats, and nucleic acids. Almost all animal cells with the exception of erythrocytes contain lysosomes. The majority appear on electron microscopy as spherical, baglike structures 0.25 to 0.5 micron in diameter with an electron-dense granular content. However, they vary greatly in appearance. They are identified by electron cytochemistry, for example, with a modified Gomori technique for acid phosphatase, and by vital staining with dyes such as neutral red and acridine orange. The specific granules of certain leukocytes also are classified as lysosomes.

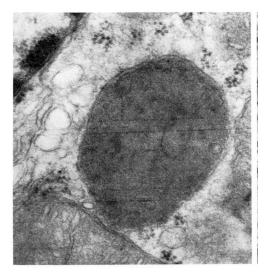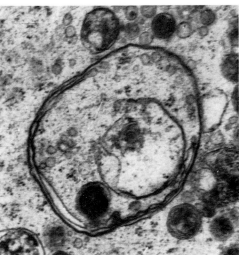

Figure 2-20. Electron micrographs of, left, a primary lysosome and, right, a secondary lysosome from a sustentacular (Sertoli) cell of the testis. Both × 44,000.

One obvious function of lysosomes is in cell necrosis and autolysis, the membranes bounding lysosomes rupturing to release the digestive enzymes when a cell is damaged, for example, by lack of oxygen. Further, other organelles such as ribosomes and mitochondria in certain conditions can become enclosed in vacuoles (autosomes or autosomal bodies) which then combine with one or more lysosomes with resulting digestion of the organelles, presumably to provide energy or to provide material essential for the life of the cell. Foreign particles such as ingested bacteria are disposed of in a similar manner.

Lysosomal enzymes probably are synthesized, like other proteins, by ribosomes of the endoplasmic reticulum and then transported to and packaged (wrapped in a membrane) in the Golgi apparatus (see page 55). The bodies so formed, termed *nascent granules*, develop into *primary lysosomes*. Some of these undoubtedly discharge their contents outside the cell but the majority remain quiescent until they are required for intracellular digestion. The fusion of a primary lysosome with a particle brought into the cell from outside (a phagosome) or with an autosome produces a *secondary lysosome* (respectively, a heterolysosome or an autolysosome) with a pleomorphic content. This, after digestive activity is completed, may remain in the cell as a *residual body*.

Microtubules

Microtubules are thin, elongated, tubular structures of only about 270 Å overall diameter which run a straight course in the cytoplasm. They are not very obvious in tissue fixed in osmium tetroxide but are well seen after glutaraldehyde or acrolein fixation. The tubules have a core of about 170 Å diameter, with a wall thickness there-

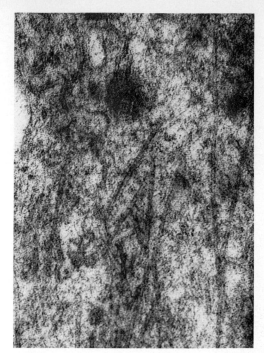

Figure 2-21. Electron micrograph of cytoplasmic microtubules from an intestinal epithelial cell. × 70,000.

fore of about 50 Å. The wall is composed of longitudinal subunits, which are beaded fibrils with a center to center spacing of about 50 Å. Probably there are 13 such subunits in the wall of a microtubule. This appearance is very similar to that of the tubular elements in cilia and flagella, where the double microtubule probably is composed of two standard microtubules which share three or four subunits along their line of fusion.

In interphase (nondividing) cells, microtubules are not very prominent but in mitosis they become associated with the centrioles and chromosomes to form the mitotic spindle and asters. They probably also function to maintain cell shape, forming a cytoskeleton, and it is possible that they are capable of contraction to change the shape of a cell or to initiate cell movement. Further, it has been suggested that they form diffusion channels throughout the cytoplasm for water and metabolite transport.

Inclusions

Cytoplasmic inclusions are structures present in the cytoplasm which are not living components of the protoplasm. They include stored foods, secretion granules, pigments, and crystals.

Stored Foods. During times of complete starvation, the human body maintains metabolism from food material stored within cell cytoplasm. All three types of food (protein, fat, and carbohydrate) are involved in this.

PROTEIN. Protein is rarely stored as an inclusion although it occurs, for example, in the liver. The body store or reserve of protein exists in the general cytoplasm, i.e., the matrix, and to a certain extent cells can maintain metabolism by consuming a portion of their own cytoplasm.

FAT. Fat is stored mostly in connective tissue fat cells, which together form adipose tissue, and is present also in many other cells, e.g., the liver and some types of muscle cells. During normal section preparation, fat is dissolved out and thus appears as clear spaces in the cytoplasm, which are usually smooth and circular in outline. As cells accumulate more fat, the droplet becomes larger until finally the cell cytoplasm remains only as a slender strip enclosing the fat droplet. After osmium tetroxide fixation, fat remains in sections as dark brown or black masses, and fat can be demonstrated also by using special stains (for example, Sudan black or Scharlach red) on frozen sections. Other types of lipid are present in cytoplasm and can be demonstrated only by chemical extraction. These types usually are called masked or bound fat.

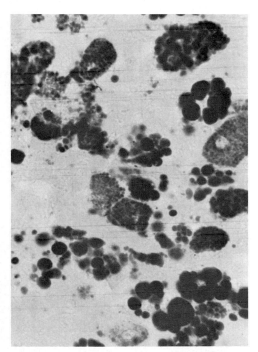

Figure 2-22. Photomicrograph of lipid inclusions in liver cells, showing a marked difference in the content of lipid material from cell to cell. Osmic acid. × 450. See filmstrip I, frame 4.

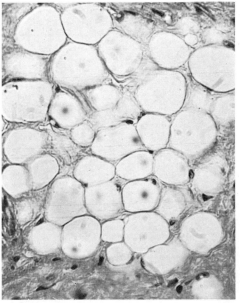

Figure 2-23. Photomicrograph of adipose tissue. Individual fat cells lose their content of lipid during preparation, and each cell in this section contained so much lipid that only a thin rim of cytoplasm and nucleus remains. This "chicken-wire" appearance is typical of adipose tissue. × 250.   See filmstrip I, frame 5.

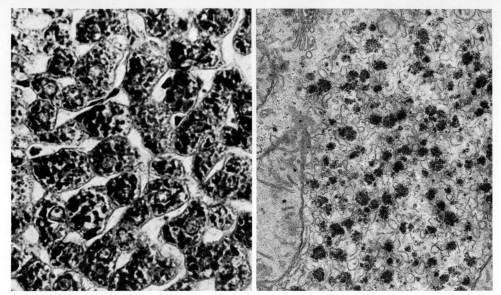

Figure 2-24. Left: Photomicrograph of a section of the liver to show glycogen. Best's carmine, × 350. Right: Electron micrograph of particulate glycogen in a liver cell. × 24,000. (Courtesy of J. Steiner.)   See filmstrip I, frame 2.

CARBOHYDRATE. Carbohydrate is absorbed from the intestine mainly in the form of glucose and then is converted to glycogen for storage, particularly in the liver although glycogen can be demonstrated in many other cells. In ordinary H and E preparations, glycogen has been removed but leaves a characteristic pattern of irregular, ragged spaces between strands of cytoplasm giving the cell a moth-eaten appearance. A positive demonstration can be obtained after staining with the periodic acid–Schiff reagent, which imparts a brilliant red color to glycogen. By electron microscopy, glycogen appears as dark amorphous areas in the cytoplasm and, if in sufficient quantity, it pushes most of the organelles into a paranuclear position. With staining techniques, glycogen has a particulate appearance, the granular material varying in size from about 150 to 400 Å in diameter. Glycogen may also appear as rosettes about 950 Å in diameter, each being a complex of several smaller particles.

Secretion Granules. In secretory epithelial cells, digestive enzymes and other fluids are synthesized within the cytoplasm from raw materials and often form small globules or droplets of fluid, lying in the cytoplasm and bounded by a membrane. These usually are precipitated by fixation to form granules. Such inclusions are present within the cytoplasm only for a limited period of time between synthesis and secretion or release from the cell. In many cases, these granules can be stained specifically by special histochemical techniques.

Pigments. Pigments are materials which possess color. They do not have to be stained by dyes as do other cell ingredients in order to be visible. Usually pigments are classified as either exogenous, being formed outside the body and later taken into it, or as endogenous, being formed within the body.

Exogenous pigments include carotin, a yellowish pigment found in vegetables, lipochromes of similar origin, dusts, e.g., carbon, and minerals such as lead and silver. Tattooing is a process whereby exogenous pigments are introduced into the deeper layers of the skin.

Endogenous pigments are mainly

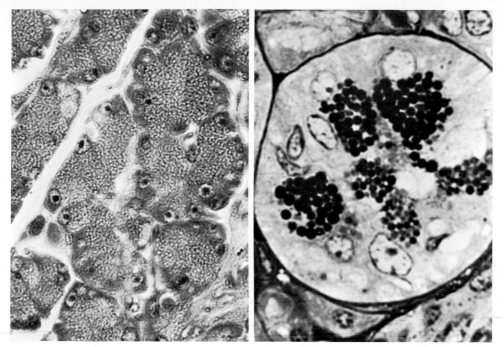

Figure 2-25. Left: Photomicrograph of pancreatic acinar (enzyme-secreting) cells showing secretion granules. The nucleoli are large. × 550. Right: secretion granules in Paneth (sero-zymogenic) cells of the duodenum. Epon section. × 1500.   See filmstrip I, frame 6.

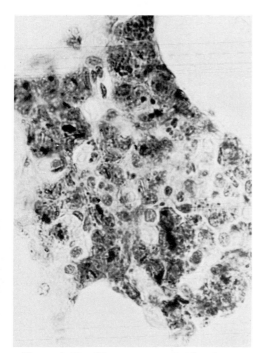

Figure 2-26. Photomicrograph of carbon, an exogenous pigment, in lung tissue. × 550.

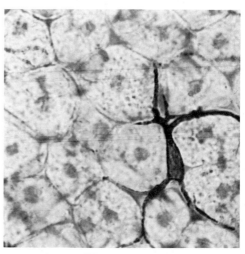

Figure 2-27. Photomicrograph of a pigment cell from salamander skin. The pigment is melanin, and the cell has a characteristic shape with long cytoplasmic processes extending between epithelial cells. × 550.

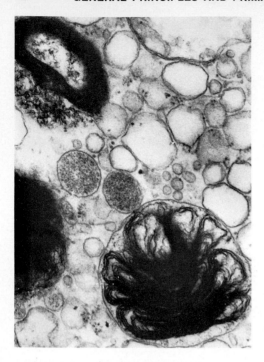

Figure 2-28.　Electron micrograph of pigment (fuchsin) granules from the pigment epithelium of the rat retina. × 40,000.

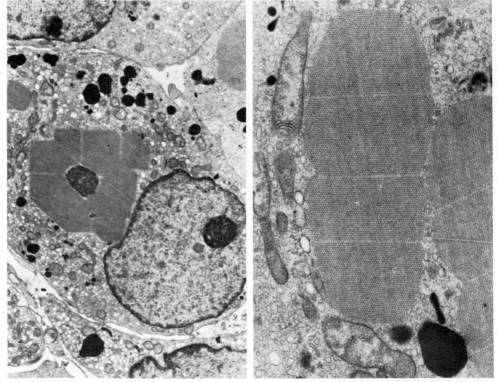

Figure 2-29.　Left: survey electron micrograph of an interstitial cell of the human testis. Contained in the cytoplasm near the nucleus is a large crystalloid (gray) and several lipid inclusions (black) × 4200. Right: a higher magnification of a crystalloid from a similar cell. The crystalloid shows a regular lattice pattern. There also is a lipid inclusion (bottom right). × 28,000.

of two types, hemoglobin and its breakdown products such as hemosiderin, which contains iron, and bilirubin (hematoidin), which does not, and melanin. The latter, a dark brown or black pigment found in the skin and the eye, is the pigment of suntan. It appears in large amounts in the epidermis of the Negroid races.

Crystals.   Crystalline material, probably proteinaceous, is found in a few cells, for example, the Sertoli and interstitial cells of the testis. The nature and significance of such material is unknown.

NUCLEUS

The nucleus (or nuclei if multiple) of a cell is a spherical or ovoid blue-staining body in an H and E preparation, situated usually toward the center of the cell. It is limited by a thin nuclear membrane or envelope and contains within its karyoplasm or nuclear sap darker-staining irregular chromatin strands or granules. Also visible may be one or more spherical or ovoid bodies, the nucleolus, or nucleoli. This description is of the nucleus of an interphase cell, viz., a cell which is resting and not undergoing cell division. It can be shown by the Feulgen technique, by ultraviolet microscopy, and by histochemical studies after enzyme digestion that the karyoplasm and chromatin contain DNA and the nucleolus RNA, the latter often appearing pink in an H and E preparation.

Nuclear Envelope

This structure, separating nucleus from cytoplasm, is visible by light microscopy as a thin, darkly staining membrane. It is shown by electron microscopy to be composed of two parallel membranes separated by a *perinuclear space* or *cisterna* of 500 Å width. The nuclear envelope shows continuity of the outer membrane with the membranes of the endoplasmic reticulum, both being studded on their outer surfaces with ribosomes. The perinuclear space thus is considered to be a cistern of the reticulum and the nuclear envelope an essential part of the reticulum.

In many sections *pores* are present in the nuclear membrane. A pore or annulus is circular in outline, about 700 to 1200 Å in diameter, and at its circumference inner and outer nuclear membranes are continuous. The pore, however, is closed by a single thin membrane or diaphragm. In tangential sections annuli are seen in surface view and may show a ring structure composed of small subunits. It is known that there is a nuclear-cytoplasm interchange of material across the nuclear envelope, perhaps mainly through the nuclear pores.

On the inner aspect of the nuclear envelope of some cells there is a *fibrous lamina* formed by a layer of fine filaments. Its significance is not known, but it may be a mechanical support.

Karyoplasm

The karyoplasm or *nuclear sap* was so termed to describe those areas of the nucleus not occupied by nucleolus or chromatin. This area appears lightly staining by light microscopy; electron microscopy reveals that it contains dispersed chromatin and small granules. It certainly contains proteins and probably exists in a colloidal state, presumably as a gel during interphase and as a sol during mitosis and DNA duplication when a sol state would be necessary to permit free movement of other nuclear structures.

Nuclear Chromatin

Chromatin granules or strands, which stain strongly with basic dyes, contain DNA and basic and acidic

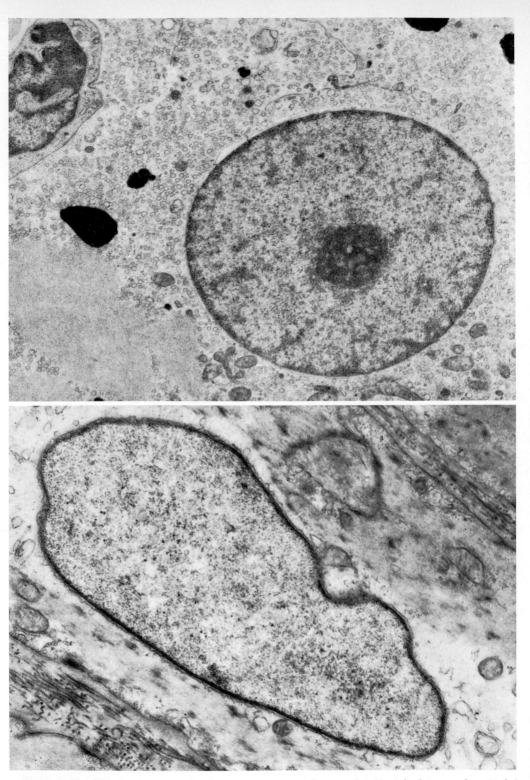

Figure 2-30. Electron micrographs demonstrating interphase nuclei. Top: the large nucleus (right) is of an interstitial (Leydig) cell of the human testis and shows a spherical profile with nuclear envelope, central nucleolus, chromatin granules and karyoplasm. The nucleus (top left) of a connective tissue cell is of highly irregular outline. × 12,500. Bottom: the elongated nucleus of a smooth muscle cell shows nuclear envelope and fibrous lamina internal to it. No nucleolus or chromatin granules are seen. × 17,000.

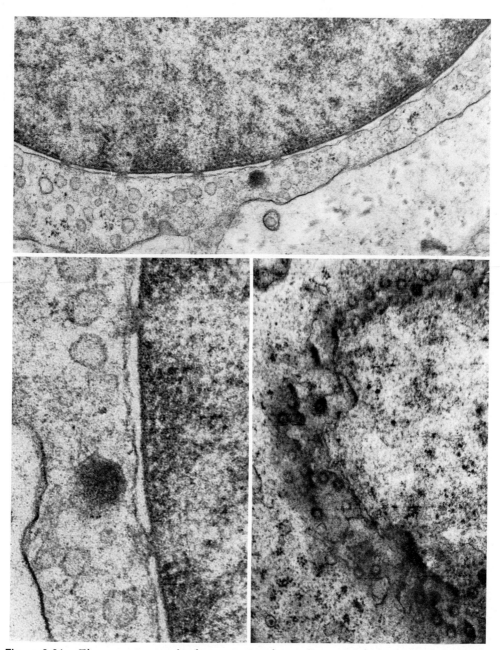

Figure 2-31.   Electron micrographs demonstrating the nuclear envelope and nuclear pores. Top: the nucleus lies above and four pores are shown. × 22,000. Bottom left: higher magnification showing two pores. × 68,000. Bottom right: tangential section of nuclear envelope showing nuclear pores as circular profiles, nucleus on the right. × 18,000.

proteins. These granules vary in number and size not only from cell type to cell type but also from species to species. Chromatin particles, for example, are not obvious in nerve cell nuclei and are larger and more numerous in rodent cells than they are in the human. They represent those parts of the chromosomes (DNA) which remain in a nondispersed phase during interphase, i.e., those segments which retain a tight coiling. (The segments of chromosomes which are dispersed, i.e., have uncoiled during interphase, are present in the nuclear sap and are not identifiable as chromosomes.) By electron microscopy, chromatin masses show a fine dense granularity with individual particles 50 Å or more in diameter. Interspersed between them, thin coiled filaments can be seen occasionally.

Nucleolus

Each nucleus contains one or more nucleoli, the number in any nucleus being variable from time to time as nucleoli can fuse or new ones can be formed. They are denser, larger, and more regular in outline than chromatin granules and can be situated either within the nuclear sap or seemingly attached to the inner aspect of the nuclear membrane. Their coloration by dyes varies, and they may be acidophil or basophil, this being related to their content of basic and acid proteins and RNA and to their relation to protein of the karyoplasm, which may surround them intimately and impart thereby a distinct coloration. They are very obvious in the large, clear nuclei of nerve cells but are more difficult to identify in the darkly staining nuclei

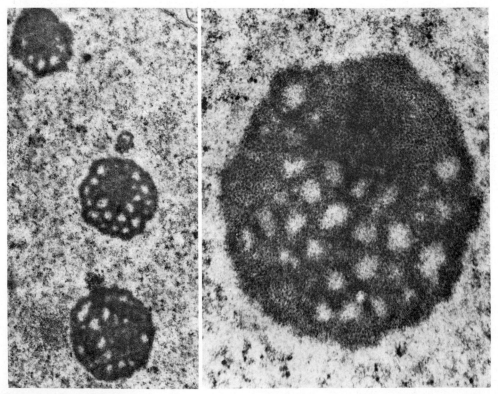

Figure 2-32.   Electron micrographs showing nucleoli; left, a portion of a nucleus containing three nucleoli and, right, a single nucleolus showing the branching, coiled network of the nucleolonema composed of granules and fine filaments. Left, × 10,000; right, × 28,000.

of lymphocytes. There is a relation between the number and size of nucleoli and cell growth and protein synthesis; in cells which are actively growing and dividing and in cells actively synthesizing protein, nucleoli are large and often multiple. The nucleolus is a site of active RNA synthesis.

The use of special techniques reveals that the nucleolus possesses a definite internal structure, consisting of a coiled, thick filament called the nucleolonema embedded in an amorphous component. This is confirmed by electron microscopy, which demonstrates that the nucleolus consists of a mass of tiny granules about 150 Å in diameter and fine filaments arranged to form a coiled cord embedded within a structureless material.

Recent work has made possible a classification of the morphological and biochemical components of the nucleolus. The nucleolar body itself or the nucleolonema consists of a fibrillar component (50 to 70 Å in diameter) and a granular component (120 to 150 Å in diameter), which probably are ribosomes. Also present is a non-nucleolonemal portion containing spherical areas of low density and irregular spaces containing nucleoplasm (karyoplasm) and chromatin, this second component being equivalent to the pars amorpha of light microscopy. A third component is nucleolus-associated chromatin consisting of nuclear histones. The first two components are composed of protein and RNA. The variable staining reactions of the nucleolus thus are explained by a variation in its biochemical components.

CELL CYCLE

In a cell population which constantly is being renewed, e.g., in the epithelium lining the intestinal tract, individual cells divide periodically. This process of mitosis and interphase

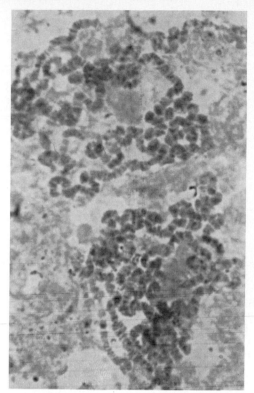

Figure 2-33. Photomicrograph of a giant chromosome from a salivary gland of the fruit fly (*Drosophila*). A smear preparation. × 850.

(the period between cell divisions) is termed the cell cycle. The duration of this cycle for any particular cell type now can be estimated accurately. Toward the end of interphase, DNA is synthesized. This stage is called the DNA duplication or the S (synthesis) stage. After the S stage, the cell enters a relatively quiescent period prior to mitosis called the post-duplication or G2 stage, and then passes through prophase, metaphase, anaphase, and telophase (see page 51). At the termination of mitosis, the daughter cells enter the preduplication or G1 stage of interphase, which lasts until DNA duplication occurs prior to the succeeding mitosis. Obviously the length of the cell cycle varies with the cell type, being, for example, short in the case of the epithelium lining the gut and much longer in liver cells.

CHROMOSOMES

Fine Structure of Chromosomes.
The great majority of nuclear DNA is located in the chromosomes. It should be emphasized that chromosomes exist as individual bodies in interphase as well as in mitosis.

In metaphase cells, chromosomes have indistinct outlines and are fibrous structures, being formed by numerous fibers. Each fiber contains DNA and nuclear histone and in sectioned material is about 200 Å in diameter. Special techniques have demonstrated that the actual fiber is only 100 Å in diameter, supercoiled to form a thread 200 to 250 Å thick. The 100 Å fiber in turn is composed of two fibrils of 30 Å, probably the DNA molecules, connected by material which holds them together and perhaps is the nuclear histone.

Chromosome Numbers

Human male somatic (body or non-germ) cells have 46 chromosomes arranged in 23 pairs, of which 22 pairs are called *autosomes* and one pair is formed by the X and Y or *sex chromosomes*. In females there are 22 pairs of autosomes plus two X chromosomes. This number, i.e., 46, is called the diploid or double number. In the gonads, the sex cells (ova or spermatozoa) contain half this number, or 23 chromosomes. This is called the haploid number, and involves a special type of cell division called meiosis or reduction division. Thus, each ovum or female sex cell contains 22 autosomes and one X chromosome, and each spermatozoon or male sex cell contains 22 autosomes and one X or one Y chromosome. After fertilization, i.e., after union of the sex cells, the fertilized ovum or gamete will contain either 44 autosomes plus two X chromosomes (a combination that develops into a female) or 44 autosomes plus one X and one Y chromosome (a combination that develops into a male).

In some cases, human somatic cells may not have the correct number of chromosomes. *Polyploidy* is a condition in which cells contain a multiple of the haploid number, e.g., tetraploidy, in which four times the number of haploid chromosomes are present (double the diploid number), i.e., 92. Polyploidy is quite common in liver cells, for example, and is characterized by a very large nucleus. It results, of course, from an abnormal mitosis. *Aneuploidy* is a condition in which a cell contains either less than the normal diploid number of chromosomes or a greater number which is not a multiple of it. Such a variation may result in an individual with a disease condition, for example, a congenital condition called mongolism. Such children are imbecilic, and the somatic cells contain one extra chromosome. Chromosome abnormalities of the aneuploid type also quite commonly involve the sex chromosomes and are associated with varying degrees of abnormality involving particularly the sex organs, e.g., Klinefelter's syndrome.

Sex Chromatin

Chromosomes both in interphase and during mitosis may show irregular densities of staining along their lengths. The parts which stain darkly, the so-called heterochromatic parts, probably are regions where the chromosomal threads are tightly coiled. This density of staining is marked in the case of one X chromosome in the female and is responsible for the sex chromatin being visible in female somatic interphase nuclei. The sex chromatin is a small body about 1 micron in diameter, frequently of planoconvex shape, located against the inner aspect of the nuclear membrane. In normal people, and in many animals, the presence of the sex chromatin is indicative of the presence of two X chromosomes, i.e., female sex, and its absence indicates XY chromosomes (the male sex). This small body

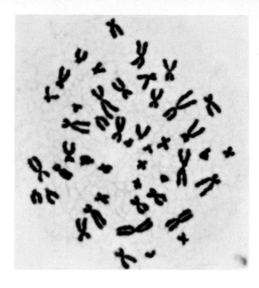

Figure 2-34. Photomicrograph of human (male) chromosomes from a squash preparation. Notice the various positions of the centromeres. × 1250. (Courtesy of Dr. M L. Barr.)

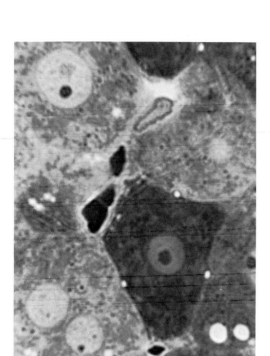

Figure 2-35. Photomicrograph of rat liver showing polyploidy. The cell at top left has a single, large polyploid nucleus; that at bottom left has two nuclei. Epon section, × 1200.

See filmstrip I, frame 2.

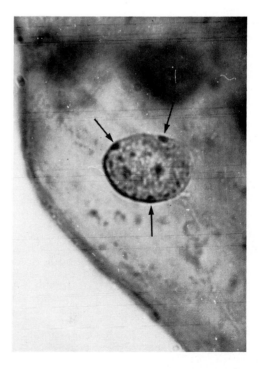

Figure 2-36. Photomicrograph of cells from the buccal smear of a 2 month old, mentally retarded child. The somatic cells of this child, presumably a Klinefelter syndrome, contain 22 times 2 autosomes plus XXXXY. The nucleus illustrated contains three female sex chromatin bodies. × 1200. (Courtesy of Dr. B. Smith.)

is seen particularly well in the nuclei of squamous epithelial cells scraped from the inside of the cheek and is easily seen after special staining, e.g., with aceto-orcein. In neutrophil granular leukocytes (a type of white blood cell) of females the sex chromatin is visible as a "drumstick" or a small body connected to one lobe of the nucleus by a fine thread. The sex chromatin is seen in nerve cell nuclei of cats as a small body associated with the nucleolus (the "nucleolar satellite"). It was in such cells of female cats that it first was recognized and its association with sex described by Barr and Bertram in 1949.

Originally it was believed that sex chromatin is formed by the presence of two X chromosomes lying closely apposed to each other and remaining tightly coiled and heterochromatic in interphase nuclei. It now appears that the first X chromosome in females (and the sole X of males) is present in an extended or dispersed state and

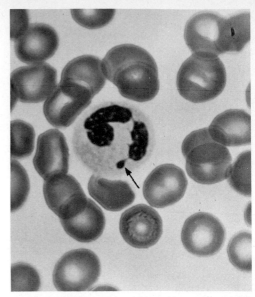

Figure 2-38. Photomicrograph of a polymorph (white blood cell) from a human female. Sex chromatin appears as a nuclear "drumstick" (arrow). × 1600. (Courtesy of Dr. M. L. Barr.)

thus is invisible. The second X of normal females, and any other which may be present in cases of sexual abnormality (aneuploidy), can assume a tightly coiled or heterochromatic state, and it is this one which appears as the sex chromatin.

DNA Structure and Duplication

DNA is a polymer (macromolecule) composed of units of the sugar deoxyribose, each with a base and a phosphate group. DNA has the form of a double-stranded ladder twisted into a helix or spiral. Before or during mitosis or cell division, obviously the DNA content of the parent cell must double if each daughter cell is to have a DNA (i.e., chromosome) content identical in quantity and quality to that of the parent. This process is termed *DNA duplication*.

CELL DIVISION

Even in adult tissues, with the notable exception of the central nervous

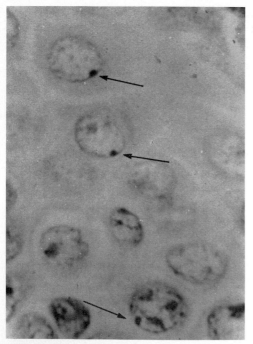

Figure 2-37. Photomicrograph of sex chromatin (arrows) in epidermal nuclei from the cheek of a human female. × 1800.

system, cells divide and reproduce themselves, this process involving both division of the cytoplasm (cytokinesis) and of the nucleus (karyokinesis). The rate at which divisions occur varies from tissue to tissue but is rapid in the epithelium of the gut tract, in the epidermis, in the blood-forming tissues, and in the generative organs. Division of the nucleus is accomplished by an indirect method called mitosis, and not by direct division or amitosis.

Mitosis

Mitosis is the process whereby the two daughter nuclei receive a chromosome complement identical to that of the mother nucleus. This process, then, involves, first, a doubling of the chromosome content of the parent nucleus and, second, an equal distribution of this content between the two daughter nuclei. For descriptive purposes, mitosis is divided into four stages, but it must be emphasized that all four are part of a continuous process.

Prophase. Prophase is characterized by the appearance within the nucleus of small granules which become lined up to form threads, these becoming in turn shorter, denser, and rodlike. These rods are the chromosomes. At the same time, the centrosome either already contains or forms two centrioles, and these separate from each other and move toward

Stages of Mitosis

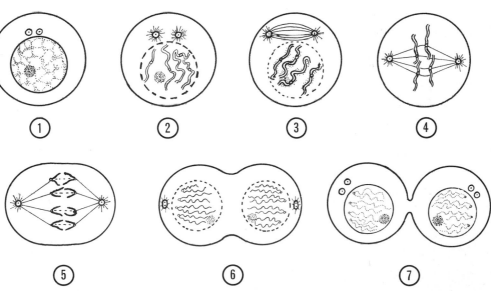

Figure 2-39. Diagram of the stages of mitosis. (1) Interphase: Nuclear envelope, nucleolus, chromatin, and a pair of centrioles are illustrated. (2) Early prophase: Two centrioles are forming asters, nuclear envelope and nucleolus are dispersing, and chromosomes are becoming visible. (3) Late prophase: A spindle is formed between the two centrioles. Nuclear envelope virtually has disappeared and the nucleolus is broken up and dispersed over the chromosomes, four of which are illustrated, each split into two chromatids, and each joined only at a centromere. (4) Metaphase: The chromosomes (pairs of chromatids) are arranged at the equator of the spindle. (5) Anaphase: The chromosomes have split, and the chromatid of each pair is moving toward one pole of the cell. (6) Early telophase: The chromatids (now chromosomes) of each daughter cell are becoming uncoiled: a nuclear envelope and nucleolus are re-forming and the centriole is duplicating. (7) Late telophase: The plasma membrane is constricting, and two new daughter cells are formed.

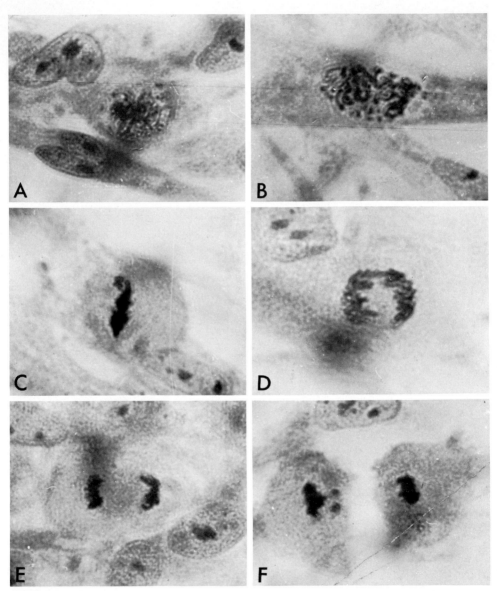

Figure 2-40.   Photomicrographs of stages of mitosis obtained from cells in tissue culture. *A,* Interphase and early prophase. *B,* Late prophase. *C,* Metaphase. *D,* Anaphase. *E,* Early telophase. *F,* Late telophase. × 950.   **See filmstrip I, frame 7.**

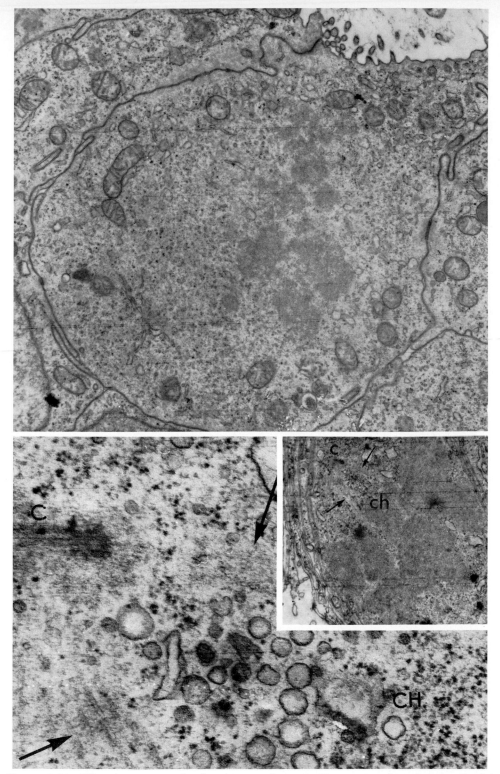

Figure 2-41. Electron micrographs demonstrating mitosis. Top: a jejunal epithelial cell of the mouse in late prophase. The cell has rounded up, chromosomes are apparent, and the nuclear envelope has disappeared. × 10,000. Bottom: inset (× 4200), a fibroblast in metaphase, and a higher magnification of a portion of the same cell. In each illustration, C = centriole, ch = chromosome and the arrows point to spindle fibers (microtubules). × 38,000.

opposite poles of the cell, each producing or organizing the formation of fine fibrils which extend from each centriole. These fibrils, as shown by electron microscopy, are microtubules. Between the centrioles, after they have reached opposite poles of the cell, the microtubules extend toward the center of the cell to form a spindle. At the same time, the nucleolus and nuclear membrane break down and no longer are visible as discrete structures. The early stages of prophase are difficult to detect in sections, but a late prophase is quite obvious.

Metaphase. At metaphase the spindle is fully formed and the chromosomes move toward its center and come to lie at the equator of the spindle. At this stage, it usually is apparent that each chromosome has become split longitudinally to form two chromatids, which, however, remain attached at one point along their length. This point is called the centromere, and it is here that the chromosome is attached in turn to one of the spindle fibers. A cell in metaphase is easily recognized if seen, as it were, from the side, because the chromosomes form a darkly staining linear mass at the equator of the spindle. However, if the cell is seen "end-on," the chromosomes appear as an irregular, darkly staining disk, and this appearance has to be distinguished, for example, from pyknosis (one form of cell death).

Anaphase. In anaphase, one chromatid (daughter chromosome) moves to each pole of the cell, i.e., toward a centriole. This is accomplished by a splitting of the centromere, and possibly by a process which involves repulsion between the two halves and contraction of the spindle fibers. In moving toward a cell pole, the chromosome travels with the centromere leading, and the remainder of the chromosome appearing to be dragged behind.

Telophase. During telophase, the final stage, each group of daughter chromosomes fuses, the chromosomes losing their identity since they become drawn out again into long threads so fine as to be beyond the resolution of the light microscope. However, some segments remain tightly coiled and are visible as chromatin granules. At this time, a nuclear membrane is formed around each chromosome mass, probably from elements of the endoplasmic reticulum, and a nucleolus (or nucleoli) forms in each. In the cytoplasm, the centriole at each pole reduplicates in readiness for the subsequent division, and the parent cell becomes constricted about its equator and eventually completely divided by the formation of discrete cell membranes around the daughter cells. Cytoplasmic organelles are distributed between the two daughter cells.

Effect of Colchicine on Mitosis. If the drug colchicine is given to experimental animals, it has the effect of arresting mitosis at metaphase. This effect occurs because colchicine delays or prevents division of the centromeres. Also, colchicine inhibits the formation of spindle fibers. Thus, in a section obtained from an animal after colchicine administration, all cells which started division during the time between drug administration and sacrifice of the animal will be in the metaphase stage. This has proved to be a valuable method of investigation of the mitotic rate, i.e., the frequency of cell division of tissues, and also is useful in preparing squash preparations for chromosome study (see page 47).

Cell Differentiation

During development, a single cell, the fertilized ovum, divides and multiplies eventually to form all the cells of the body. This process involves not only cell proliferation but also cell differentiation, different types of cells being specialized for different functions. Because all the many cell types evolve from a common cell, we assume that they possess identical chromosome (and, therefore, gene) sets. Why then do they not all synthesize the same proteins and perform identical functions? In all probability, the genetic potentialities of different cells have not been altered, but some genes, although present in the cell, do not express themselves. This may occur because the means whereby a gene can express itself are not present in the cell. Perhaps these means are associated with the cytoplasm or a part of it, for during development there is an unequal distribution of some cytoplasmic components between daughter cells. Whatever the factors in cell differentiation are, a pancreatic acinar cell, for example, will produce a particular enzyme or enzymes (protein) and, if it divides, will form two daughter cells capable of producing the same enzyme or enzymes.

PROTEIN SECRETION

The preceding description of the cell mainly is morphological in emphasis, but it must not be forgotten that the cell is a living, dynamic entity. As an example of cell function and its relation to various cellular components, a brief description of protein secretion is now presented.

Cells which are specialized for protein secretion usually show the presence of one or more large nucleoli and a mass of basophil material, i.e., granular endoplasmic reticulum, in the cytoplasm. The generally accepted

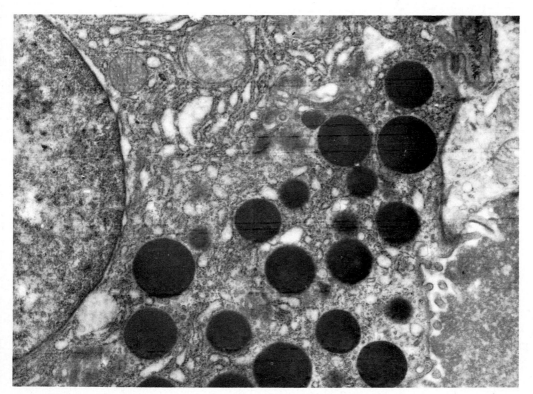

Figure 2-42. Electron micrograph of the apical portion of a pancreatic acinar cell to demonstrate the dynamic process of protein secretion (see text above). Part of the nucleus limited by the nuclear envelope lies to the left. Above it, i.e., to the right, is a mass of granular endoplasmic reticulum with mitochondria, a Golgi apparatus (top center), and secretion (zymogen) granules. The last are very dense and membrane-bounded. To the right is a portion of the lumen of the acinus containing discharged secretory material. × 18,000.

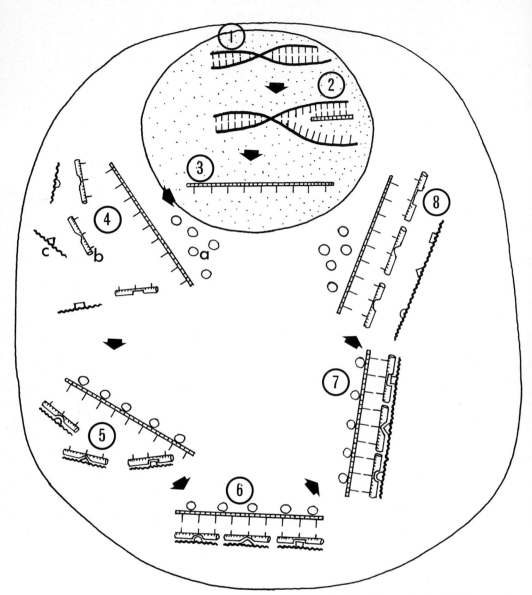

Figure 2-43.   Diagrammatic representation of the steps involved in the synthesis of a three-amino-acid protein. 1. DNA molecule. 2. Synthesis of a messenger RNA molecule from the DNA. 3. Release of the messenger RNA molecule and its transfer from nucleus to cytoplasm. 4. Messenger RNA molecule in the cytoplasm and its association with (a) ribosomes, (b) three transfer RNA molecules, and (c) three aminoacids. 5. Linkage of aminoacids to transfer RNA molecules and association of ribosomes with the messenger RNA molecule. 6. Transfer of aminoacids by transfer RNA to messenger RNA and correct alignment. 7. Linkage of aminoacids to form a polypeptide. 8. Release of the polypeptide and dissociation of ribosomes from messenger RNA. The newly synthesized protein (polypeptide) then is transported in the channels of the endoplasmic reticulum to the Golgi region where it is membrane-wrapped and either stored or transported to the cell surface for release.

theory of protein (e.g., enzyme) secretion is as follows:

The structure of a protein, or polypeptide chain, is determined by a particular deoxynucleotide sequence of a nuclear chromosome, i.e., by a gene. This sequence produces as a primary product a ribonucleic acid copy of the gene, which is called messenger RNA. The amino acids in any particular messenger RNA molecule are combined in a sequence in a manner similar to that used for DNA duplication, the bases present being adenine, guanine, cytosine, and uracil, the latter replacing thymine of DNA. When completed, messenger RNA is detached from the DNA and passes into the cytoplasm where it becomes associated with pre-existing, nonspecialized ribosomal particles. Its information is transferred to the ribosome. The process whereby this transference of information occurs is not well understood, but it is theorized that the ribosomes are strung together on one continuous strand of messenger RNA, each particle containing a reading head or groove through which the strand must pass to deliver its message. Elsewhere in the cytoplasm, amino acids become activated and attach to a molecule of soluble or transfer RNA. There are twenty types of transfer RNA, each being specific for one particular amino acid. The transfer RNA then combines with its complementary sequence of nucleotides on the ribosome, which acts as a template. By this means, the amino acids are lined up in correct sequence and, with the aid of two or more enzymes and energy derived from guanosine triphosphate, combine with the ribosome. When this process is complete, the chain of amino acids, i.e., a polypeptide, is detached from the ribosomal particle, which is then free to start another cycle, the transfer RNA molecules also becoming available for a subsequent cycle. The messenger RNA, although short-lived, may synthesize several molecules of the protein before it is destroyed.

The ribosomes, then, are nonspecific as to which type of protein they produce. They are, as it were, for hire. The specificity is determined by messenger RNA which carries the message directly from DNA of the nucleus. Transfer RNA acts simply as a carrier of amino acids used in the synthesis of the protein.

Recently it has been shown that ribosomes often work in groups, such a group being called a polyribosome or polysome. The number of individual ribosomes in any polysome appears to be related to the type of protein produced, e.g., in the manufacture of hemoglobin, groups of five ribosomes are usual.

After synthesis, the newly formed protein passes from the ribosomes into the canals of the endoplasmic reticulum whence it passes to the Golgi complex. Here the protein is concentrated and isolated from the cytoplasm by segregation into membrane-bounded vacuoles or granules. These are stored in the apical cytoplasm until released by the cell. The role of mitochondria in this process of protein secretion probably is as an energy source.

Finally, the relation of nucleoli to protein secretion should be mentioned. In all probability, the cytoplasmic ribosomes are derived from nuclear RNA, probably that of the nucleolus. (See diagram, p. 56.)

REFERENCES

Barr, M. L.: Sex chromatin and phenotype in man. Science, *130*:679, 1959.

Brachet, J., and Mirsky, A. E. (editors): The Cell. New York, Academic Press, 1959.

Cairns, J.: The form and duplication of DNA. Endeavour, 22:141, 1963.

De Duve, C.: The lysosome. Sci. Amer., *208*:64, 1963.

De Reuck, A. V. S., and Cameron, M. P. (editors): Lysosomes. London, J. & A. Churchill Ltd., 1963.

De Robertis, E. D. P., Nowinski, W. W., and Saez, F. A.: Cell Biology. Philadelphia, W. B. Saunders Co., 1965.

Fawcett, D. W.: The Cell: Its Organelles and Inclusions. Philadelphia, W. B. Saunders Co., 1966.

Gall, J. G.: Microtubule Fine Structure. J. Cell Biol., *31*:639, 1966.

Giese, A. C.: Cell Physiology, ed. 3. Philadelphia, W. B. Saunders Co., 1968.

Haggis, G. H.: The Electron Microscope in Molecular Biology. London, Longmans, 1966.

Harris, R. T. C. (editor): The Interpretation of Ultrastructure. New York, Academic Press, 1962.

Hayaski, T. (editor): Subcellular Particles. New York, Ronald Press, 1959.

Ito, S.: The enteric surface coat on cat intestinal microvilli. J. Cell Biol., *27*:475, 1965.

Kessel, R. G.: Fine Structure of Annulate Lamellae. J. Cell Biol., *36*:658, 1968.

Korn, E. D.: Structure of biological membranes. Science, *153*:1491, 1966.

Lehninger, A. L.: The Mitochondrion. New York, W. A. Benjamin, Inc., 1964.

Locke, M. (editor): Cytodifferentiation and Macromolecular Synthesis. New York, Academic Press, 1963.

Northcote, D. H.: Structure and function of plant-cell membranes. Brit. Med. Bull., *24*, No. 2, 1968.

Sjöstrand, F. S.: Electron Microscopy of Cells and Tissues. Vol. I: Instrumentation and Techniques. New York, Academic Press, 1967.

Sorokin, S. P.: Reconstructions of centriole formation and ciliogenesis in mammalian lungs. J. Cell Science, *3*:207, 1968.

Toner, P. G., and Carr, K. E.: Cell Structure. Edinburgh, E. & S. Livingstone Ltd., 1968.

CHAPTER 3

THE CELLULAR ENVIRONMENT

Any tissue in the body has three components: cells, intercellular substances, and fluids. This chapter is concerned with the latter two.

INTERCELLULAR SUBSTANCES

These have greater strength than the colloidal protoplasm of cells and greater consistency than tissue fluid. They are nonliving and form the matrix or mold in which cells live. It is important that the student appreciate the difference between the intercellular substances and connective tissue (described in Chapter 6), the latter including both the living cells and the nonliving intercellular substances. Intercellular substances, then, provide the strength and support of tissues and act as a medium for the diffusion of tissue fluid between blood capillaries and cells to permit cellular metabolism. They also have an important role in tissue differentiation. From these functions listed, it is an obvious deduction that the intercellular substances are widely distributed throughout all tissues of the body.

There are two main types of intercellular substances, fibrous (formed) and amorphous (nonformed).

Fibrous Intercellular Substances

The function of providing strength and support for tissues is performed mainly by the fibrous intercellular substances, which include three types of fibers, collagenous, reticular, and elastic, distinguished by their appearance and chemical reactions. All are complex proteins formed by long chains of amino acids with peptide linkages, i.e., polypeptide chains, and all are comparatively insoluble in neutral solvents, which explains their ability to exist as formed fibers in the fluid internal environment of the body. The characteristics of each type of fiber will be considered in more detail later in this chapter.

Amorphous Intercellular Substances

Some of the amorphous intercellular substances are in the form of stiff gels and thus help to provide strength and support for tissues, but their main function is that of providing a medium through which tissue fluid containing nutrients and waste products can diffuse between cells and capillaries. Amorphous intercellular materials, in the form of sols and gels, permit such

59

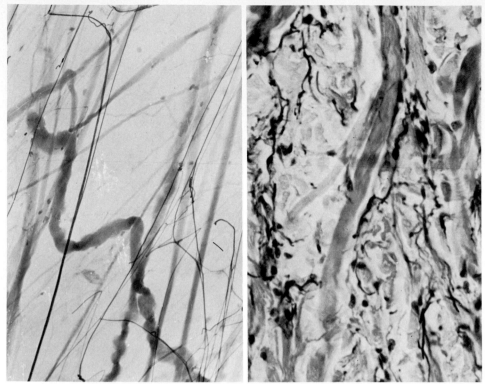

Figure 3-1. Left: Photomicrograph to illustrate collagenous fibers (lighter, wavy) and elastic fibers (darker, thinner, straight, and branching) in loose areolar connective tissue. This is a "spread" preparation, not a section, of rat mesentery. × 900. Right: Photomicrograph of a section of dense, irregular connective tissue showing elastic (black) and collagen (gray) fibers. × 900.   See filmstrip I, frame 8.

a diffusion from capillaries to cells and from cells to capillaries much more readily than do the fibrous kinds, which are embedded in the amorphous materials. Usually two kinds of amorphous material are recognized, *ground substance*, which is relatively soft, and *cement substance*, which is firmer. These materials probably are formed by connective tissue cells and contain some protein, including collagen in molecular dispersion, glycoproteins, carbohydrates, lipids, and water. The glycoproteins and mucopolysaccharides consist of complex mixtures of hexosamines and hexuronic acids combined with protein, and chemically fall into two groups distinguished by their esterification or nonesterification with sulfuric acid. The nonesterified mucopolysaccharides include hyaluronic acid, which is a polymer of glucuronic acid and acetylglucosamine, and chondroitin (which is a polymer of hyaluronic acid). The esterified group includes chondroitin sulfuric acid (a polymer of galactosamine, glucuronic acid, and sulfate) and keratohyalin. All of this group exist as gels and are more viscid than hyaluronic acid. This probably is because the sulfuric acid component permits a firm union with protein. Being firm gels, they can act as cementing substances and, when present in association with formed fibers, as in cartilage matrix, they provide considerable support.

Hyaluronic acid is a viscous, fluid-like mucopolysaccharide found in the connective tissue of most organs, Wharton's jelly of the umbilical cord, synovial fluid, and humors of the eye. It readily binds water, i.e., becomes hydrated, and is responsible for changes in the viscosity and permeability of ground substance, thus having an important influence on the exchange of material between tissue cells and blood plasma. The enzyme hyaluronidase hydrolyzes it, reducing its viscosity, and thus increases permeability of the tissue. Chondroitin sulfuric acid is found in cartilage and bone matrix, in the aorta and heart valves, in the cornea of the eye and in the umbilical cord, and, as mentioned previously, is sulfated.

Amorphous intercellular substance has the same refractive index as water and thus is invisible in fresh preparations but can be seen in tissue spreads mounted in a medium of different refractive index, e.g., serum or a sugar solution. Generally, the ground substances, particularly chondroitin sulfuric acid, stain more readily if some-

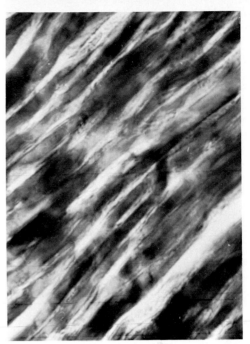

Figure 3-3. Photomicrograph of the ligamentum nuchae (an elastic ligament) of the ox showing broad, intermeshing fibers of elastin. The cells are unstained. Weigert's elastic stain. × 450.

what erratically with hematoxylin. Both types of mucopolysaccharide stain *metachromatically*, for example, with a dilute solution of toluidine blue.

Fibrous Intercellular Substances

Collagenous Fibers. Collagenic or collagenous fibers are found in all types of connective tissue and consist of the protein collagen. They are extremely tough and in bulk in the fresh state, e.g., in muscle tendons, appear white and hence also are termed "white" fibers. Chemically, collagen is composed of three polypeptide chains, each composed of about a thousand amino acid units linked together. Each chain is twisted into a left-handed helix or spiral, and three such chains are twisted around each other to form a right-handed superhelix. This superhelix is called the

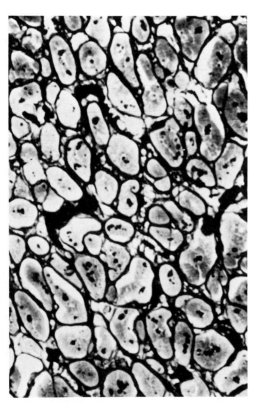

Figure 3-2. Photomicrograph of reticular fibers (black) in cardiac muscle (unstained). × 450.

tropocollagen* molecule (or proto-fibril) and is 2800 Å in length and 14 Å in diameter. From this tropocollagen, all types of collagen are formed. In natural collagen, the tropocollagen molecules are lined up in parallel rows, all molecules facing the same direction, and between rows there is an overlap of one quarter of the length of the tropocollagen molecule. Such a collection of molecules forms a micro-fibril or unit fiber of collagen which on electron microscopy has a diameter varying from about 425 to 1000 Å. It is probable that fiber diameter increases with age. Along the unit fiber, a peri-odicity or cross banding is visible with the electron microscope, the major cross bands occurring at intervals of about 640 Å, with several finer bands between the major periods (see Figure 3-4). It is deduced that the cross band-ing is caused by the one-quarter length overlap of the tropocollagen mole-cules (four times 640 is 2560, approxi-mately the length of a tropocollagen molecule).

The finest strand of collagen visible by light microscopy is the fibril, which is about 0.3 to 0.5 of a micron thick and does not branch. In turn, bundles of fibrils in parallel array form collage-nous fibers which in loose fibrocon-nective tissue appear as long, straight or slightly wavy threads or ribbons about 1 to 12 microns in diameter. These fibers run in all directions in loose connective tissue and are of indeterminate length. They are color-less and show a longitudinal striation because they are formed by numerous parallel fibrils. The fibrils forming a fiber are held together by a cementing substance of a protein nature which can be digested by trypsin. The fibers may branch and recombine owing to the interchange of clusters of fibrils between one fiber and another.

In boiling water, collagenous mate-rial becomes hydrated and softens, forming gelatin. Weak acids and alkalis cause swelling of collagenous fibers; the fibers can be digested by pepsin in acid solution and by the enzyme col-lagenase. Collagen, after treatment with salts of heavy metals or tannic acid, forms an insoluble product. This is the basis of the "tanning" process for the preparation of animal hides (leather), which consist chiefly of col-lagen. Collagen in tissue sections is colored pink to red in H and E prep-arations, but can be stained more specifically by van Gieson's picro-fuchsin (red), by aniline blue of Mallory's connective tissue stain (blue-purple), and by Masson's trichrome (green). Collagenous fibers can be identified also by their birefringence under polarized light.

In addition to the unit fiber with the periodicity of 640 Å characteristic of native collagen, collagen can exist also in a long-spacing form with a periodicity of about 2400 Å. There are two varieties of this long-spacing form: the fibrous long-spacing (FLS) variety, in long fibrils with a periodicity of 2400 Å, which is found in a natural state in the trabecular meshwork of the eye and recently has been de-scribed in aging cartilage, and the segment long-spacing (SLS) variety, in short segments, with a length of 2400 Å or multiples thereof, and vary-ing width. Each form can be dissolved readily and reprecipitated into either of the other two forms. It is hypothe-sized that FLS collagen is formed by rows of tropocollagen units lying end to end in parallel-antiparallel array without overlap and that SLS collagen is formed by lateral and lengthwise aggregation of similar particles.

Reticular Fibers. Reticular fibers are of small diameter and branch to form a netlike supporting framework or reticulum. They occur as fine net-works around small blood vessels, muscle fibers, nerve fibers, and fat cells, in the fine partitions of the lung and, particularly, at boundaries be-tween connective tissue and other

*Tropocollagen is a term derived from the Greek *tropos*, turning: i.e., turning into col-lagen.

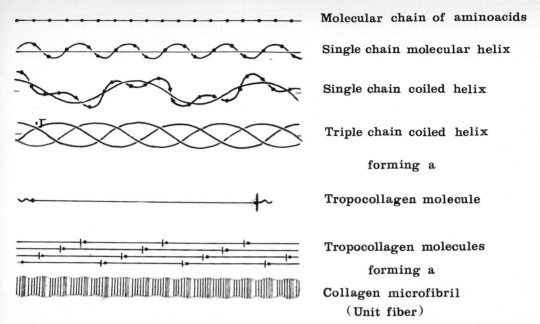

Molecular chain of aminoacids

Single chain molecular helix

Single chain coiled helix

Triple chain coiled helix

forming a

Tropocollagen molecule

Tropocollagen molecules
forming a
Collagen microfibril
(Unit fiber)

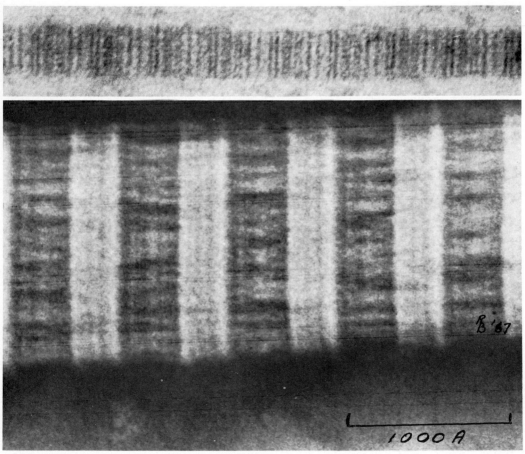

Figure 3-4. The diagrams (after Gross) illustrate the formation of a collagen microfibril. The electron micrograph (center) is of a single collagen microfibril stained positively with uranyl acetate. × 185,000. The lowest micrograph is a single microfibril stained negatively by phosphotungstic acid × 430,000. (Photograph courtesy of Dr. R. Borasky.)

types of tissue. Beneath epithelial membranes, for example, reticular fibers form dense networks as components of basal laminae. Reticular fibers are continuous with collagenous fibers, and there appears to be a gradual transition from one to the other. They are not seen easily in H and E sections but can be demonstrated by silver impregnation methods, e.g., Bielschowsky's method, when they become visible as thin dark lines, collagenous fibers being colored yellow or brown. The coloration of reticular fibers by silver impregnation has led to the term "argyrophil." They stain more darkly with the PAS technique (see below, this page) than do collagenous fibers, and are not birefringent, but on electron microscopy show the periodicity of 640 Å characteristic of collagenous fibers. It may be that reticular fibers are young or immature collagenous fibers. The staining differences between the two types may be due to physical size, for reticular fibers usually are of smaller diameter, or may be dependent upon differences in the amorphous intercellular material which surrounds individual fibers.

Elastic Fibers. Elastic fibers are present in loose fibrous connective tissue and are seen as long, thin, highly refractile, cylindrical threads (Figure 3-1) or flat ribbons, ranging in size from less than a micron to 4 microns in diameter, although in some elastic ligaments they may reach a diameter of 10 to 12 microns. In contrast to collagenous fibers, by light microscopy they appear homogeneous and not fibrillar in nature. They may form extensive, perforated sheets, e.g., around blood vessels. In the fresh state adult elastic tissue in bulk has a yellowish color. Elastic fibers stain erratically with eosin but can be stained selectively with orcein (brown) and resorcin-fuchsin (dark blue-purple). If fresh tissue is treated with dilute acid solutions, collagen fibers swell and become transparent, but

elastic fibers become visible as highly refractile, homogeneous, shining threads.

Elastic fibers are composed of the albuminoid elastin which shows a remarkable resistance to most agents. It is not affected by hot or cold water or by dilute solutions of acids or alkalis but is digested enzymatically by pancreatin. As indicated by the name, elastic fibers yield easily to stretching and return to their former length when tension is released.

By electron microscopy, elastic fibers have been shown to consist of peripheral collections of thin tubular fibrils of 100 Å diameter with a central amorphous component (Figure 3-5). Recent studies have shown that the amorphous component is elastin and that the 100 Å fibrils are composed of an as yet unidentified protein.

The Periodic Acid–Schiff Reaction in Connective Tissue. Collagenous and elastic fibers in general are colored only faintly by the PAS technique, whereas reticular fibers are strongly positive. The Schiff reagent, as explained in Chapter 1, is basic fuchsin which has been bleached with sulfurous acid. In the presence of free aldehyde, the magenta (pink-purple) color of unbleached basic fuchsin is produced. Periodic acid is an oxidizing agent and can be used on tissue sections to produce aldehydes from polysaccharides. In the PAS technique, tissue sections are exposed to periodic acid which forms aldehydes from polysaccharides, and the sections then are treated with the Schiff reagent which colors the sites of aldehyde production magenta. The PAS technique is a good method for the demonstration of the polysaccharide glycogen, and it might be expected that all connective tissue mucopolysaccharides also would give a positive reaction. However, recent studies have indicated that both pure hyaluronic acid and purified chondroitin sulfate are PAS negative. The positive reaction of reticular fibers pre-

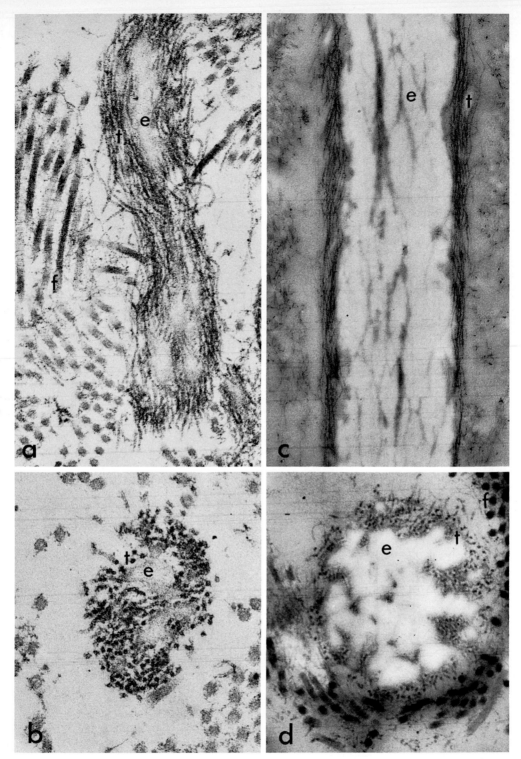

Figure 3-5. Electron micrographs of elastic fibers; *a* and *b* respectively are longitudinal and transverse sections from the ligamentum nuchae of a three month fetal calf, and *c* and *d* from a calf at term (nine months). Note the tubular fibrils (t) surrounding a core of amorphous material (e). With increasing age the amorphous component increases in amount. There is evidence that the central amorphous component is elastin, the tubular fibrils being an as yet unidentified protein. Unit fibrils of collagen (f) also are present. *a*, × 50,000; *b*, × 80,000; *c*, × 25,000, and *d*, × 45,000. (Courtesy of Russell Ross.)

sumably is due to the presence of sugars intimately associated with the fibers.

Basal Laminae. Basal laminae or basement membranes* are sheets of extracellular material present under the basal surface of epithelial cells and around muscles or nerves and situated between these elements and the underlying or surrounding connective tissue. They thus are distributed widely and, indeed, the connective tissue elements within many organs virtually are limited by basal laminae.

---

*Note on terminology: Basal lamina refers to an acellular structure and probably is preferable to the term "basement membrane," for the latter term is confusing in that "membrane" has come to mean a unit or trilaminar membrane, i.e., a cellular structure. Also, confusion exists between "basement membrane" and such terms as "boundary tissue or membrane" used to designate a layer including connective tissue, e.g., around the seminiferous tubules of the testis, or in lung and renal glomeruli. The term basement membrane has been used synonymously with "boundary membrane" or "zona densa" for such areas.

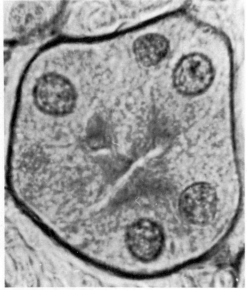

Figure 3-6. Photomicrograph of a cross section of a renal tubule lined by low columnar epithelium to illustrate the homogeneous basal lamina (dark) surrounding the tubule. PAS stain. × 1500.   See filmstrip I, frame 9.

Basal laminae probably are a secretion of epithelial cells, at least in part. They are rich in mucopolysaccharides and stain intensely with the PAS and silver techniques but are not well demonstrated in H and E preparations. The thickness of basal laminae varies and even after PAS or silver staining they may be so thin as to be scarcely discernible by light microscopy. By electron microscopy two layers usually are recognized. One is a layer of relatively high electron density of 300 to 3000 Å thickness composed of a feltwork or mat of fine fibrils of about 40 Å diameter. Between this layer and the cell surface is a narrower layer of low electron density. This layer appears to blend with material between cells on one surface and with the fibrillar layer on the other. On the outer, noncellular surface, the fibrillar layer blends gradually with fine reticular fibers and unit fibers of collagen of the connective tissue. Some studies have indicated that the fine fibrils are tropocollagen molecules and that the zone of low density immediately adjacent to plasma membranes is occupied by polysaccharide. The PAS technique probably stains both these layers and also the reticular fibers of connective tissue associated with its outer surface. Basal laminae, interposed between epithelial and other cells and their blood supply, probably play an important role in diffusion of oxygen and metabolites in addition to serving as limiting membranes beneath epithelia. Also, the mingling between the fibrillar elements of the basal lamina and unit fibrils of collagen of connective tissue provides for strong connection between epithelia and underlying connective tissue, and between muscle and connective tissue.

Origin of Fibers. There have been two views concerning the origin of connective tissue fibers, although both argue that fibers are formed by the fibroblast cells. One view has held that fibers arise intracellularly within fibroblasts and then pass into the ground substance of the extracellular spaces.

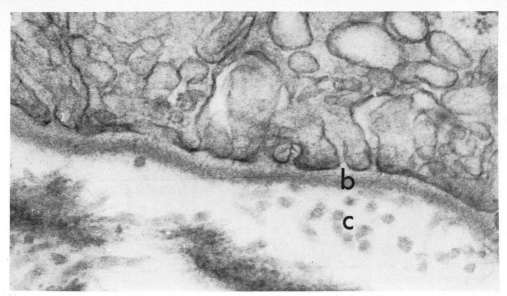

Figure 3-7. Electron micrograph showing the bases of epithelial cells above, beneath which is the basal lamina (b) and unit fibers of collagen (reticular fibers) (c). × 80,000.

The other view, for which there is much recent evidence from electron microscopy, suggests that fibers form extracellularly, i.e., outside the cell, but in close association with the fibroblast plasma membrane. By light microscopy and silver impregnation methods, it is possible to show that fibers first appear as very fine, delicate networks at the surface of fibroblasts and between cells. These fibers by electron microscopy may be only 50 to 500 Å in diameter, but all show the characteristic periodicity of 640 Å. Later the fibers become arranged in parallel bundles, increase in thickness, and lose their ability to be impregnated with silver. At this stage, they show the staining characteristics of collagenous fibers.

The currently held view of fiber formation, then, is that the first fibrils arise at the cell surface following polymerization of material into protofibrils within the cell. Incidentally, fibroblasts active in fibrillogenesis show an extensively developed endoplasmic reticulum. Formation of collagenous fibers is dependent on the presence of vitamin C, and they do not form in scurvy, a disease caused by a deficiency of this vitamin. The amount of collagen increases with age. It is well known that meat from old animals is tough, and this is due mainly to an increased amount of collagen.

Little is known about the formation of elastic fibers, but they probably develop in a manner similar to collagenous fibers.

TISSUE FLUID

It is the blood vascular system which is responsible for transporting oxygen and food materials to, and removing waste products from, the cells but it must be appreciated that the great majority of cells are situated external to and some distance removed from blood vessels. Thus it is necessary for oxygen and nutritive materials to leave the blood, pass through the thin walls of small blood vessels called capillaries, and enter the intercellular spaces to reach the cells. Waste materials follow a similar route in the reverse direction. The capillaries have walls which permit the ready passage through them of a watery fluid containing crystalloids, dissolved oxygen, and food materials. This fluid is called *tissue fluid*. The capillary wall, however, permits passage of colloid materials, e.g., protein, less readily or not at all. This filtrate of the blood, the tissue fluid, is formed by simple *diffusion* and occurs at the arterial end of a capillary, i.e., toward the heart. The drainage of tissue fluid back into a capillary is accomplished by *osmosis*, the thin endothelial lining of the blood capillary functioning as a living, semipermeable membrane.

In the intercellular spaces, tissue fluid is related to the intercellular substances, and this relationship varies with the type of intercellular material. In tissues where the amorphous type of intercellular substance is in the form of a sol, and fluid or semifluid in nature, it is the tissue fluid which functions as the dispersion medium. In sites where intercellular substance is present in the form of a rigid or semirigid gel, there is a high content of bound water which is obtained from tissue fluid at the time of formation of the intercellular substance. Such a gel is readily permeable because diffusion can occur through the bound water. In sites where the intercellular substance not only is gelled but becomes impermeable because of impregnation with calcium and other salts, e.g., in bone matrix, tiny channels exist in the matrix to permit passage of tissue fluid. Thus cellular metabolism, although dependent on the blood vascular system, occurs by the exchange of material with tissue fluid. Tissue fluid sometimes is called "extracellular fluid" or "intercellular fluid," as opposed to "intracellular fluid" within the cells.

Composition of Tissue Fluid

Tissue fluid contains those constituents of the blood that can diffuse readily through capillary walls. Blood consists of a fluid component, the *plasma*, which is a fluid containing both crystalloids and colloids, and cellular elements. Only the crystalloid component of plasma can diffuse readily through the capillary walls to enter the tissue fluid, the cells and the great majority of the colloids remaining inside the blood vessels. The volume of tissue fluid varies from tissue to tissue and within any tissue there are physiological and pathological variations also. One common pathological condition, *edema*, occurs when there is an increase in the volume of tissue fluid.

Formation

As stated earlier, the capillary wall, consisting only of a single layer of very thin, attenuated, endothelial cells supported by a basal lamina, acts as a semipermeable membrane. If diffusion of tissue fluid through the capillary wall is to occur, there must be a powerful hydrostatic pressure inside the capillary. This pressure, of course, is derived from the heart and although the hydrostatic pressure is comparatively low in a capillary, it is of sufficient magnitude to cause diffusion of fluid through the capillary wall. In spite of the fact that hydrostatic pressure is much greater in the arteries, diffusion of fluid does not occur here due to the thickness of the arterial wall. It is important to appreciate also that hydrostatic pressure decreases along the length of the capillary from arterial to venous end, and thus the formation of tissue fluid occurs mainly at arterial ends of capillaries. In general, veins do not act as a source of tissue fluid because, although there is some hydrostatic pressure, the walls are too thick to allow production of tissue fluid.

Absorption

It is obvious that there must be some mechanism for the absorption of tissue fluid; otherwise, the tissues rapidly would become swollen with excess

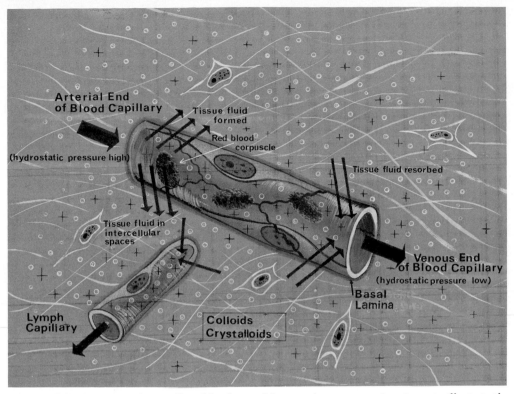

Figure 3-8. Diagram of a capillary blood vessel lying in loose connective tissue to illustrate the formation and resorption of tissue fluid.

fluid. There are two mechanisms for absorption and together they balance the rate of formation of tissue fluid.

Capillary Absorption: Osmosis. Osmosis can be defined as the diffusion of water (or fluid) through a membrane in response to a concentration gradient. Crystalloids in solution give a relatively high osmotic pressure to the solution. This means that if such a fluid is separated from a weaker one (e.g., water) by a semipermeable membrane, then the crystalloid solution will exert an osmotic or "suction" force and attract water through the membrane. Both blood and tissue fluid contain crystalloids and are separated by a semipermeable membrane, viz., the endothelium lining the blood capillary. However, they cause little flow of fluid because the osmotic pressures due to the crystalloid content are approximately equal on both sides and

cancel out. Blood does contain, however, more colloids than tissue fluid. Although colloidal solutions have low osmotic pressures, those present in blood are in sufficient quantities to cause a concentration gradient, and tissue fluid will pass through the capillary endothelium into the blood, the endothelial lining permitting the passage of crystalloids but not colloids. The osmotic pressure of the blood colloids, then, attracts tissue fluid into the capillaries, but this force in part is canceled by the hydrostatic pressure of the capillaries which tends to force fluid out. At the arterial end of a capillary, the hydrostatic pressure is greater than the osmotic pressure of the blood, and fluid passes out through the capillary wall to become tissue fluid. At the venous end of a capillary, however, the osmotic pressure exceeds the hydrostatic pressure, and tissue fluid returns through the capillary wall to the blood. This results in a circulation of tissue fluid, as explained diagrammatically in Figure 3-8. The actual mechanism of fluid transport across endothelium lining blood capillaries is discussed in Chapter 11, page 217.

Transport of fluid occurs either between endothelial cells, i.e., at cell interfaces, or across endothelial cytoplasm by a process termed *pinocytosis*. Pinocytosis involves the formation of small pits or caveolae in the plasma membrane which then pinch off to form small vesicles (pinocytotic vesicles) containing fluid. These vesicles pass through the endothelial cytoplasm to reach the opposite cell surface where they fuse with the plasma membrane and release their fluid contents. It is possible that colloids may also be transported via pinocytosis.

Lymphatic Absorption. In most regions of the body there are capillaries which start blindly in the tissues and drain ultimately into the venous system. These are the lymphatic capillaries. Tissue fluid can pass through the endothelial walls of these lymphatics and, once inside, is called *lymph* and not tissue fluid. These small vessels drain to larger ones which finally open into veins near the heart to return the contained lymph to the vascular system.

There probably is some slight leakage of blood colloids through the endothelium of blood capillaries into tissue spaces. It is important that this colloid be removed or obviously it would retain water in the tissues by its osmotic pressure, upsetting the mechanism of osmosis in capillary absorption described previously. The escaped colloid can pass through the endothelial lining of lymphatic capillaries, and thus is drained from the tissues. The lymphatic capillaries not only regulate the quantity of tissue fluid, but, by removing colloid, also regulate its quality.

Diffusion of fluid into lymphatic capillaries probably occurs both by pinocytosis and by passage of material through endothelial interfaces. The latter mechanism particularly is important in relation to lymphatics of the intestine where small fat particles (chylomicrons) move into lymphatics (called *lacteals*) by passing between endothelial cells (see page 308).

Demonstration of Tissue Fluid

In histological preparations, tissue fluid is removed and therefore cannot be seen as such under the microscope. However, in all organs there are small, empty spaces and slits, and although most of these are caused by shrinkage of tissues in preparation and therefore are artifactual, they do represent to some extent the tissue spaces which in life are occupied by tissue fluid.

Types of Edema

As indicated previously, edema is a condition producing an excess of tissue fluid. Microscopically, the cells and intercellular fibers are spread apart more widely than usual, but this varies with the tissue. Loose fibrous connective tissue, for example, can accumulate a considerable amount of fluid, whereas more solid tissues, like tendons, will show little effect. Excess fluid obviously causes an increased hydrostatic pressure in the tissue, and when this pressure balances that within the capillaries, the production of more tissue fluid ceases. Edema, therefore, is to some extent self-limiting.

The types and causes of edema, which basically represents upsets in the normal balance between the formation and absorption of tissue fluid, are illustrated diagrammatically in Figure 3-9 and can be summarized as follows:

Increased Formation of Tissue Fluid

INCREASED HYDROSTATIC PRESSURE IN THE BLOOD CAPILLARIES. This usually is due to venous obstruction and not to increased arterial pressure. In heart failure, for example, venous re-

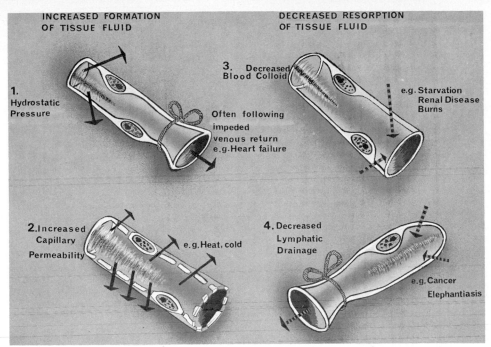

Figure 3-9. Diagrammatic representation of capillary blood vessels to illustrate the four main mechanisms involved in edema.

turn to the heart is impeded and edema often results, first appearing in the dependent parts of the body, i.e., ankles and lower legs. Localized edema due to venous obstruction may be a sequel to venous thrombosis.

INCREASED PERMEABILITY OF THE ENDOTHELIUM OF BLOOD CAPILLARIES. This results in the leaking of blood colloids into the tissue spaces, causing a raised osmotic pressure of the tissue fluid and consequent lowering of the resorption gradient. Increased capillary permeability can be caused by heat (burns and scalds) or by excessive cold (frostbite).

Decreased Absorption of Tissue Fluid

LYMPHATIC OBSTRUCTION. This may be a result of pressure on, or internal occlusion of, lymphatics because of cancer, which commonly spreads by lymphatic vessels, or by a small parasite (elephantiasis). If lymphatics are blocked, drainage of lymph (tissue fluid) along them ceases, resulting in edema.

LOWERED BLOOD COLLOID. Starvation, particularly of protein, if severe enough, causes a lowering of the content of plasma proteins, which are colloids, and consequently there is a diminished osmotic pressure of the blood. This, of course, in turn diminishes the resorption of tissue fluid at the venous ends of the blood capillaries. In some kidney diseases, blood colloids may leak through the kidney and be eliminated in the urine, and edema is a common symptom of renal disease. It also can occur in extensive burns, for an increased capillary permeability causes loss of colloids into tissue spaces, and colloids can also leak through the burnt skin surface, thus resulting in a lowered blood colloid.

REFERENCES

Asboe-Hansen, G. (editor): Connective Tissue in Health and Disease. Copenhagen, E. Munksgaard, 1954.

Banga, I.: Structure and Function of Elastin and Collagen. Budapest, Akademiai Kiado, 1966.

Borasky, R.: Amino acids distribution profiles of collagen fibrils. Jour. of the Amer. Leather Chemists Assn., Vol. LXII, No. 12, 1967.

Davies, D. V.: Specificity of staining methods for mucopolysaccharides of the hyaluronic acid type. Stain. Techn., 27:65, 1952.

Drinker, C. K., and Field, M. E.: Lymphatics, Lymph and Tissue Fluid. Baltimore, Williams & Wilkins Co., 1933.

Edds, M. V., Jr.: Origin and structure of inter-cellular matrix. *In* The Chemical Basis of Development, edited by W. C. McElory and B. Glass. Baltimore, Johns Hopkins Press, 1958.

Greenlee, T. K., Jr., and Ross, R.: The development of the rat flexor digital tendon, a fine structure study. J. Ultrastructure Res., 18: 354, 1967.

Greenlee, T. K., Jr., Ross, R., and Hartman, J. L.: The fine structure of elastic fibers. J. Cell Biol., 30:59, 1966.

Gross, J.: The structure of elastic tissue as studied with the electron microscope. J. Exp. Med., 89:699, 1949.

Gross, J.: The collagen fibril and its building

block, tropocollagen. J. Biophys. Biochem. Cytol., 2:261, 1956.

Hodge, A. J., and Schmitt, F. O.: The tropocol-lagen macromolecule and its properties of ordered interaction. *In* Macromolecular Com-plexes, edited by M. V. Edds, Jr. New York, Ronald Press, 1961.

Jackson, S. F.: Connective tissue cells. *In* The Cell, edited by J. Brachet and A. E. Mirsky. New York, Academic Press, 1964, Vol. 6, pp. 387-520.

Kramer, H., and Little, K.: Nature of reticulin. *In* Nature and Structure of Collagen, edited by J. T. Randall and S. F. Jackson. New York, Academic Press, 1953.

Porter, K. R., and Pappas, G. D.: Collagen for-mation by fibroblasts of the chick embryo dermis. J. Biophys. Biochem. Cytol., 5:153, 1959.

Porter, K. R.: Morphogenesis of connective tissue. *In* Cellular Concepts in Rheumatoid Arthritis, edited by C. A. L. Stephens and A. B. Stanfield. Springfield, Charles C Thomas, 1966.

Yoffey, J. M., and Courtice, F. C.: Lymphatics, Lymph and Lymphoid Tissue. Cambridge, Harvard University Press, 1956.

CHAPTER 4

THE FOUR PRIMARY TISSUES

As explained previously, the body is composed of three different elements, i.e., cells, intercellular substances, and body fluids. During development, there is a stage when the embryo consists of three simple cellular layers, each of which is specialized with respect to function, future development, and differentiation. These three primitive layers are the ectoderm, which covers the body surface and gives rise to the epidermis and to the nervous system, the endoderm, which lines the gut tube, and the mesoderm, which lies between the other two. It is from these three layers that the body develops. In the adult, there are only four primary tissues, each differing in appearance and function from the others, and, obviously, these four basic tissues all are derived from the three primitive germ layers. A primary or basic tissue may be defined as a group of similar cells specialized in a common direction and able to perform a common function. The four primary tissues are epithelium, connective tissue, muscle, and nervous tissues.

In turn organs are formed from these tissues, and usually all four types are present in any single organ. If the student learns to recognize these four basic tissues, he will have taken a large step toward the understanding of histology and the identification of tissues. It is important to emphasize that under the microscope, the tissue section may at first appear complex and confusing but, in fact, is composed of only four types of tissue, each easily identified after a little practice. A few characteristics usually will prove sufficient for identification.

Epithelium. The cells are closely apposed with very little cementing substance between, and they are arranged as sheets covering or lining surfaces or as masses of cells in glands.

Connective Tissue. The cells usually are widely separated by a relatively large amount of intercellular substance. This group includes certain specialized tissues such as blood and blood-forming tissues, bone, and cartilage.

Muscle. There are three types; cells are elongated, contain cytoplasmic filaments, are relatively closely associated, and are separated by fine, vascular connective tissue.

Nervous Tissue. This consists of cells, some of which are very large, and their elongated processes, which are usually grouped as relatively isolated masses or bundles.

The subdivisions and varieties of these four primary tissues can be classified according to structure and function:

Classification of Tissues

PRIMARY TISSUE	SUBDIVISIONS			EXAMPLES
Epithelium	a. Covering external body surface or limiting internal surface	1. Simple	Squamous	Bowman's capsule (kidney), endothelium, mesothelium
			Cuboidal	Collecting tubule (kidney)
			Columnar	Gallbladder (nonciliated) / Uterine tube (ciliated)
		2. Pseudostratified columnar		Male urethra (nonciliated) / Trachea (ciliated)
		3. Stratified	Squamous	Skin (keratinizing) / Vagina (nonkeratinizing)
			Squamous	Without connective tissue papillae—cornea. With connective tissue papillae—skin (keratinizing), vagina (nonkeratinizing)
			Cuboidal	Sweat glands
			Columnar	Male urethra
			Transitional	Urinary tract
	b. Multicellular glands	1. Exocrine	Simple	Gastric, sweat
			Compound	Salivary
		2. Endocrine		Thyroid, pituitary
	c. False (derived from mesoderm)		Endothelium	Lining of blood and lymph channels
			Mesothelium	Pleura, pericardium, peritoneum
Muscle	a. Smooth (involuntary)			Intestinal tract, blood vessels
	b. Striated (voluntary)			Skeletal muscle
	c. Striated involuntary			Heart

Classification of Tissues (Continued)

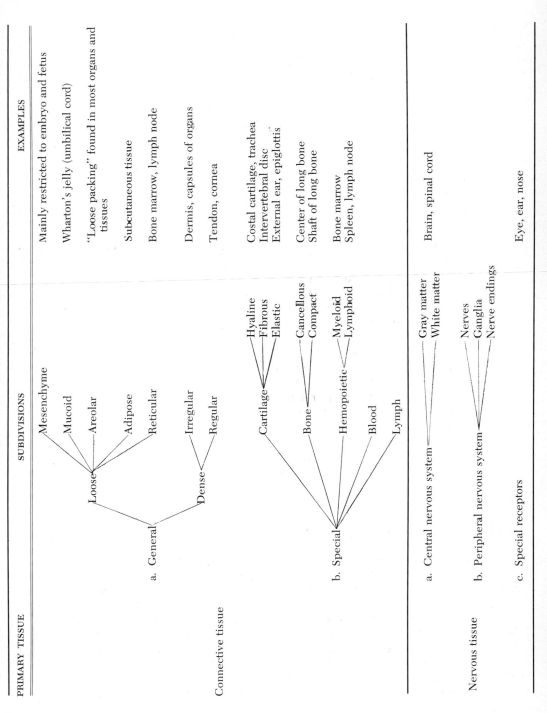

PRIMARY TISSUE	SUBDIVISIONS		EXAMPLES
		Mesenchyme	Mainly restricted to embryo and fetus
		Mucoid	Wharton's jelly (umbilical cord)
	Loose	Areolar	"Loose packing" found in most organs and tissues
		Adipose	Subcutaneous tissue
		Reticular	Bone marrow, lymph node
a. General		Irregular	Dermis, capsules of organs
	Dense	Regular	Tendon, cornea
Connective tissue			
	Cartilage	Hyaline / Fibrous / Elastic	Costal cartilage, trachea / Intervertebral disc / External ear, epiglottis
	Bone	Cancellous / Compact	Center of long bone / Shaft of long bone
b. Special	Hemopoietic	Myeloid / Lymphoid	Bone marrow / Spleen, lymph node
	Blood		
	Lymph		
	a. Central nervous system	Gray matter / White matter	Brain, spinal cord
Nervous tissue	b. Peripheral nervous system	Nerves / Ganglia / Nerve endings	
	c. Special receptors		Eye, ear, nose

CHAPTER 5

EPITHELIUM

MEMBRANES

Epithelial membranes are sheets of epithelial cells arranged either in single or multiple layers; these are called *simple* and *stratified* respectively. Basically there are only three types of epithelial cells: *squamous* cells, which are very flat with a height much less than the width and which in profile show a thickening at the site of the nucleus; *cuboidal* cells, whose height and width approximately are equal and which appear many-sided in cross section due to close packing; and *columnar* cells, whose height is greater than width and which also are many-sided in cross section, i.e., they are polygonal. However, all three types may be of very irregular shape.

In membranes, the epithelial cells are held together firmly and are supported by and lie upon a *basal lamina* (see page 66), which separates the epithelium from underlying connective tissue. Basal laminae stain poorly in ordinary light microscopic preparations but can be well shown—for example, by the PAS technique. They are composed of mucopolysaccharide and probably are of epithelial origin, at least in part. By electron microscopy, they appear as fine electron dense laminae closely subjacent to the basal surfaces of epithelial cell membranes.

Epithelial membranes, then, consist of cells arranged in sheets with a minimal amount of intercellular substances, the whole lying upon a basal lamina, which in turn separates the epithelium from underlying connective tissue. There are no blood or lymph vessels in epithelium; it derives its nutrition by diffusion of tissue fluid from the vessels of the underlying connective tissue. Epithelial cells thus are kept moist mainly by fluid from beneath, although in many sites the epithelium lines a moist cavity, e.g., the lining of the cheek, where epithelium is kept moist by saliva. Numerous small nerve fibers are located in the connective tissue immediately beneath epithelial membranes, the fine terminal branchings of which may penetrate the basal lamina to run between epithelial cells.

Epithelia thus, as mentioned before, are classified basically as either simple, consisting of a single layer of cells, or stratified, consisting of more than one layer. In stratified epithelia, the subgroups are termed according to the nature of the superficial (surface) layer of cells, e.g., squamous, cuboidal, or columnar. It is not feasible to classify them according to their embryological origin as, in fact, all three

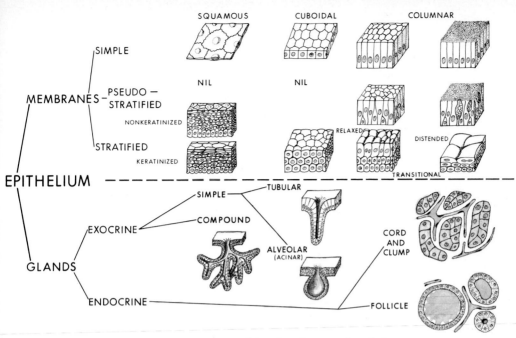

Figure 5-1. Diagram of the classification of epithelia.

layers, i.e., ectoderm, endoderm, and mesoderm, give rise to epithelia.

lining pulmonary alveoli, and in the inner and middle ear.

SIMPLE EPITHELIA

Simple Squamous Epithelium

Simple squamous epithelium is composed of very thin, flat cells of irregular outline fitted closely together to form a continuous sheet. From the surface, this epithelium has the appearance of a tiled floor, but with grossly irregular outlines, whereas in section the cells show attenuated cytoplasm with local protuberances where the cytoplasm contains the nuclei. Structurally, this description also includes endothelium lining blood and lymph vessels and mesothelium lining the serous cavities (pleura, pericardium, and peritoneum), these being derived from mesoderm. Other examples of simple squamous epithelium are found in the parietal layer of Bowman's capsule and the loop of Henle in the kidney,

Simple Cuboidal (Cubical) Epithelium

Simple cuboidal (cubical) epithelium is so termed because of its appearance in sections at right angles to the surface of the membrane, each cell appearing box- or cubelike. From the surface, the cells appear as polygons. Such an epithelium is found in many glands, both in secreting units and ducts, and, for example, covering the surface of the ovary.

Simple Columnar Epithelium

Simple nonciliated columnar epithelium has a similar appearance in surface view to the simple cuboidal type, but in perpendicular sections is seen to be composed of tall cells, the nuclei of which usually are all approximately at the same level and situated nearer to the basal than to the apical

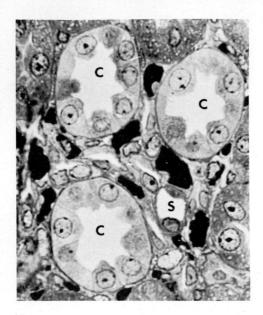

Figure 5-2. Photomicrograph of kidney to show tubules lined by simple cuboidal (C) and by simple squamous (S) epithelium. Epon section. × 650.   See filmstrip I, frame 10.

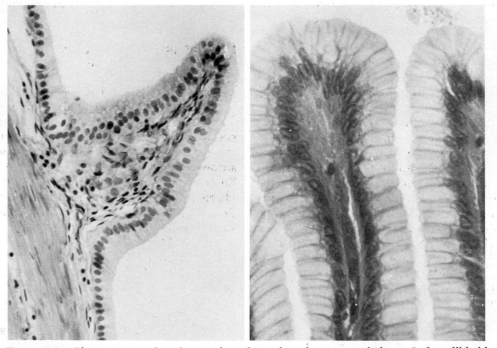

Figure 5-3. Photomicrographs of examples of simple columnar epithelium: Left, gallbladder. × 250. Right, stomach. × 650.   See filmstrip I, frame 11.

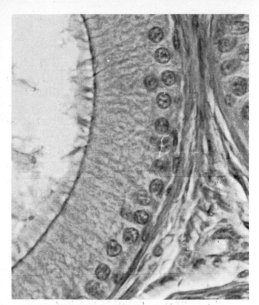

Figure 5-4. Photomicrograph of simple columnar epithelium with stereocilia from the epididymis. × 450. See filmstrip I, frame 7.

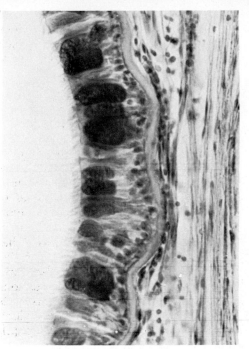

Figure 5-5. Photomicrograph of pseudostratified ciliated columnar epithelium with goblet (mucous) cells from the trachea. Nuclei are at various levels; cilia, the very dark goblet cells, and the basal lamina are obvious. The goblet cells are unicellular glands. × 650.

(luminal) surface. Such an epithelium usually is associated with secretion or absorption and thus is found lining much of the digestive system and the larger ducts of many glands. In such sites, there may be more than one cell type present; e.g., interspersed among the columnar cells often are mucus-secreting cells which are "goblet" shaped. Each "goblet" cell is regarded as a unicellular gland and will be discussed in more detail later.

Simple ciliated columnar epithelium has an appearance identical to simple nonciliated columnar epithelium on low power, but high magnification shows that the free surface of the cells is covered with cilia (see page 86). This type of epithelium lines the uterus and uterine tubes, the ductuli efferentia of the testis, small intrapulmonary bronchi, and the central canal in the spinal cord.

PSEUDOSTRATIFIED EPITHELIA

Pseudostratified columnar epithelium is composed of more than one type of cell with the cell nuclei lying at different levels in a perpendicular section, thus giving the impression that the membrane is composed of more than one layer of cells. Some of the cells may not reach the lumen although all are adjacent to the basal lamina. Such an epithelium lines the larger excretory ducts of many glands and parts of the male urethra. This type of epithelium may be ciliated, usually in association with goblet cells, and found lining the larger respiratory passages and some of the excretory ducts of the male reproductive system.

STRATIFIED EPITHELIA

All stratified epithelia can withstand more trauma than the simple types and thus are located in sites where they are subjected to friction and shearing forces, but because of their thickness they are not membranes through which absorption can occur readily.

Stratified Squamous Epithelium

Stratified squamous epithelium is a thick membrane, only the more superficial cells being flat. The deeper layers of cells vary from cuboidal to columnar, and often the basal layer, i.e., that adjacent to the basal lamina, shows considerable irregularity. That covering the cornea of the eye lies upon connective tissue with a smooth, regular surface, but in other locations the underlying connective tissue is raised into ridges and folds which appear as finger-like processes (papil-

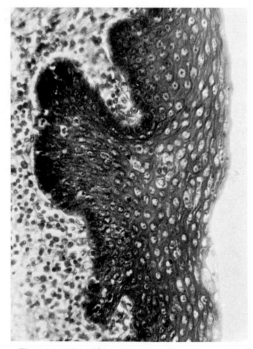

Figure 5-6. Photomicrograph of stratified squamous nonkeratinizing epithelium from the tongue. The underlying connective tissue (left) is irregular and is raised into a papilla. The corneal epithelium is similar to that illustrated, but rests upon a smooth connective tissue which shows no papillae. × 450. See filmstrip I, frame 12.

lae) in perpendicular section. Such an arrangement is found in, for example, the vagina, the esophagus, and the skin. In the vagina and esophagus, the surface of the epithelium is moist, and here the epithelium is nonkeratinized, whereas in the skin the surface is dry, and the surface cells undergo a transformation into a tough, resistant, nonliving layer of material called keratin. Hence the name of stratified squamous keratinizing epithelium. Keratin will be discussed in detail later (see Chapter 13), but it is important to appreciate that this material is resistant to friction, is relatively impervious to bacterial invasion, and is waterproof.

Stratified Cuboidal Epithelium

Stratified cuboidal epithelium is found only in the ducts of sweat glands in the adult and consists of two layers of cuboidal cells. As this type lines a tube, it is obvious that the cells of the superficial layer or layers are smaller as seen in cross section than those of the basal layer.

Stratified Columnar Epithelium

Stratified columnar epithelium also is relatively rare, and usually the basal layer or layers consist of relatively low, irregularly polyhedral cells and only the cells of the superficial layer are of the tall columnar type. Such an epithelium lines part of the male urethra and is found also in some larger excretory ducts.

Transitional Epithelium

Transitional epithelium is so termed because originally it was believed to represent a transition between the stratified squamous nonkeratinizing and stratified columnar types. It is found lining the urinary system from the renal pelvis down to the urethra,

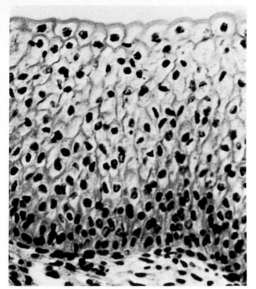

Figure 5-7. Photomicrograph of transitional epithelium lining the ureter. The surface cells stain more deeply, have a luminal convex border, and often are binucleate. × 350.

See filmstrip I, frame 13.

sites where it is subject to considerable variations in internal pressure and capacity. Hence its appearance varies with the degree of distention. The basal layer is cuboidal or even columnar in type, the intermediate levels are cuboidal and polyhedral, and the superficial layers vary from cuboidal to squamous depending upon the degree of distention. The superficial cells lining a nondistended organ characteristically have a convex free border and are often binucleate; i.e., they exhibit polyploidy.

ENDOTHELIUM, MESOTHELIUM

Endothelium lines all blood and lymph channels, and mesothelium is the lining of the serous body cavities (pericardial, pleural, and peritoneal). Structurally, both are simple squamous epithelia but they differ in their origin and potentialities, being capable of many functions not shown by ordinary simple squamous epithelium. For example, endothelial and mesothelial cells are actively phagocytic, can form fibroblasts by cell division, and are responsible for a variety of interesting tumors. They formerly were called false epithelia or pseudoepithelia.

CELL ADHESION IN EPITHELIAL MEMBRANES

Cells of an epithelial membrane are held together very firmly and indeed can resist considerable trauma which would tend to separate them, e.g., in the stratified squamous nonkeratinizing epithelium lining the oral cavity and the esophagus. In such sites, relatively hard masses of food material pass over the epithelial surface and yet do not separate cells. Several

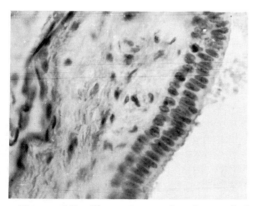

Figure 5-8. Photomicrograph of stratified columnar epithelium from a large lactiferous duct of the mammary gland. × 450.

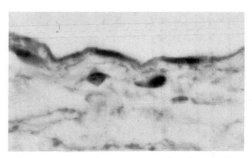

Figure 5-9. Photomicrograph of mesothelium (peritoneum) lining the abdominal cavity. Parts of two cells with their dark, flattened nuclei are shown. × 350.

factors are concerned in such resistance.

It has been emphasized already that the space between adjacent epithelial cells is very narrow, the adjacent plasma membranes of opposing cells being separated by a distance of only 100 to 150 Å. Occupying this space is a small amount of mucopolysaccharide which possibly acts as a kind of plastic cement. This material has a high content of cations, particularly calcium and perhaps also strontium. The former ion has been considered important in cell adhesion for a long time. Its actual role still is uncertain.

Cell Junctions

In some epithelia, e.g., of the epidermis, by light microscopy small cytoplasmic processes, the *intercellular bridges,* appear to extend between cells, with small intercellular spaces between the bridges. Present in these cells are fine cytoplasmic filaments, the tonofibrils, and these appear to pass through a bridge between ad-

jacent cells. Electron microscopy demonstrates that there is no cytoplasmic continuity between such cells and that at the sites of intercellular bridges there are small dense bodies called *desmosomes.* Desmosomes are scattered along epithelial and other cell interfaces also, and are not confined to the sites of intercellular bridges.

Desmosomes, visible only by electron microscopy, are small, discrete, bipartite ellipsoidal discs, about 4100 Å by 2500 Å. They usually are orientated with their long axes perpendicular to the basal lamina, i.e., along the long axis of the cells. At a desmosome, the plasma membranes of opposing cells appear dense and thickened by the presence of a thin dense layer on their cytoplasmic surfaces (Figures 5-10 and 5-12) with a thicker layer of fine cytoplasmic fibrils arranged in a feltwork more distant from the interface. If present, tonofilaments in the cytoplasm converge upon the desmosome and may terminate within it. In the intercellular space at a desmosome, a thin intermediate lamina may be seen running parallel to and midway be-

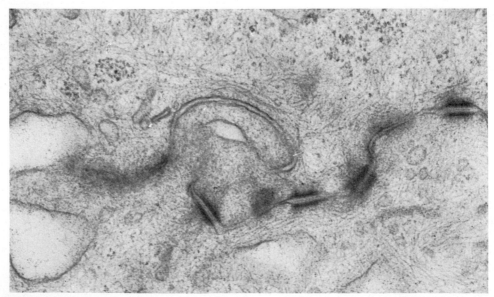

Figure 5-10.   Electron micrograph of parts of two epithelial cells to show desmosomes and the irregularity of the cell interface. × 55,000.

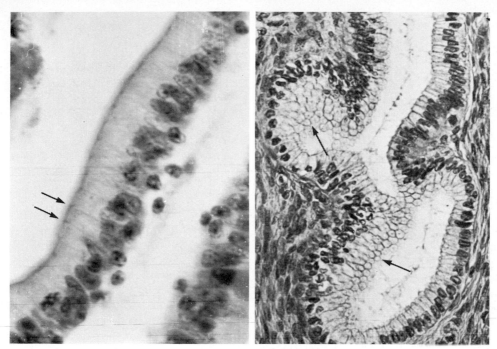

Figure 5-11. Left, photomicrograph of the simple columnar epithelium of the small intestine in vertical section to show terminal bars (arrows). × 750. Right, terminal bars in oblique section of columnar epithelium of cervical glands (arrows). × 250.

tween the plasma membranes (Figure 5-12). In some epithelia, half desmosomes sometimes are present on the basal plasma membrane adjacent to the basal lamina. Recently the term *"macula adherens"* (adherent spot) has been used instead of desmosome to indicate its function and shape.

Terminal bars are found on lateral epithelial cell interfaces near the free (luminal) surface and are seen particularly well after staining with iron hematoxylin. In grazing sections near the cell surface or in whole mounts, terminal bars outline cells in a hexagonal pattern (Figure 5-11, right) and are seen as dense dots near the luminal surface in perpendicular sections (Figure 5-11, left). By electron microscopy, lateral cell interfaces in this region show an area of specialization termed the *junctional complex,* consisting of three distinct parts. Immediately beneath the free surface, plasma membranes of adjoining cells

converge and the two external laminae of the unit membranes appear to fuse, thus completely obliterating the intercellular space. This region, the *zonula occludens* or tight junction, surrounds the entire cell perimeter, extends deeply for about 0.5 micron and passes into a middle zone, the *zonula adherens,* where the intercellular space is about 150 to 200 Å. The inner aspects of the plasma membranes are supported by some dense filamentous material often continuous with the terminal web. Deep to the zonula adherens is the third part of the complex, the *macula adherens* or desmosome. It is probable that the zonula occludens and the zonula adherens form what is seen as the terminal bar by light microscopy, only these two parts forming a continuous corona or crown around the apical portion of the cell.

In addition to the features mentioned, lateral cell interfaces commonly do not run in a parallel fashion

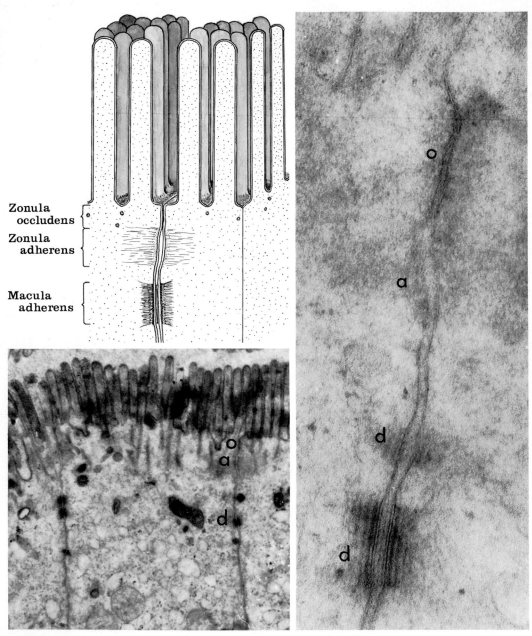

Figure 5-12. Junctional complex. The diagram at upper left illustrates appearance on electron microscopy of the apical cell interface between two epithelial cells with microvilli on the apical surfaces. The electron micrograph at lower left shows the apical portion of one such cell (× 18,000), and that on the right shows the features of the junctional complex at high magnification (× 105,000). o = zonula occludens, a = zonula adherens, d = macula adherens or desmosome.

but show interdigitation, termed "jig-saw" or "zipper" interlocking, often associated with desmosomes. They are developed extensively, for example, in the epithelium lining the proximal convoluted tubule of the kidney and in that of the rete testis. Presumably all these specializations of cell junctions function to maintain cell adhesion, with the zonula occludens in addition preventing passage of fluid between the lumen and the intercellular space. This implies that material passing across the epithelium must do so through the apical cytoplasm.

At the basal surface of epithelial cells the plasma membrane may show numerous infoldings, which are presumed to be a method of increasing surface area. For example, these infoldings are well developed in the convoluted tubules of the kidney. In a few instances, half desmosomes may be present on the basal plasma membrane of epithelial cells. As described in Chapter 3 previously, nearly all epithelia are supported by, and rest upon, a basal lamina or basement membrane.

SPECIALIZATIONS OF THE CELL SURFACE IN EPITHELIA

Many of these specializations have been described briefly in Chapter 2. Such specializations are developed to different degrees in different sites, and these will be indicated later during description of the organ systems.

Microvilli

Microvilli are small, slender, finger-like projections of the apical cell surface consisting of tubelike evaginations of the plasma membrane of the apical surface containing a core of cytoplasm. Individually, they are too small to be seen with the light microscope. In many epithelia, particularly high cuboidal and columnar types, they are numerous and of regular dimensions and form a brush or striated border, visible by light microscopy. In such cells there often is a condensation of fibrillar material in the apical cytoplasm extending into the cores of

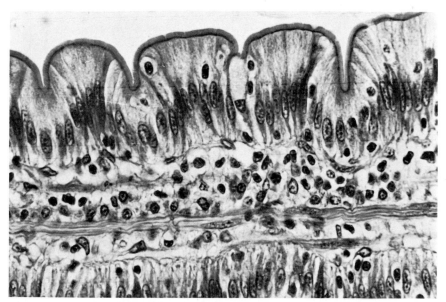

Figure 5-13. Photomicrograph of the simple columnar epithelium lining the small intestine to show the brush or striated border. × 400.   See filmstrip I, frame 14.

the microvilli and continuous at the circumference of the cell with the fibrillar material of the terminal bar. This network of fibrils is called the "terminal web." It is evident, for example, in the columnar epithelium of the intestine after staining with the tannic acid, phosphomolybdic acid, and amido black technique.

In epithelial cells lining part of the male generative tract, so called *stereocilia* are present on the apical surface (see Figure 5-4). By light microscopy they appear as long, slender, sometimes branching processes which are nonmotile. By electron microscopy, it can be demonstrated that stereocilia bear no resemblance to true cilia but are composed of groups of extremely long and slender microvilli.

Cilia

Cilia project from the free apical surfaces of some epithelial cells and may be very numerous; for example, some 270 cilia are on each ciliated cell lining the trachea. Cilia and flagella have a similar structure. By light microscopy, each cilium appears as a

long, slender process in which an axial filament may be visible. In the cytoplasm at the base of each is a small, dense, highly refractile basal body which stains black with iron hematoxylin. By electron microscopy each cilium is seen to contain nine peripheral longitudinal filaments or microtubules and two central filaments. In cross section, each peripheral filament is composed of two microtubules, the wall of one being more dense than that of its partner and bearing two short projecting arms extending into the core of the cilium toward the adjacent filament. The central filaments are single microtubules. The basal body at the base of a cilium appears as a hollow cylinder containing in its wall nine peripheral filaments. This appearance is similar to that of a centriole, and there may be rootlets extending from it into the apical cytoplasm. In movement, each cilium undergoes a rapid forward beat with a slower recovery stroke, the beat appearing as a wave of movement in a ciliated epithelial membrane, transporting material (e.g., mucus) in one direction along the surface of the membrane. The mechanism of cilial beat is not known,

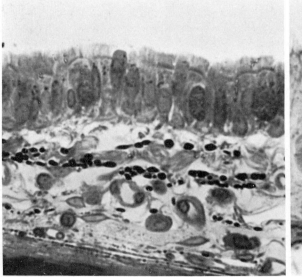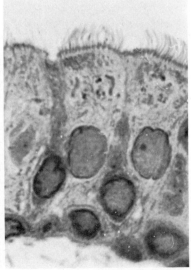

Figure 5-14.   Photomicrographs to show ciliated columnar epithelium of trachea. Epon sections. Left, × 450; right, × 1200.   See filmstrip I, frame 15.

but its direction is associated with the orientation of cilial filaments.

Cilia occur also in the maculae and cristae of the inner ear and in a modified form as retinal rods of the eye; in such sites they appear to be nerve receptors. In other sites single cilia have been considered chemoreceptors. The single flagellum of spermatozoa is of similar structure and, of course, is motile.

GLAND EPITHELIUM

As has been noted on page 73, cells of epithelial membranes in many instances secrete materials in addition to their other functions such as protection and absorption. However, this function of secretion is often of secondary importance in that a cell highly specialized for protection or absorption cannot also be highly specialized for secretion. In addition, the epithelial surfaces of the body are of inadequate surface area to accommodate the numbers of secretory cells required. Thus, a system of multicellular glands is present, each composed of masses of epithelial cells highly specialized for secretion. The secretory product of these cells is passed into a system of tubes or ducts which then transport it to a surface. The glandular secretion consists of an aqueous fluid containing the secretory product, e.g., a hormone, an enzyme, or mucin. This process of synthesis involves interaction of cell organelles and the expenditure of energy.

Classification of Glands

Glands usually are divided into two main groups, exocrine and endocrine. A gland of the exocrine type passes its secretion to a duct system and thus to a body surface; i.e., there is an external secretion. An endocrine gland passes its secretion directly into the blood or into the lymph; i.e., it is an internal secretion or hormone, which is transported throughout the body and thus to the target organ or organs where its actions are performed. Both types of glands develop in the embryo in a similar fashion by an invagination of epithelial cells into the connective tissue underlying an epithelial membrane. In exocrine glands the site of the original invagination persists as the duct system, whereas connection with the epithelial membrane is lost in endocrine glands, the secretion then passing into the vascular system.

In some glands the secretion characteristically contains intact, living cells, e.g., the sex glands, which secrete living germ cells. Three other types of secretory cells are described according to the manner in which their secretory product is elaborated. In some glands the entire secretory cell, having formed and accumulated secretory products within its cytoplasm, dies, disintegrates, and is discharged from the gland as the secretion. Such a gland, where the entire cell is secreted, is called *holocrine,* and obviously cell division in such a gland must be rapid to replace cells lost in secretion. Examples of this type are sebaceous and tarsal glands. In *apocrine* glands the secretory product accumulates in the apical portion of the cell, which is then pinched off, the cell losing some of its apical cytoplasm together with the specific secretory product. The cell then passes through another secretory cycle after a short recovery period. An example of an apocrine gland is the mammary gland. The great majority of glands are of the *merocrine* type whose secretory product is formed in and discharged from the cell without the loss of any cytoplasm. Examples of this type are the salivary glands and pancreas.

Unicellular Glands

Unicellular glands, in which a single cell forms a gland, are represented by

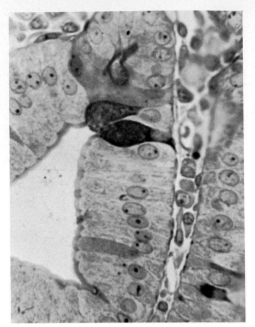

Figure 5-15. Photomicrograph of the columnar epithelium lining an intestinal crypt to show two unicellular glands (goblet cells, darkly staining). Epon section, × 850.

mucous or goblet cells, mentioned previously in relation to epithelial membranes. These cells, for example, in the epithelia lining the trachea and the large and small intestines, characteristically resemble a goblet or wine glass in shape, the dilated, oval apical portion being filled with a mass of mucigen droplets which are pale staining in an H and E preparation but which can be stained specifically by other methods. The mucin which is secreted by these cells is a protein-polysaccharide complex that forms mucus in water, mucus being a slimy, lubricating fluid. It should be emphasized that not all mucin-secreting cells are goblet cells. The stomach epithelium, for example, contains three different type of columnar, mucin-secreting cells, none of which is of the goblet shape, and each of which is a little different from the others both in structure and chemical composition of the mucin secreted.

Multicellular Glands

Multicellular glands are represented most simply by an epithelial sheet composed of secretory cells, but the majority arise as an invagination of an epithelial sheet into underlying connective tissue. Thus, a gland consists of epithelial elements lining its duct system, epithelial elements of the secretory units, and the supporting fibroconnective tissue. The latter contains an extensive network of blood vessels and nerve terminals of the autonomic nervous system. In exocrine glands the epithelial cells of the secretory elements are supported by a basal lamina which separates them from the blood capillaries, but a basal lamina usually is not demonstrable in endocrine glands, e.g., the thyroid.

Exocrine Glands

The various types of multicellular exocrine glands are classified according to whether the duct branches and according to the shape of the secretory unit (tubular, alveolar, or mixed). As indicated in Figure 5-1, the duct may be unbranched or branched, and this distinction provides two large groups of simple and compound glands. In simple glands the duct may be straight or coiled. The secretory unit situated at the termination of a duct, or a small branch of a duct in a compound gland, may be tubular or flask-shaped, the latter being called alveolar or acinar (like a hollow vessel or like a berry). In many glands the secretory units are mixed and the gland is then termed tubuloalveolar. The nature of the secretion may be either mucous or serous, the latter being a clear, watery fluid usually containing enzymes. The cells responsible for the production of these two types of secretion differ greatly in their appearance. Often both serous and mucous alveoli or acini are found in the same gland, which then is called a mixed gland. An acinus which contains cells of both types is called a mixed acinus. It is by these three characteristics that exocrine glands are classified; thus we describe, for example, simple tubular serous glands and compound alveolar mucous glands.

Connective Tissue Elements. During development of both exocrine and endocrine glands, invagination of cells from an epithelial membrane extends into the connective tissue (mesenchyme) underlying that membrane. This connective tissue forms the fibroconnective tissue capsule and supporting framework of the gland. The amount of such tissue varies, being, for example, relatively profuse and dense in salivary glands but much thinner and finer in the pancreas. From the capsule, septa of connective tissue extend into the center of the gland but are never complete in that they are pierced by blood vessels. The major septa subdivide the glands into lobes, and each lobe is subdivided by finer connective tissue into lobules. The supporting tissue of the lobule is fine reticular connective tissue, containing within its mesh the secretory units and ducts, and connected at the periphery of the lobule to the more substantial fibroconnective tissue surrounding the lobule.

Blood vessels, lymphatics, and nerves are carried in the connective tissue of the gland, entering the gland through its capsule and then being distributed along interlobar and interlobular septa, the small arteries passing from interlobular septa into the lobule where they break up into a capillary network in the intralobular reticular tissue between secretory units.

Epithelial Duct Elements. Usually one major duct supported and surrounded by connective tissue leaves a gland, and, to use an analogy, this is like the trunk of a tree whose branches and twigs are the smaller ducts and whose leaves are the secretory units. The smallest ducts are the intercalary or intercalated ducts, the term indicating that they are inserted between

(and therefore connect) secretory units and intralobular ducts. The intralobular ducts are supported by fine reticular connective tissue and are lined by small cuboidal cells, the nuclei of which resemble a necklace of beads when the duct is cut in cross section. Several of these intralobular ducts join to form a larger lobular duct, this also lying between acini, and in turn, several lobular ducts unite to form an interlobular duct which is situated in the fibroconnective tissue of an interlobular septum. At the apex of a lobe, the interlobular ducts of that lobe unite to form a lobar duct, this being surrounded by relatively dense fibroconnective tissue. Finally, the lobar ducts unite to form the (usually) single duct which drains the entire gland and terminates by opening onto a surface.

The epithelium lining the duct system varies from the squamous or low cuboidal type of the intercalated duct through cuboidal and columnar to, usually, stratified columnar or stratified squamous in the main duct. Although the duct epithelium mainly functions as a passive lining of the drainage system of a gland, there is evidence that in many glands it can modify the nature and concentration of the secretion. In passing from smaller to larger ducts (i.e., from twigs to branches of the tree) not only does the lining epithelium become more robust, but the supporting elements of the duct change from fine reticular to fibroconnective tissue, usually with an outer smooth muscle coat, the muscle cells often being arranged in inner circular and outer longitudinal layers.

Glandular Units. As indicated previously, exocrine glands generally are classified into serous, mucous, or mixed glands, each being identified on a histological slide by the appearance of its secretory units. In all instances, the units of a lobule will be cut in different planes, some showing a lumen and occasionally continuity with an intercalated duct, and others appearing as a solid clump of cells, the plane of section having missed the lumen. The following features should serve to distinguish the types of exocrine glands.

SEROUS GLANDS. Usually the cytoplasm is darkly staining, being pink or pinkish purple with H and E stain, and somewhat darker toward the cell base. Cell membranes often are not easily defined. Nuclei are regularly round or oval and situated near, but not at, the base of the cell. In the apical cytoplasm, zymogen (secretory) granules are present and may be stained specifically. The lumen of the acinus is usually definite and smaller in diameter than that of a mucous acinus. By electron microscopy, an extensive granular endoplasmic reticulum is present in the basal cytoplasm with quite numerous mitochondria scattered throughout the cell. The Golgi apparatus is well developed and situated on the apical side of the nucleus. Zymogen granules of varying density, each surrounded by a single membrane, are present in the apical cytoplasm. In serous cells it is easy to visualize the cycle of secretion as outlined on page 55.

MUCOUS GLANDS. The cytoplasm stains much lighter in an H and E preparation and may have a foamy, "moth-eaten" appearance. Specific stains for mucoprotein, e.g., alcian blue, mucicarmine, and the PAS reaction stain, demonstrate mucous acini well. The nuclei are usually small, dark, and thin and are flattened against the basal plasma membrane of the cells. Normally the lumen is small and irregular. By electron microscopy the cytoplasm usually is seen to be filled with large "mucigen" droplets between which are strands of cytoplasm containing sparse organelles.

MIXED GLANDS. As explained pre-

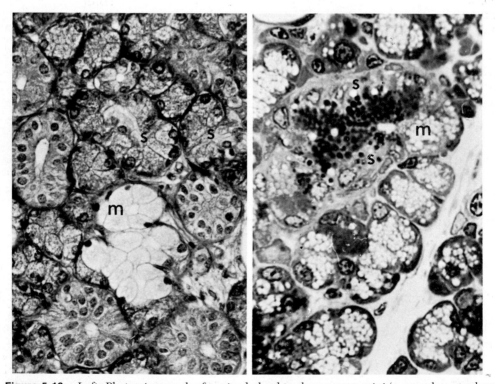

Figure 5-16. Left: Photomicrograph of a mixed gland to show serous acini (s, granular cytoplasm, small lumen) and mucous acini (m, nuclei flattened at the bases of cells, pale "foamy" cytoplasm). × 550. Right: Photomicrograph to show a mixed acinus (top, center) with mucous (m) and serous (s) cells. Epon section, × 650.   See filmstrip I, frame 16.

viously, a mixed gland is one in which both mucous and serous acini are present or one in which component acini contain both mucous and serous cells. In a mixed acinus the majority of cells are the mucous type but to one side is a collection of serous cells arranged in a crescent or half-moon fashion. The cells of these serous demilunes pass their secretion into tiny intercellular canals between adjacent mucous cells and thus into the lumen of the acinus.

Myoepithelial Cells. Each acinus, of whatever type, is surrounded by a fine extracellular basal lamina. Surrounding the acinar cells are the myoepithelial or basket cells, which usually are seen as small dark nuclei surrounded by a small amount of cytoplasm lying just within the basal lamina. From the central mass of cytoplasm containing the nucleus, long thin arms of cytoplasm extend around the cells of the acinus to grasp it rather in the fashion of an octopus or in the form of a basket. These cells, although epithelial in origin, contain fibrillar cytoplasmic elements and show many of the features of smooth muscle cells. They can be clearly demonstrated by the alkaline phosphatase technique. They are thought to be contractile and thus to aid in expelling secretion from the gland. Myoepithelial cells can be demonstrated also in relation to the smaller ducts of mucous, serous, and mixed glands—for example, around the secretory units of sweat glands.

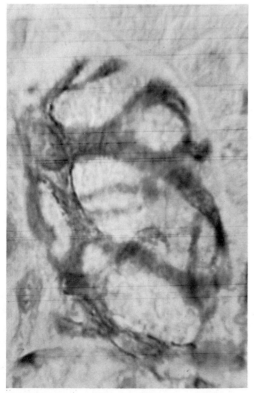

Figure 5-17. Photomicrograph of a myoepithelial or "basket" cell (dark), with nucleus (top, left) and cytoplasmic "arms" surrounding a glandular acinus. This myoepithelial cell lies *within* the basal lamina of the acinus. Alkaline phosphatase technique. × 1500.

Endocrine Glands

These will be discussed in detail in a later chapter, but they are much simpler histologically than exocrine glands. Usually they are surrounded by a thin connective tissue capsule from which incomplete septa extend into the glands to divide them into lobes. The main supporting tissue, however, is composed of very fine reticular (connective tissue) fibers associated with a very rich blood capillary or sinusoidal meshwork. Between the fine blood channels are clumps and cords of epithelial cells which elaborate the specific hormone or hormones of the gland, each cell closely associated with a fine blood vessel into which it passes its secretion. Storage of hormones is intracellular in most cases, but in some glands, the thyroid for example, a group of cells may pass their secretion centrally to form a vesicle or follicle surrounded by the secretory cells. When required, the hormone passes back peripherally through the cells and into blood capillaries situated between follicles.

Many glands are mixed, having both

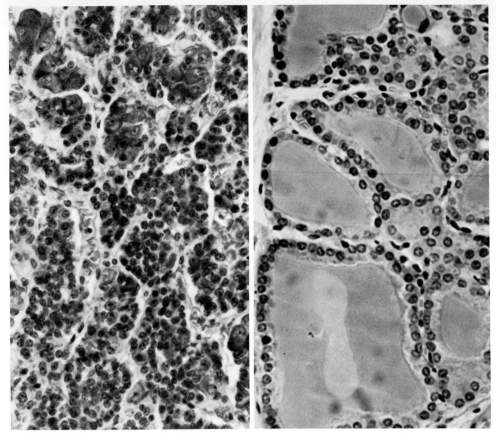

Figure 5-18. Photomicrographs of endocrine glands: Left, of the "cord and clump" type (anterior pituitary). × 250. Right, of the "follicle" type (thyroid). × 350.

exocrine and endocrine functions. Liver cells not only formulate bile as an exocrine secretion, passing it into a duct system, but also secrete internal secretions directly into the blood system. In other mixed glands, i.e., pancreas, testis, and ovary, one group of cells secretes into a duct system and another group secretes directly into the blood system.

REFERENCES

Bennett, H. S.: Morphological aspects of extra-cellular polysaccharides. J. Histochem. & Cytochem., 11:2, 1963.

Farquhar, M. G., and Palade, G. E.: Junctional complexes in various epithelia. J. Cell Biol., 17:375, 1963.

Fawcett, D. W.: Structural specializations of the cell surface. In Frontiers in Cytology, edited by S. L. Palay. New Haven, Yale University Press, 1958, p. 19.

Fawcett, D. W.: Cilia and flagella. In The Cell: Biochemistry, Physiology, Morphology, edited by J. Brachet and A. E. Mirsky. New York, Academic Press, 1961, Vol. 2, p. 217.

Fawcett, D. W.: Physiologically significant specializations of the cell surface. Circulation, 26:1105, 1962.

Fawcett, D. W.: Surface specializations of absorbing cells. J. Histochem. & Cytochem., 13:75, 1965.

Gabe, M., and Arvy, L.: Gland cells. In The Cell: Biochemistry, Physiology, Morphology, edited by J. Brachet and A. E. Mirsky. New York, Academic Press, 1961, Vol. 5, p. 1.

Leeson, C. R.: Localization of alkaline phosphatase in the submaxillary gland of the rat. Nature, 178:858, 1956.

Puchtler, H., and Leblond, C. P.: Histochemical analysis of cell membranes and associated structures as seen in the intestinal epithelium. Amer. J. Anat., 102:1, 1958.

Revel, J. P., and Ito, S.: The surface components of cells. In The Specificity of Cell Surfaces, edited by B. D. Davis and L. Warren. Englewood Cliffs, New Jersey, Prentice-Hall, Inc., 1967, pp. 211-234.

CHAPTER 6

CONNECTIVE TISSUE PROPER

Early during embryological development, the ectoderm and endoderm become separated by the third germ layer, the mesoderm. The tissue formed by the cells of this layer is known as *mesenchyme* (*mesos*, middle; *enchyma*, infusion), and it is from mesenchyme that the connective tissues of the body develop. These include the connective tissue proper, cartilage, bone, and blood.

Mesenchyme is typically a loose spongy tissue which in early embryonic life is found as packing between structures developing from other germ layers. It is composed of stellate and fusiform cells forming a network and of an amorphous intercellular substance which contains a few scattered fibers.

Mesenchymal cells have multiple developmental potentialities. They are able to differentiate along several different lines to produce many different kinds of connective tissue cells. Thus the tissues which have a common origin from mesenchyme are known as *mesenchymal tissues* or the *connective tissues*.

Connective tissues differ from epithelium by the presence of abundant intercellular material or matrix. Matrix is composed of fibers and an amorphous ground substance. The proportions of cells and intercellular substance show considerable variation and form the basis of classification. The classification is inexact since various types are linked by transitional forms.

In any type of connective tissue there are three elements to consider: the cells, the fibers, and the amorphous ground substance. The fibers and the ground substance have been described previously in Chapter 3. The cells will be discussed in detail before consideration is given to the features of the various types of connective tissue. The description of the cells is based upon their appearance in areolar (loose) connective tissue, which is the chief "packing" material in the adult, and which may be considered as the prototype of the connective tissues.

CONNECTIVE TISSUE CELLS

Fibroblasts

These are one of the two most numerous cells of areolar connective tissue, the other being *macrophages* (or *histiocytes*). Fibroblasts, as their name suggests, are considered to be responsible for the formation of the fibers and also are thought to elaborate most, if not all, of the amorphous component of the matrix. They are large, flat, branching cells which appear fusiform or spindle-shaped in profile. The branching processes are slender. The nucleus is oval or elongated and has a delicate nuclear membrane, one or two distinct nucleoli, and a small amount of finely granular chromatin. In connective tissue spreads the nucleus appears pale, but in sectioned material it usually appears shrunken and deeply stained with basic dyes. In most histological preparations the outlines of the cells are indistinct, and the nuclear characteristics are of considerable value in identification. The cytoplasm stains palely and is relatively homogeneous. After suitable staining, mitochondria appear as slender rods and are most numerous near the nucleus, where the Golgi apparatus also is located. Granular endoplasmic reticulum, as seen by electron microscopy, is scattered throughout the cytoplasm. The scant cytoplasm of fully differentiated fibroblasts is weakly basophil. In sections such fibroblasts appear as well stained nuclei surrounded by pale, poorly defined cytoplasm. Such mature fibroblasts are sometimes called *fibrocytes.* In young fibroblasts, which are actively engaged in protein synthesis for the production of intercellular substance, the cytoplasm is more strongly basophil.

Fibroblasts are regarded as fixed cells of connective tissue but they re-

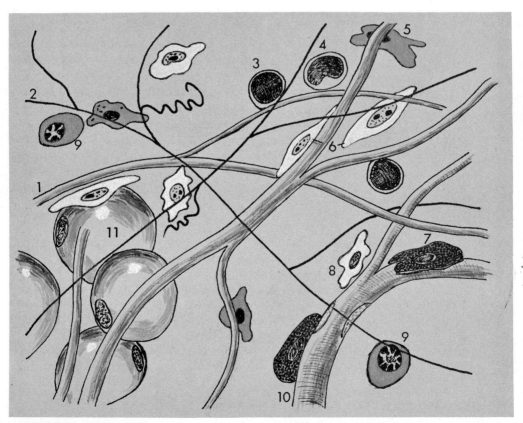

Figure 6-1.   Diagram of a section through subcutaneous, loose areolar connective tissue. (1) Collagenous fiber. (2) Elastic fiber. (3) Lymphocyte. (4) Monocyte. (5) Macrophage. (6) Fibroblasts. (7) Mast cell. (8) Undifferentiated mesenchymal cell. (9) Plasma cell. (10) Capillary. (11) Fat cell.

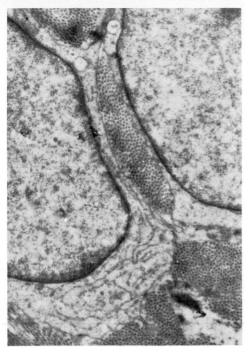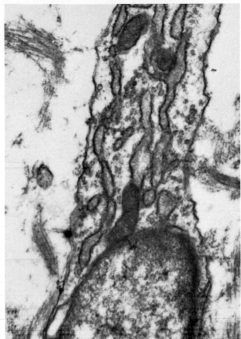

Figure 6-2. Left: Electron micrograph of portions of two fibroblasts and collagenous fibrils of the dense connective tissue of the penis. The collagenous fibrils are associated closely with the cell membrane of fibroblasts. Osmium fixation. × 13,500. Right: Single fibroblast from loose connective tissue covering the ureter. × 15,000.

tain throughout adult life a capacity for growth and regeneration, and when stimulated, as on the periphery of healing wounds or in inflamed tissues, they are capable of a slow gliding movement.

Undifferentiated Mesenchymal Cells

Some embryonic cells are thought to persist in the adult. They are difficult to distinguish from active fibroblasts but in general are smaller. Whereas fibroblasts are seen usually in close association with collagen fibers, undifferentiated mesenchymal cells are located along the walls of blood vessels, particularly capillaries. Their recognition comes not with the microscope but from numerous observations of their responses to certain stimuli, when they are capable of differentiation into various cell types. Probably they are similar to the *primi-*

tive reticular cells of the blood-forming tissues (see Chapter 8).

Macrophages

Often termed histiocytes, macrophages are almost as numerous as fibroblasts in loose connective tissue and are most abundant in richly vascularized areas. They are irregularly shaped cells with processes which usually are short and blunt. Occasionally they may exhibit long, slender branching processes. When stimulated, macrophages are capable of ameboid movement and in this phase they are very irregular in outline with pseudopodia extending in numerous directions. The nucleus is ovoid, sometimes indented, and smaller and more densely staining than that of the fibroblast. Nucleoli are not conspicuous. The cytoplasm stains darkly and may contain a few small vacuoles which

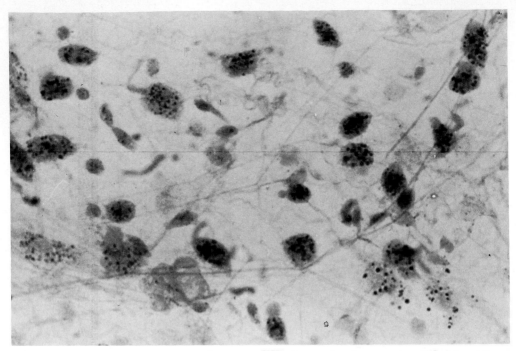

Figure 6-3. A spread preparation of rat omentum after vital staining with trypan blue. Macrophages contain numerous particles of ingested dye. × 425.

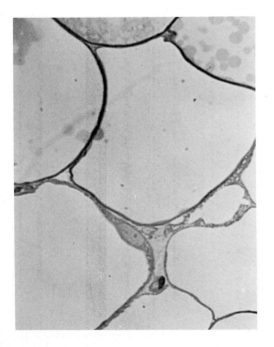

Figure 6-4. Photomicrograph of fat cells in the omentum. Note the nucleus and the thin rim of cytoplasm surrounding the large fat globule, which has been dissolved in preparation. Epon section, × 650.

stain supravitally with neutral red. These cells, when they are activated, can be distinguished readily from fibroblasts, owing to their ability to ingest particulate matter. Then the cells appear much larger and the cytoplasm is filled with granules and vacuoles containing ingested material. Sections of tissue from animals which have received injections vitally of colloidal carbon or of colloidal dyes such as trypan blue show macrophages with accumulations of the dye within vacuoles in the cytoplasm. Fibroblasts contain little or none of the dye.

Macrophages are important agents of defense. Because of their mobility and phagocytic activity, they are able to act as scavengers, engulfing extravasated blood cells, dead cells, bacteria, and foreign bodies. Ingested organic material is destroyed by the action of intracellular proteolytic enzymes, but inert foreign matter which resists digestion may remain in the cytoplasm indefinitely. An example of the latter is the inhaled carbon particles which accumulate within macrophages of the lung.

Macrophages are a component of the reticuloendothelial system, which will be discussed in more detail on page 107.

Fat Cells

These conspicuous cells are a normal component of areolar tissue. They occur singly or in clumps along small blood vessels. If they accumulate in large numbers, the tissue is transformed into *adipose tissue*. In fresh tissue they appear as glistening droplets of oil surrounded by an exceedingly thin rim of cytoplasm. Each fat cell contains a single large droplet of oil, and the thin rim of cytoplasm contains in one area the flattened nucleus. In fresh or formalin-fixed tissue the fat droplet can be stained with osmic acid or with Sudan dyes, but in most histological preparations the lipid has been extracted leaving only the delicate protoplasmic envelope. Individual cells are surrounded by a fine network of reticular (argyrophil) fibers.

Fat cells are fully differentiated cells and are incapable of mitotic division. New fat cells therefore, which may develop at any time within connective tissue, arise as a result of differentiation of more primitive cells. Although fat cells, before they store fat, resemble fibroblasts, it is likely that they arise directly from undifferentiated mesenchyme cells present within the body. Initially small droplets of fat make their appearance within the cytoplasm. The droplets increase in size and finally coalesce to form a single large droplet, and the cytoplasm is reduced to a thin encompassing layer. The nucleus is compressed and flattened.

When fat is utilized it leaves the cell as soluble components (the same form in which it enters) and the cell takes on a wrinkled appearance.

Mast Cells

These elements are widely distributed in connective tissues but tend to occur in small groups in relation to

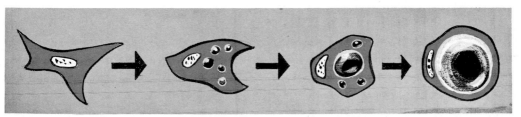

Figure 6-5. Diagram to illustrate the development of a fat cell.

blood vessels. They are particularly common in connective tissue of rodents. Mast cells are identified easily by their content of cytoplasmic granules. They are irregularly oval in outline and occasionally have short pseudopodia, an indication of their slow mobility. The nucleus is small and inconspicuous, often masked by the crowded granules. In most preparations many mast cells are ruptured and their granules escape into the surrounding· tissue. The granules are refractile and water soluble and stain with basic dyes. Neutral red stains them supravitally a dark red-brown and they exhibit metachromasia with basic aniline dyes such as methylene blue or azure A. The granules also show a positive staining reaction with the periodic acid–Schiff reagent.

Mast cells are thought to produce an *anticoagulant* similar to, if not identical with, *heparin*. Chemically, heparin is a sulfated polysaccharide, which gives a metachromatic staining reaction with basic aniline dyes, as do mast cell granules. Quantitative studies have shown that tissues and organs in which mast cells are most numerous contain more heparin-like substance than do structures containing few mast cells. Mast cell tumors possess a heparin-like content many times greater than that of liver, which is used as a commercial source of the anticoagulant. Other evidence indicates that mast cells also may contain *histamine* and *serotonin*, a vasoconstrictor.

Blood Leukocytes

Although leukocytes are transported by the blood stream, they perform their chief functions extravascularly, and thus it is not surprising that they are encountered within connective tissue.

Lymphocytes are the smallest of the free cells of connective tissue, the majority being only 7 to 8 microns in diameter. They have a spherical, darkly staining nucleus which occupies most of the cell. Around the nucleus is a thin rim of homogeneous

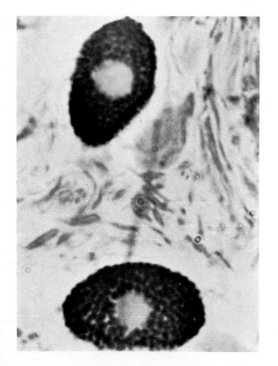

Figure 6-6. Photomicrograph of mast cells in loose connective tissue. Note the pale nuclear area devoid of granules. Toluidine blue stain, Epon section. × 1000. **See filmstrip I, frame 17.**

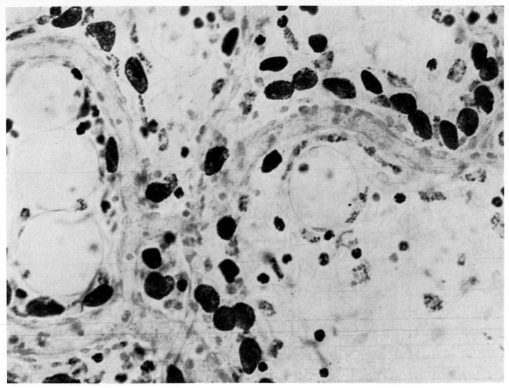

Figure 6-7. A spread preparation of rat omentum after vital staining with trypan blue and supravital staining with neutral red. A small quantity of vital dye was injected, with the result that macrophages contain only small qualities of the dye (compare with Figure 6-3). Mast cells are stained densely with neutral red and are aligned along the capillary network. Unstained fat cells are present also. × 425.

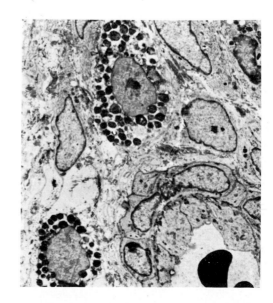

Figure 6-8. Low power electron micrograph of two mast cells in relation to a small blood vessel. Compare with Figure 6-7. × 2500.

cytoplasm which is basophil. Lymphocytes are not seen in large numbers in
connective tissue generally but are
numerous in the connective tissue
which supports the epithelial lining
of the respiratory and alimentary
tracts. They accumulate in sites of
chronic inflammation, and it is thought
by some authorities that they are concerned with antibody production. The
majority of lymphocytes present in
the loose connective tissue are thought
to emigrate there from the blood
stream. In tissue cultures lymphocytes
appear to be actively ameboid; it is
thought that they egress from the
circulation between lining cells of
the blood vessels. Some lymphocytes,
however, originate in the connective
tissue and they remain there. They
may, however, enter or re-enter the
circulation at any time.

Recent radioautographic studies
have indicated that there are two
distinct populations of lymphocytes,
one with a brief life span and the other
living for months or years. It is the
latter group which is migratory in the
connective tissues.

Eosinophil Cells

Eosinophil cells also may emigrate
from the blood stream into the connective tissue. They are not numerous
in human connective tissue generally
but are plentiful in connective tissue
of the lactating breast and of the respiratory and alimentary tracts. They
are a marked feature of the loose connective tissue of rat, mouse, and guinea
pig. The nucleus is usually reniform
or bilobed, and the cytoplasm contains
spherical granules which are highly
refractile and stain with acid dyes.
Eosinophils accumulate in the blood
and in the tissues in certain allergic
and subacute inflammatory conditions, and the suggestion has been
made that they may be related in some
way to the phenomenon of hyper-
sensitivity.

Other white blood cells which may

be found in connective tissue are
neutrophils, but generally these escape
into the connective tissue from capillaries only in regions of inflammation.
They may be recognized by the multi-
lobation of the nucleus. *Monocytes*
are seen rarely.

Plasma Cells

These cells bear a resemblance to
lymphocytes. They possess more cytoplasm which, like that of the lymphocytes, is basophil, and a nucleus which
usually is eccentric in position. Within
the nucleus, chromatin occurs in
coarse clumps peripherally and often
is arranged in a pattern suggestive of
the spokes of a wheel or the hours on a
clock. Accordingly, the nucleus is described as having a cartwheel or clock-
face appearance. The cytoplasm contains a clear, rounded area which is
the site of the centrosphere and the
Golgi apparatus. An extensive endoplasmic reticulum with associated
ribosomes is a fine structural feature
of the cytoplasm.

Plasma cells are rare in connective

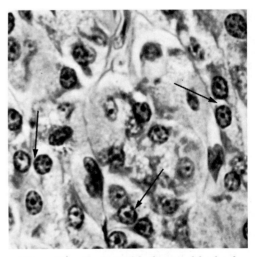

Figure 6-9.   Section of the lining of the fundus
of the stomach, in which numerous plasma cells
are present (arrows). The nuclei of these cells
show the typical peripheral condensations of
chromatin. × 1025.

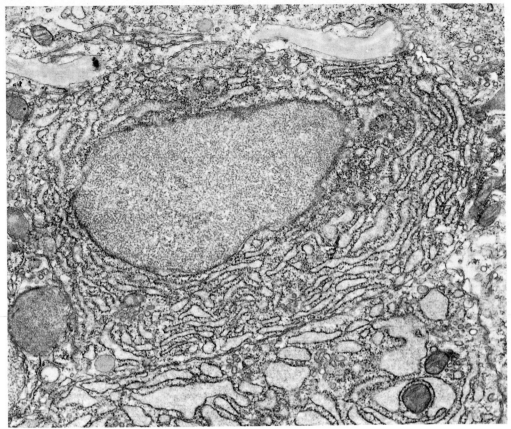

Figure 6-10. Electron micrograph of a plasma cell in the red pulp of mouse spleen. Note the extensive development of granular endoplasmic reticulum. × 12,500. (Courtesy of T. K. Shnitka.)

tissues generally but are found frequently in serous membranes and lymphoid tissue and are plentiful in sites of chronic inflammation. They probably represent a special differentiation of the lymphocyte, and like the lymphocyte they have been implicated as a possible site of antibody production.

Occasionally acidophil inclusions called *Russell bodies* are present in the cytoplasm of plasma cells. They probably represent products of degeneration rather than of secretion.

Pigment Cells

Cells containing pigment are rare in loose connective tissue but are found commonly in the dense connective tissue of the skin, in pia mater, and in the chorioid coat of the eye. These cells are derived from neural crest, however, and do not arise directly from mesenchyme. Typically such cells have irregular cytoplasmic processes which, like the general cytoplasm, contain small granules of pigment. The pigment is *melanin,* which has a role in the absorption of light rays, and the cells which produce it are referred to as *melanocytes.* Thus the pigment is endogenous (see Chapter 13).

CONNECTIVE TISSUE FIBERS AND GROUND SUBSTANCE

Collagenous, reticular, and elastic fibers and ground substance (amor-

phous intercellular material) have
been discussed in detail in Chapter 3
and should be reviewed before proceeding to study the types of connective tissue.

TYPES OF CONNECTIVE
TISSUE PROPER

The character of connective tissue
varies greatly in different parts of the
body. The appearance depends upon
the relative proportions and arrangement of the cellular, fibrous, and
amorphous components. The major
subdivision in the classification of connective tissues is determined by the
concentration of fibers. The connective tissues which are characterized
by a loose arrangement of fibers are
referred to as *loose connective tissues*.
In *dense connective tissues* there is
an abundance of compactly arranged
fibers. A further division of loose connective tissues into those which are
present only in the embryo and those
which are found in the adult can be
made.

Loose Connective Tissues

Mesenchyme. Mesenchyme, as
mentioned in the introduction to this
chapter, is the typical, unspecialized
connective tissue of the early weeks
of embryonic life. Subsequently it
disappears as such when component
cells undergo differentiation. It is composed of mesenchymal cells, whose
branching processes appear to join
although they do not form a true
syncytium, and of a ground substance
which is a coagulable fluid in the
earliest stages but later contains fine
fibrils.

Mucous Connective Tissue. This
is a transient type of tissue which appears in the normal development and
differentiation of the connective tissues. It occurs also as *Wharton's jelly*
in the umbilical cord, where it does
not differentiate further.

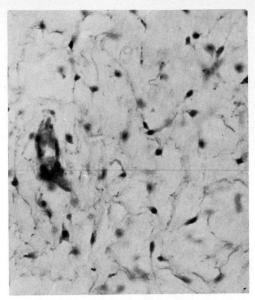

Figure 6-11. Section of mesenchyme, containing a small blood vessel, from subcutaneous
tissue of a 10 mm. pig embryo. × 425.
See filmstrip I, frame 18.

Component cells are large, stellate
fibroblasts whose processes often appear to fuse with those of neighboring
cells. A few macrophages and wandering lymphocytes are encountered occa-

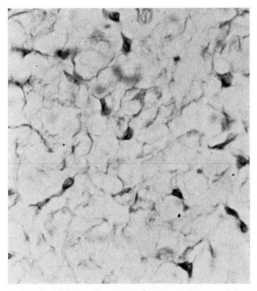

Figure 6-12. Section of mucous connective
tissue of the umbilical cord. × 425.

sionally. The ground substance is soft and jelly-like, gives a mucin reaction, and stains metachromatically with toluidine blue. It contains a few collagenous fibers.

Loose (Areolar) Connective Tissue. Loose connective tissue is formed by the direct differentiation of mesenchyme. It is a loosely arranged, fibro-elastic connective tissue, which is encountered in almost every microscopic section of the body, since it is the packing and anchoring material and is the embedding medium of many structures, including blood vessels and nerves.

All the structural elements, cells, fibers, and ground substance, previously described, are present within it. The two commonest cell types are fibroblasts and macrophages. Collagenous fibers are most prominent; elastic fibers, which form a continuous branching network, are relatively in-conspicuous. Reticular fibers are represented also but are abundant only where areolar tissue borders upon other structures. The ground substance is relatively fluid-like and occupies many little areas (*areolas*) in which no structure ordinarily can be seen.

Areolar connective tissue is studied usually in two different types of preparation. It can be found in most sectioned material and can be examined also in spread preparations of subcutaneous tissue and of mesentery. The distinction between these two types of preparation is important. Study of sectioned material alone, although it reveals many cytological details, does not easily demonstrate the three dimensional organization of areolar connective tissue. In spread preparations, unlike sectioned material, whole cells are viewed and the pattern of the fiber networks can be discerned.

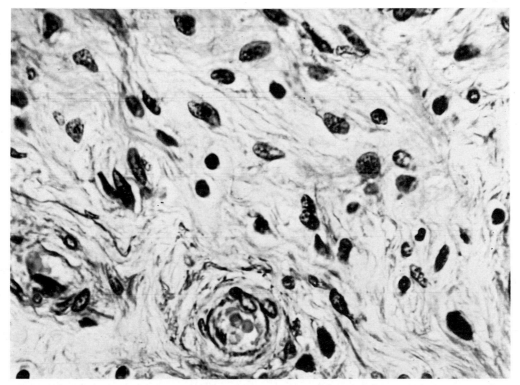

Figure 6-13. Section of loose (areolar) connective tissue of the epididymis. At lower center there is a small arteriole. Aldehyde fuchsin stain. × 825.

Adipose Tissue. Fat cells are scattered in areolar connective tissue. When fat cells form large aggregations and are the principal cell type, the tissue is designated adipose tissue. Each fat cell is surrounded by a web of fine reticular fibers; in the spaces between are fibroblasts, lymphoid cells, eosinophils, and some mast cells. The closely packed fat cells form *lobules*, separated by fibrous septa. There is a rich network of blood capillaries in and between the lobules. The richness of the blood supply is indicative of the high metabolic activity of adipose tissue, a fact which has been recognized only recently.

It should be appreciated that adipose tissue is not static. There is a vital balance between deposits and withdrawals. Fat contained within fat cells may be derived from three sources. Fat cells, under the influence of the hormone insulin, can synthesize fat from carbohydrate. They can also produce fat from fatty acids which are derived from the breakdown of dietary fat. Fatty acids may also be synthesized from glucose in the liver and transported to the fat cells as serum lipo-protein. Fats from different sources differ chemically. Dietary fat may be unsaturated or saturated depending upon the individual diet. Fat which is synthesized from carbohydrate is mostly saturated. Withdrawals of fat result from enzymatic hydrolysis of stored fat and release of free fatty acids into the blood stream. If there is a continuous supply of glucose, withdrawals are negligible. The normal balance is affected by hormones, principally insulin, and by the autonomic nervous system. The latter is necessary for the mobilization of fat from adipose tissue.

Adipose tissue may develop almost anywhere areolar tissue is plentiful, but in man the commonest sites of fat accumulation are in the subcutaneous and retroperitoneal connective tissues, in the mesenteries, and in bone marrow. In addition to the primary function of storage and metabolism of neutral fat, in the subcutaneous tissue adipose tissue also acts as a good shock absorber and insulator to prevent excessive heat loss or gain through the skin.

Brown Fat Tissue. Brown fat tissue should be distinguished from common,

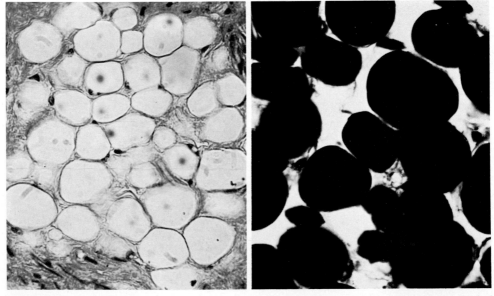

Figure 6-14. Left: Section of adipose tissue of human dermis. × 240. Right: Fat cells in which the content of fat has been preserved. Osmic acid. × 350.   See filmstrip I, frame 19.

or white, fat tissue. It is a peculiar type of fat found in certain locations in various mammals, particularly rodents. The brown fat contains a pigment which gives the tissue its color. The fat occurs as numerous, discrete droplets distributed throughout the cytoplasm. Unlike white fat, it is not readily affected by changes in the nutritional state of the animal. However, it is depleted rapidly after hypophysectomy or adrenalectomy. It is not present in adult man and the significance of it is not well understood.

Reticular Tissue. This is a primitive type of connective tissue which is characterized by the presence of a network of reticular fibers associated with *primitive reticular cells.* These cells are stellate and have long cytoplasmic extensions which appear to join with those of other cells. In appearance they are not unlike mesenchymal cells. They have large, pale nuclei and abundant basophil cytoplasm.

Reticular cells are believed to retain certain of the developmental potentialities of primitive mesenchymal cells. Those associated with the fibrous elements of reticular tissue have fibroblastic tendencies and differ from fibroblasts only in their multipotentiality. Others have phagocytic properties. Many with phagocytic properties are positioned as part of the wall of a lymphatic sinus or a blood sinusoid and constitute part of the reticuloendothelial system. Reticular cells may give rise to free macrophages, to early precursors of erythrocytes and leukocytes, and perhaps to other cell types.

Although reticular fibers are distributed widely in the body in association with fibroblasts, reticular fibers in association with reticular cells (i.e., reticular tissue) are limited to certain sites. Reticular tissue forms the framework of lymphoid organs, bone marrow, and liver. In appearance it resembles embryonic mesenchyme, but it is largely inconspicuous since the interstices of the tissue normally are crowded with other cell types, principally lymphocytes and other blood cells.

Dense Connective Tissues

Dense connective tissues are characterized by the close packing of their fibers. Cells are proportionally fewer than in loose connective tissues and there is less amorphous ground substance. In areas where tensions are exerted in all directions, the fiber bundles are interwoven and without regular orientation and the tissues are termed *irregularly arranged.* In structures subject to tension in one direction, the fibers have an orderly parallel arrangement and the tissues are designated *regularly arranged.* In most regions collagenous fibers are the main component, but in a few ligaments elastic fibers predominate.

Dense Irregularly Arranged Connective Tissue. This tissue occurs in sheets, its fibers interlacing to form a coarse, tough feltwork. Although coarse collagenous fibers are the main component, elastic and reticular fibers are present also in small numbers. Dense irregularly arranged connective tissue forms the basis of most fascias, the dermis of the skin, the fibrous capsules of some organs, including testis, liver, and lymph nodes, and the fibrous sheaths of bone (periosteum) and cartilage (perichondrium).

Dense Regularly Arranged Connective Tissue. This tissue contains fibers which are densely packed and lie parallel to each other forming structures of great tensile strength. This group includes tendons, ligaments, and aponeuroses. The latter two are less regularly arranged than tendons but in general have a similar organization.

In *tendons*, the collagenous fibers, or *primary tendon bundles*, run parallel courses. Each fiber or bundle is composed of a large number of fibrils. Fibroblasts, or *tendon cells*, are the only cell type present and in longi-

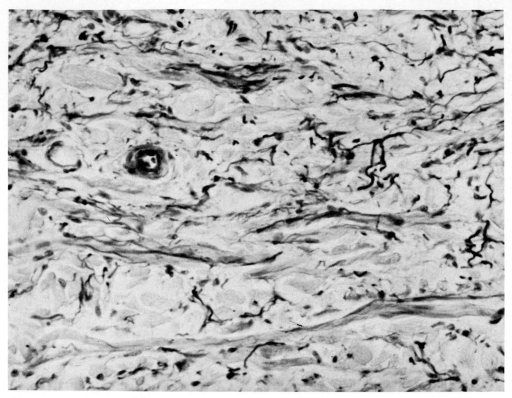

Figure 6-15.   Section of dense irregular connective tissue of human scalp. Elastic fibers are stained darkly, collagenous fibers more lightly. Note the relative lack of cells. Weigert's elastin stain and hematoxylin and eosin. × 425.

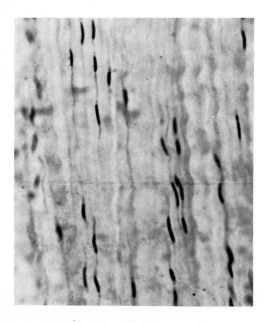

Figure 6-16.   Longitudinal section of tendon. Fibroblasts, or tendon cells, are flattened and aligned in rows between the bundles of collagenous fibers. × 350.

tudinal sections of tendon they are aligned in rows between the collagenous fibers. Cytoplasm of the cells is often indistinct. In cross sections, the cells appear stellate in shape with cytoplasmic processes extending between the collagenous bundles. Each primary bundle is covered by a small amount of loose areolar (fibroelastic) connective tissue, termed the *endotendineum*. Generally, several primary bundles are grouped together into secondary bundles or fascicles bounded by a coarser type of connective tissue, the *peritendineum*. The tendon, composed of a number of fascicles, is ensheathed by thick connective tissue called the *epitendineum*.* Nerves and blood vessels course in the major connective tissue septa but do not invade the fascicles.

Aponeuroses have the same composition as tendons but are broad and flat. Most ligaments have a similar composition but a few are composed almost entirely of elastic fibers.

In *yellow elastic ligaments*, coarse parallel fibers of elastic tissue are bound together by a small amount of delicate connective tissue, in which typical fibroblasts are present. The elastic fibers branch frequently and fuse with one another. Individual fibers are surrounded by a network of reticular fibers. Yellow elastic ligaments show numerous oval or elongated nuclei of fibroblasts between the parallel elastic fibers. This is one feature of elastic ligaments which distinguishes them histologically from tendons and collagenous ligaments, in which fibroblasts are sparse and their nuclei markedly flattened. The most typical form of yellow elastic ligament is found in the ligamentum nuchae of quadrupeds. In the human, examples are found in the ligamenta flava of the vertebrae, the suspensory

*Note on terminology: The prefixes "endo-," "peri-," and "epi-" indicate a progression in size. They are also used in reference to muscle with the word stem "-mysium," and to nerve with the word stem "-neurium."

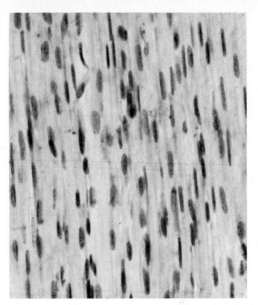

Figure 6-17. Longitudinal section from ligamentum nuchae of ox. Fibroblast nuclei are present between the elastic fibers. Compare with Figure 6-16. × 425.

ligament of the penis, and the true vocal cords.

THE RETICULOENDOTHELIAL (MACROPHAGE) SYSTEM

The use of the word "system" here is somewhat unfortunate since it refers to physiological and pathological considerations rather than to a discrete anatomical entity. It is a collective term for a widespread system of highly phagocytic cells. The term *macrophage system* is more appropriate since the cells do not form a true endothelium and many of them have no direct relationship to a reticulum. However, the term reticuloendothelium has received considerable usage among workers in the field.

All highly phagocytic cells of the body, with the exception of blood cells, belong to this system. They are present in large numbers in the body in certain situations. They possess no morphological characteristics that distinguish them with certainty from other cells. They are identified by their marked affinity for nontoxic colloidal dyes and for inert particulate matter. The macrophages take up the dye or inert particles and segregate them into vacuoles, and thus can be identified easily. True endothelial cells, fibroblasts, lymphocytes, and certain other cells may phagocytose small amounts of the dye but can be distinguished from cells of the reticuloendothelial system by a marked quantitative difference.

Cells of the reticuloendothelial system are found in the following situations: (1) In connective tissues, where they correspond to the macrophages or histiocytes just described. They occur in large numbers in relation to small blood vessels and lymphatics of the subserous connective tissue of the pleura and peritoneum. Here, often they are aggregated into small patches known as *milky spots*. (2) In the liver, lining the sinusoids, where they are known as *Kupffer's cells*. (3) Lining the blood sinuses of the spleen, lymph nodes, and bone marrow, where often they are referred to as large reticular cells. (4) Lining blood sinuses of the suprarenal gland and the hypophysis. (5) In the *microglia* of the central nervous system, which are phagocytic and of mesodermal origin.

The source of the cells has not been determined fully. Many arise from undifferentiated mesenchymal cells. Others may arise from lymphocytes and monocytes.

The functional importance of the macrophages of the reticuloendothelial system is considerable. On account of their phagocytic and ameboid properties, they are active in the defense of the body against microorganisms. They may be involved, along with other cells, in the production of antibodies. In the spleen and liver they phagocytose broken down erythrocytes and store iron-containing pigment within their cytoplasm. Foreign particulate matter in the blood stream is removed by the macrophages of the spleen, liver, and bone marrow, and foreign particulate matter in lymph is removed by macrophages of the lymph nodes. There is evidence to suggest that macrophages are concerned with the metabolism of lipids. Lipid inclusions are common within macrophages, and macrophages are involved extensively in certain disorders of lipid metabolism.

REFERENCES

Asboe-Hansen, G. (editor): Connective Tissue in Health and Disease. Copenhagen, E. Munksgaard, 1954.

Baker, B. L., and Abrams, G. D.: The physiology of connective tissue. Ann. Rev. Physiol., *17*:61, 1955.

Bloom, G. D.: Electron microscopy of neoplastic mast cells: A study of the mouse mastocytoma mast cell. Ann. N.Y. Acad. Sci., *103*:53, 1963.

Clark, E. R., and Clark, E. L.: Microscopic studies of the new formation of fat in living adult rabbits. Amer. J. Anat., *67*:255, 1940.

Cohn, Z. A., Fedorko, M. E., and Hirsch, J. G.: The *in vitro* differentiation of mononuclear phagocytes. IV. The ultrastructure of macrophage differentiation in the peritoneal cavity and in culture. V. The formation of macrophage lysosomes. J. Exper. Med., *123*:747, 757, 1966.

Daniels, J. C., Ritzmann, S. E., and Levin, W. C.: Lymphocytes: Morphological, developmental, and functional characteristics in health, disease, and experimental study—an analytical review. Texas Rep. Biol. Med., *26*:5, 1968.

Della Porta, G., and Muhlback, O. (editors): Structure and control of the melanocyte. New York, Academic Press, 1966.

de Petris, S., Karlsbad, G., and Pernis, B.: Localization of antibodies in plasma cells by electron microscopy. J. Exper. Med., *117*:849, 1963.

Fawcett, D. W.: A comparison of the histological organization and cytochemical reactions of brown and white adipose tissues. J. Morph., *90*:363, 1952.

Fernando, N. V. P., and Movat, H. Z.: The fine structure of connective tissue. III. The mast cell. Exp. Mol. Pathol., *2*:450, 1963.

Gersh, I., and Catchpole, H. R.: The organization of ground substance and basement membrane and its significance in tissue injury, disease and growth. Amer. J. Anat., *85*:457, 1949.

Jackson, S. F.: Connective tissue cells. *In* The Cell: Biochemistry, Physiology, Morphology, edited by J. Brachet and A. E. Mirsky. New York, Academic Press, 1964, Vol. 6, p. 387.

Jacoby, F.: Macrophages. *In* Cells and Tissues

in Culture, edited by E. N. Willmer. London, Academic Press, 1967.

Kautz, J., Demarsh, Q. B., and Thornburg, W.: A polarizing and electron microscope study of plasma cells. Exp. Cell Res., *13*:596, 1957.

Leduc, E., Avrameas, S., and Bouteille, M.: Ultrastructural localization of antibody in differentiating plasma cells. J. Exper. Med., *127*:109, 1968.

Maximow, A. A.: The macrophages or histiocytes. *In* Special Cytology, ed. 2, edited by E. V. Cowdry. New York, Paul B. Hoeber, 1932, Vol. 2, p. 709.

Movat, H. Z., and Fernando, N. V. P.: The fine structure of connective tissue. I. The fibroblast. II. The plasma cell. Exp. Mol. Pathol., *1*:509, 535, 1962.

Porter, K. R.: Cell fine structure and biosynthesis of intercellular macromolecules. Biophysic. J., *4*:167, 1964.

Riley, J. F.: The Mast Cells. Edinburgh and London, E. and S. Livingston, Ltd., 1959.

Sacks, B.: The reticuloendothelial system. Physiol. Rev., *6*:504, 1926.

Smith, D. E.: Electron microscopy of normal mast cells under various experimental conditions. Ann. N.Y. Acad. Sci., *103*:40, 1963.

West, G. B.: Function of mast cells. J. Pharm. Pharmacol., *14*:618, 1962.

Wislocki, G. B., Bunting, H., and Dempsey, E. W.: Metachromasia in mammalian tissues and its relationship to mucopolysaccharides. Amer. J. Anat., *81*:1, 1947.

Wood, E. M.: An ordered complex of filaments surrounding the lipid droplets in developing adipose cells. Anat. Rec., *157*:437, 1967.

CHAPTER 7

SPECIALIZED CONNECTIVE TISSUE: CARTILAGE AND BONE

Cartilage and bone, the skeletal tissues, are specialized connective tissues and, like all connective tissues, are composed of three elements: cells, fibers, and ground substance, the latter two constituting the intercellular substance or matrix. They differ from the connective tissues discussed previously in the rigidity of their matrices. In cartilage the ground substance is composed principally of chondromucoid, a glycoprotein which is rich in chondroitin sulfate. In bone the ground substance is impregnated with certain inorganic salts, principally calcium phosphate.

CARTILAGE

In early fetal life, cartilage temporarily forms most of the skeleton and it persists in adult mammals over the articular surfaces of bones and as the sole skeletal support in the respiratory passages and parts of the ear. The matrix contains collagenous or elastic fibers which increase the tensile strength and the elasticity respectively and adapt the tissue to the mechanical requirements of the different regions of the body. The differences in the kind and abundance of fibers incorporated within the matrix form the basis of classification. There are three common types: *hyaline cartilage, elastic cartilage*, and *fibrocartilage*. Of these, hyaline cartilage is the most widely distributed and the most characteristic.

Development and Growth of Cartilage. Cartilage, like other connective tissues, develops from mesenchyme. In an area where cartilage will develop, mesenchymal cells round up and become closely packed, and collagenous fibrils are deposited within the intercellular substance. As the cells elaborate ground substance, the collagenous fibrils become masked and the cells gradually become more separated, as a result of the elaboration of matrix around them. The cells, now embedded in cartilage matrix, soon acquire the characteristics of chondrocytes (see page 111). They accumulate vacuoles, lipid, and glycogen. Mesenchyme surrounding the enlarging mass of cartilage is compressed and forms a fibrous envelope, the *perichondrium*. This merges gradually into the cartilage on one side and into the surrounding connective tissue on the other.

Continued growth of cartilage occurs by two methods. Young chondrocytes, which retain the ability to divide, proliferate and lay down new matrix. This expansion of cartilage from within, called *interstitial growth*, occurs only in relatively young cartilage which is malleable enough to allow expansion. The cell groups or cell nests seen in mature cartilage are an indication of the condition that existed when interstitial growth ceased. The second method by which cartilage increases in size, known as *appositional growth*, is a process in which new layers of cartilage are added to one surface. It results from activity within the inner layer of the perichondrium. Fibroblasts in the perichondrium multiply by division and some transform into cartilage cells and surround themselves with intercellular substance. These in time become overlaid by still newer cells and matrix added from the perichondrium.

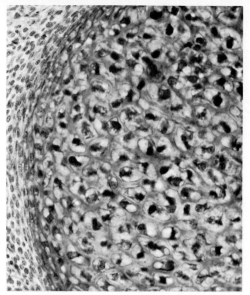

Figure 7-1. Fetal hyaline cartilage from developing human ilium. The primitive perichondrium lies to the left of the figure. × 300. (Courtesy of R. D. Laurenson.)

See filmstrip I, frame 20.

Hyaline Cartilage

The word "hyaline" is derived from the Greek *hyalos*, meaning glass. Hyaline cartilage appears as a translucent, bluish-white mass in the fresh condition. It forms the articular surfaces of bones within joints, the costal cartilages, and the cartilages of the nose, larynx, trachea, and bronchi. In the fetus nearly all the skeleton is first laid down as hyaline cartilage, which is replaced later by bone.

Cells. The *cartilage cells* or *chondrocytes* occupy small cavities or lacunae within the matrix. The cells usually are spherical, and each contains a large, spherical, centrally placed nucleus with one or more nucleoli. The cytoplasm is finely granular and moderately basophil and contains large mitochondria, vacuoles, fat droplets, and some glycogen. In living cartilage the chondrocytes completely fill their lacunae, but, owing to shrinkage resulting from fixation and dehydration, cartilage cells in paraffin sections show marked distortion and seldom conform to the shape of their lacunae. In the center of a mass of cartilage in the adult, the cells may be arranged in groups, each group representing the offspring of a single parent chondrocyte. Such a group of cells within a single lacuna is referred to as a *cell nest* or isogenous group. Toward the periphery of a mass of cartilage the cells are elliptical and flattened parallel to the surface. In fetal cartilage the cells often are flattened and cell nests are seen rarely.

The Matrix (Intercellular Substance). Although the matrix appears homogeneous in the fresh condition and after ordinary fixation, it contains considerable quantities of both formed and amorphous kinds of intercellular substance. The formed kind is represented by collagenous fibers, which are not apparent in fresh material since

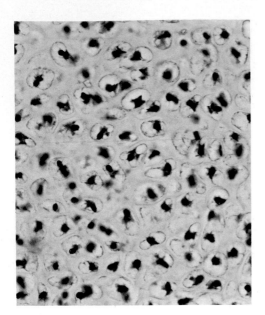

Figure 7-2. Fetal hyaline cartilage from developing human ilium. This specimen was from a fetus older than that demonstrated in Figure 7-1 and shows a greater development of ground substance. × 300. (Courtesy of R. D. Laurenson.)

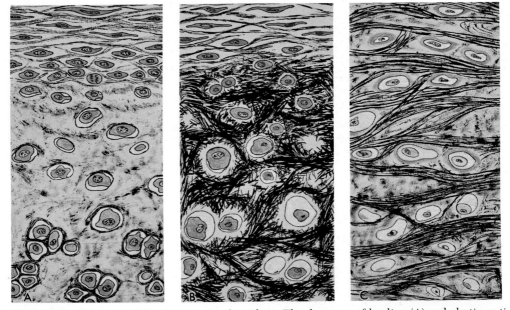

Figure 7-3. Diagram of the three types of cartilage. The diagrams of hyaline (A) and elastic cartilage (B) show perichondrium above. Note that intercellular elastic and collagenous fibers are prominent respectively in elastic (B) and fibrocartilage (C). A also illustrates both appositional (above) and interstitial (below) forms of growth.

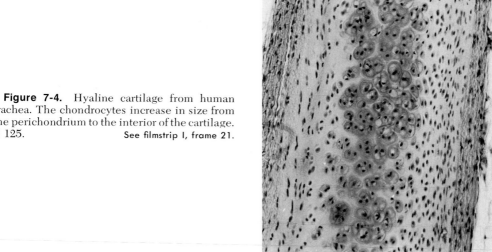

Figure 7-4. Hyaline cartilage from human trachea. The chondrocytes increase in size from the perichondrium to the interior of the cartilage. × 125.   See filmstrip I, frame 21.

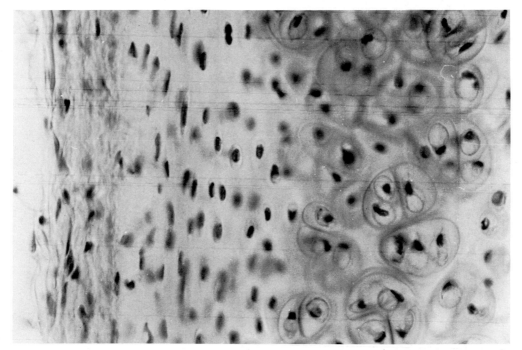

Figure 7-5. Hyaline cartilage from the same preparation as Figure 7-4. Cell nests and cartilage capsules are evident within the interior of the cartilage. The perichondrium lies to the left of the figure. × 450.

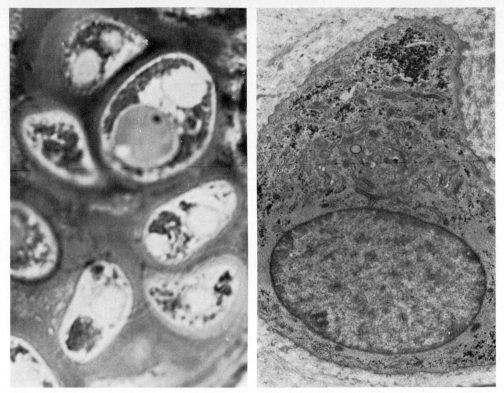

Figure 7-6. Left: Hyaline cartilage from trachea. Epon section. × 1500. Right: Electron micrograph of chondrocyte from tracheal cartilage. The dark granular mass in the cytoplasm (above) is glycogen. × 5800.

they have approximately the same refractive index as that of the surrounding ground substance. Collagenous fibers can be detected in thin sections examined with the polarizing microscope, and they can be demonstrated after digestion with trypsin or dilute alkalis. They can be seen readily in electron micrographs. They rarely occur in definite bundles but form a fine feltwork.

The ground substance of cartilage is markedly basophil owing to its content of *chondromucin,* a glycoprotein which on hydrolysis yields chondroitin sulfates. Chondromucin is abundant throughout the matrix of embryonal cartilage, but in mature cartilage it is unevenly distributed. It is concentrated around cells and cell groups where it is referred to as *territorial matrix* (or the *cartilage capsules*). The

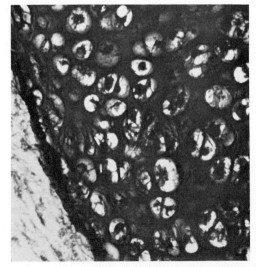

Figure 7-7. Hyaline cartilage from a preparation stained with toluidine blue to illustrate the metachromatic staining of the ground substance. × 350.

ground substance stains metachromatically with toluidine blue and gives a positive reaction with the periodic acid–Schiff reaction (PAS). Since pure chondroitin sulfate is not PAS positive, the response is thought to be due to some carbohydrate component present within the matrix, but this is not yet fully understood.

Perichondrium. Except over articular surfaces, cartilage is enclosed by a tough layer of dense connective tissue, the *perichondrium.* This is composed of spindle-shaped cells, indistinguishable from fibroblasts, and of elastic and collagenous fibers. Next to the cartilage, the perichondrium is more cellular and merges by a smooth transition into cartilage. This is due to the fact that cells in the inner zone of the perichondrium have the potentiality of being able to surround themselves with matrix and become incorporated into the cartilage as typical chondrocytes.

Nutrition. In general, cartilage is devoid of blood vessels, lymphatics, and nerves. The blood vessels that are seen occasionally in cartilage are passing to another destination. Consequently, chondrocytes are nourished by substances diffusing through the intercellular substance from blood vessels of the perichondrium. This diffusion is adequate since the requirements of cartilage are modest.

Retrogressive Changes. With old age, cartilage loses its translucency and becomes less cellular, and the matrix shows less basophilia owing to a loss of chondromucin and an increase in the amount of albuminoid. Within large masses of cartilage, closely packed coarse fibers, totally unlike collagenous fibers, may be deposited. These silky fibers may spread over large areas. Eventually this process, known as *asbestos transformation,* may lead to softening of the matrix, or even to cavity formation.

The most important retrogressive change within cartilage is *calcification.* Calcification also occurs as a temporary strengthening expedient during the replacement of cartilage by bone. Minute granules of calcium phosphate and calcium carbonate are deposited in the intercellular substance, initially in the vicinity of the cells and later in the general matrix. The granules enlarge and merge, and the cartilage becomes hard and brittle. When the intercellular substance becomes calcified in this manner, it no longer permits ready diffusion of nutrients and the cells die. With their death, the calcified matrix undergoes a slow process of resorption.

Regeneration. Injuries are repaired by a slow process which occurs primarily as a result of activity of the perichondrium. Tissue from the perichondrium proliferates and fills in the defect. This tissue gradually is converted to cartilage in a manner similar to appositional growth. A fracture of mature cartilage may be repaired not by cartilage but by dense fibrous tissue which itself may be replaced by bone.

Elastic Cartilage

This type of cartilage occurs in locations where support with flexibility is

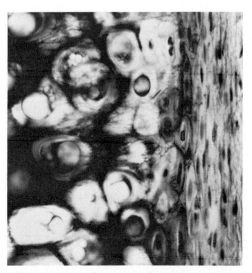

Figure 7-8. Elastic cartilage from human external ear, with perichondrium to the right. Elastic fibers within the ground substance have been stained with orcein. × 325.

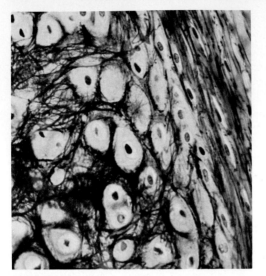

Figure 7-9. Elastic cartilage from human epiglottis. A preparation similar to Figure 7-8. There is a profusion of elastic fibers within the ground substance. × 325.

See filmstrip I, frame 22.

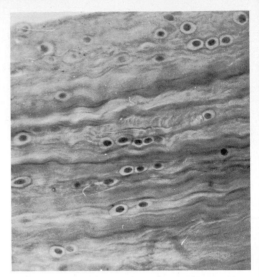

Figure 7-10. Fibrocartilage taken from a tendon close to its insertion into bone. Note that the cartilage cells lie within definite lacunae. × 375.

required, as in the external ear, auditory tube, epiglottis, and certain cartilages of the larynx. It is yellow in color, owing to the preponderance of elastic fibers, and is more opaque than hyaline cartilage, of which it is a modification. Component cells show less accumulation of fat and glycogen than do those of hyaline cartilage. The matrix contains masked collagenous fibers and, in addition, extensive networks of elastic fibers. These vary in thickness and abundance and in general are larger and more densely packed in the interior of a cartilage. The cartilage is surrounded by a perichondrium and growth occurs both interstitially and by apposition from the perichondrium.

Fibrocartilage

This type of cartilage occurs where a tough support or tensile strength is required. It occurs in association with certain joints of the body, including intervertebral discs, and where some ligaments and tendons are attached to bone. It never occurs alone, but merges gradually into neighboring

hyaline cartilage or with dense fibrous tissue. Unlike elastic cartilage, it cannot be considered a modification of hyaline cartilage. It is composed of dense collagenous connective tissue, between bundles of which there are small regions of hyaline cartilaginous matrix containing lacunae with enclosed cells. These may occur singly or in groups, but commonly are in short rows. Fibrocartilage lacks a perichondrium. It is found closely associated with the dense connective tissue of ligaments and joint capsules and should be considered a transitional form between cartilage and dense connective tissue. It develops in a manner similar to that of ordinary connective tissue, and initially only fibroblasts, separated by considerable amounts of fibrillar material, are present. Later the cells become transformed into chondrocytes and surround themselves with a thin layer of cartilaginous matrix.

BONE

Bone, or *osseous tissue*, is a rigid form of connective tissue that constitutes most of the skeleton of higher vertebrates. It consists of cells and of an intercellular matrix, or ground substance. The matrix contains an organic component, chiefly collagenous fibers, and an inorganic component which accounts for approximately two-thirds of the weight of bone. The inorganic salts which are responsible for the hardness and rigidity of bone include calcium phosphate (about 85 per cent), calcium carbonate (10 per cent), and small amounts of calcium fluoride and magnesium fluoride. Collagenous fibers contribute greatly to the strength and resilience of bone.

Macroscopically, two types of bone may be distinguished: the *spongy* (*cancellous*) and the *compact* (*dense*). Spongy bone consists of slender, irregular trabeculae or bars which branch and unite with one another to form a meshwork, the intercommunicating spaces of which are filled with bone marrow. Compact bone appears solid, except for microscopic spaces. No sharp boundary may be drawn between the two types of osseous tissue, and the differences between them depend merely upon the relative amount of solid matter and the size and

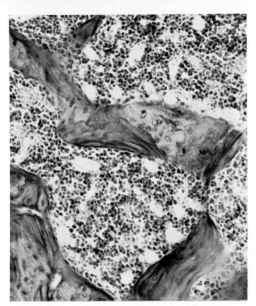

Figure 7-12. Spongy bone of the tibia. Bone marrow lies between the bony trabeculae. × 150.   See filmstrip I, frame 23.

number of spaces in each. They both contain the same histological elements. With few exceptions, both spongy and compact types are present in every bone, but the amount and distribution of each vary considerably. In typical long bones, the shaft (*diaphysis*) is chiefly compact bone surrounding a *medullary* (or bone marrow) *cavity*. Each end (*epiphysis*) consists of spongy bone covered by a thin shell of compact bone. The cavities of the spongy bone are continuous with the bone marrow cavity of the diaphysis. In flat bones, two plates of compact bone enclose a middle layer of spongy bone (diploë). Most irregular bones consist of spongy bone covered by a thin shell of compact bone.

Each bone, except over its articular surfaces, is enveloped by a specialized connective tissue coat, the *periosteum*. A similar, but less well developed, connective tissue layer, the *endosteum*, lines the marrow cavity and marrow spaces.

Microscopically, the most characteristic feature of bone is its lamellar structure, the calcified intercellular

Cementing line

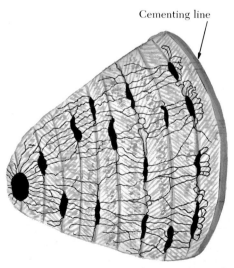

Figure 7-11. Diagram of a segment of a Haversian system in cross section to illustrate the arrangement of osteocytes, canaliculi, and lamellae.

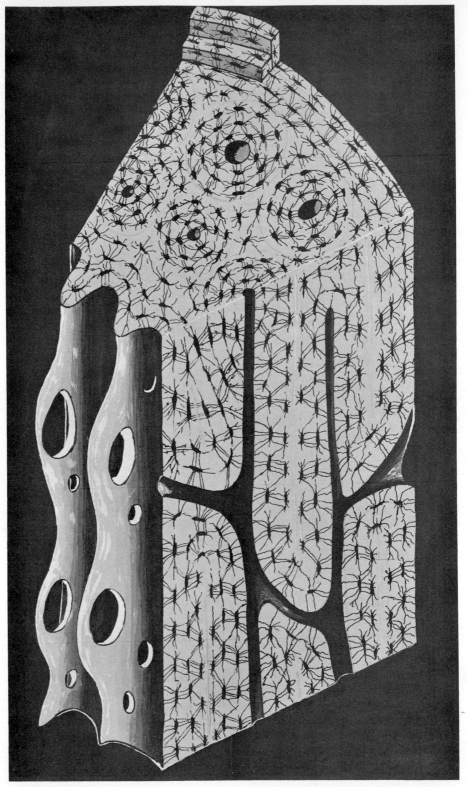

Figure 7-13. A diagrammatic representation of a small portion of compact bone.

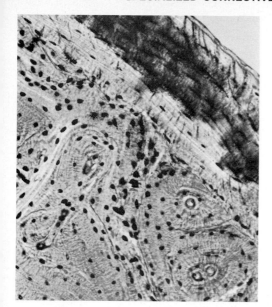

substance, or *bone matrix*, being organized into layers or *lamellae* arranged in various ways. Within the interstitial substance there are small cavities, or *lacunae*, which contain the bone cells (*osteocytes*). Radiating from each lacuna are numerous narrow channels, termed *canaliculi*, which penetrate adjacent lamellae to join with canaliculi of neighboring lacunae. Thus all lacunae are interconnected by a system of minute channels.

Figure 7-14. Low power photomicrograph of ground bone to show portions of outer (periosteal) circumferential lamellae and of Haversian systems. × 150.

Structural Elements

In a histological study of bone, it must be borne in mind that, owing to its inorganic component, bone cannot be examined in routine histological preparations. Two special methods of preparation are employed commonly. In one the cellular and organic com-

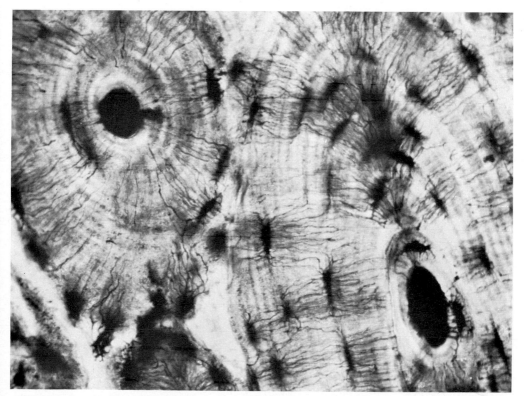

Figure 7-15. High power photomicrograph of portions of two Haversian systems transversely sectioned. Note the arrangement of lacunae and canaliculi. × 500. **See filmstrip I, frame 24.**

ponents of bone are preserved and the inorganic component is removed by *decalcification* in an acid solution. After decalcification bone can be embedded and sectioned in the normal manner. Cells in decalcified bone tend to be shrunken, and details of the matrix are blurred owing to swelling of osteocollagenous fibers by the reagents used. In *ground bone* sections, which are prepared by taking a thin piece of bone and grinding it down with abrasives until a section thin enough to be viewed under the microscope is obtained, details of matrix structure are well preserved. How-

ever, bone cells are removed by this method and lacunae appear empty.

Bone Cells

Three cell types peculiar to bone are recognized: *osteoblasts, osteocytes,* and *osteoclasts.* They are closely interrelated and transformation from one to another occurs readily.

Osteoblasts. Osteoblasts are associated with bone formation and are found in relation to the surface of bone where osseous matrix is being deposited. They vary in shape, some

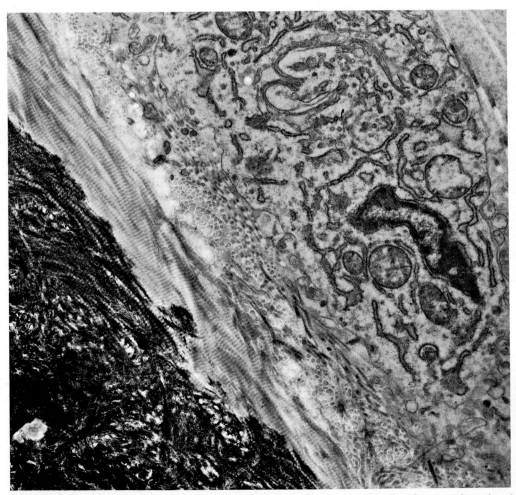

Figure 7-16. Electron micrograph of a portion of an osteoblast with abundant rough-surfaced endoplasmic reticulum. Note the unmineralized matrix, containing collagen fibrils, running obliquely across the center of the figure, and mineralized matrix at left. × 18,400. (Courtesy of R. R. Cooper.)

being cuboidal and others pyramidal, and are present frequently in a continuous layer suggestive of an epithelial arrangement. The nucleus is large and usually has a single prominent nucleolus. The cytoplasm exhibits marked basophilia, suggesting the presence of ribose nucleoprotein, which is concerned probably with the synthesis of protein components of the bone matrix. Fine granules are present in the cytoplasm of osteoblasts closely associated with sites of active deposition of matrix. Osteoblasts contain the enzyme *alkaline phosphatase,* which would suggest that they are concerned not only with the elaboration of matrix but also with its calcification.

Osteocytes. The osteocyte, or bone cell, is an osteoblast which has become imprisoned within bone matrix. It has a faintly basophil cytoplasm which can be shown to contain fat droplets, some glycogen, and fine granules similar to those present within osteoblasts. The nucleus is darkly staining. Osteocytes are often somewhat shrunken in preparation, but their normal configuration can be inferred from the shape of the lacunae which they occupy. A lacuna is irregularly oval on the flat and biconvex on edge. Fine cytoplasmic processes of osteocytes extend for some distance into the canaliculi which radiate out from the lacunae. In developing bone the processes of osteocytes extend even further so that there is direct contiguity (but not continuity) between neighboring osteocytes. In mature bone the processes are withdrawn almost completely, but the canaliculi remain to provide an avenue for the exchange of metabolites between the blood stream and the osteocytes.

Osteoclasts. Osteoclasts are multinucleated giant cells which vary greatly in size and in the number of nuclei they possess. They are found in close association with the surface of bone, often in shallow excavations known as *Howship's lacunae.* The cytoplasm is faintly basophil and gran-

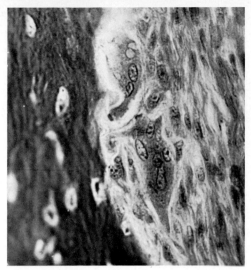

Figure 7-17. A portion of spongy bone, in immediate relationship to which are two osteoclasts. × 350.

ular. Osteoclasts arise by fusion of uninucleate cells, probably osteoblasts, although numerous opinions have been put forward as to the cell of origin. Although they are concentrated usually in areas where resorption of bone is taking place, there is no conclusive evidence that they actively erode bone.

Bone Matrix

Although the intercellular substance of bone is apparently homogeneous, it has a well-ordered structure. The organic portion, comprising about 35 per cent, is chiefly *osteocollagenous fibers* similar to the collagenous fibers of loose connective tissue. The fibers are difficult to see in ordinary preparations but can be revealed by special methods. They are united by a special *cementing substance* which consists mainly of acid mucopolysaccharides. The inorganic component is located solely in the cement between fibers and accounts for 65 per cent of the weight of a bone. The minerals are present principally as crystals of calcium phosphate with an *apatite* pattern or structure. X-ray diffraction studies have shown that more specifically the pattern is that of *hydroxyapatites*. The minerals are deposited as dense particles aligned in relation to the osteocollagenous fibers. Lacunae and canaliculi are bordered by a layer of special organic cement which differs from the rest of the intercellular substance in that it lacks fibrils.

Bone matrix is arranged characteristically in layers or lamellae 3 to 7 microns thick. The lamellae result from the rhythmical manner in which matrix is deposited. The fibers in any lamella are roughly parallel to each other and take a spiral or helical course. The pitch of the spiral changes in adjacent lamellae in such a manner that fibers in one make an angle of nearly 90 degrees with the fibers in the next. This alternating arrangement in fiber direction explains why lamellae appear to be so distinct, one from another.

Architecture of Bone

Spongy bone is simple in structure and consists of trabeculae or plates forming a network, the pattern of which is determined by the mechanical functions of individual bones. The trabeculae comprise a varying number of lamellae in which are lacunae containing osteocytes and a system of intercommunicating canaliculi.

In compact bone the lamellae are regularly arranged in a manner determined by the distribution of blood vessels which nourish the bone. The bone is traversed by longitudinal channels, the *Haversian canals*, which anastomose freely with each other by transverse and oblique connections. From the periosteal and endosteal surfaces, *Volkmann's canals* enter the bone at right angles to its long axis and communicate with the Haversian canals. Thus there is a continuous and complex system of canals which con-

tains the blood vessels and nerves of the bone.

Each Haversian canal is surrounded by a varying number (8 to 15) of concentric lamellae. The lamellae of bone matrix, the cells, and the central canal constitute the *Haversian system*, or *osteone*, the unit of structure of compact bone. Canaliculi that border upon a Haversian canal communicate with its cavity and thus bring all lacunae of a system into continuity with the canal. Since Haversian systems are orientated mainly in the long axis of the bone, in cross section the canals appear as round openings surrounded by ring-shaped concentric lamellae and in longitudinal sections the canals are long slits bordered by columns of lamellae. The intervals between Haversian systems are filled with the *interstitial lamellae*, which are the remnants of Haversian systems partly destroyed during the internal reconstruction of the bone (see page 129). At the periphery and on the internal surface in relation to the marrow cavity lamellae run parallel with the surface and are orientated circumferentially with respect to the axis of the bone. These are the outer (periosteal) and inner (endosteal) *circumferential* or *general* lamellae. Adjacent lamellar systems are delimited by a thin layer of refractile, modified matrix (*cement line, cement membrane*).

In addition to the osteocollagenous fibers contained within lamellae, coarse collagenous bundles, or *Sharpey's fibers*, are found in the outer layers of the bone. They are fibers which pass from the periosteum into the outer circumferential and interstitial lamellae and are not found in Haversian systems or in the internal circumferential lamellae. They are surrounded by a narrow zone of uncalcified or only partially calcified matrix. Sharpey's fibers serve to anchor the periosteum firmly to bone and are particularly numerous at points of insertion of ligaments and tendons.

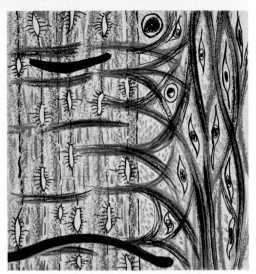

Figure 7-18. Diagram of Sharpey's fibers extending into compact bone as direct continuations of fibers of the periosteum.

Periosteum. This fibrous sheath envelops bone, except on articular surfaces. Its close connection with bone depends upon the presence of Sharpey's fibers. It consists of two layers, although these are not sharply defined. The outer layer is dense fibrous connective tissue and contains a network of blood vessels. The inner layer is composed of more loosely arranged connective tissue, some component collagenous fibers of which enter the bone as Sharpey's fibers. In the adult, the inner layer contains numerous spindle-shaped connective tissue cells which on stimulation (e.g., by fracture) become activated. Osteoblasts then reappear.

Endosteum. This delicate layer lines the marrow cavities and extends as a lining into the canal system of compact bone. It consists of a condensed reticular tissue which has both osteogenic and hemopoietic potencies.

Development and Growth of Bone

Bone has certain unique qualities which must be borne in mind when consideration is given to the methods whereby a bone develops and increases in size. First, bone has a canalicular system, the tiny canals of which extend from one lacuna to another and to bony surfaces, where they open into tissue spaces. Tissue fluid in these spaces becomes continuous with fluid within the canalicular system and thus allows for exchange of metabolites between the blood stream and the osteocytes. By this mechanism cells of bone remain alive even though surrounded by an intercellular substance that is calcified. Secondly, bone is vascular. The canalicular system cannot operate effectively if it is more than about 0.5 mm. removed from a capillary. Hence bone is richly supplied with capillaries which are carried in Haversian and Volkmann's canals. Thirdly, bone can grow only by an appositional mechanism. Interstitial growth, as in cartilage, is impossible in bone because the presence of lime salts in the matrix prevents expansion within the interior. Finally, bone architecture is not static. Bone is destroyed locally and re-formed repeatedly. There is thus a continuous process of reconstruction to consider.

According to the embryological origin there are two types of bone development, *intramembranous* and *endochondral* (or *intracartilaginous*). In the former bone develops directly on or within membrane, whereas in the latter it develops within cartilage which must be removed before ossification can occur. Some of the cartilage matrix may remain as a framework upon which bone is laid down. It must be realized, however, that the actual process of bone deposition is the same in both cases. The first bone formed is always spongy. Later some of it becomes compact, owing to internal reconstruction.

Intramembranous Bone Formation. This process can be studied best in the flat bones of the skull. In the area where bone is to develop, the mesenchyme consists of primitive connective

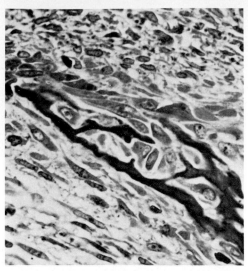

Figure 7-19. Photomicrograph of a section cut through a newly formed spicule of bone of the developing skull of a human embryo. Note that osteoblasts, which have differentiated from surrounding mesenchymal cells, lie in close relationship to the spicule. × 550.

See filmstrip I, frame 25.

tissue cells connected to one another by their processes, but without cytoplasmic continuity, and of a semifluid intercellular substance containing delicate collagenous fibers. This mesenchymal sheet or membrane becomes richly vascularized, and consequently some of the cells differentiate. They enlarge and assume a polyhedral form, and their cytoplasm becomes more basophil. They now can be identified as osteoblasts. Between such cells thin bars of dense intercellular substance appear. They mask the connective tissue fibers already present within the matrix. The bars of dense matrix increase in size and the cells become surrounded by them. At this stage the matrix is not calcified and constitutes the organic component of bone matrix, termed *osteoid.*

Later the matrix becomes calcifiable through some transformation, supposedly the result of activity by osteoblasts. The minerals are deposited in an orderly fashion as minute crystals in close association with the collagenous fibers. There often is a delay in the deposition of mineral salts in osteoid, and thus matrix at the periphery of growing bone stains less densely than the fully mineralized matrix at the center. As calcified matrix is deposited around osteoblasts and their processes, lacunae and canaliculi are formed, and since processes of adjoining cells are in contact with one another, canaliculi of adjoining lacunae connect with each other. After the initial stages of bone formation, a layer of osteoblasts appears on the surface of the developing bone. Through the activity of the osteoblasts the bone increases in thickness. Successive layers of matrix are added by apposition, and osteoblasts, which lie on the surface of bone initially, become included within it as osteocytes. The number of osteoblasts on the surface is maintained by mitosis and by formation of osteoblasts from undifferentiated cells within the surrounding connective tissue.

As growth continues at several foci of bone formation, initially the bone consists of spicules, plates, and trabeculae and it is spongy. The spaces between the plates of bone, the *primary marrow cavities,* are filled with richly vascularized connective tissue which gradually becomes transformed into myeloid, or *hemopoietic,* tissue. The connective tissue which surrounds a growing mass of bone gives rise to the periosteum.

Endochondral (Intracartilaginous) Bone Formation. This type of ossification, involving the replacement of a cartilage model by bone, is best observed in a long bone. The shape of the cartilage corresponds closely with that of the future bone. During development the cartilage is replaced by bone except at the joint surfaces, but this is a slow process which is not achieved until the bone has reached its full size and growth has ceased. Externally the cartilage is covered by a perichondrium which shows marked cellularity owing to the presence of numerous embryonic connective tissue cells.

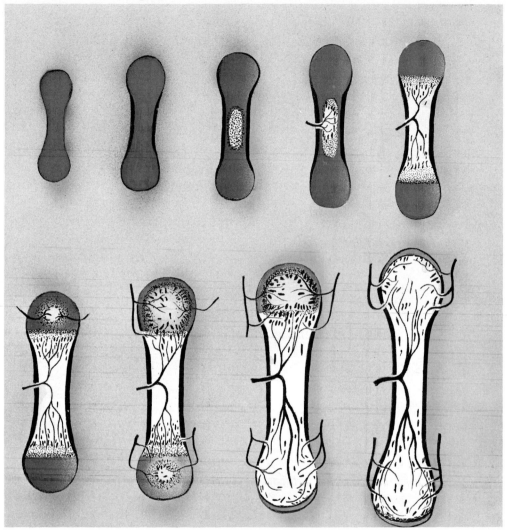

Figure 7-20. Diagram of stages in endochondral ossification. See text for description of stages, beginning on page 124.

Bone formation is initiated within a band-shaped area of perichondrium surrounding the center of the diaphysis. The perichondrium here assumes an osteogenic function. Cells of the perichondrium adjoining the cartilage hypertrophy and become osteoblasts. They begin to form bone of the intramembranous type. This is the *periosteal bone ring* or *collar* which surrounds the middle of the diaphyseal region of the cartilage. The perichondrium around this area becomes a periosteum.

Simultaneously with the appearance of the bony collar, changes become apparent in the cartilage itself. In the center of the diaphysis, the cartilage cells hypertrophy and the matrix between the lacunae becomes reduced in amount and calcified. Through apertures in the bony collar, connective tissue sprouts, together with blood vessels, grow into the region of the changed cartilage matrix. These are the *periosteal buds*, which penetrate the partitions between the enlarged cartilage cells and open up cavities.

The cavities thus formed are the *primary marrow spaces,* which contain thin-walled blood vessels and embryonic connective tissue cells. Some of the embryonic cells become osteoblasts and enclose the calcified cartilage matrix, first with osteoid and then with calcified bone, just as in intramembranous bone formation. The fate of the cartilage cells in this region is not known, but many undoubtedly die and some may become osteoblasts. The deposition of bone in the center of the diaphysis constitutes the *primary ossification center.*

The zone of endochondral ossification extends toward the ends of the cartilage by a sequence of changes similar to that which took place in the establishment of the primary ossification center. At the same time the periosteal bone collar becomes thicker and widens toward the epiphyses. It assists in maintaining the strength of the shaft, which otherwise would be weakened by the dissolution of carti-

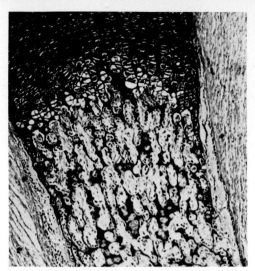

Figure 7-22. Endochondral ossification in longitudinal section through the zone of epiphyseal growth of the proximal end of the radius of a rat (epiphysis above). × 65.

lage within the diaphysis. Thus the periosteal bone collar acts as a buttress to support the central zone of resorbing cartilage prior to its replacement by bone.

With the continued growth of cartilage in the epiphyses, the entire cartilage model increases in size. As a result of this and of the extension of the primary ossification center, definite zones become apparent within the cartilage. Of course, each zone changes character as ossification advances toward it. Beginning at the ends of the cartilage and passing toward the ossification center, the following zones, which illustrate the continuing process of endochondral bone formation, can be recognized:

QUIESCENT OR RESERVE ZONE. This zone, composed of primitive hyaline cartilage, is present nearest to the ends of the bone. Initially it is a relatively long zone but shortens progressively as ossification encroaches upon it. It is a zone which shows growth in all directions.

ZONE OF PROLIFERATION. This is an active zone showing numerous mitoses. Cells of the quiescent zone divide

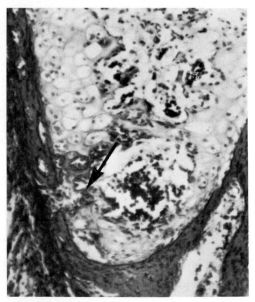

Figure 7-21. Ossification of the human ilium. The periosteal cuff of bone is well developed and a periosteal bud (arrow), comprising bone forming and vascular elements, has entered the cartilage model. × 160. (Courtesy of R. D. Laurenson.)

and produce daughter cells which align themselves in distinct rows or columns parallel with the long axis of the cartilage model. Each row consists of a number of cells which are crowded, flattened, and separated by little matrix. A row grows principally by the addition of cells at the distal, free end in relation to the quiescent zone. By this mechanism the cartilage increases in length more than in breadth.

MATURATION ZONE.   Mitoses no longer occur and the cells and lacunae enlarge, becoming cuboidal in shape. This enlargement adds further to the length of the cartilage in this region.

ZONE OF CALCIFICATION.   In this zone the matrix surrounding the enlarged lacunae stains deeply basophil owing to the deposition of minerals within it.

ZONE OF RETROGRESSION.   The cartilage cells die and undergo dissolution as does the matrix between cells. The thicker plates of matrix between rows of cells remain virtually intact. Thus this zone on cross section has the appearance of a honeycomb. Vascular primary marrow extends into the spaces resulting from the destruction of cells and matrix.

ZONE OF OSSIFICATION.   Here osteoblasts differentiate from mesenchymal cells of the marrow tissue and gather on the exposed plates of calcified cartilage, where they commence to lay down bone. The remnants of calcified cartilage form a supporting framework.

ZONE OF RESORPTION.   As ossification advances toward the ends of the cartilage, the marrow cavity increases in size, owing to resorption of bone in the center of the diaphysis. As a result, the length of spongy bone remains nearly constant. The cavity which forms is the *secondary marrow cavity.*

While all these changes are taking place, there is further activity in the periosteum. The periosteal collar of bone thickens and extends at each end. The increase in extent of the periosteal collar compensates for the loss, by

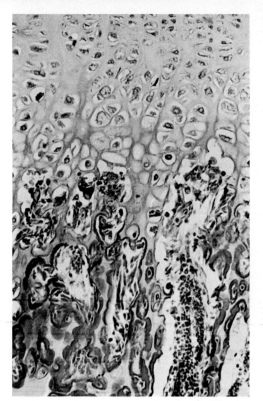

Figure 7-23. High power photomicrograph of a longitudinal section through the proximal end of the radius. Notice the zones of activity within the epiphyseal disc. × 375.

See filmstrip I, frames 26 and 27.

resorption, of endochondral bone centrally. The zone of reserve cartilage is maintained by cell division, but it becomes reduced in length as ossification of the diaphysis proceeds.

At about the time of birth, *secondary centers of ossification (epiphyseal centers)* appear in both ends of most long bones. The sequence of changes in the cartilage of these centers is identical with that observed in the diaphysis. Cartilage cells proliferate and hypertrophy, and vascular osteogenic buds enter from the periphery or through tunnels from the diaphysis. Cartilage removal and bone deposition follow. Ossification spreads peripherally in all directions until there is replacement of cartilage by bone except in two regions. Cartilage remains over the free end as articular cartilage and as a plate between the epiphysis and the diaphysis. This is the *epiphyseal plate* or *disc*.

The epiphyseal disc continues to form new cartilage at the proximal surface facing the diaphysis. The formation of cartilage columns, the calcification of cartilage, and the deposition of bone continue here as earlier in the shaft. These processes cause an increase principally in the length of the bone. Proliferation of cartilage and bony replacement occur at about the same rate so that the thickness of the epiphyseal disc remains constant. When growth ceases, there is no further proliferation of cartilage and the epiphyseal disc is replaced by bone. The epiphysis and diaphysis are united by bone, a union which is visible in the adult, the *epiphyseal line*. Henceforth increase in length is impossible.

Increase in diameter of long bones occurs by the deposition of new periosteal bone, which forms intramembranously by appositional growth. The thickness of bone does not increase at the same rate since, as bone is added progressively to the periosteal surface, bone in lesser amounts is

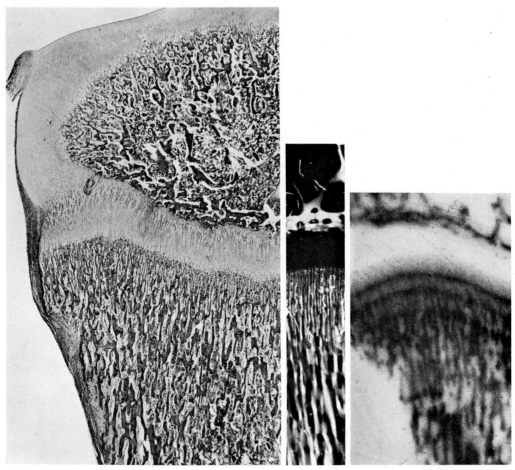

Figure 7-24.   Left: Upper tibial epiphysis of two week old rabbit, showing secondary center of ossification and epiphyseal disc. Undecalcified section. × 12. Center: Contact microradiograph of a thin slice of upper tibial epiphysis in which the arterial system was injected with Micropaque. The epiphyseal bony plate, cartilage, and metaphysis are set at the same levels as adjacent figures. Right: Radioautograph to illustrate growth of epiphysis. Radioactive calcium injected, 9, 8, 3, 2, and 1 day prior to sacrifice. (Courtesy of F. W. Fyfe.)

resorbed from the endosteal surface. Thus the secondary marrow cavity increases in extent.

Remodeling and Reconstruction of Bone

As a bone enlarges in size, its structure is complicated by internal reconstruction and by remodeling. Remodeling results from resorption in certain areas and deposition of new bone elsewhere. Resorption is associated with the appearance of osteoclasts although the significance of their presence is unknown. A relationship between the appearance of osteoclasts and active sites of erosion led to the widely accepted belief that osteoclasts play a major role in bone resorption. An alternative interpretation is that osteoclasts arise by the coalescence of osteocytes liberated during the process of resorption. At the interface between osteoclasts and bone there is evidence of surface activity in the form of cytoplasmic striations. On electron microscopy they appear as irregular, deep infoldings of the cell membrane. However, there is little evidence that the cells are capable of a mechanical form of erosion or of active phagocytosis. Any reconstruction of bone occurs in response to local mechanical stresses to which the bone is subjected.

In growth of bone, we have been concerned so far with the deposition of spongy bone. In certain areas this is replaced by compact bone. In this process osteoblasts produce layer after layer of bone inward on the surface of longitudinal cavities within spongy bone until the cavities are reduced to narrow canals containing the blood vessels. The system of concentric lamellae with its canal and blood vessels is called a *primitive Haversian system.*

The majority of Haversian systems develop in compact bone by a more complicated process. Bone substance may be dissolved by vascular buds

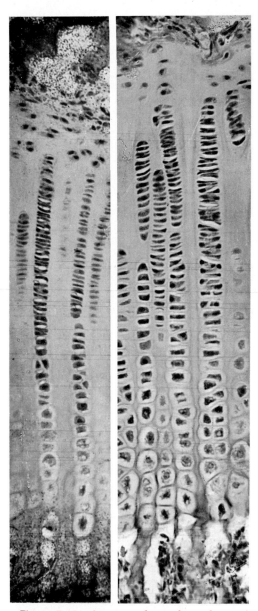

Figure 7-25. Sections of growth cartilages of upper end of tibias of two month old (left) and three month old (right) rabbits. Radioactive calcium was injected 30 hours before sacrifice, and the undecalcified sections were dipped in photographic emulsion and developed after several weeks. Silver grains overlie the secondary ossification center (above) and the calcifying ends of the cartilage columns (below), in continuity with the primary bony trabeculae. × 250. (Courtesy of F. W. Fyfe.)

from endosteal or periosteal surfaces. Recent evidence suggests that the normal mechanism of internal bone resorption occurs under the influence of mature osteocytes. This process is referred to as *osteolysis*. The cells responsible for this activity are able to produce both alkaline phosphatase and protease. They are surrounded by a matrix which has a low concentration of both salts and organic matter. The lytic process, which is hormonally controlled (see page 132), results in the formation of wide cylindrical cavities containing blood vessels and embryonic marrow tissue. The tunnel resulting from the erosion process becomes lined by osteoblasts which differentiate from the primitive cells present within the marrow. Successive lamellae of bone are deposited progressively inward until the tunnel is reduced to a narrow canal around the blood vessels. The reconstruction of bone does not terminate, however, with the replacement of primary bone by secondary bone, but continues throughout life. Resorption cavities appear continuously and are replaced by third, fourth, and higher orders of Haversian systems. In this process portions of former Haversian systems may escape destruction and become interstitial lamellae which fill in between new systems. As growth nears completion, the periosteum and endosteum lay down successive layers of basic or circumferential lamellae, which persist as concentric lamellae.

In a mature bone, therefore, the majority of the matrix is of intramembranous origin. Bone of endochondral origin persists only as narrow trabeculae in the diaphysis and the metaphyses and as the central spongy bone of the epiphyses.

Development of Irregular Bones. The foregoing description is based upon conditions in a typical long bone. Irregular bones develop in a manner similar to the epiphyses of long bones. Ossification begins in the center and extends out in all directions. Cartilage at the periphery serves as a prolifera-

tive zone until growth within it ceases, when it is replaced by bone. Further bone may be added by apposition from the periosteum.

Repair of Bone

After a fracture there is hemorrhage from torn vessels and clotting. Proliferating fibroblasts and capillaries invade the clot and form granulation tissue, the *procallus*. The granulation tissue becomes dense fibrous tissue and later transforms into a mass of cartilage. This is the *temporary callus* that unites the fractured bones. Osteoblasts develop from the periosteum and endosteum and lay down spongy bone which progressively replaces the cartilage of the temporary callus in a manner similar to endochondral ossification. Bony union of the fracture is achieved. The bony callus, initially spongy, undergoes reorganization into compact bone and excess bone is resorbed.

The sequence of callus formation after bony injury illustrates the multipotentiality of cells of the periosteum and of the endosteum. After injury the nature of cell differentiation is dependent upon the blood supply. Initially the blood supply to the area is poor, and differentiation of cells is in the direction of fibroblasts and of chondroblasts. After the ingrowth of blood vessels, osteoblasts make their appearance.

Histophysiology of Bone

Both vitamins and hormones play an important role in ossification and the maintenance of bone. In vitamin D deficiency there is a faulty absorption of calcium from foods and a diminished concentration of phosphate in the blood plasma. In children this results in *rickets*. The cartilage matrix and the osteoid tissue fail to calcify completely, and the epiphyseal discs become thick and irregular. In

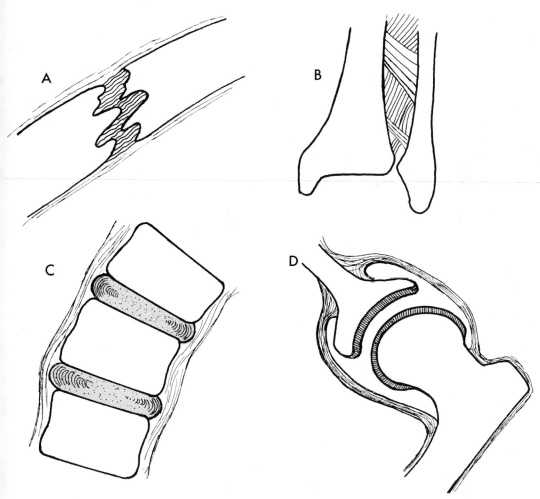

Figure 7-26.   Types of joints. *A*, Synarthrosis: syndesmosis (suture). *B*, Synarthrosis: syndesmosis (interosseous membrane). *C*, Synarthrosis: synchondrosis (intervertebral disc). *D*, Diarthrosis.

adults the deficiency causes a diminution in calcium content of the bones, a condition known as *osteomalacia.* Vitamin C deficiency results in a condition known as *scurvy,* which is characterized by an inability of tissues of mesenchymal origin to produce and maintain fibers and ground substance. This causes a destruction of osteocollagenous fibers and a diminished production of organic matrix in bones. In vitamin A deficiency there is a diminution in the rate of growth of the skeleton and interference with the process of remodeling.

Hormones profoundly influence the growth and maintenance of bones. The *growth hormone* of the anterior pituitary is essential for normal bone growth. Lack of growth hormone results in *dwarfism;* excessive production leads to *gigantism.* Parathyroid hormone regulates the resorption of bone and controls the release of calcium to the blood. The action of parathyroid hormone appears to be in direct opposition to that of thyrocalcitonin, which inhibits resorptive activity. The appearance and closure of epiphyseal centers of ossification are related to the production of sex hormones by the gonads.

THE JOINTS

Bones are connected at joints, or *articulations.* Two principal types of joints are distinguished: *synarthroses,* which are immovable or only slightly movable, and *diarthroses,* which are freely movable joints with a joint cavity interposed between the bones.

In synarthroses, the union may be by dense fibrous tissue, either collagenous or elastic *(syndesmosis),* as in the sutures of the skull and the ligamenta flava, or by cartilage, either hyaline or fibrocartilage *(synchondrosis).* Examples of the latter include the pubic symphysis and the intervertebral discs. A synchondrosis may be transformed into a *synostosis* as a result of gradual replacement of the cartilage by bone.

In *diarthroses* articular (hyaline) cartilage covers the ends of the bones and the articulation is enveloped by a joint capsule. The outer layer of the capsule is dense fibrous tissue, which is continuous with the periosteum over the bones and is thickened in various places to form the ligaments of the joint. The inner layer of the capsule, the *synovial membrane,* lines the joint cavity, except over articular cartilage and, when present, intra-articular discs. The synovial membrane is a loose vascular layer without a complete layer of cells at the surface. The surface comprises both cells, thought to be flattened fibroblasts, and fibers. The membrane commonly is thrown into folds *(synovial villi).* The *synovial fluid* probably is in part secreted by the cells of the synovial membrane. It acts as a lubricating fluid to facilitate free movement of the articular surfaces.

REFERENCES

Barland, P., Novikoff, A. B., and Hermermann, D.: Electron microscopy of the human synovial membrane. J. Cell Biol., *14*:207, 1962.

Bélanger, L. F., Semba, T., Tolnai, S., Copp, D. H., Krook, L., and Gries, C.: The two faces of resorption. *In* Third European Symposium on Calcified Tissues, edited by H. Fleisch, H. J. J. Blackwood, and M. Owen. Berlin, Springer-Verlag, 1966, p. 1.

Bourne, G. H. (editor): The Biochemistry and Physiology of Bone. New York, Academic Press, 1956.

Brookes, M.: Cortical vascularization and growth in foetal trabecular bones. J. Anat., 97:597, 1963.

Cabrini, R. L.: Histochemistry of ossification. *In* Int. Rev. Cytol., *11*:283, 1961.

Clark, E. R., and Clark, E. L.: Microscopic observations on new formation of cartilage and bone in the living mammal. Amer. J. Anat., 70:167, 1942.

Cooper, R. R., Milgram, J. W., and Robinson, R. A.: Morphology of the osteon. J. Bone Joint Surg., 48:1239, 1966.

Davies, D. V.: The structure and functions of synovial membrane. Brit. Med. J., *1*:92, 1950.

Dudley, H. R., and Spiro, D.: The fine structure

of bone cells. J. Biophys. Biochem. Cytol., 11:627, 1961.

Fell, H. B.: Skeletal development in tissue culture. In The Biochemistry and Physiology of Bone, edited by G. H. Bourne. New York, Academic Press, 1956, p. 409.

Fernández-Morán, H., and Engström, A.: Electron microscopy and x-ray diffraction of bone. Biochim. Biophys. Acta, 23:260, 1957.

Godman, G. C., and Lane, N.: On the site of sulfation in the chondrocyte. J. Cell Biol., 21:353, 1964.

Gomori, G.: Calcification and phosphatase. Amer. J. Path., 19:197, 1943.

Gonzales, F., and Karnovsky, M. J.: Electron microscopy of osteoclasts in healing fractures of rat bone. J. Biophys. Biochem. Cytol., 9:299, 1961.

Ham, A. W.: Cartilage and bone. In Special Cytology, edited by E. V. Cowdry. New York, Paul B. Hoeber, 1932, Vol. 2, p. 979.

Lacroix, P.: Bone and cartilage. In The Cell: Biochemistry, Physiology, Morphology, edited by J. Brachet and A. E. Mirsky. New York, Academic Press, 1961, Vol. 5, p. 219.

Leblond, C. P., Bélanger, L. F., and Greulich, R. C.: Formation of bones and teeth as visualized by radioautography. Ann. N.Y. Acad. Sci., 60:629, 1955.

Meyer, K.: The mucopolysaccharides of bone. In Ciba Foundation Symposium on Bone Structure and Metabolism, edited by Wolstenholme and O'Connor. Boston, Little, Brown and Co., 1956.

Owen, M., and MacPherson, S.: Cell population kinetics of an osteogenic tissue, II. J. Cell Biol., 19:33, 1963.

Palfrey, A. J., and Davies, D. V.: The fine structure of chondrocytes. J. Anat. Lond., 100:213, 1966.

Pritchard, J. J.: General anatomy and histology of bone. In The Biochemistry and Physiology of Bone, edited by G. H. Bourne. New York, Academic Press, 1956, p. 1.

Schenk, R. K., Spiro, D., and Wiener, J.: Cartilage resorption in the tibial epiphyseal plate of growing rats. J. Cell Biol., 34:275, 1967.

Silverberg, R., Silverberg, M., and Feir, D.: Life cycle of articular cartilage cells: An electron microscope study of the hip joint of the mouse. Amer. J. Anat., 114:17, 1964.

Streeter, G. L.: Developmental horizons in human embryos (fourth issue): A review of the histogenesis of cartilage and bone. Contributions to Embryology No. 220, Carnegie Institution of Washington Publ. No. 583, 33:149, 1949.

CHAPTER 8

SPECIALIZED CONNECTIVE TISSUE: BLOOD

Blood is a specialized form of connective tissue consisting of formed elements (principally cells) and a fluid intercellular substance, the *blood plasma*. The volume of blood in the healthy adult human is about 5 liters, and quantitatively blood constitutes about 8 per cent of the body weight. Because of the fluidity of plasma, blood cells have no definite spatial relationship. Cells of blood are designated according to their appearance in the fresh, unstained condition and are of two main types: red (*erythrocytes*) and white (*leukocytes*). Other formed elements present in blood are the *blood platelets*.

ERYTHROCYTES

The erythrocytes, or *red blood corpuscles*, are highly differentiated cells which functionally are specialized for the transportation of oxygen. In mammals the erythrocyte is a cell which has lost its nucleus and its cytoplasmic organelles during development. Each cell is shaped like a biconcave disc and when observed on the flat has a circular outline. In certain diseases human erythrocytes of

altered shape are found in the circulation. The corpuscles are elastic and are capable of considerable distortion as is evident in their ability to pass through capillaries of small caliber. They average about 7.6 μ in diameter in dried smears. The living undehydrated corpuscle has a diameter larger than this (about 8.5 μ), and in sectioned material the diameter is smaller (about 7 μ). (These figures, which show remarkable uniformity, should be remembered since they form a convenient means of estimating the size of adjacent cells in blood smears or in sections.)

The erythrocytes are much more numerous than any of the other formed elements of blood. In human males there are 5,000,000 to 5,500,000 erythrocytes per cubic millimeter; in females, 4,500,000 to 5,000,000. Prolonged residence at high altitude is accompanied by an increase in the number of erythrocytes. The figure for the total surface area of all the red blood corpuscles in the human body is impressive. It amounts to about 3500 square meters. This enormous area is available for exchange between the corpuscles on the one hand and the plasma and air on the other.

134

A single, fresh erythrocyte is pale greenish yellow in color. In dense masses of red blood corpuscles the color turns red. In a dry smear of peripheral blood the erythrocytes stain red (i.e., are acidophil) with the Wright or Giemsa stain. The cytoplasm appears homogeneous and no nucleus is present. Each erythrocyte is bounded by a delicate plasma membrane which is a lipoprotein complex (i.e., a typical "unit" membrane). Normally about 1 per cent of the corpuscles encountered in peripheral blood are not fully mature. These immature elements, the *reticulocytes*, representing a stage in red cell maturation, appear a little larger than the red cells, and when stained supravitally with brilliant cresyl blue, exhibit an internal network, or reticulum.

Erythrocytes have a tendency to adhere to each other along their concave surfaces, thus forming columns or rows like piles of coins. This phenomenon is termed *rouleaux formation* and occurs spontaneously in a stagnant circulation or in blood removed from the circulation. Although the exact cause is not known, it is thought by many to be due to surface tension.

Chemically the content of the erythrocyte consists of a lipoid and protein colloidal complex, principally *hemoglobin*, which is responsible for the color of red blood corpuscles. Hemoglobin has the property of binding oxygen, which it does in the capillaries of the lung. In the tissues the oxygen is distributed in exchange for carbonic acid.

The contents of the corpuscle normally are in osmotic equilibrium with the plasma. If plasma is concentrated

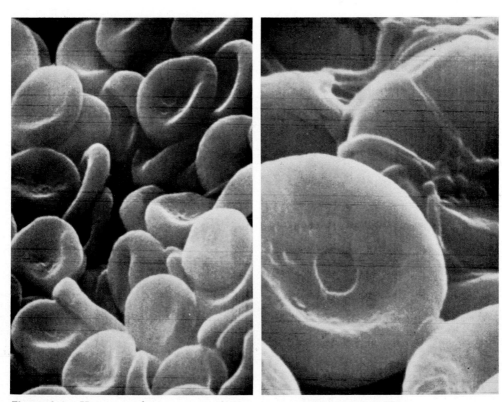

Figure 8-1.   Human erythrocytes in a plasma clot. This picture, taken with a scanning electron microscope, illustrates well that the cells are biconcave discs. The strands visible at higher magnification (right) are of fibrin. Left, × 4000. Right, × 13,000. (Courtesy of T. L. Hayes.)

by evaporation or if hypertonic solutions are added to the blood, *crenation* of the corpuscles occurs. This is the result of the passage of water from the corpuscles into the plasma, causing shrinkage of the corpuscles and so producing a scalloped contour. On the other hand, if the plasma is diluted, water enters the corpuscles and they swell, becoming spherical in shape. If this continues, hemoglobin escapes into the plasma and the corpuscles lose their color, becoming *blood shadows* or *blood ghosts*. The outward passage of hemoglobin is called *hemolysis* or *laking*. Hemolysis is accomplished also by agents that damage the plasma membrane, and the substances which effect it are known as *hemolysins* or *hemolytic agents*.

Agglutination or clumping of corpuscles is induced by various agents. It may occur in the circulating blood in a variety of pathological conditions. *Agglutinins* present in the plasma of some individuals may cause agglutination of erythrocytes in others. The agglutinins form the basis for the four main blood groups.

In certain pathological conditions not only the number, but also the size, shape, and hemoglobin content of the erythrocytes may vary enormously. A variation in size, *anisocytosis*, may occur. Cells smaller then 6 μ in diameter are termed *microcytes* and cells larger than normal, found commonly in some types of anemia, are known as *macrocytes* or *megalocytes*. Distortions in shape are termed *poikilocytosis*. When the rate of red cell formation is greater than the rate of hemoglobin synthesis, red cells are produced which contain a concentration of hemoglobin less than the normal. Such cells appear paler (*hypochromic*) than the normal erythrocytes (*normochromic*).

LEUKOCYTES

Leukocytes, or *white blood corpuscles*, are cells which contain nuclei.

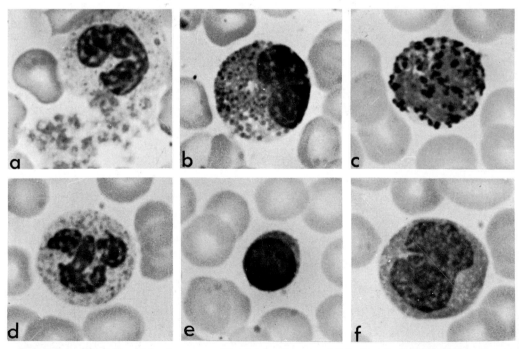

Figure 8-2.   Peripheral blood smear. *a*, Platelets and neutrophil leukocyte. *b*, Acidophil leukocyte. *c*, Basophil leukocyte. *d*, Neutrophil leukocyte. *e*, Small lymphocyte. *f*, Monocyte. Wright's stain. All × 1350.   See filmstrip I, frames 28 and 29.

There is an average of 5000 to 9000 leukocytes per cubic millimeter in normal human blood. The count in children is much higher and marked variations from the normal number occur pathologically. If the number is increased above 12,000, the condition is referred to as *leukocytosis*; if decreased below 5000, it is called *leukopenia*.

Leukocytes are of two main types, *agranular* and *granular*. Agranular leukocytes have a cytoplasm which appears homogeneous and nuclei which are spherical to reniform in shape. Granular leukocytes contain abundant specific granules (which in life are semifluid droplets) within their cytoplasm and possess nuclei which exhibit considerable variation in shape. There are two types of agranular leukocytes: *lymphocytes*, which are small cells with a scanty cytoplasm, and *monocytes*, which are slightly larger cells containing somewhat greater amounts of cytoplasm. The granular leukocytes are of three types: *neutrophil*, *basophil*, and *acidophil* (or *eosinophil*), distinguished by the affinity of their respective granules for neutral, basic, and acid stains.

It must be appreciated that leukocytes seen in the living state or in routine histological sections appear quite different from the same cells seen in dried smears. In sectioned material the leukocytes appear rounded as they do within the circulation, but their diameters are less than in the living condition owing to shrinkage. In smear preparations cells flatten and appear larger than in life and many structural details are altered or distorted; for instance, the nucleolus of granular leukocytes is obscured. Thus the type of preparation must be borne in mind when consideration is given to the histological appearances of the various cells.

Agranular Leukocytes

Lymphocytes. In human blood the lymphocytes are spherical cells which vary from 6 to 8 μ in diameter, although a few may be larger. Most are only a little larger than erythrocytes. They constitute from 20 to 35 per cent of the leukocytes of normal blood. The most striking feature of the small lymphocyte is that it has a relatively large nucleus surrounded by a narrow rim of cytoplasm. The nucleus appears spherical and generally shows a small indentation to one side. The densely packed chromatin of the nucleus stains intensely, and the nucleolus is invisible in stained dry smears. The cytoplasm stains basophil, owing to a concentration of ribosomes throughout the cytoplasm, as is evident on electron micrographs. Purplish, azurophil granules occasionally may be seen within the cytoplasm, but unlike the specific granules of the granular leukocytes, they are not a constant feature.

A few of the lymphocytes of normal circulating blood may be as large as 10 to 12 μ. Their larger size is due chiefly to a greater amount of cytoplasm. These cells sometimes are referred to as *medium-sized lymphocytes*. Some of the larger cells may appear to be intermediate between lymphocytes and monocytes. None of these large cells should be confused with the *large lymphocytes* which reside in the lymph nodes and appear in the blood only in pathological conditions. The latter are distinguished by the presence of a vesicular nucleus with prominent nucleoli.

Monocytes. Monocytes are large cells which constitute only from 3 to 8 per cent of the leukocytes of normal blood. They measure 9 to 12 μ in diameter but in dry smears may flatten out to achieve a diameter of 20 μ or more. The nucleus usually is eccentrically placed within the cell and is ovoid or kidney-shaped. It may show a deep depression or be horseshoe-shaped in older cells. The chromatin material within it is disposed in a delicate network, and thus the nucleus does not stain as deeply as that of the lymphocyte. The cytoplasm is relatively abundant and with Wright's stain is pale grayish-blue in color in dry smears. Electron micrographs of monocytes reveal an abundance of endoplasmic reticulum within the cytoplasm but fewer free ribosomes than are found in lymphocytes.

Rarely one may find intermediates between monocytes and medium-sized lymphocytes, and in such cases positive identification is difficult.

Granular Leukocytes

In contrast to lymphocytes and monocytes, granular leukocytes always contain specific granules. They are further characterized by the presence of a many-lobed (polymorphous) nucleus. For this reason sometimes they are referred to as *polymorphonuclear leukocytes*.

Neutrophils. The neutrophil, polymorphonuclear leukocytes are 7 to 9 μ in diameter in the fresh condition and 10 to 12 μ in dry smears. They are the most numerous of the leukocytes in human blood and constitute 65 to 75 per cent of the total. The nucleus is highly polymorphous and shows a variety of forms. It usually consists of from three to five irregularly oval lobes connected by fine threads of chromatin. The number of lobes increases with age. No nucleoli can be seen. In dry smears of the peripheral blood of human females one can see a small nuclear appendage attached to the remainder of the nucleus by a fine strand of chromatin in about 3 per cent of the neutrophils. This "drumstick," first noted by Davidson and Smith, probably represents the sex chromosome. Presumably it is present in all the cells of females, but it is closely packed within one of the lobes of the nucleus in most cells and thus is obscured.

The abundant cytoplasm is filled

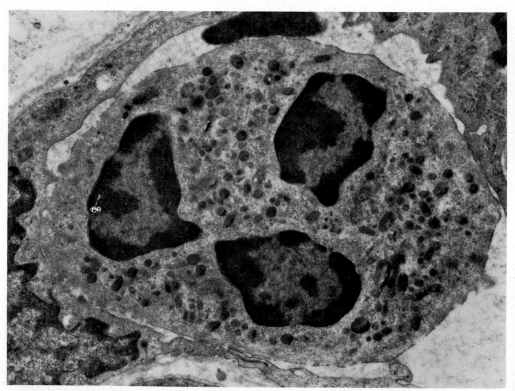

Figure 8-3. Electron micrograph of a neutrophil within a capillary. Three lobes of the nucleus may be seen. Numerous specific granules lie within the finely granular cytoplasm. × 14,500.

with fine granules which are neutrophil. In other mammals the granules have a variable size and staining reaction. In the rabbit and guinea pig the granules accept the acid stain, and thus in these animals the cells may be called *pseudoeosinophils*. Since the cells vary in their staining reactions in different species, sometimes they are called *heterophil* leukocytes rather than neutrophils. The granules are a special type of lysosome which contains principally hydrolytic enzymes. The enzymes are liberated following ingestion by neutrophils of particles such as carbon, bacteria, and other microorganisms.

Eosinophils. The eosinophil, or acidophil, leukocytes are somewhat larger than the neutrophils and in the fresh condition are 9 to 10 μ in diameter. In dry smears the size of the flattened cells varies from 12 to 14 μ. They normally constitute about 2 to 4 per cent of the white blood cells. The nucleus is usually bilobed. The cytoplasm characteristically is filled with coarse, refractile granules of uniform size, which stain intensely with acid dyes. The specific granules

have a striking appearance in electron micrographs. The granules appear banded because of the presence within them of dense cylindrical crystals.

Basophils. These cells are difficult to find in human blood since they constitute only about 0.5 to 1 per cent of the total number of leukocytes. They are about the same size as neutrophils, 7 to 9 μ in diameter in the fresh condition and 10 μ or a little more in dry smears. The nucleus often is irregular in outline and partially constricted into two lobes. The cytoplasmic granules are round, coarse, and variable in size. Some characteristically overlie the nucleus and tend to obscure its outline. The granules are soluble in water and therefore are partly dissolved or absent in routine preparations. They are basophil and metachromatic.

Functions of Leukocytes

Little is known about the functions of leukocytes while in the blood stream, where they appear to be largely inactive. They perform most of their functions outside the vascular

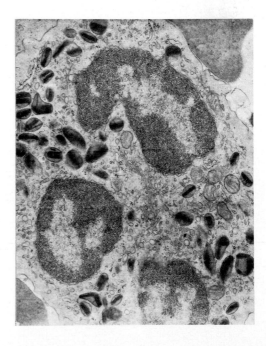

Figure 8-4. Electron micrograph of a portion of an eosinophil within a capillary. Three lobes of the nucleus may be seen. An element of the Golgi apparatus lies in the central region of cytoplasm. Note the large specific granules, each containing a dark, angular mass. × 13,500.

system, where they show active movement and some exhibit phagocytosis. The movement they exhibit is a crawling or ameboid process on a substrate. Neutrophils are the most active, followed in order by monocytes and basophils. Lymphocytes generally appear the most sluggish but in certain conditions may become remarkably active. There is a constant migration of leukocytes out of the vessels into the tissues. Some cells may return into the blood or lymph vessels. Emigration is greatly increased toward the site of local injury or inflammation. This is a specific response to chemotactic stimulation. The first cells to respond to such a stimulus are granulocytes and later monocytes. Lymphocytes accumulate in the tissues at sites of chronic inflammation.

Neutrophils possess the capacity to ingest by a phagocytic process small particles such as carbon or bacteria. The other granular leukocytes rarely exhibit phagocytosis and lymphocytes are not known to be phagocytic. Monocytes are able to engulf particulate matter under suitable conditions.

Some leukocytes contain certain enzymes. Peroxidases are present in granular leukocytes and in monocytes. Phosphatases and certain proteolytic enzymes are found in neutrophils. Neutrophils constitute the first line of defense against invading organisms, but they are not equally effective against all types of bacteria. The granules within eosinophils, like those within neutrophils, are lysosomal in nature. The number of eosinophils is greatly increased in certain allergic conditions and in parasitic infestations, and the number is decreased following the administration of adrenal corticosteroids. Basophils increase in number in relatively few pathological conditions, but there is some evidence to support the view that they elaborate the heparin and histamine of circulating blood.

Monocytes migrate readily through vessel walls and develop into phagocytic cells which cannot be distinguished from macrophages already present within the connective tissues. They are effective in combating tubercle bacilli.

The exact functions of lymphocytes are not clearly understood. Some investigators believe that they are responsible for the formation of antibodies. They are abundant beneath the epithelial lining of the digestive and respiratory systems, and they accumulate in relation to grafts of foreign material. They appear to have a protective function but the mechanism is yet to be determined.

BLOOD PLATELETS

Blood platelets are small protoplasmic discs which are colorless in circulating blood. They are 2 to 4 μ in diameter and their number varies considerably, but usually it is given as 200,000 to 300,000 per cubic millimeter of blood. Their number is extremely difficult to count since they adhere to each other and to all surfaces as soon as blood is removed from a vessel. Lower vertebrates lack platelets; instead they possess small nucleated cells, the *thrombocytes*.

Platelets are round or oval on the flat; when seen in profile they appear spindle- or rod-shaped. Blood stains demonstrate two regions of the platelet, a deeply basophil zone (the *chromomere*), usually centrally located, and a pale, homogeneous peripheral zone (the *hyalomere*). No nucleus is present. Electron micrographs of platelets reveal the presence of numerous small granules within the cytoplasm. The fine structural appearance of the granules and recent biochemical evidence indicate that the granules contain a catecholamine.

Platelets arise as detached portions of peculiar giant cells of bone marrow, the *megakaryocytes*. Platelets play several roles in hemostasis. They adhere to injured regions of blood vessels, producing a *white thrombus*

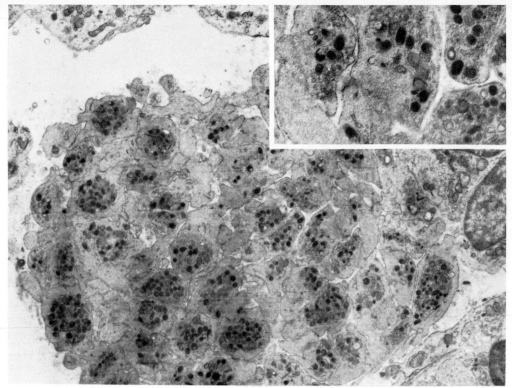

Figure 8-5. Electron micrograph of a clump of platelets within a small blood vessel. Each contains a group of dense granules within the finely granular cytoplasm. × 5750. Inset: Portions of five platelets at higher magnification. × 17,500.

which covers injured surfaces and plugs deficiencies within the vessel walls. They are presumed to produce an enzyme, *thromboplastin*, which is of importance in the clotting mechanism. Thromboplastin aids in the transformation of *prothrombin* into *thrombin*, and thrombin in turn transforms *fibrinogen* into *fibrin*.

A decrease in the number of circulating platelets is seen clinically in a condition known as *thrombocytopenia*.

PLASMA

Plasma is the fluid which transports all nutritive materials. In it are found the nutritive substances derived from the digestive system, the waste substances produced in the tissues, and the hormones. It constitutes 55 per cent of blood; cellular elements account for 45 per cent. Plasma is a homogeneous, slightly alkaline fluid which contains, in addition to the materials already mentioned, dissolved gases, inorganic salts, proteins, carbohydrates, lipids, and certain other organic substances. Suspended particles can be demonstrated within it by phase and by dark-field microscopy. These are *chylomicrons*, minute fat globules which are more numerous after a fatty meal.

When the circulation ceases, or when blood is exposed to air, one of the globulins of plasma (fibrinogen) precipitates as a network of fine filaments, the fibrin. The contraction of clotted blood or plasma *(syneresis)* expresses a clear, yellowish fluid, *serum*.

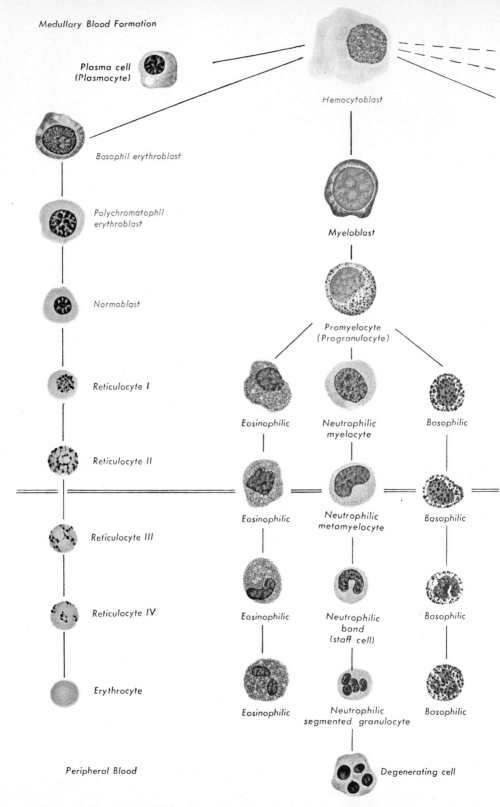

Figure 8-6.   (*See legend on opposite page.*)

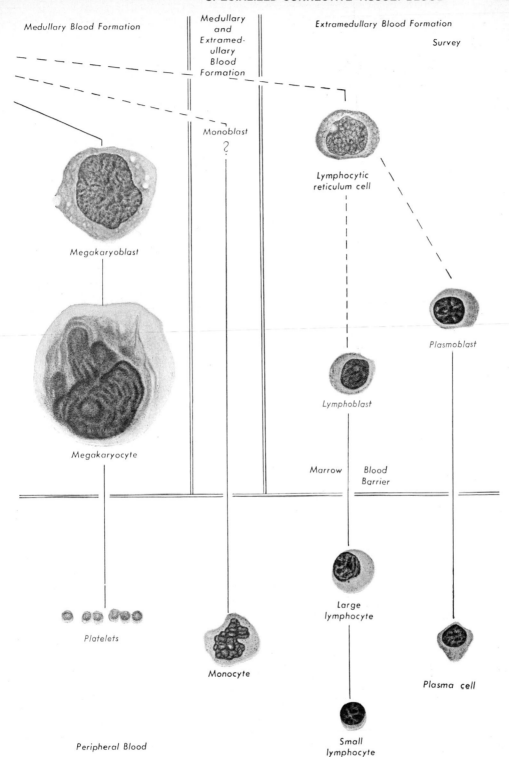

Medullary Blood Formation

Medullary and Extramedullary Blood Formation

Extramedullary Blood Formation

Survey

Monoblast
?

Lymphocytic reticulum cell

Megakaryoblast

Plasmoblast

Megakaryocyte

Lymphoblast

Marrow | Blood Barrier

Platelets

Large lymphocyte

Monocyte

Plasma cell

Peripheral Blood

Small lymphocyte

Figure 8-6. (*Continued*) Development of blood cells. This plate comprises a survey of all blood cells. The horizontal double line separates the cells that are found in the marrow and lymphoid tissue from the mature cells below the line seen normally in peripheral blood. (Plate from Heilmeyer, L., and Begemann, H.: Atlas der Klinischen Hamatologie und Cytologie. Berlin, Springer, 1955.)

LYMPH

Lymph is the fluid which is collected from the tissues and returned to the blood stream. Its composition varies considerably. There are no cellular elements within the lymph of the smallest lymph vessels. Cells, the majority of them lymphocytes, are added to the lymph as it passes through the lymph nodes. Lymph draining from the walls of the small intestine is milky because of the fat globules which it contains, and in this situation it is referred to as *chyle*. Lymph coagulates but the process occurs much more slowly than in blood and the clot is soft.

LIFE SPAN AND DISPOSAL OF BLOOD CELLS

In contrast to many cells, red and white blood cells live for only a relatively short period of time. The life span of the human erythrocyte is approximately 120 days. This may be determined by several methods. Differential agglutination, in which the length of time compatible donor cells survive in a recipient, is cumbersome and largely has been superseded by methods tagging red cells with isotopes. Of the latter, chromium tagging, utilizing Cr^{51}, now is most commonly used. A small quantity of washed red cells simply is mixed with a solution of $Na_2Cr^{51}O_7$ and this is reinjected into the subject from whom the blood was removed. The life span is estimated by the persistence of radioactivity.

It is believed that the reticuloendothelial elements, particularly in the spleen and liver, remove most of the aging erythrocytes from the circulation. After destruction of red blood cells by the phagocytic cells, hemoglobin is broken down into an iron-containing portion (*hematin*) and an iron-free portion (*globin*). The hematin is further broken down into iron, which is reutilized or stored, and into bilirubin, which is transported to the liver and excreted in the bile.

The life span of the various types of white blood cells is difficult to determine since these cells leave the blood vascular system to enter the tissue spaces, but it appears to be quite variable. There is evidence that the white blood cells remain in the circulation only for about 24 hours. However, many lymphocytes undoubtedly return to the lymphoid organs and recirculate. How long white cells remain viable after leaving the circulation is unknown. Granulocytes appear to remain alive in the tissue spaces only a few days. Senile and dead cells are thought to be removed by phagocytes within the liver and spleen and locally within the connective tissues. There is a considerable loss of white blood cells owing to migration through the lining epithelia of mucous membranes, particularly into the lumina of the digestive and respiratory systems.

Platelets are believed to survive for four to five days in circulating blood. They are thought to be removed from the circulation similarly to erythrocytes, i.e., by phagocytic activity of macrophages in the spleen and liver.

HEMOPOIESIS

Formed elements of blood are short-lived and continuously are being destroyed. The number of formed elements within blood is kept at a constant number by the formation of new cells. The process by which blood cells are formed is called *hemopoiesis*, and this occurs in the *hemopoietic tissues*. The formed elements of blood are divided into two groups according to the sites of their development and differentiation in the adult. Lymphocytes and monocytes are developed chiefly in the lymphoid tissues and are termed *lymphoid elements*. Erythrocytes and granulocytes normally

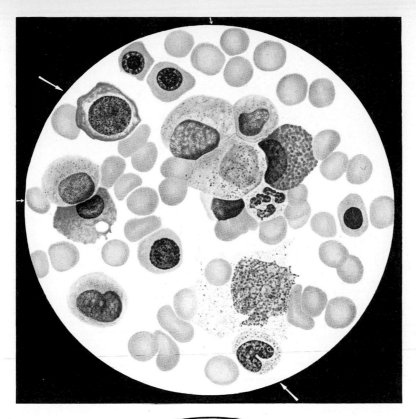

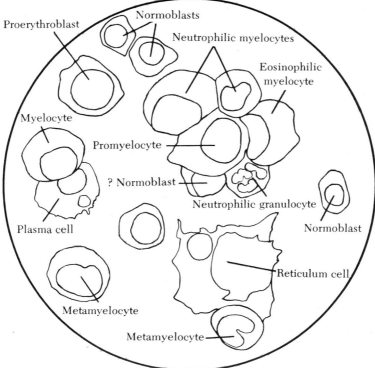

Figure 8-7. Normal marrow smear and diagram of a representative area. Leishman stain. (Plate from Heilmeyer, L., and Begemann, H.: Atlas der Klinischen Hamatologie und Cytologie. Berlin, Springer, 1955.)

are produced within the bone marrow (*myeloid tissue*) and are referred to as *myeloid elements*. This separation is not absolute since it does not occur in the fetus, where blood cells are formed in different sites at different ages and appear successively in the yolk sac, mesenchyme and blood vessels, liver, spleen, and lymph nodes. Also, it does not occur in the adult in certain pathological conditions in which myeloid elements may be formed again in the spleen, liver, and lymph nodes, a condition known as *extramedullary hemopoiesis*.

Hemopoiesis is one of the greatest areas of controversy in the field of histology. The two major points of disagreement concern the nature of the stem cell or cells of the several lines of differentiation and the sites of development of blood cells in relation to the vascular channels. Concerning the sites of development of blood cells, two diametrically opposed theories are presented: (1) that erythrocytes develop intravascularly and (2) that they develop outside the vascular channels. With regard to the nature of the stem cell and its differentiation, one theory, the *unitarian* or *monophyletic* theory of hemopoiesis, holds that all blood cells, red and white, arise from a common stem cell, the *hemocytoblast*. The *dualistic* or *diphyletic theory* holds that lymphocytes and monocytes derive from one stem cell (called the *lymphoblast* by many authors) and granular leukocytes and erythrocytes from a separate cell (the *myeloblast*). According to a further theory (*trialistic* or *polyphyletic*), three distinct stem cells give rise to (1) lymphocytes, (2) monocytes, and (3) erythrocytes and granular leukocytes. There has been considerable misunderstanding in the past with regard to these theories, and much of this has been the result of the use of different terminologies by proponents of the different theories. Today the unitarian theory appears to be accepted by the majority of hematologists. The following account is based

upon this interpretation, and it should be emphasized that the controversies do not affect the factual descriptions of the structural features of the cells of various developmental stages. The controversies essentially center around the relationships between cells of the earliest stages.

Development of Myeloid Elements

Myeloid tissue, under normal conditions, is confined to the marrow cavities of bone, where it is termed *bone marrow*. Bone marrow is the largest organ in the body, constituting about 4.5 per cent of the total body weight. In the adult there are two types of bone marrow, *red* and *yellow*. Red bone marrow is actively hemopoietic, whereas in yellow bone marrow most of the hemopoietic tissue has been replaced by fat. In the adult, red bone marrow occurs principally in the sternum, ribs, vertebrae, skull, and proximal epiphyses of some of the long bones.

Myeloid tissue consists of a frame-

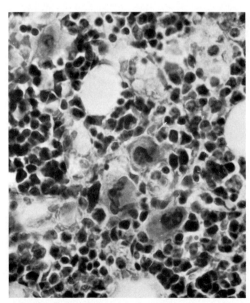

Figure 8-8. Section of active human bone marrow from the cranium. Three megakaryocytes and portions of three fat cells are present. × 400.   See filmstrip I, frame 23.

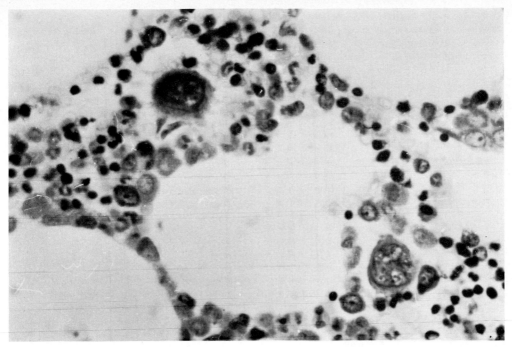

Figure 8-9. Section of human bone marrow in which there is considerable invasion of fat. Strands of myeloid elements lie between the fat cells. Note the two megakaryocytes present. × 600.

work or *stroma*, blood vessels, and the free cells lying within the meshwork of the stroma.

Stroma. The framework is a loose latticework of reticular (argyrophil) fibers in close association with primitive and phagocytic reticular cells. Fat cells are scattered singly within the stroma, unlike yellow bone marrow in which the fat cells are so concentrated as to exclude nearly all other elements.

Blood Vessels. The characteristic feature of the circulation of myeloid tissue is the presence of large, tortuous sinusoids, lined by flattened, phagocytic reticular cells (fixed macrophages, *littoral cells*). These cells do not form a complete lining to the vessels and may detach and become free within the sinusoidal blood. The deficiencies within the walls of the sinusoids allow newly formed blood cells ready access into the circulation. The manner in which arteries connect into the sinusoids is not clear, but it is thought that small arterioles break

up into a capillary network prior to entry. Sinusoids drain into venules which leave the bone marrow at numerous sites. No lymph vessels have been demonstrated within bone marrow.

Free Cells. Cells lying free within the meshes of the stroma represent all stages in the maturation of red and white blood cells. Mature erythrocytes and the three types of granular leukocytes are found between the immature elements.

The Stem Cell: The Hemocytoblast

The hemocytoblast (or myeloblast of the dualistic theory) is an ameboid cell of lymphoid nature. It is a large cell, approximately 15 μ in diameter, which is characterized by a deeply basophil cytoplasm. The nucleus is relatively undifferentiated and contains one or two nucleoli. In dried smears the nucleus shows dense accumulations of chromatin material. In sectioned material of bone marrow the nucleus appears vesicular and the nucleoli are distinct. Azurophil granules are seen occasionally within the cytoplasm.

Hemocytoblasts arise chiefly by mitotic divisions of their own type, but new ones can differentiate from the primitive reticular cells which detach from the reticulum of the stroma and become free, rounded cells. They give rise to all myeloid elements and in addition, according to the unitarian theory of hemopoiesis, to lymphoid elements.

Erythrocytes

The stages of erythrocyte development, in order of differentiation from the hemocytoblast, are: *basophil erythroblast, polychromatophil erythroblast, normoblast,* and *erythrocyte.* It should be borne in mind that the principal processes involved in the differentiation of erythrocytes are reduction in size, loss of nucleus and cellular organelles, and acquisition of hemoglobin.

Basophil Erythroblast. This is a smaller cell than the hemocytoblast and contains a nucleus with a coarser network of chromatin material. The cytoplasm shows intense basophilia, more so than that of the hemocytoblast, owing to an increased content of ribonucleic acid (RNA). Some authors describe an intermediate cell between the hemocytoblast and the basophil erythroblast. This cell is intermediate both in the size and degree of the basophilia of its cytoplasm and is termed the *proerythroblast.*

Polychromatophil Erythroblast. The basophil erythroblasts undergo numerous mitotic divisions and produce cells which acquire a small amount of hemoglobin. After staining with Wright or Giemsa stain, the cytoplasm varies in color from a purplish-blue to a lilac or gray owing to the presence of varying amounts of pink-staining hemoglobin within the baso-phil cytoplasm of the erythroblasts. Thus they are *polychromatophil.* The nucleus of the polychromatophil erythroblast has a denser chromatin network than that of the basophil erythroblast and the cell is smaller.

Normoblast. The polychromatophil erythroblasts undergo numerous mitotic divisions. Some remain in a resting condition as a reservoir of cells. In others the basophilia of the cytoplasm decreases and the amount of hemoglobin increases to such an extent that the cytoplasm stains approximately as acidophil as that of the mature erythrocyte. Cells which exhibit this degree of acidophilia within their cytoplasm are referred to as normoblasts. The normoblast is smaller than the polychromatophil erythroblast and contains a smaller nucleus which stains densely basophil. Gradually the nucleus becomes pyknotic. There is no further mitotic activity. Finally the nucleus is lost by a process thought to be simple extrusion from the cell, although a few investigators believe the process to be one of *karyolysis.*

The young erythrocytes (reticulocytes) contain a delicate network which can be demonstrated by supravital staining with dyes such as neutral red or cresyl blue or by phase microscopy. The majority of the reticulocytes lose their reticular structure before leaving the bone marrow, the reticulocyte count of peripheral blood normally being less than 1 per cent of the erythrocytes.

The stages just described in the process of *erythropoiesis* are, in the main, morphological manifestations of the synthesis of hemoglobin. The concentration of ribonucleic acid (RNA) in the ribosomal clusters (polyribosomes) that are synthesizing hemoglobin is responsible for the marked basophilia of the cytoplasm. This basophilia is most marked in the basophil erythroblast. The presence of RNA can be correlated with the active synthesis of nucleotides and hemoglobin.

The normal development of erythrocytes is dependent upon many different factors, including the presence of the parent substances (principally globin, heme, and iron) of hemoglobin. Additional factors, such as ascorbic acid, vitamin B_{12}, and the *intrinsic factor* (normally present in gastric juice), which function as coenzymes or as precursors of coenzymes in the synthetic process, also are necessary for the normal maturation of erythrocytes.

Granulocytes

The stages of granulocyte development, in order of differentiation from the hemocytoblast (myeloblast) are: *promyelocyte, myelocyte, metamyelocyte*, and granular leukocyte. It should be emphasized that myelocytes of the three types (neutrophil, eosinophil, and basophil) contain their characteristic granules and cannot be transformed into myelocytes of another type.

Promyelocytes. These are large cells, sometimes larger than the hemocytoblast. They have a rounded or oval nucleus with coarser chromatin than that of the hemocytoblast. Generally the cytoplasm is basophil, but it often shows localized acidophil areas. A few specific granules may be present, usually situated in the acidophil areas, but they are so sparse that normally no attempt is made to classify them. Some nonspecific, azurophil granules also may be present within the cytoplasm but later these disappear.

Myelocytes. Promyelocytes proliferate and differentiate into myelocytes. In the process of differentiation, the cells show decreased basophilia of the cytoplasm, an increase in the number of specific cytoplasmic granules, and an increase in the density of the nuclear chromatin. The specific granules, present in large numbers, can be identified easily. The nucleus indents and begins to assume a horseshoe shape.

Metamyelocytes. After repeated divisions of the myelocytes, the cells become smaller and cease dividing. The cells which are a product of the final division are metamyelocytes. They are juvenile forms of granular leukocytes and have a characteristic granular content. The nucleus, at first horseshoe-shaped, gradually indents further and acquires its typical lobation. As the cells age, the nucleus increases in lobation, the number of lobes usually varying from three to five. The mature cells enter the sinusoids and thus reach the blood stream.

In each of the aforementioned myelocyte stages, the neutrophils far outnumber the eosinophils and basophils. The granular leukocyte precursors far outnumber the progenitors of the erythrocytes. This preponderance of early leukocyte forms over erythrocyte progenitors is in contrast to the opposite relationship in blood. The difference in numerical relationship can be explained partly by the fact that erythrocytes survive for a much longer time in the circulation than do the leukocytes.

Megakaryocytes and Platelet Formation

The megakaryocytes are giant cells (30 to 100 μ or more in diameter) which are thought to be derived from the hemocytoblast. They are characteristic of all adult mammalian bone marrow, and they may be found also in the hemopoietic tissues (liver, spleen) during embryonic development. The nucleus is complexly lobed, and individual lobes may be closely packed or connected by fine strands of chromatin material. The cytoplasm is finely granular and exhibits a patchy basophilia. The cell outline often is indistinct since pseudopodial cytoplasmic processes extend through the walls of the sinusoids.

Megakaryocytes arise from hemocytoblasts by a peculiar form of nuclear division in which the nucleus undergoes multiple mitotic divisions

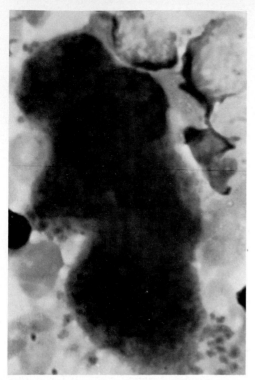

Figure 8-10. Bone marrow smear. A megakaryocyte, which exhibits active platelet formation, occupies the majority of the field. Leishman stain. × 450.

without cytoplasmic division. The number of mitoses is not known. After their formation, megakaryocytes extend cytoplasmic processes which become pinched off as platelets. Electron microscopic studies have revealed an extensive development of smooth surfaced membranes within the cytoplasm, thus dividing it up into small compartments and delineating the extent of future platelets. Megakaryocytes are short-lived and stages of degeneration are seen commonly. After the peripheral cytoplasm is shed as platelets, the megakaryocytes become shrunken and their nuclei fragment.

Development of Lymphoid Elements

The development of lymphocytes and monocytes occurs in the lymphoid tissues but cannot be followed as readily as that of the myeloid elements. Morphological evidence of differentiation is not marked. The appearance of definitive characteristics such as nuclear disappearance or lobation, cytoplasmic granulation, and loss of cytoplasmic basophilia does not occur in lymphocytes and monocytes, which retain the cytoplasmic basophilia and generally primitive nuclear shape of the stem cell.

The stroma of lymphoid tissue, like that of myeloid tissue, contains a framework of reticular fibers closely associated with primitive reticular cells and fixed macrophages. The sinuses present within lymphoid tissue are lined by *littoral cells* of the reticuloendothelial system. The meshes of the stroma contain the free cells, megakaryocytes, and some fat cells.

Free Cells

LYMPHOCYTES. Some of the undifferentiated reticular cells present within the stroma differentiate into *large* and *medium-sized lymphocytes* characterized by basophil cytoplasm and pale staining nuclei with distinct nucleoli. These immature lymphocytes resemble the hemocytoblasts of bone marrow and, according to the unitarian theory of development, they are the same cells in a different location. (Proponents of the dualistic theory claim that the large lymphocytes differ slightly from the hemocytoblasts and can differentiate only into lymphoid elements; thus they are called *lymphoblasts.*) These primitive cells, both large and medium-sized lymphocytes, are a direct differentiation of the primitive reticular cells and proliferate actively. They, in turn, differentiate into small lymphocytes which enter the circulation via the lymphatics.

In postnatal mammals most lymphocytes arise by proliferation of preexisting lymphocytes within the lymphoid tissues, principally within lymph nodes and the spleen. Only when such a production is unable to

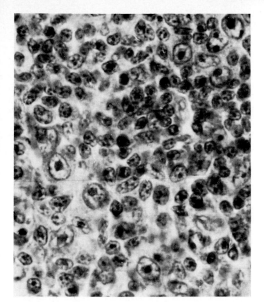

Figure 8-11. A small portion of a sectioned germinal center of a lymph nodule. A few large lymphocytes (lymphoblasts), distinguished by the presence of a large pale nucleus containing a distinct nucleolus, lie between the small lymphocytes. × 650.

supply the demand for lymphocytes is it likely that there is any marked differentiation from primitive reticular cells. It is apparent that small lymphocytes retain the ability to divide mitotically and must be considered as multipotential cells with regard to hemopoiesis.

It should be noted that radiographic studies, aimed principally at determining the life span of lymphocytes, have indicated that they represent a heterogeneous collection of cells. There are at least two distinct populations of lymphocytes: one group has a life span of months and possibly years; the other group lives for a matter of a few days only. In the main, it is the former group which recirculates between blood and lymph and which may be a transient inhabitant of connective tissue. The latter group is found principally in the thymus and in bone marrow.

MONOCYTES. The main site of development of monocytes is said to be within the spleen although in addition many authorities claim that monocytes develop in large numbers within the liver and bone marrow. Numerous theories exist as to their origin, and macrophages, hemocytoblasts, *monoblasts,* and lymphocytes have all been implicated as parent cells. The unitarian view recognizes that monocytes develop from hemocytoblasts directly or via a lymphocyte stage since the latter cell is thought to retain developmental potencies identical with those of the hemocytoblast. That monocytes may develop from lymphocytes appears most plausible if one studies the two cell types in a blood smear, where it is impossible to separate many monocytes as a cell type distinct from lymphocytes. Many transitional forms between the two cell types exist. There has been much confusion in the past with regard to the origin of monocytes and the question is best summarized by stating that they appear to be lymphocytes which have developed in a phagocytic direction. Monocytes are not actively phagocytic, but they acquire the ability to store vital dyes as they develop into macrophages in response to some stimulation such as is provided at a site of inflammation.

Embryonic Development of Blood Cells

The initiation of hemopoiesis is the same in all sites and consists of a rounding up of mesenchymal cells into free cells whose cytoplasm acquires a definite basophil character. These cells (hemocytoblasts) proliferate actively and then become transformed into *primitive erythroblasts* by the elaboration and accumulation of hemoglobin within their cytoplasm. Such a process occurs initially within the yolk sac during the third week of development. Blood formation begins in the liver at about six weeks and hemocytoblasts present here probably are brought in part by the circulation; in part they may develop from mesenchymal cells present between the strands of liver cells. The hemocytoblasts proliferate and differentiate into nucleated and nonnucleated red cells, leukocytes, and megakaryocytes. The formation of nucleated red cells gradually diminishes prior to the middle of fetal life. Hemopoiesis occurs within the spleen between the second and eighth months, and myelopoiesis ceases at or just after birth although lymphocytes and monocytes continue to be produced within the spleen postnatally. Lymph nodes develop relatively late during fetal life and production of myeloid elements is never a marked activity within them. However, they continue to function throughout life, like the spleen, in the production of lymphocytes.

The myeloid tissue of bone marrow appears in the third fetal month when the cartilaginous primordia of the bones become invaded by mesenchyme during the process of ossification. Again mesenchymal cells round off and become hemocytoblasts, which

give rise to erythroblasts, myelocytes, monocytes, and megakaryocytes. With the appearance of bone marrow, production of nucleated red cells ceases.

INTERRELATIONSHIPS BETWEEN CELLS OF BLOOD AND CONNECTIVE TISSUES: DEVELOPMENTAL POTENTIALITIES

Mesenchymal cells have great potentiality. They are able to differentiate along any one of several lines leading to the formation of many different kinds of cells in the connective tissues (Figure 8-13). The process of cellular differentiation implies the acquisition of a property or properties not possessed previously and leads to specialization.

It is important to realize that complete differentiation is not achieved by all cells. Maximow originated the concept that in the development of any kind of adult connective tissue from mesenchyme some undifferentiated cells remain as a reservoir of multipotential cells. It should be appreciated that there is a tendency for the process of differentiation to be halted somewhere along the line of differentiation. Thus in any connective tissue there may be cells which are undifferentiated, cells which are partially differentiated, and cells which have achieved complete differentiation.

Two further concepts with regard to the process of cellular differentiation remain to be considered. In general, the more differentiated a cell becomes, the more restricted its developmental potencies. Once a cell has achieved a certain degree of differentiation along a particular line, further differentiation is possible only along the original line of differentiation. The second point is that once differentiation has been completed cellular proliferation becomes markedly restricted. Many specialized cells are incapable of division.

Interrelationships between cells of

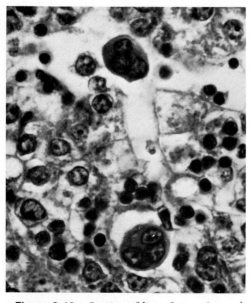

Figure 8-12. Section of liver from a 6 month old human fetus. Note the presence of extramedullary hemopoiesis. Numerous myeloid elements, principally of the erythrocyte series, lie between the plates of liver cells. Note the two megakaryocytes. × 650.

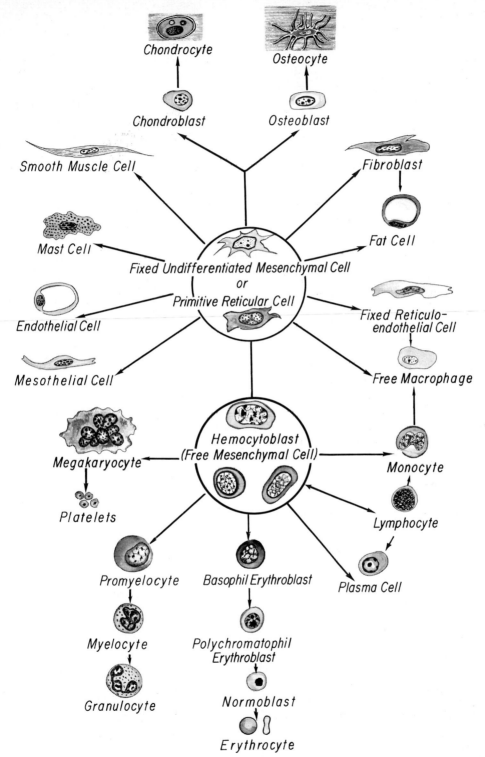

Figure 8-13. Diagram to illustrate the interrelationships between cells of blood and connective tissues.

blood and connective tissues appear confusing and somewhat tenuous at first sight, but become apparent under certain conditions in tissue culture, in response to disease processes, and in extramedullary hemopoiesis. Studies of such conditions demonstrate that hemocytoblasts (lymphocytes) possess fibrocytic and phagocytic potencies as well as hemopoietic potencies. One can summarize the relationship by saying that lymphocytes represent a mobile reserve of mesenchymal cells which, together with the fixed undifferentiated mesenchymal cells present in adult connective tissues, constitute a group of multipotential cells. None of these tissues is stable. Cell loss is balanced by replacement, a process which involves multiplication of undifferentiated cells and their differentiation.

Metaplasia is a process which illustrates well the concepts of cellular differentiation just described. It occurs under certain pathological conditions when one specialized type of connective tissue appears to transform into another. This, in fact, is not the case since specialized cellular elements are unable to differentiate. Actually metaplasia represents a replacement of one type of connective tissue by another from undifferentiated cells present within the tissue. It occurs in response to altered environmental factors.

REFERENCES

Archer, G. T., and Hirsch, J. C.: Motion picture studies of degranulation of horse eosinophils during phagocytosis. J. Exp. Med., *118*:287, 1963.

Bessis, M.: The blood cells and their formation. *In* The Cell: Biochemistry, Physiology, Morphology, edited by J. Brachet and A. E. Mirsky. New York, Academic Press, 1961, Vol. 5, p. 163.

Braunsteiner, H., and Zucker-Franklin, D.: The Physiology and Pathology of Leucocytes. New York, Grune & Stratton, 1962.

Cronkite, E. P., Bond, V. P., Fliedner, T. M., Paglia, D. A., and Adamik, E. R.: Studies on the origin, production and destruction of platelets. *In* Blood Platelets, edited by S. A. Johnson, R. W. Monto, I. W. Rebuck, and R. C. Horn. Boston, Little, Brown and Co., 1961, p. 595.

Custer, R. P.: Atlas of the Blood and Bone Marrow. Philadelphia, W. B. Saunders Co., 1949.

Daniels, J. C., Ritzmann, S. E., and Levin, W. C.: Lymphocytes: Morphological, developmental and functional characteristics in health, disease, and experimental study—an analytical review. Texas Rep. Biol. Med., *26*:5, 1968.

Davidson, W. M., and Smith, D. R.: A morphological sex difference in the polymorphonuclear leucocytes. Brit. Med. J., *2*:6, 1954.

Diggs, L. W., Sturm, D., and Bell, B. A.: The Morphology of Human Blood Cells. Philadelphia, W. B. Saunders Co., 1956.

Downey, H.: Handbook of Hematology. New York, Paul B. Hoeber, 1938.

Elves, M. W.: The Lymphocytes. London, Lloyd Luke Ltd., 1966.

Hirsch, I. G., and Cohn, Z. A.: Degranulation of polymorphonuclear leucocytes following phagocytosis of microorganisms. J. Exp. Med., *112*:1005, 1960.

Low, F. N., and Freeman, J. A., Sr.: Electron Microscopic Atlas of Normal and Leukemic Human Blood. New York, Blakiston Division of McGraw-Hill, 1958.

Miller, F., de Harven, E., and Palade, G. E.: The structure of eosinophil leukocyte granules in rodent and in man. J. Cell. Biol., *31*:349, 1966.

Pease, D. C.: An electron microscopic study of red bone marrow. J. Hemat., *2*:501, 1956.

Rebuck, J. W. (editor): The Lymphocyte and Lymphocytic Tissue. New York, Paul B. Hoeber, 1960.

Rodman, N. F., Painter, J. C., and McDevitt, N.B.: Platelet disintegration during clotting. J. Cell Biol., *16*:225, 1963.

Sabin, F. R.: Studies of living human blood cells. Bull. Johns Hopkins Hosp., *34*:277, 1923.

Sabin, F. R.: Bone marrow. Physiol. Rev., 8:191, 1928.

Simpson, C. F., and Kling, J. M.: The mechanism of denucleation in circulating erythroblasts. J. Cell Biol., *35*:237, 1967.

Skutelsky, E., and Danon, D.: An electron microscopic study of nuclear elimination from the late erythroblast. J. Cell Biol., *33*:625, 1967.

Sorenson, G. D.: An electron microscopic study of hematopoiesis in the liver of the fetal rabbit. Amer. J. Anat., *106*:27, 1960.

Weiss, L.: The structure of fine splenic arterial vessels in relation to hemoconcentration and red cell destruction. Amer. J. Anat., *111*:131, 1962.

Yoffey, J. M., and Courtice, F. C.: Lymphatics, Lymph and Lymphoid Tissue. Cambridge, Harvard University Press, 1956.

CHAPTER 9

MUSCLE

Muscle tissue is specialized for producing movement both of the body as a whole and of the many parts with respect to one another. Muscle cells show great development of the function of contractility and, to a lesser extent, of conductivity. This specialization involves elongation of the cells in the axis of contraction and because of this the cells often are referred to as muscle fibers.*

In muscle tissue, muscle cells or fibers usually are grouped into bundles, but muscle tissue consists of more than just muscle fibers. Muscle fibers, because they perform mechanical work, require a rich blood supply to provide food materials and oxygen and to eliminate toxic waste products. The blood vessels are carried in fibroconnective tissue which also serves to bind together the muscle fibers and to provide a harness for them so that their pull may be exerted usefully. Nerves also run in the connective tissue.

There are three types of muscle and these are classified on both a struc-

tural and a functional basis. Regular transverse bands along the length of the fibers are present in *striated* muscle and absent in *smooth* muscle. Functionally, muscle either is under the control of the will (*voluntary* muscle) or is not (*involuntary* muscle). The three types of muscle are smooth involuntary muscle, present chiefly in hollow organs; striated voluntary or skeletal muscle, attached to bones or fascia and constituting the flesh of the limbs and body wall; and striated involuntary or cardiac muscle, forming the wall of the heart and extending into the major veins opening into the heart.

For histological study of muscular tissue, sectioned material (for light and electron microscopy) is used mainly but useful additional information may be obtained from *macerated tissue*. Small pieces of muscle are immersed in a solution of 10 per cent hydrochloric acid in physiological saline for 24 to 48 hours. After rinsing in water, individual muscle fibers can be teased out on a microscope slide using two mounted needles, covered with a glass coverslip, and examined under the microscope.

---

*Note on terminology: There is a special terminology associated with muscle tissue: protoplasm is called sarcoplasm (*sarcos* = muscle) and the cell membrane complex is the sarcolemma. Other terms used are sarcoplasmic reticulum (endoplasmic reticulum), sarcosome (mitochondrion), and sarcomere (a linear unit); myofilaments and myofibrils are contractile elements.

SMOOTH MUSCLE

This type also is called unstriped, nonstriated, or involuntary muscle.

Individual cells are fusiform, elongated, and closely associated with connective tissue. Smooth muscle mainly is visceral in distribution, forming the contractile portion of the wall of the digestive tract from the midpoint of the esophagus to the anus, including the ducts of glands associated with the system. It is found in the respiratory, urinary, and genital systems and in arteries, veins, and larger lymphatic ducts. In addition it is present in the dermis and in the iris and ciliary body of the eye.

Shape and Size

Smooth muscle fibers are elongated, spindle-shaped cells with fine tapering ends and a wider central region in

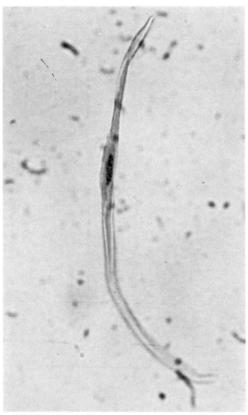

Figure 9-1. Photomicrograph of a single teased smooth muscle cell from the tunica muscularis of the human duodenum. × 660.

which the nucleus is situated. In size, they vary with location, being only 20 microns or less in length around small ducts and blood vessels, but reaching 0.5 mm. in the pregnant uterus. Generally throughout the intestinal tract and in association with larger blood vessels, they are about 0.2 mm. long and about 6 microns in diameter at the midpoint of the cell. The sarcoplasm of a smooth muscle cell in a stained preparation is acidophil and usually appears homogeneous but may show small, clear areas which probably indicate the location of glycogen. In special preparations—for example, after gentle maceration in acid—fine longitudinal striations can be demonstrated. These are the myofibrils or contractile elements. Cytoplasmic organelles are few and are grouped near the nucleus. The nucleus in cross section of the fiber is central or slightly eccentric in position. Owing to the length of the fibers, nuclei are seen in only a few cells in cross section. The nucleus is elongated, oval, or cylindrical, has a fine chromatin network, and thus does not stain darkly. It contains one or more nucleoli. In cells fixed during contraction, nuclei characteristically show a folded or twisted shape.

Organization

In many regions of the body, particularly in the dermis, smooth muscle cells are scattered singly or in small groups and are associated intimately with connective tissue. Individual cells are embedded in bundles of reticular or thin elastic fibers, and small groups of cells, e.g., in association with hairs, often are held in a small cylindrical mass or fascicle, covered by a fine envelope or sheath of fibroelastic tissue. The other common arrangement is in sheets, the fibers all being orientated in the same direction in each sheet. Often two such sheets form the contractile wall

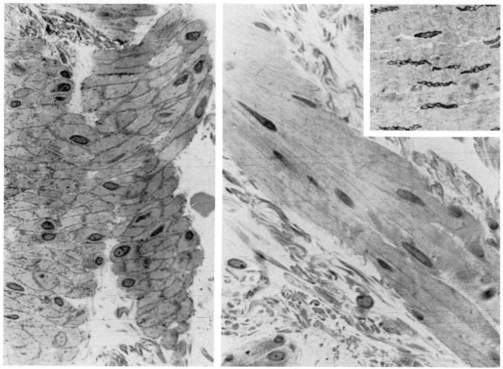

Figure 9-2.   Left: Photomicrograph of a cross section of smooth muscle from the tunica muscularis of the human duodenum. × 650. Right: Longitudinal section. × 650. Epon sections. Insert (top right): Wrinkled nuclei of smooth muscle cells in contraction. × 550. Note the appearance of extracellular collagen around the muscle cells.   See filmstrip I, frame 30.

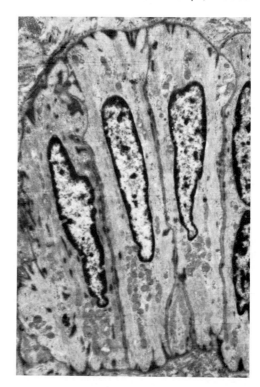

Figure 9-3.   Survey electron micrograph of smooth muscle from the artery of a rat. These cells are curved around the blood vessel; the section is tangential. × 3500.

a myofibril as seen by light microscopy, are a few mitochondria and small dense, oval bodies. Similar dense areas are present along the inner aspect of the plasma membrane. The dense bodies, which resemble Z bands of striated muscle (see later), and the dense areas at the plasma membrane represent points for attachment of the myofilaments. Between attachment areas the plasma membrane shows numerous small vesicular inpocketings or *caveoli*, presumably indicative of micropinocytosis.

In striated muscle two types of myofilament can be identified, actin and myosin, but while both chemically are present in smooth muscle, only the type of myofilament composed of actin is readily seen. Recently small lateral processes protruding from the actin myofilaments have been demonstrated and these probably are myosin, present in a relatively nonaggregated form. In striped muscle contraction occurs by a sliding filament mechanism (see later); in contraction of smooth muscle also, the actin myofilaments do not change their length. Thus it is theorized that here too contraction is achieved by actin filaments sliding with respect to one another and driven by small units of myosin.

Around the plasma membrane of smooth muscle cells is a basal lamina closely associated with unit fibers of collagen, which constitute the fine, argyrophil reticular fibers of light microscopy. Over limited areas basal laminae of adjacent smooth muscle cells may be lacking, with very close apposition of adjacent plasma membranes. In such regions the outer laminae of opposing unit membranes appear to fuse in a similar manner to the zonula occludens of epithelial cell junctions. Such a region is termed the fascia occludens or *nexus*. Probably nexi represent regions of low resistance for rapid spread of excitatory impulses from one cell to its neighbor. In the wall of the small intestine, in the esophagus, and in the uterus, actual cytoplasmic bridges between adjacent cells have been described. In addition, the dense areas of plasma membranes where myofilaments attach, described previously, often are opposite one another. This suggests cell cohesion at such sites.

Origin, Growth, and Regeneration

The great majority of smooth muscle develops by the differentiation of mesenchymal cells. However, in association with some glands and their ducts, e.g., salivary, sweat, and lacrimal glands, cells with many of the characteristics of smooth muscle differentiate from ectoderm and are called myoepithelial cells (see Chapter 5). Smooth muscle cells can increase in size in response to physiological stimuli (e.g., in the uterus in pregnancy) and pathological stimuli (e.g., in arterioles in hypertension). There also is evidence that although the increase in bulk (for example, of the uterus in pregnancy) is due mainly to an increased size of individual muscle cells, there also may be an increase in the number of cells following differentiation of mesenchymal cells present in the uterus. There is some evidence that smooth muscle cells themselves can divide by mitosis.

Differentiation Between Smooth Muscle and Collagen Fibers

One of the most common difficulties in identification of tissues is that of distinguishing between smooth muscle and connective tissue. Muscle fibers are cellular and usually stain more intensely with eosin than do collagen fibers. Nuclei are situated *within* the fibers, may be wrinkled, and are larger than the nuclei of fibroblasts which are situated *between* collagen fibers. Certain staining techniques, e.g., Mallory and van Gieson, readily distinguish between the two.

STRIATED MUSCLE

Striated or skeletal muscle is that which the layman recognizes as muscle and comprises the flesh or meat of animals. In the fresh state, human striated muscle has a pink color owing partly to a pigment in the muscle fibers and partly to the rich vascularity of the tissue, but there is some variation in color and "red" and "white" muscles have been recognized. The individual striated muscle fiber or cell is long, cylindrical, and multinucleate, the ends tapering to a point or being somewhat rounded or notched at the junction of muscle and tendon. Each fiber is independent and may be of great length, e.g., in the sartorius muscle of the thigh where the fibers are arranged in parallel fashion and extend from the muscle origin on the innominate bone to the insertion on the upper medial aspect of the tibia. In many muscles, however, individual fibers are shorter than the overall length of the muscle, one end being attached to tendon and the other to a connective tissue septum within the muscle. Variations in arrangement are described in textbooks of gross anatomy, but it is accepted generally that the power of a muscle is dependent not upon the length of the component muscle fibers but upon the total number of fibers present in the muscle.

In teased preparations of fresh or macerated muscle, individual fibers have a faint yellow coloration and are striated in both longitudinal and transverse directions. Fibers vary from 1 to 40 mm. in length, and from 10 to 100 microns in diameter. Nuclei are numerous in each fiber, there being about 35 per mm. of length. They are ovoid, situated peripherally in the fiber, and orientated lengthwise. An individual fiber is limited by a thin, structureless membrane, the sarcolemma, which is seen to advantage in regions where muscle fibers have been crushed with consequent retraction of sarcoplasm within the sarcolemma.

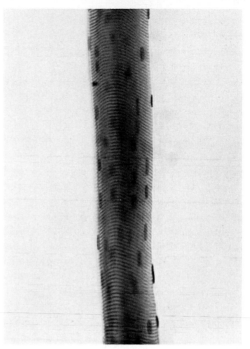

Figure 9-6. Photomicrograph of a single teased skeletal (striated) muscle fiber from human gastrocnemius muscle. × 275.

See filmstrip I, frame 31.

The sarcolemma of light microscopy is seen by electron microscopy to consist of a complex of the plasma membrane of the muscle cell, the supporting extracellular basal lamina and a fine network of associated reticular fibers. In the sarcoplasm there are numerous sarcosomes (mitochondria) and a small Golgi apparatus near each nucleus. Both lipid and glycogen are present as inclusions, together with the pigment myoglobin. Lying in the sarcoplasm are the myofibrils, composed of bundles of myofilaments.

Myofibrils and Striation

By light microscopy, the cytoplasm of each striated muscle fiber in longitudinal section shows alternating thin discs or bands of light and dark material, the dark bands being anisotropic (birefringent) and the light ones isotropic when seen with polarized light. Hence, the dark and light bands

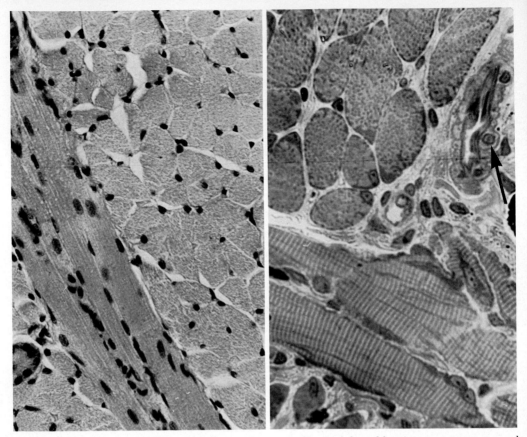

Figure 9-7.   Photomicrographs of the striated muscle fibers of the rabbit tongue cut in cross and longitudinal section. Left, × 250. Right, epon section, × 450. Note the smooth muscle fibers in the wall of the arteriole cut in cross section (arrow).

are called respectively "A" and "I" bands. The lighter I band is intersected by a thin dark line, the "Z" band. Although the A, I, and Z bands appear to cross the entire muscle fiber, in a good preparation all three are seen to be limited to the myofibrils and do not extend across the sarcoplasm lying between them. Other bands in the myofibril are visible occasionally. These are the pale, thin H bands bisecting the dark A band and, within this, a very fine, dark M or middle stripe. The N band, only rarely visible, is a dark band lying in the I band between the Z and A bands.

In a cross section of a striated muscle fiber, the various bands are not seen, but the myofibrils are seen as small spherical or polygonal dots and are separated from adjacent bundles by clear sarcoplasm. The separation of myofibrils by areas of sarcoplasm reveals the so-called areas or fields of Cohnheim. The peripheral nuclei are obvious also in cross section.

In longitudinal section, the cross bands are distinct in *relaxed* muscle, and it is customary to consider the muscle fibril as composed of structural units. Each unit extends between adjacent Z lines and is termed a *sarcomere*. In muscle fixed in a *contracted* state, the fibrils are thicker and the sarcomeres shorter, the distance between Z lines progressively shortening with the extent of contraction. As the I bands become shorter, the ends of the A bands approach the Z lines. Eventually A and I bands are indis-

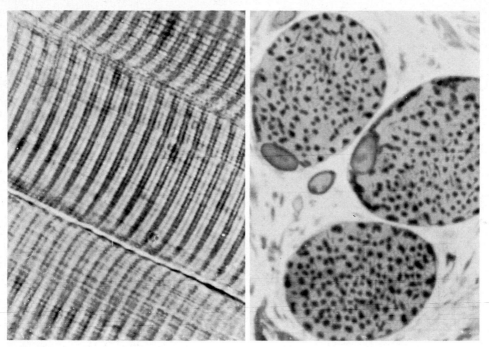

Figure 9-8. Left: Photomicrograph of striated muscle fibers from human gastrocnemius in longitudinal section showing A, I, Z, and H bands. × 1250. Right: Striated muscle of rabbit tongue in transverse section. Note the numerous mitochondria. Epon section. × 1000. See filmstrip I, frame 32.

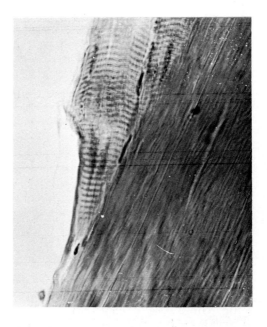

Figure 9-9. Photomicrograph of a striated muscle fiber of rabbit gastrocnemius inserting into its tendon. × 670.

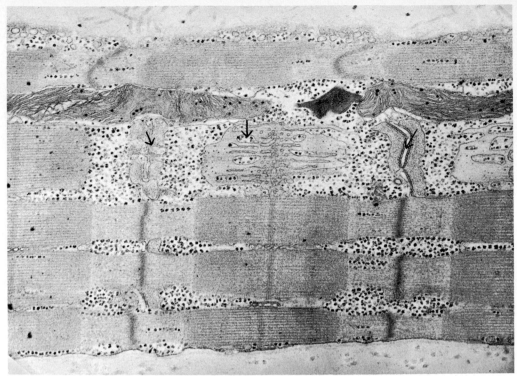

Figure 9-10. Electron micrograph of a longitudinal section of frog sartorius muscle. In the top center, a sheet of the sarcoplasmic reticulum (center arrow) at the level of the A band is grazed by the plane of section. Triads (left and right arrows) are visible at the level of the two Z lines. The dark granules between myofibrils are glycogen. Note also mitochondria and a lipid droplet (dark, angular mass). × 24,000. (Courtesy of Dr. H. E. Huxley.)

tinguishable, *but the length of the A band in contraction remains constant.* The explanation for this is discussed on page 167.

Fine Structure

The *sarcolemma* is too thin to be resolved clearly with the light microscope, but electron microscopy shows it to consist of the plasma membrane of the muscle cell covered by a fine extracellular basal lamina with which a few unit fibrils of collagen are associated. Fine slips of elastic tissue also are present between adjacent muscle fibers.

In the sarcoplasm, the mitochondria or *sarcosomes* are numerous and large, each with closely packed cristae. This is to be expected in view of the high energy requirements for muscle contraction. Sarcosomes lie subjacent to the sarcolemma, concentrated near the poles of the elongated nuclei, and in parallel rows between the myofibrils: in all sites they lie with their long axes along the length of the fiber. Also in a paranuclear position is a small Golgi apparatus. Scattered throughout the sarcoplasm may be small dense granules 200 to 400 Å in diameter, which probably are glycogen, and small masses of lipid also may be present.

Sarcoplasmic reticulum corresponds to the endoplasmic reticulum of other cell types, but its membranes are not associated with ribosomes. The sarcoplasmic reticulum comprises an extensive, continuous system of membrane-limited sarcotubules enclosing each myofibril as in a net. Over the

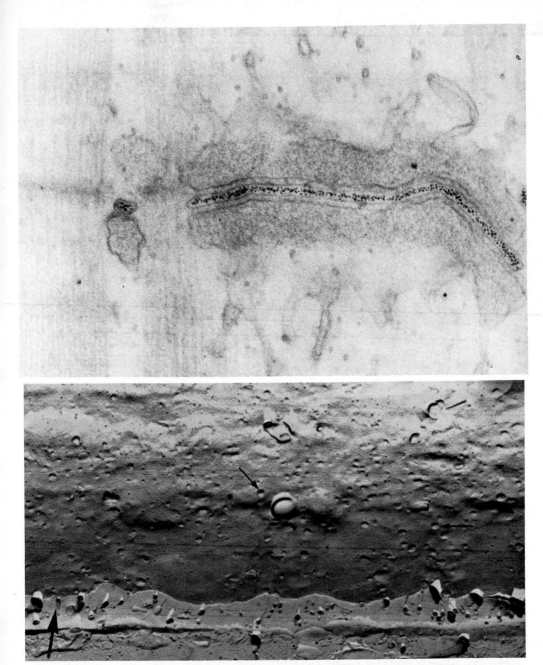

Figure 9-11.   Top: Electron micrograph of frog sartorius muscle after bathing in ferritin. The ferritin particles (small, dense granules) have penetrated from the exterior into the transverse tubule of a triad, thus demonstrating continuity of the system with the exterior. × 145,000. (Courtesy of Dr. H. E. Huxley.) Bottom: Electron micrograph of a freeze-etch preparation of striated muscle. The fracture has exposed the outer surface of the plasma membrane in which numerous pits or depressions are visible (thin arrows). These are believed to represent apertures of transverse tubules or of caveolae (micropinocytotic vesicles). Myofibrils run longitudinally across the cell. The direction of metal shadowing is indicated by the broad arrow. × 14,800 longitudinally. (Courtesy of Dr. D. G. Rayns.)

length of the A band, the sarcotubules are arranged longitudinally with frequent cross connections in the region of the H band. A similar arrangement covers the I band. As longitudinal tubules approach the A-I junction from each side, they are connected to dilated, transverse cisternae called terminal cisternae. The two terminal cisternae of a pair are separated by a central, smaller transverse tubule, the T tubule, located at the A-I junction. This arrangement of two outer terminal cisternae of sarcoplasmic reticulum and a central T tubule is called a *triad*, and there are two triads to each sarcomere in mammalian muscle. (In amphibian muscle, a triad encircles each I band at the Z line.) The T tubule is not part of the sarcoplasmic reticulum and its lumen is not continuous with that of the reticulum. T tubules are tubular invaginations from the surface sarcolemma, their lumina being continuous with the extracellu-lar space (see Figure 9-11). Collectively, the T tubules are referred to as the *T system*.

Myofibrils, which on light microscopy appear as long, parallel, unbranching threads 2 to 3 microns in diameter, by electron microscopy are found to be bundles of more slender units, the myofilaments. These are of two types differing in dimensions and chemical composition. The cross banding seen on light microscopy is simply a reflection of the distribution of the two types of myofilaments. The thicker *myosin* filaments are 100 Å in diameter and 1.5 microns long. They are confined to the A band, in parallel array and about 450 Å apart. They show slight thickening at their centers and taper at the extremities. At the central thickenings, they are held by slender cross connections, thus giving rise to the transverse M line. In cross section, they are seen to be arranged in a regular hexagonal pattern. The thinner

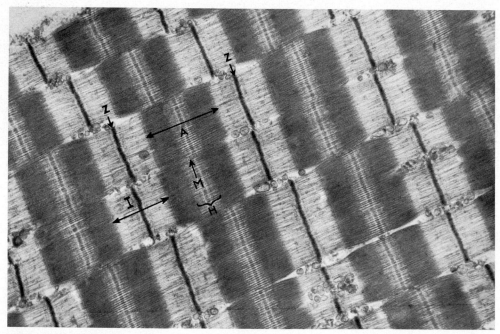

Figure 9-12. Electron micrograph, showing portions of seven myofibrils cut longitudinally from the noncontracted (i.e., relaxed) psoas muscle of a rabbit. The dark A (anisotropic) bands are bisected by the lighter H bands in which there is a thin, dark M band. The I (isotropic) bands are bisected by very dark Z lines. A single sarcomere extends from one Z line to the next Z line. × 13,000. (Courtesy of Dr. H. E. Huxley.)

actin filaments are 50 Å in diameter and 2 microns long with their midpoints at the Z line and extending for about 1 micron on each side of it. Thus, they form the I band but are not confined to it, extending into the A bands between myosin filaments for a short distance in a relaxed fiber. In cross section at the periphery of the A band, six actin filaments surround each myosin filament. The extent of the overlap and interdigitation of the two types of myofilaments varies with the state of contraction and determines the width of the H band. The H band is simply the central area of the A band free of actin filaments. In cross sections in the regions of overlap, small cross bridges extend radially from

myosin filaments toward surrounding actin filaments. The nature of the Z line remains undecided. It often shows a zigzag pattern on longitudinal section. As actin filaments approach it from adjacent sarcomeres, four fine strands leave each filament and form interlacing loops. This arrangement may be responsible entirely for the formation of the Z line, or the zigzag mesh may be formed by the addition of tropomyosin.

Mechanism of Contraction

The theory of the "sliding filament mechanism" now is accepted generally. It is evident by phase contrast

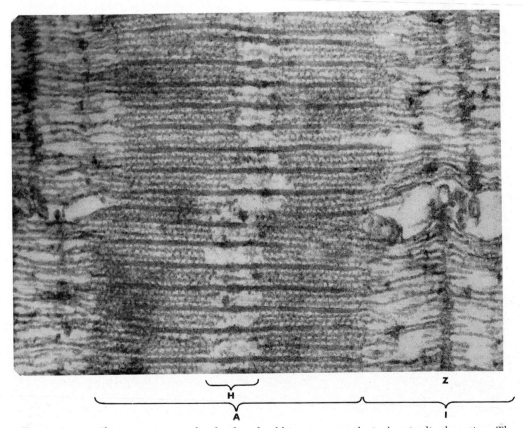

Figure 9-13. Electron micrograph of relaxed rabbit psoas muscle in longitudinal section. The thick myosin filaments extend throughout the length of the A band; the thin actin filaments are found in the I band and extend into the A band as far as the H band. There are two actin filaments between every two myosin filaments. Cross linkages between actin and myosin filaments are visible. × 74,000. (Courtesy of Dr. H. E. Huxley.)

and interference microscopy that in contraction the A band remains constant in length while the I band and the H band both diminish. The sliding filament mechanism involves a change in relative position of the two sets of myofilaments although neither the myosin nor the actin filaments are altered in length. During contraction, the thin actin filaments slide past the thick myosin filaments so that the ends of the former extend further into the A band, with consequent narrowing and, eventually, obliteration of the H band. Naturally, the I band decreases in width, the thick myosin filaments approach the Z lines, and the sarcomere is shortened. This mechanism involves a change in the site of attachment of the spines of the thick fila-

ments to the thin actin filaments, each spine breaking one attachment and making others successively further along the actin filament. This slides the filaments past each other in the manner of an animated cogwheel. Energy for the process is derived from the breakdown of adenosine triphosphate (ATP) to adenosine diphosphate (ADP) by ATPase localized in the bridges.

The role of the T system and the sarcoplasmic reticulum in contraction and relaxation has been clarified recently. Following stimulation, all myofibrils contract simultaneously and instantaneously. It is known also that contraction in a myofibril commences at the A-I junction, i.e., at the site of the triad. Further, calcium

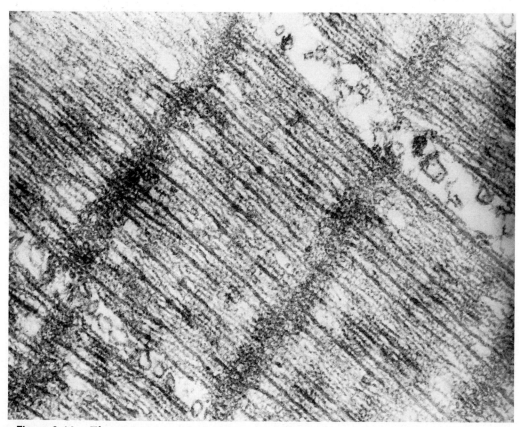

Figure 9-14.   Electron micrograph of contracted rabbit psoas muscle in longitudinal section. Compare with Figure 9-13: The I and H bands have disappeared. × 74,000. (Courtesy of Dr. H. E. Huxley.)

in the fluid around myofibrils is known to be necessary for muscle contraction and it is believed that the great majority of calcium in muscle is concentrated in the sarcoplasmic reticulum. Following ι stimulation, membrane depolarization of the sarcolemma spreads to the interior of the fiber by the T system. This depolarization, by some mechanism, causes release of calcium ions from the sarcoplasmic reticulum to the myofibrils. In turn, the calcium ions activate myosin ATPase to break down ATP to ADP, with energy release and contraction of the actomyosin system as just described. At the end of contraction, calcium ions return to the sarcoplasmic reticulum and relaxation occurs.

Organization of Striated Muscle Fibers into Muscles

In a muscle, muscle fibers lie in a parallel arrangement held together by fibroconnective tissue. The entire muscle is wrapped in a substantial envelope of connective tissue, the *epimysium*. On cross section of a muscle, finer partitions of connective tissue, the *perimysium*, lie around bundles or fascicles of muscle fibers, and still finer connective tissue extends from the perimysium into a muscle bundle, penetrating between individual muscle fibers. This tissue is the *endomysium*, and it consists of a network of reticular fibers carrying fine blood capillaries and a few con-

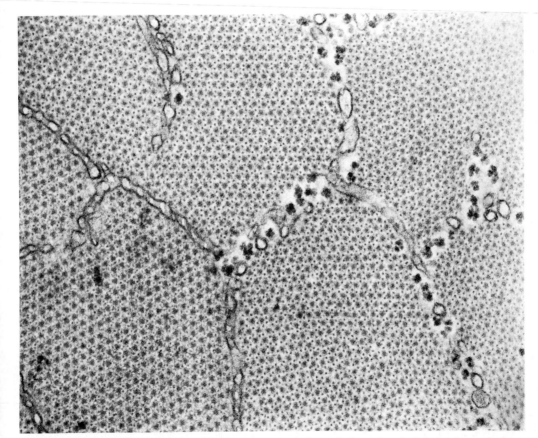

Figure 9-15.   Electron micrograph of a cross section through the A band of skeletal muscle from the frog sartorius. The thin actin filaments have a hexagonal arrangement around the thicker myosin filaments. × 50,000. (Courtesy of Dr. H. E. Huxley.)

nective tissue cells. The content of elastic fibers varies with the muscle but is prominent in the small muscles of the eye, face, and tongue. The total amount of fibroconnective tissue varies with the muscle. Some, e.g., gluteus maximus, have a large content and are coarse and relatively tough. Others, e.g., psoas major, have very little connective tissue and are tender: "filet mignon" is the psoas. Toughness of muscle thus is dependent on the amount of connective tissue and increases with age.

At the extremity of a muscle where it is attached, whether to a tendon, periosteum, aponeurosis, raphe, or dermis of the skin, the perimysium blends with, and is continuous with, the connective tissue of the attachment. Here the muscle fibers are cone-shaped and fit into the connective tissue like fingers into a glove, the sarcolemmal sheaths being the material of the gloves in the analogy. At the extremities of a muscle fiber, the myofibrils are connected to the sarcolemma. Thus there are physical and mechanical forces attaching muscle fibers to the muscle origins and insertions so that the pull of contraction may be employed usefully and without separation of muscle from tendon. Indeed, from a clinical point of view, such a separation rarely occurs, and it is more usual for a tendon to pull off a flake of bone at its attachment after a too powerful contraction.

Blood and Lymph Supply

Arteries pierce the epimysium to reach the substance of the muscle and branch, and smaller vessels run in the perimysium, finally to terminate as capillaries which lie in the endomysium between individual muscle fibers. Most of these lie longitudinally along fibers but cross anastomoses are common, forming an extremely rich plexus. Lymphatic vessels, to drain tissue fluid, are quite numerous, but are not found in close association with fibers. They lie in epimysium and perimysium, but are not present in endomysium.

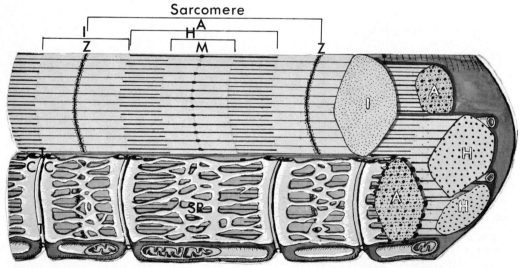

Figure 9-16.   Three-dimensional diagram of a portion of a mammalian striated muscle fiber with five myofibrils as seen by electron microscopy. The cut surfaces of the myofibrils show the appearances in cross section of A, I, and H bands. The sarcoplasmic reticulum (SR) surrounds the lowest myofibril with triads opposite A-I junctions, each composed of a central tubule (T) and two lateral cisternae (C). Mitochondria are shown within the sarcolemma.

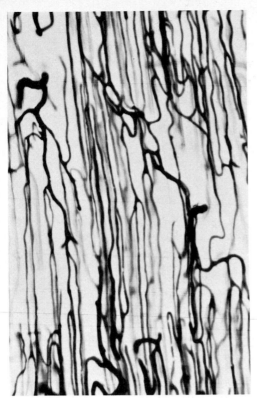

Figure 9-17. Photomicrograph of a thick section of human skeletal muscle after injection of the vascular system with colored gelatin. Muscle fibers unstained. × 170.

Nerve Supply

The nerve supply to a muscle enters through the epimysium at a point which is fairly constant—the so-called "motor point." It then branches, the branches lying in the perimysium. The number of muscle fibers supplied by one nerve fiber varies and is related to the delicacy of movement required. In the eye muscles, there is a nerve fiber supplying each muscle fiber, but in the larger muscles of the trunk and limbs, one nerve fiber may supply 100 or more muscle fibers. A single nerve together with the muscle fibers which it supplies is called a *motor unit*. This arrangement is important from the physiological point of view, for an individual muscle fiber cannot contract at different degrees of intensity.

It either contracts completely to maximum capacity or not at all: this is called the *all or none law*. Thus, the power of contraction of a muscle depends not upon the degree of contraction of its component muscle fibers but on the number of its fibers which contract.

As a terminal nerve fiber approaches the muscle fiber it supplies, it loses its myelin sheath and enters into a close association with the muscle fiber. This complex is termed a *motor end plate* or a *myoneural junction*. Here the endoneurium of the nerve blends with the endomysium of the muscle fiber. By electron microscopy it can be seen that the nerve axon, covered by the neurolemma, shows a terminal dilation which contains many small cytoplasmic vesicles, the synaptic vesicles. Beneath the nerve ending, the sarcoplasm—here called the soleplasm—shows a small moundlike protuberance in which sarcosomes and nuclei are numerous. In this region the sarcolemma is intact but shows irregularly grooved indentations in which amorphous ground substance is obvious. Silver impregnation techniques demonstrate the coarser features of the motor end plates for light microscopy.

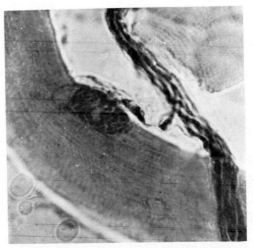

Figure 9-18. Photomicrograph of a neuromuscular junction. Gold chloride preparation. × 670.   See filmstrip II, frame 91.

Functional Correlations

Striated muscle has a more rapid contraction than smooth muscle. Two types of striated muscle fiber have been described: red and white. Red fibers are smaller, contain numerous mitochondria and proportionally fewer myofibrils, and are capable of a rapid rate of contraction without fatigue. The white fibers are larger and contain less mitochondria and proportionally more myofibrils. They are capable of a more powerful contraction but fatigue more rapidly. Many individual muscles (e.g., extraocular muscles) show a mixture of the two types of fiber. There is also a species difference and, in general, the smaller the animal, the higher the content of red fibers.

Muscles, as is well known, show an increase in size with exercise. This is due to an increase in the size of each individual muscle fiber (hypertrophy) and is not due to an increase in the number of fibers (hyperplasia).

Regeneration

After damage, degenerated muscle fibers can regenerate to a limited extent, but gross damage is repaired by connective tissue which thus leaves a scar. If the nerve or blood supply is interrupted, the muscle fibers degenerate and are replaced by fibrous tissue.

CARDIAC MUSCLE

Cardiac muscle, which is involuntary but striated, contracts rhythmically and automatically. It is found only in the myocardium (muscle layer of the heart) and in the walls of the large vessels joining the heart. A cardiac muscle fiber by light microscopy is a linear unit composed of several cardiac muscle cells joined end to end at specialized junctional zones called *intercalated discs*. The fibers in any region run mainly in parallel fashion, but "cross beams" are numerous and

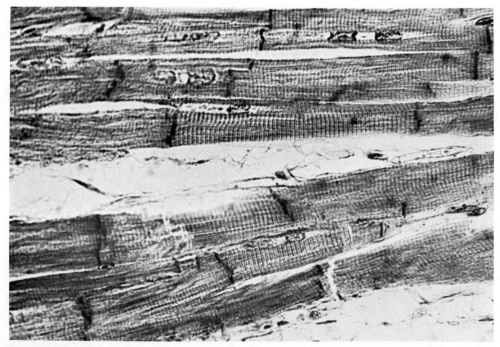

Figure 9-19. Photomicrograph of a longitudinal section of human cardiac muscle, showing intercalated discs. Iron hematoxylin and eosin. × 660.　　　See filmstrip I, frame 33.

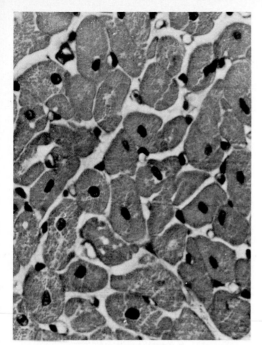

Figure 9-20. Photomicrograph of cardiac muscle fibers in transverse section. Note the central nuclei and the numerous capillaries between muscle fibers. × 400.

See filmstrip I, frame 34.

this gives the false impression of a syncytial network. Between the fibers is fine connective tissue, the endomysium, containing small blood vessels and lymphatics.

The cardiac muscle fiber is enveloped by a thin sarcolemma similar to that of skeletal muscle, and sarcoplasm is abundant with numerous mitochondria. Myofibrils are separated by mitochondria arranged in rows between them, with consequent obvious longitudinal striation. A pattern of cross striations of the myofibrils, with A, I, Z, M, and H bands identical to those of skeletal muscle, also is obvious. Nuclei are elongated and situated centrally in the fiber between diverging myofibrils. Around the nuclei are fusiform areas of sarcoplasm containing many mitochondria, a small Golgi apparatus at one pole of the nucleus, a few lipid droplets, and, with increasing age, some deposits of lipofuchsin pigment. This pigment may be so extensive as to give a

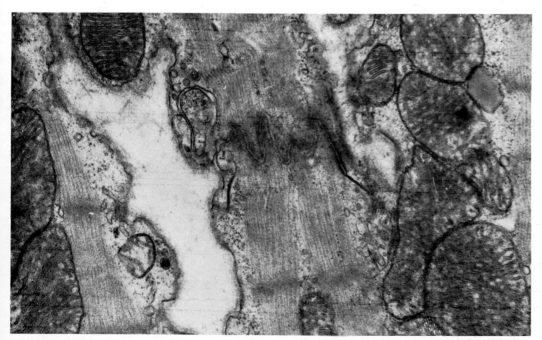

Figure 9-21. Electron micrograph of rat cardiac muscle. Note the large, numerous mitochondria, myofilaments, and the intercalated disc running transversely in the center of the picture. × 38,000.

brownish tinge to the fresh myocardium, a condition known as "brown atrophy of the heart." The sarcoplasm also contains larger deposits of glycogen than are found in skeletal muscle. By light microscopy, intercalated discs appear as dark lines which pass in an irregular, zigzag, or steplike manner transversely across the fibers at irregular intervals. They always cross fibers at the level of the Z lines and are more obvious in adult tissue, first appearing in late fetal life. Intercalated discs are areas of cell adhesion between adjacent cardiac muscle cells, specialized to transmit tension of the myofibrils along the axis of an entire fiber.

Fine Structure

Myofilaments of actin and myosin are identical to those of skeletal muscle and show a similar arrangement. They are limited to individual muscle cells and do not cross cell junctions. However, grouping of myofilaments into myofibrils is not complete as it is in skeletal muscle, and cross sections show that myofibrils are incompletely surrounded and delineated by sarcoplasmic reticulum and sarcoplasm. Mitochondria characteristically are large, about 2.5 microns long (the length of a sarcomere), and show closely packed cristae.

The *T tubules* of cardiac muscle resemble those of skeletal muscle in that they are invaginations of the sarcolemma but differ in that they are of greater diameter and lie at the Z lines and not at A-I junctions. The tubules are an extension of the extracellular space and contain extracellular basal lamina material continuous with that of the sarcolemma. The *sarcoplasmic reticulum* consists of longitudinal, interconnected tubules which expand into small terminal sacs to contact a T tubule at the Z line, but no large terminal cisternae are present. Thus the total area of contact between the sarcoplasmic reticulum and the T tubules is less than in skeletal muscle.

The *intercalated discs* are areas of extensive cell contact. If two cells could be separated at a disc, the opposing surfaces would show a complex pattern of ridges and papillae and reciprocal grooves and pits. Opposed plasma membranes show areas comparable to the macula adherens (desmosome), zonula adherens, and zonula occludens of junctional complexes of epithelia (page 83). Generally, in regions where the intercalated disc runs transversely across the fiber, extensive and irregular maculae adherentes (desmosomes) are separated by small areas similar to the zonula occludens: the latter here are called *maculae occludentes*. At desmosomes actin filaments from adjacent cells terminate in the associated dense material. Between transverse areas the opposed cell membranes run longitudinally to give a steplike pattern to the whole disc. In these regions, where cells are joined side by side, there is obliteration of the intercellular space: these areas are called *fasciae occludentes*. They are believed to permit rapid spread of excitation from cell to cell while the other specializations in the transverse parts probably maintain cell cohesion and transmit the pull of the contractile elements from cell to cell along the length of the cardiac muscle fiber.

Purkinje Fibers

Purkinje fibers are composed of specialized cardiac muscle cells which form part of the impulse conducting system of the heart (see Chapter 11). They are located just beneath the endocardium on the internal surface of the heart, particularly in relation to the interventricular septum. As with cardiac muscle, the Purkinje fibers form a network composed of separate cellular units. By light microscopy, in comparison to cardiac muscle fibers, Purkinje fibers are larger, thicker, and more palely staining, with abundant central sarcoplasm and relatively few myofibrils, which usually are found in

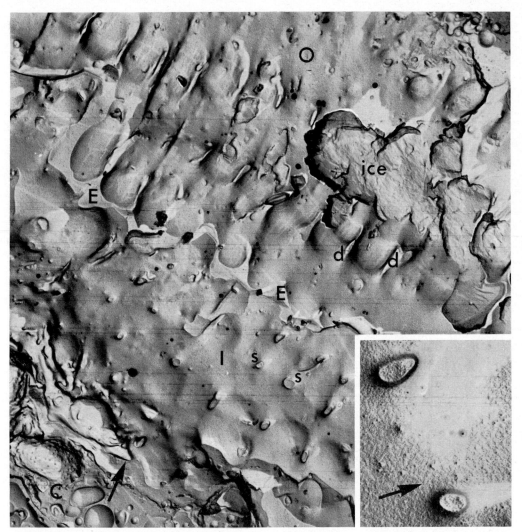

Figure 9-22. Electron micrograph of a freeze-etch preparation of cardiac muscle. Portions of two muscle cells are shown running obliquely from upper left to lower right. The upper cell (O) has fractured to show the outer surface of the plasma membrane with depressions or pits (d) as apertures of transverse tubules. In this cell also is an ice crystal as an artifact. In the lower cell (I) the fracture has exposed the inner, cytoplasmic surface of the plasma membrane with stumps (s) of transverse tubules. A capillary (C) is present at lower left. × 8300. Insert (lower right) shows the stumps of two transverse tubules at higher magnification. × 55,400. The broad arrows indicate the direction of metal shadowing. (Courtesy of Dr. D. G. Rayns.)

a peripheral position. Purkinje fibers contain large quantities of glycogen. Intercalated discs are present but not seen commonly. Regions exist where there is a gradual transition between Purkinje and ordinary cardiac muscle fibers.

Purkinje fibers form part of a system of impulse conducting tissue which regulates the coordinated contractions of cardiac muscle in various chambers of the heart.

Connective Tissue

Connective tissue is not prominent in cardiac muscle but extends between fibers as a delicate endomysium containing a very rich capillary network, more extensive than that of skeletal muscle. Lymphatic capillaries also are numerous, and fine autonomic nerves may be seen occasionally.

Regeneration

Cardiac muscle is more resistant to injuries than are the other types of muscle but shows very little evidence of regeneration after injury. Damaged cardiac muscle is repaired by fibro-connective scar tissue.

REFERENCES

Bergman, R. A.: Uterine smooth muscle fibers in castrate and estrogen-treated rats. J. Cell Biol., 36:639, 1968.

Bourne, G. H. (editor): The Structure and Function of Muscle. New York, Academic Press, 1960, Vols. 1-3.

Fawcett, D. W.: The sarcoplasmic reticulum of skeletal and cardiac muscle. Circulation, 24:336, 1961.

Hagopian, M., and Spiro, D.: The sarcoplasmic reticulum and its association with the T system in an insect. J. Cell Biol., 32:535, 1967.

Hanson, J., and Huxley, H. E.: The structural basis of contraction in striated muscle. Sympos. Soc. Exp. Biol., No. 9:228, 1955.

Huxley, H. E.: The contractile structure of cardiac and skeletal muscle. Circulation, 24:328, 1961.

Huxley, H. E.: The mechanism of muscular contraction. Sci. Amer., 213:18, 1965.

Kelly, D. E.: Models of muscle Z-band fine structure based on a looping filament configuration. J. Cell Biol., 34:827, 1967.

Kelly, R. E., and Rice, R. V.: Localization of myosin filaments in smooth muscle. J. Cell Biol., 37:105, 1968.

Knappeis, G. G., and Carlsen, F.: The ultrastructure of the Z disc in skeletal muscle. J. Cell Biol., 13:323, 1962.

Leeson, C. R.: The electron microscopy of the myoepithelium in the rat exorbital lacrimal gland. Anat. Rec., 137:45, 1960.

Panner, B. J., and Honig, C. R.: Filament ultrastructure and organization in vertebrate smooth muscle. J. Cell Biol., 35:303, 1967.

Philpott, C. W., and Goldstein, M. A.: Sarcoplasmic reticulum of striated muscle: Localization of potential calcium binding sites. Science, 155:1019, 1967.

Porter, K. R., and Franzini-Armstrong, C.: The sarcoplasmic reticulum. Sci. Amer., 212:72, 1965.

Robertson, J. D.: Electron microscopy of the motor end-plate and the neuromuscular spindle. Amer. J. Phys. Med., 39:1, 1960.

Shafiq, S. A., Gorycki, M., Goldstone, L., and Milhorat, A. T.: Fine structure of fiber types in normal human muscle. Anat. Rec., 156:283, 1966.

Simpson, F. O., and Oertelis, S. J.: The fine structure of sheep myocardial cells; sarcolemmal invaginations and the transverse tubular system. J. Cell Biol., 12:91, 1962.

Simpson, F. O., and Rayns, D. G.: The relationship between the transverse tubular system and other tubules at the Z disc levels of myocardial cells in the ferret. Amer. J. Anat., 122:193, 1968.

Smith, D. S.: Reticular organizations within the striated muscle cell. An historical survey of light microscopic studies. J. Biophys. Biochem. Cytol., 10:61, 1961.

Sommer, J. R., and Johnson, E. A.: Cardiac muscle: A comparative study of Purkinje fibers and ventricular fibers. J. Cell Biol., 36:497, 1968.

Stromer, M. H., Hartshorne, D. J., and Rice, R. V.: Removal and reconstitution of Z-line material in a striated muscle. J. Cell Biol., 35:C23, 1967.

Thaemert, J. C.: Intercellular bridges as protoplasmic anastomoses between smooth muscle cells. J. Biophys. Biochem. Cytol., 6:67, 1959.

Thaemert, J. C.: Ultrastructural interrelationships of nerve processes and smooth muscle cells in three dimensions. J. Cell Biol., 28:37, 1966.

Veratti, E.: Investigations on the fine structure of striated muscle fiber. J. Biophys. Biochem. Cytol., 10:1, 1961.

Walker, S. M., and Schrodt, G. R.: Connections between the T system and sarcoplasmic reticulum. Anat. Rec., 155:1, 1966.

Zadunaisky, J. A.: The location of sodium in the transverse tubules of skeletal muscle. J. Cell Biol., 31:C11, 1966.

CHAPTER 10

NERVOUS TISSUE

The nervous system includes the total mass of nervous tissue in the body. Nervous tissue is widely distributed and with a few minor exceptions all organs of the body include a nervous element. Basically, the nervous system consists of tissue which collects stimuli from the environment, transforms such stimuli into nervous impulses, and passes them to a large, highly organized reception and correlation area. Here the impulses are received and interpreted and, in turn, are issued to effector organs to institute appropriate responses. The nervous system also includes structural areas for all conscious experience. All these functions are performed by a highly specialized collection of cells called *neurons* which, together with their supporting cells and associated extracellular material, form the nervous system.

Anatomically, the nervous system can be divided into the *central nervous system* and the *peripheral nervous system*. The central nervous system is composed of the brain and spinal cord located in the cranium and vertebral canal; the peripheral nervous system includes all other nervous structures. The central nervous system receives all nervous impulses from the body (interoceptive) and all impulses following stimuli originating outside the body (exteroceptive). The peripheral nervous system serves to interconnect all other tissues and organs with the central nervous system. Functionally, the nervous system is divided into *somatic* and *autonomic* parts, each with central and peripheral divisions.* The somatic portion is concerned with structures derived from the embryological somites, i.e., muscles, bones, and skin. Muscles derived from branchial arches are included in this part because, histologically, the muscles of the two groups are identical. The autonomic nervous system is concerned with the innervation of smooth and cardiac muscle and the glands of the body. To a great extent its functions are independent of the rest of the nervous system.

In the neuron, two properties of protoplasm are developed to a great degree. These are *irritability*, which is the capacity for response to physical and chemical agents with the initiation of an impulse, and *conductivity*, the ability to transmit such an impulse from one locality to another. The extreme degree to which these two properties of protoplasm are developed in neurons, together with the great diversity of shape and size of the cell bodies and the length of their processes, distinguishes neurons from all

---

*Note on terminology: *soma* = body; *autos* = self, *nomos* = control, i.e., automatic.

177

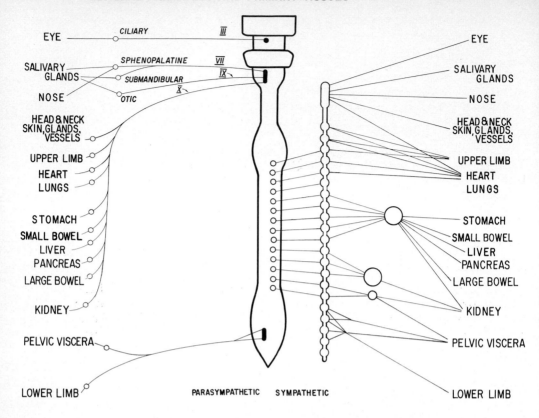

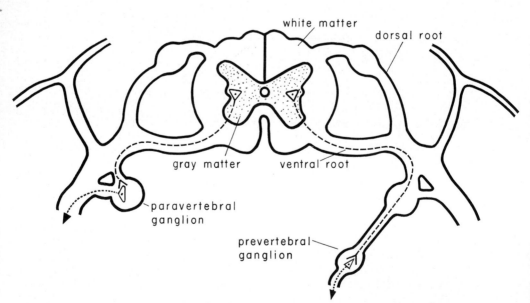

Figure 10-1. Top: Diagram of the peripheral distribution of components of the autonomic system; parasympathetic division on the left, sympathetic division on the right. The three peripheral or prevertebral ganglia represented by circles on the right are the celiac, superior mesenteric, and inferior mesenteric. Bottom: Diagram of a cross section of the spinal cord to show two possible courses taken by preganglionic (- - - -) and postganglionic (. . . .) fibers of the sympathetic nervous system.

other cell types. Most of the nerve cell bodies are collected in or near the central nervous system. Their processes, which are capable of transmitting impulses, may lie totally within the central nervous system, may extend from the central nervous system for great distances, or may lie entirely outside the central nervous system. All neurons are capable of exciting other neurons in contact with them. Such specialized contacts between neurons are called *synapses*. The term neuron, then, refers to a complete nerve cell, including the nucleus and its surrounding cytoplasm (the perikaryon) and one or more protoplasmic extensions or processes. The latter usually comprise several *dendrites* and one *axon* or *axis cylinder*. Connections with other neurons at synapses are by contact only. Thus, the neuron is the structural and functional unit of the nervous system.

(The student may experience some confusion in terminology. The nerve cell body of a neuron often is called the nerve cell and its threadlike processes the nerve fibers, both being constituent parts of the neuron.)

THE REFLEX ARC

The basic unit of the nervous system is the neuron, but the integrative unit is the reflex arc. Any nervous activity involves the activity of many neurons with numerous potential interconnections by their synapses. However, the basic pattern is best exemplified by the simple reflex arc. Most of the actions in man involve such reflex arcs. The simplest reflex arc involves only two neurons, and is illustrated in Figure 10-2 (top). One example of this is the *knee jerk*, commonly used clinically in the examination of patients. With the knees crossed in a sitting, relaxed patient, the patellar tendon of the uppermost leg is tapped sharply but gently. Normally the quadriceps muscle contracts to kick forward the foot. This reflex response involves one

afferent or sensory neuron and an efferent, motor neuron. A peripheral process (a dendrite) of the afferent neuron lies in the substance of the patellar (quadriceps) tendon and passes centrally to the cell body lying in a posterior root ganglion near the spinal cord. From the cell body, a second nerve process (an axon) passes into the substance of the spinal cord. Here it synapses with an efferent (motor) neuron cell body from which a nerve fiber (an axon) passes in a peripheral nerve to terminate by supplying muscle fibers in the quadriceps muscle. This is a very simple mechanism and, of course, most reflex arcs in the body are more complex. By inserting a third neuron (a connector, association, or internuncial neuron) between the afferent and efferent neurons, potentially numerous connections within the central nervous system are established (Figure 10-2, bottom). Thus more complex reflex arcs can be built. It must be emphasized that once a nervous impulse reaches the central nervous system in an intact animal, there is widespread activity within the central nervous system and that, in fact, the simple reflex arc as just described does not exist. It is a simplification of a basic principle that such activity involves inflow to the central nervous system (by the afferent neuron), modification and integration (by the internuncial neuron), and outflow to an effector organ (by the efferent neuron).

STRUCTURE OF THE NEURON

Neurons vary greatly in size and shape but each consists of a cell body, or *perikaryon*, and one or more processes. These processes are of two types, the *axon*, always a single process, and the *dendrites*. A neuron with just one process, which branches beyond the cell body into an axon and a dendrite, is termed unipolar. A neuron with two processes is *bipolar*; with more than two it is multipolar. For

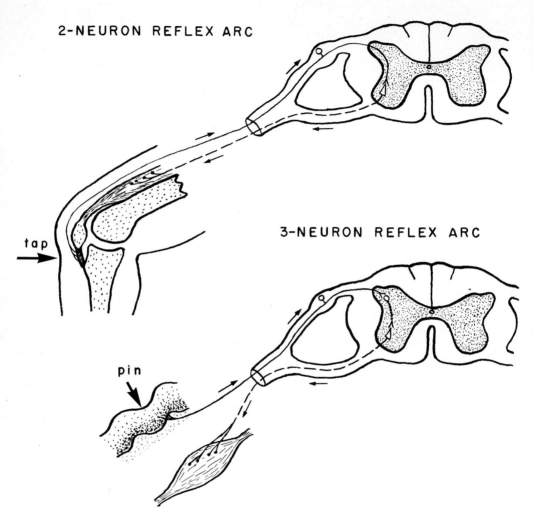

2-NEURON REFLEX ARC

tap

3-NEURON REFLEX ARC

pin

Figure 10-2. Diagrams illustrating two-neuron reflex arc (knee-jerk, above) and three-neuron reflex arc (pain withdrawal reflex, below). The afferent (sensory) nerve cell body is situated in the posterior root ganglion, and its processes are indicated by a solid line; the efferent (motor) neuron is in the anterior horn of gray matter, and its axon is indicated by a broken line. The internuncial neuron lies within the gray matter and has its axon indicated by a dotted line.

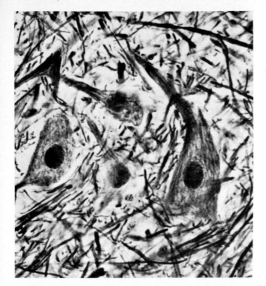

Figure 10-3. Photomicrograph of a multipolar ganglion cell from the spinal cord. Neurofibrils are seen. Cajal silver method. × 500.

convenience, the cell body, or perikaryon, and the processes will be described separately.

PERIKARYON

The cell body usually is large in comparison to other cells and varies from 4 to 135 microns in diameter. The shape is variable in the extreme and is dependent upon the number and orientation of cell processes. Unipolar cells are globular in shape and have a single process which bifurcates. They are found in the cranial and spinal ganglia (a ganglion being a collection of nerve cell bodies situated outside the central nervous system). A bipolar cell is elongated, spindle-shaped, and with a process at each end or pole of the cell. Examples are found in organs of special sense, e.g., in the retina of the eye, in the olfactory epithelium, and in the acoustic ganglion. Multipolar cells, by far the most common, have numerous processes and vary from stellate to pyramidal to pear-shaped. They are found throughout the central nervous system and in

autonomic ganglia. The total number of nerve cells in the body never has been estimated accurately, but there are probably 14 billion in the cerebral cortex alone.

Nucleus

This usually is large, spherical, and situated centrally in the cell body and has a distinct nuclear membrane. Nuclear chromatin is scanty, nuclear sap is abundant, and usually there is a single, prominent nucleolus. The total effect is that the nucleus is pale-staining with a dark prominent nucleolus, and this appearance often results in the inexperienced mistakenly identifying the nucleus as the entire cell and the nucleolus as the nucleus. This type of nucleus is called vesicular. Sex chromatin, as described in Chapter 2, often is prominent as a nucleolar satellite.

Cytoplasmic Organelles

The protoplasm of the nerve cell body is termed the *neuroplasm*. The cell membrane by light microscopy is a thin, somewhat indefinite line limiting the perikaryon and by electron microscopy shows the typical structure of a plasma membrane. Mitochondria and the Golgi apparatus are present but neither is remarkable in extent. The former usually are small. By electron microscopy, one can see small collections of the Golgi complex scattered throughout the cytoplasm. Centrosomes are prominent in young, developing neurons (neuroblasts) but are seen rarely in adult neurons. One characteristic feature is the presence of *neurofibrils*. These are best developed and most numerous in large neurons but probably are present in all. They form a complicated network in the perikaryon and extend into the nerve cell processes, both dendrites and axon. They can be demonstrated in living cells from tissue culture and

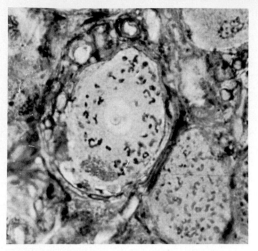

Figure 10-4. Photomicrograph of a nerve cell body from a spinal ganglion stained to demonstrate the Golgi apparatus. Note the pale-staining nucleus with darker nucleolus. × 550.

are stained vitally by methylene blue. With silver impregnation techniques, neurofibrils are seen as branching and anastomosing threads. Electron microscopy demonstrates that there is a network of filaments and microtubules (neurotubules) throughout the cytoplasm and extending into nerve cell

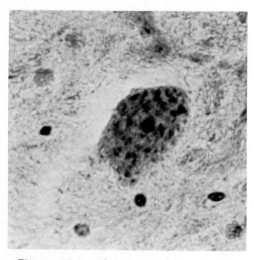

Figure 10-5. Photomicrograph of a nerve cell body from the spinal cord stained to demonstrate the granular chromophil substance or Nissl bodies. × 500.   See filmstrip I, frame 35.

processes. This network corresponds to the neurofibrils seen by light microscopy, which, it should be emphasized, are not demonstrated in an ordinary H and E preparation. The microtubule has a lumen of about 100 Å diameter with a wall about 60 Å thick. The wall appears to be composed of longitudinally orientated filaments: in cross section of a microtubule, the wall is seen to be composed of circular densities resembling filaments in cross section. The cytoplasmic filaments, approximately 60 Å in diameter, appear to have a dense periphery with a lighter core.

A second characteristic feature of the perikaryon is the extent of the ergastoplasm or basophil component. It is present in nerve cell bodies in bulk and appears as *Nissl bodies*. These are demonstrated as discrete clumps of material by phase contrast microscopy of living or fresh material. They are stained in fixed preparations by toluidine blue, thionine, and other basic aniline dyes. Such stains indicate that Nissl bodies contain nucleoprotein (RNA), and by electron microscopy they are seen to be composed of parallel, flat sacs of ergastoplasm with numerous attached ribosomes, and with many free ribosomes between the sacs. The regularity of arrangement varies in different kinds of nerve cell bodies, being most regular in large motor neurons and less regular in other smaller neurons. Although Nissl bodies are distributed widely in the perikaryon, they are not found in the extreme peripheral cytoplasm (ectoplasm), or in the axon or *axon hillock*, which is a clear, conical area at the origin of the axon from the perikaryon. It is accepted generally that this extensive development of the ergastoplasm is correlated with protein synthesis, as it is also, for example, in pancreatic acinar cells.

The reaction of the Nissl bodies to injury of the neuron is characteristic, the Nissl bodies apparently breaking up and diffusing generally throughout the neuroplasm. This results in a general, dark staining of the entire neuroplasm. If such an effect follows injury of the axon, it is termed the Nissl reaction or primary irritation of the nerve cell. The dissolution of the Nissl bodies after damage to the nerve cell itself is termed *chromatolysis*.

Cytoplasmic Inclusions

Fat droplets commonly are seen in the perikaryon and represent either reserve material or are a product of normal or pathological metabolism. Glycogen, although present in embryonic nerve cells, is not present in adult neurons. Pigment granules of various types are widespread. Lipochrome pigment, visible as yellow or brownish granules, is found chiefly in large neurons, and the amount increases considerably with age. Its significance is unknown, but it may represent a metabolic product which is useless but nonharmful. Melanin,

as brownish-black granules, is present particularly in cells of certain regions, for example, in the substantia nigra of the midbrain, in spinal and sympathetic ganglia, and in the locus ceruleus in the floor of the fourth ventricle. Its significance is unknown. Iron-containing granules, demonstrable by the Prussian blue technique, are found in nerve cells in various regions, for example, the globus pallidus. Like granules of lipochrome, such iron-containing granules tend to increase in number with age.

NERVE CELL PROCESSES

The processes, or nerve fibers, of neurons are a remarkable feature developed to provide conduction pathways and to provide greater surface areas for contact. These processes, as explained previously, are cytoplasmic extensions of the nerve cell body, there being one axon and one or more dendrites to each cell. The dendrites conduct impulses toward the cell, and the single axon or axis cylinder conducts impulses away from the cell.

Dendrites. The number of dendrites or dendrons varies, but in unipolar and bipolar cells there is only one dendrite, atypical in structure and resembling an axon. In multipolar cells, dendrites leave the perikaryon like the branches of a tree and each dendrite itself branches into primary, secondary, tertiary, and even more arborizations. Just as in a tree, the dendrites are thick where they leave the nerve cell body and become more slender with branching. In the more stout parts, i.e., in the proximal portions, both neurofibrils and chromidial substance are present and the neurofibrils extend into the finest branches. Also present in many dendrites are numerous, regularly spaced tubules or canaliculi about 200 Å in diameter and of indefinite length. These tubules probably are not continuous with the endoplasmic reticulum. In Golgi prep-

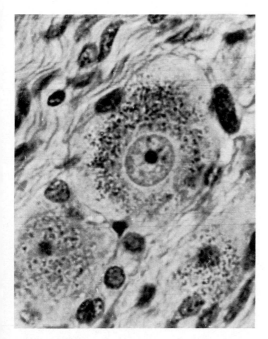

Figure 10-6. Photomicrograph of a nerve cell body from a spinal ganglion to demonstrate lipochrome pigment. Note the vesicular nucleus with nucleolus. × 750.   See filmstrip I, frame 37.

arations, the dendrites are not smooth, but are contorted with numerous spinelike processes, the "gemmules" (spiny spicules), which often are expanded and bulbous at their tips. The fine terminal twigs and the gemmules serve as synaptic organs whereby their parent neuron makes contact with, and receives impulses from, many functionally related neurons. The number, extent of branching, and length of dendrites vary from neuron to neuron and are not dependent upon the size of the perikaryon. It is the dendrites which constitute much of the feltlike "neuropil" of the central nervous system (see page 199).

Axon. The axon, or axis cylinder, is single and arises usually from the periphery of the nerve cell body at a region termed the axon hillock. This area contains no chromophil substance but passing through it is a concentration of neurofibrils which then enters the axon. There is no chromophil substance in the axon. An axon is more slender and usually much longer and straighter than the dendrites of the same neuron. Axons vary from less than a micron to several microns in diameter and from a fraction of a millimeter to a meter or more in length. Along the course of an axon, there may or may not be a series of branches, called collaterals, which usually leave the axon at right angles. The surface of the axon is smooth and its diameter constant, unlike a dendrite. Terminally, an axon ends in twiglike branchings, the *telodendria*, which touch the cell body, dendrites or axons of one or more neurons. In some cases, the telodendria are so numerous as to surround the neuron on which they terminate in a basket-like arrangement. As will be described later in more detail, axons are covered with accessory sheaths.

It now is accepted generally that the nerve cell body, with its extensive ergastoplasm, continuously synthesizes new protoplasm which flows down the nerve cell processes to replace protoplasm used in metabolism, protoplasm which cannot be synthesized in the cell processes themselves. This newly synthesized protein probably is distributed via the neurotubules. The rate of flow has been estimated at about 1 mm. per day.

TYPES OF NEURONS

As indicated earlier, neurons can be uni- or multipolar depending on the number of dendrites. They also vary considerably in size and shape. Some of these neuron types are described here in more detail.

Golgi Type I. The majority of these neurons have very long axons, which leave the cell body in the gray matter of the central nervous system, and pass in white matter, some of them leaving the central nervous system to become peripheral nerve fibers. This type includes neurons whose axons contribute to peripheral nerves and those whose axons form the main fiber tracts of the brain and spinal cord.

Golgi Type II. These are stellate neurons which have short axons. They

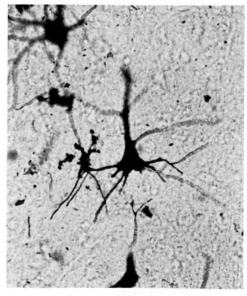

Figure 10-7. Photomicrograph of a pyramidal cell from the cerebral cortex showing cell body and branching dendrites. Golgi method. × 225.

See filmstrip I, frame 36.

are numerous in the cerebral and cerebellar cortices and in the retina. These neurons vary greatly in size and shape. Spherical, oval, piriform, fusiform, and polyhedral types are described, but all have many radiating processes which give them a stellate or star-shaped appearance.

Unipolar Neurons. True unipolar neurons have only an axon, and although they are of limited distribution in the adult, they are common in the developing nervous system. More common are the *pseudounipolar* neurons. These are originally typically bipolar but, during development, axon and dendrite come together, leave the cell body at the same site, and run together for some distance before separating. Such neurons are found in cranial and spinal ganglia.

Bipolar Neurons. These have an axon and a single dendrite at opposite poles of the cell body. They are found in olfactory epithelium, in the retina, and in certain special sensory ganglia.

Multipolar Neurons. Multipolar neurons, the commonest type, vary

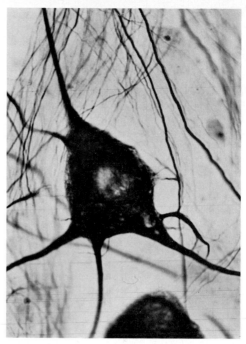

Figure 10-9. Photomicrograph of a multipolar neuron in the myenteric plexus of the cat jejunum. Silver impregnation. × 550. (Courtesy of Dr. G. Schofield.)

in shape depending on the arrangement of their multiple dendrites. Pyramidal and star shapes are common.

Purkinje Cells. These cells, found only in the middle layer of the cerebellar cortex, have a unique shape with a treelike dendrite arising from the pointed pole of a flask-shaped cell body. The single dendrite sometimes bifurcates into two. The branching of the dendrites is extensive but limited to a single plane, somewhat in the manner of a pear tree growing against a wall. A small axon leaves the opposite broader pole.

In addition to the types just listed, there are many other named types of neurons of varying shape and size.

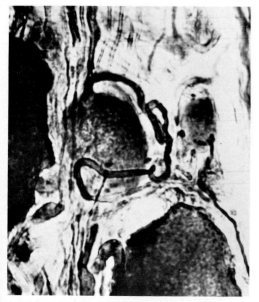

Figure 10-8. Photomicrograph of a unipolar cell from a spinal ganglion. Note the glomerulus formed by the coiled cell process. Golgi method. × 550. (Courtesy of W. R. Ingram.)

GANGLIA

A collection of nerve cell bodies located outside the central nervous system is called a *ganglion*, although

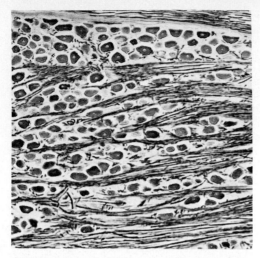

Figure 10-10. Photomicrograph of a sensory ganglion (nodose ganglion of vagus), showing groups of nerve cell bodies intermingled with groups of nerve fibers. Golgi method. × 110.

all ganglia do not lie outside the CNS. A similar collection in the substance of the central nervous system is termed a *nucleus*. Ganglia are of two main types: those of the craniospinal group (sensory ganglia) and those of the autonomic nervous system (visceral, motor ganglia).

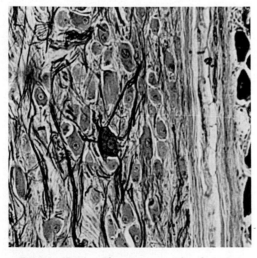

Figure 10-11. Photomicrograph of an autonomic ganglion (cervical sympathetic ganglion), showing nerve cell bodies intermingled with nerve fibers. Compare with Figure 10-10. Golgi method. × 110.

General Features. Ganglia vary greatly in size, ranging from very small ones containing only a few nerve cell bodies to very large ones with 50,000 or more cells. Each ganglion has a connective tissue capsule, which may be quite dense around large ganglia. Continuous with the capsule is a fine connective tissue network. This network, found throughout the substance of the ganglion, is composed of fine slips of collagenous and reticular fibers. Blood vessels run in the connective tissue, between the meshes of which are situated the nervous elements. In addition to nerve cell bodies, nerve fibers (axons and dendrites) are present, with their supporting sheaths (see page 187), and each ganglion cell has a capsule composed of a single layer of small, cuboidal cells called the capsule or *satellite cells.*

Craniospinal Ganglia. The spinal ganglia are fusiform or globular swellings situated on the posterior roots of the spinal nerves (Figure 10-1, bottom). Cranial ganglia are similar swellings found on some of the cranial nerves. The ganglion cells are pseudounipolar in type and spherical in shape, having a single process, an axon which, on leaving the nerve cell body, becomes somewhat convoluted to form a "glomerulus." At some distance from the nerve cell body, the nerve cell process enters a fiber bundle and splits in a T or Y fashion, one process being somewhat thicker and passing in a spinal or cranial nerve to the periphery where it originates in a receptor organ. The other, more slender process passes into the central nervous system. Histologically, both processes have an identical structure. The nerve cell bodies, usually arranged in groups at the periphery of the ganglia, are separated by fiber bundles. These nerve cell bodies may be only 15 to 25 microns in diameter and the processes of these cells are unmyelinated (see page 187). Larger cells of up to 100 microns in diameter have processes

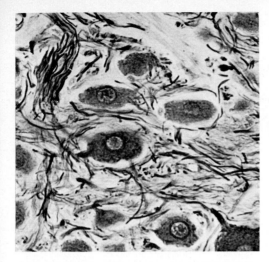

Figure 10-12. Photomicrograph of ganglion cells in a dorsal root (spinal) ganglion. Golgi method. × 250.

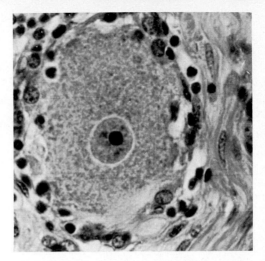

Figure 10-13. Photomicrograph of a ganglion cell from a sympathetic ganglion. Note nucleus and nucleolus of the ganglion cell and nuclei of satellite cells. × 550.

See filmstrip I, frame 37.

which are myelinated. Each cell body is surrounded by a single layer of small, flattened, low cuboidal cells, the satellite cells or *amphicytes*, which are analogous to neuroglia cells of the central nervous system. They are continuous with the neurolemma sheath of the nerve cell process and are derived embryologically from the neural crest, as also are the neurons.

Autonomic Ganglia. These are situated as swellings along the sympathetic chain and its ramifications and within the walls of the organs supplied by the autonomic system. In the latter sites, the ganglia may be very small. The majority of the nerve cells are multipolar and stellate in shape, although a few unipolar and bipolar cells may be present. Generally, the cells are smaller than those of the craniospinal ganglia, ranging from 15 to about 45 microns in diameter. The dendrites of these cells may be coiled to' form a glomerulus situated either within or outside the capsule, although in some cells a capsule is lacking, particularly in the small ganglia situated in the walls of viscera. In such situations, the capsule cells may be replaced by small,

spindle-shaped cells similar in appearance to small fibroblasts. In autonomic ganglia, the axons usually are unmyelinated and, unlike the axons of craniospinal ganglia, do not show a tendency to group into distinct fiber bundles.

NERVE FIBERS

Nerve fiber is a term applied particularly to long axons. All nerve fibers, i.e., nerve cell processes, both within the central nervous system and outside it, have one or more sheaths. In the central nervous system, fibers may be partially covered only by glial cells, the small supporting cells of the central nervous system, or they may be covered also by a layer of myelin. These two types are called *unmyelinated*, or *nonmyelinated*, and *myelinated*. In the peripheral nervous system, unmyelinated fibers (*Remak's fibers*) are common as small sensory fibers and numerous in the autonomic system; they have a sheath of *neurolemma* (neurilemma), also called the *sheath of Schwann*. Myelinated fibers of the peripheral nervous system have a sheath of myelin and a sheath of

Osmium Ordinary fixation

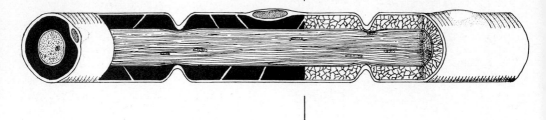

Figure 10-14. Three-dimensional diagram of a single myelinated nerve fiber. Note the clefts of Schmidt-Lanterman seen in the osmium-fixed material and the neurokeratin network seen after ordinary fixation.

Schwann. A description of the characteristics of the axon, myelin, and the sheath of Schwann of peripheral nerves follows.

Axon. The axon is cylindrical, of smooth outline, and uniform in thick-

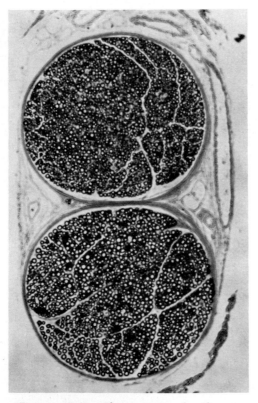

Figure 10-15. Photomicrograph of nerves in cross section. Note epineurium and perineurium. Osmic acid fixation. × 110.

ness along its length. It is bounded by the axolemma, which is continuous with the plasma membrane of the parent nerve cell body. Within its protoplasm (axoplasm), neurofibrils, continuous with those of the cell body, and mitochondria are present, but no Nissl bodies are found.

Myelin. In myelinated nerves, the axon is surrounded by a tubular sheath of myelin, which in the fresh state is highly refractile and white. The myelin is responsible for the color of the white matter of the brain and spinal cord. After ordinary fixation methods, myelin is dissolved because it largely is composed of lipid, but a protein material is precipitated and remains around the axon as *neurokeratin*. If nerves are fixed and stained in osmium tetroxide, myelin becomes black, and after bichromate fixation, myelin stains well with hematoxylin. In osmium tetroxide-fixed material, myelin shows small clefts or fissures extending through its diameter to the axon; these are termed the *Schmidt-Lanterman* clefts. Their significance is unknown, but these funnel-shaped dislocations in the myelin sheath have been demonstrated also by electron microscopy. By light microscopy, the myelin sheath is seen to be an incomplete cylinder, for at intervals of about 0.1 to 0.6 mm. it is interrupted, and at these regions the neurolemmal sheath comes into contact with the appearance of concentric layers of dark material, the major dense lines, of about 25 to 30 Å separated by light intervals about 100 Å thick. Between each two major dense lines in the center of the light material is a finer dark line called the *intraperiod line.* The theory concerning the method of formation of the myelin sheath now accepted generally is illustrated in Figure 10-21. This hypothesis involves the axon first indenting the Schwann cell to lie longitudinally in a trough in its cytoplasm. Then, theoretically, the Schwann cell rotates around the axon so that its plasma membrane comes to form a spiral around the axon. (Although this process is easily understood, in fact, the site of invagination of the Schwann cell, the *mesaxon,* probably itself grows, resulting in a spiral invagina-

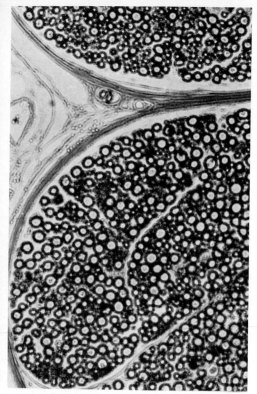

Figure 10-16. Higher magnification of Figure 10-15. Myelin is stained black; axons are unstained. × 500.

axolemma. These constricted areas are called the *nodes of Ranvier.* Covering the myelin of each segment between two adjacent nodes of Ranvier, i.e., an internode, there is a single neurolemma cell.

Electron microscopy has demonstrated that myelin is not a structureless material secreted either by the axon or by the neurolemmal sheath (or by neuroglia in the central nervous system) but is in fact a series of lamellae formed by, and continuous with, the plasma membrane of the neurolemma cells. X-ray diffraction has indicated that myelin is composed of concentric lamellae of lipid interspersed with thin layers of protein of a neurokeratin nature. Formation of myelin from plasma membrane explains its lipoprotein nature. By electron microscopy, myelin has the

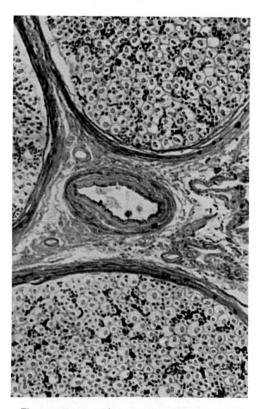

Figure 10-17. Photomicrograph of nerve in cross section. Axons are stained; myelin is unstained. Ordinary fixation, silver stain. × 170.
See filmstrip I, frame 38.

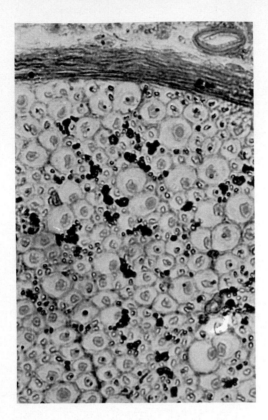

Figure 10-18. Higher magnification of Figure 10-17. Myelinated and unmyelinated fibers are present. × 750.

Figure 10-19. Photomicrograph of myelinated nerve fibers in longitudinal section. Note the node of Ranvier. Osmic acid fixation, Epon section. × 1000.   See filmstrip I, frame 39.

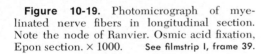

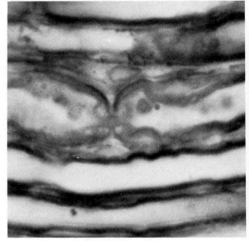

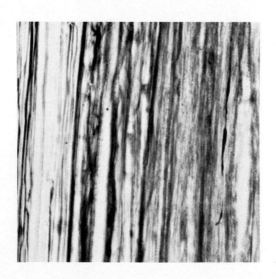

Figure 10-20. Photomicrograph of normal (left) and degenerating (right) nerve fibers. Osmium fixation. × 250.

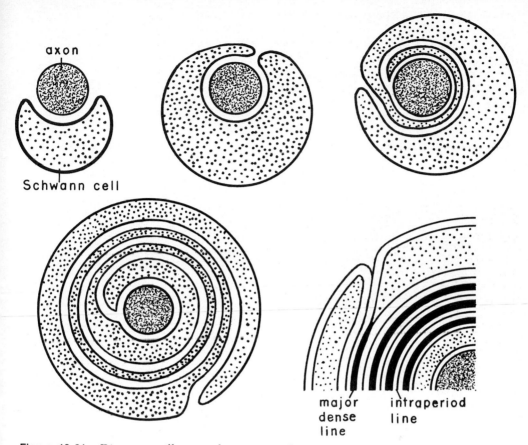

Figure 10-21. Diagram to illustrate the stages in the formation of a myelin sheath (the "jelly-roll" hypothesis) and the formation of major dense and intraperiod lines in the myelin.

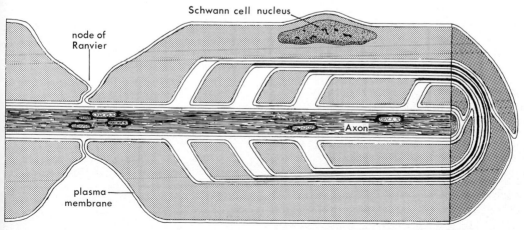

Figure 10-22. Diagram to illustrate the appearance of a myelinated nerve fiber and a node of Ranvier in longitudinal section as seen with the electron microscope.

tion into the depths of the Schwann cell. Thus this process does not involve rotation of the Schwann cell around the axon.) The diagram (Figure 10-21) shows that where the inner cytoplasmic surfaces of the plasma membrane come together, a major dense line is formed in the myelin. An intraperiod line is formed by the opposition of outer surfaces of the Schwann cell membrane.

This hypothesis explains the formation of myelin as seen in cross section of a nerve, but it also is necessary to demonstrate the process in the third dimension to understand the appearance of nodes of Ranvier as seen in longitudinal section. In longitudinal section, the lamellae of myelin are seen to be progressively of shorter length from the external to the internal lamellae, as shown in Figure 10-22, the juxta-axonal lamella being the shortest. As each lamella bends toward the axon, the major dense line splits to enclose a small area of

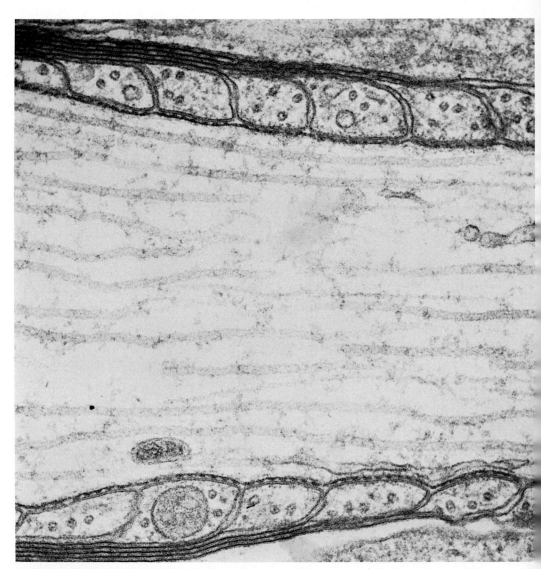

Figure 10-23. Electron micrograph of a longitudinal section of a myelinated axon near a node of Ranvier from a rat brain. × 100,000. (Courtesy of Dr. A. Hirano. Reproduced by permission from the Editors, The Journal of Cell Biology, 34:561, 1967.)

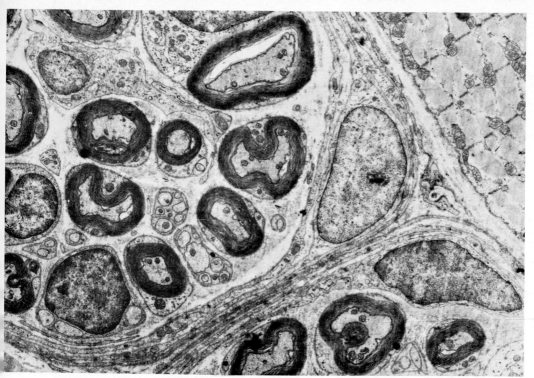

Figure 10-24. Low power electron micrograph of parts of two bundles of myelinated and unmyelinated nerve fibers cut in cross section. Note that each bundle is enveloped in perineurium consisting of concentric layers of flattened cells and collagen fibrils. × 4200.

Schwann cell cytoplasm. In peripheral nerves, the axon surface is not bare, as is shown in Figure 10-22, for the two adjacent Schwann cells interlock. In smaller, less well-myelinated fibers the "bare area" at a node of Ranvier may be 2 to 3 microns in length.

In the central nervous system, there are no Schwann cells, but the myelinated fibers bear a similar intimate relationship with oligodendrocytes. In general, however, there are fewer lamellae of myelin, and the internodes between nodes of Ranvier are of shorter length.

Neurolemma. Schwann's cells, or the neurolemma, envelop all axons of peripheral nerves and extend from their attachment to the spinal cord or brain stem almost to their terminations. The individual cells of the Schwann sheath have a single flattened nucleus, located toward the center of

an internode in myelinated fibers, and attenuated cytoplasm in which a Golgi apparatus and mitochondria can be identified. In unmyelinated fibers, several axons may be surrounded by one Schwann cell and occupy indentations in the cytoplasm. There is one point in each axon where the plasma membranes of the Schwann cells fail to envelop the axon, thus leaving a pair of parallel membranes to form a mesaxon (Figures 10-21 and 10-22). In myelinated fibers, as explained previously, one Schwann cell covers an axon between two nodes of Ranvier. Schwann cells are ectodermal in origin and are essential to the vitality and function of peripheral axons. Not only do they produce myelin but they are necessary for regeneration of axons. After division an axon is regenerated from the central stump, i.e., from the part continuous with the nerve cell

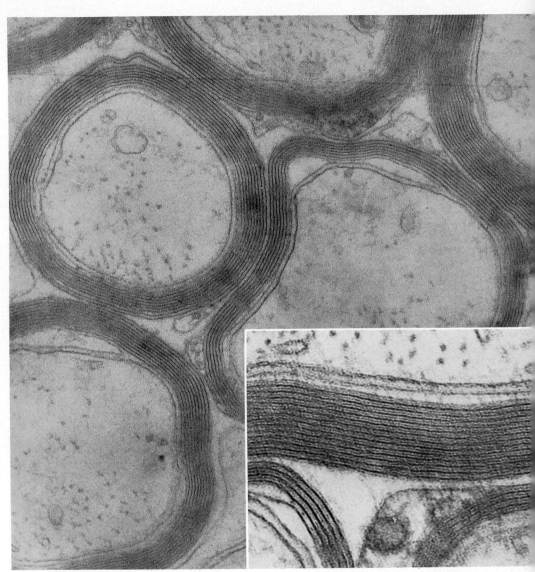

Figure 10-25.   Electron micrograph of myelinated nerve fibers in a cross section of the rat optic nerve. × 70,000. Inset, bottom right: Higher magnification to show major dense and intraperiod lines. × 125,000. (Preparation by A. Peters.)

body, and grows peripherally to its termination along a channel formed by Schwann cells. Schwann cells also can become phagocytic after nerve injury, removing cellular debris. In the central nervous system, the sheath of Schwann is not present but is replaced by neuroglial cells, particularly the oligodendroglia.

Staining of Nerve Fibers. Myelinated fibers are highly refractile in fresh preparations. In fixed preparations, myelin is darkened by osmium tetroxide or Weigert's method. The axon remains unstained. Myelin, being a lipoprotein complex, is dissolved by fat solvents. Silver impregnation and methylene blue vital staining methods are used to demonstrate axons and are of particular value for unmyelinated fibers which are not easily seen in routine histological preparations.

PERIPHERAL NERVES

Peripheral nerves are composed of many nerve fibers held together by connective tissue. There is a sheath of relatively strong connective tissue surrounding the entire nerve and this is termed the *epineurium*. It is composed of fibroblasts and collagenous fibers orientated mainly in a longitudinal manner and also contains blood vessels. Inside or deep to the epineurium are bundles or fascicles of nerve fibers, each surrounded by a sheath of connective tissue finer than that of the epineurium. Within this *perineurium* are strands of fine connective tissue extending between individual nerve fibers. These strands comprise the *endoneurium*. The perineurium is composed of concentric layers or sleeves of flattened cells, each sleeve being one cell thick. Externally, between perineurium and epineurium, and internally, between perineurium and endoneurium, are continuous basal laminae. In the perineurium between concentric layers of cells are discontinuous basal laminae. Between individual cells in a sleeve there are tight junctions so that each sleeve is a complete cylinder around the nerve bundle. The number

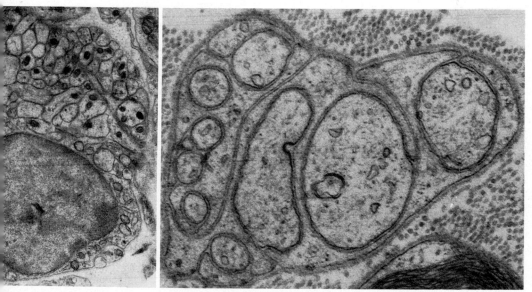

Figure 10-26. Electron micrographs of unmyelinated nerve fibers. Left: Schwann cell with nucleus and numerous axons in the cytoplasm. × 6000. Right: Axons with well defined mesaxons at higher magnification. × 40,000.

of sleeves decreases as the nerve branches and becomes smaller, and the last sleeve terminates just before the termination of the nerve. Thus there is an open end where endoneurium and epineurium are in continuity. The perineural sheath can be traced back along the nerve trunk to its point of attachment to the central nervous system where the perineurium is continuous with the pia arachnoid membrane of the central nervous system (see page 204). It is possible that the perineural sheath cells, like those of the pia arachnoid, are derived embryologically from ectoderm and thus the perineural sheath should be considered an epithelium. The perineural epithelium probably functions as a metabolically active diffusion barrier and serves to protect the peripheral nervous system. The endoneurium is composed of delicate collagenous and reticular fibers, amorphous ground substance, and flattened fibroblasts; it is closely adherent to the neurolemma, and it is difficult to distinguish one from the other.

The blood supply to a peripheral nerve is rich. Numerous branches from adjacent arteries enter the epineurium, freely anastomose, and run mainly longitudinally. From these, smaller vessels extend into the perineurium, and there is an extensive capillary network in the coarser parts of the endoneurium. Lymphatic vessels also are present in the epineurium.

Most peripheral nerves contain a mixture of both myelinated and unmyelinated fibers. The myelinated fibers vary greatly in size, the larger diameter fibers conducting more rapidly than the smaller.

THE SYNAPSE

A synapse is the site of junction of neurons where the termination of an axon of one neuron is in contact with the nerve cell body, dendrites or axon of another neuron. Rarely, a synapse is between axon and axon. Physiologically, a synapse is the site of transneuronal transmission of an impulse.

The structure of the synapse is variable, but usually the axon terminals or branches end in minute bulblike expansions called *end bulbs*, *end feet*, or *boutons terminaux*, closely applied to the cell body or dendrites of the receiving neuron. In some cases the axon terminals form a basket-like arrangement around the cell body or dendrites, or run parallel and adjacent to dendrites or cell body for considerable distances. In some cases the synapse is between an axon and small,

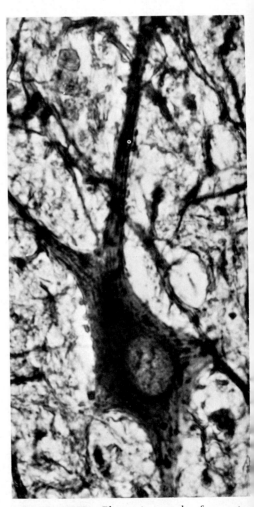

Figure 10-27. Photomicrograph of an anterior horn cell to show boutons terminaux on the cell body and its dendrites. × 1100. (Preparation by E. G. Bertram.)

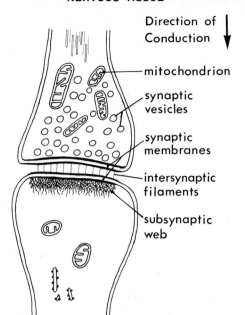

Direction of
Conduction

mitochondrion

synaptic
vesicles

synaptic
membranes

intersynaptic
filaments

subsynaptic
web

Figure 10-28.   Diagram of a typical synaptic region as seen with the electron microscope.

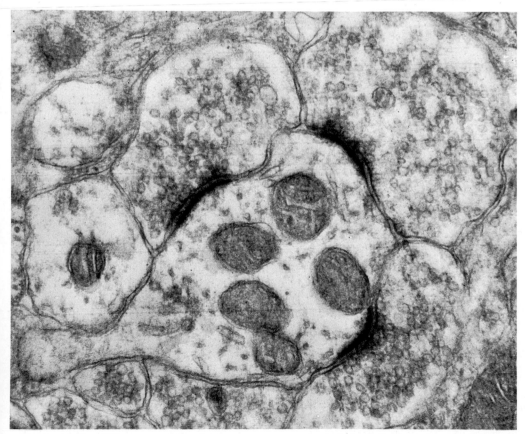

Figure 10-29.   Electron micrograph of synapses on a dendrite from the lateral geniculate body of a cat. Note the thickenings of the adjacent plasma membranes and collections of presynaptic vesicles in the terminal synaptic processes surrounding the centrally placed dendrite. × 60,000. (Preparation by A. Peters.)

spiny processes or gemmules of a dendrite. By its terminals, one axon may make contact with several neurons and, conversely, a neuron can receive impulses from the axons of many other neurons.

By electron microscopy, a bouton or end bulb lies in close apposition to the dendrite, perikaryon, or axon on which it terminates. Neurotubules and neurofibrils extend up to the axon terminal, which contains numerous mitochondria and a collection of so-called "*synaptic vesicles.*" These are about 500 Å in diameter and remarkably uniform in size. There is strong evidence that they contain transmitter substances, e.g., acetylcholine, which are released at the synapse by the action of a nerve impulse. Larger vesicles of 1000 Å diameter with a dense central core may be present, especially in postganglionic endings, where presumably they are associated with catecholamines. The mitochondria in an axon terminal probably are concerned in energy release for transmitter formation. The apposed plasma membranes of a synapse are separated by a cleft of only 60 to 200 Å and these regions show specializations which may be called the *synaptic complex*. The two synaptic membranes show thickenings, and there are intersynaptic filaments joining the two membranes across the cleft. A system of filaments arranged in a network projecting into the postsynaptic region is termed the *subsynaptic web*. No Schwann or glial cell processes extend into the cleft between the synaptic membranes.

Unlike a nerve fiber which is capable of conduction in either direction, a synapse is dynamically polarized and can conduct only from the axon to the dendrites or perikaryon of the receiving neuron.

AUXILIARY TISSUES OF THE NERVOUS SYSTEM

As stated at the beginning of the chapter, the nervous system includes all nervous tissue of the body, the basic functional unit of which is the neuron. However, like other tissues in the body, nervous tissue includes associated connective and supporting elements. Some of these, e.g., the neurolemma of the peripheral nervous system and the capsule cells of peripheral ganglia, have been described already. Others will be described in this section.

NEUROGLIA

As the name suggests (neuron, nerve, and glia, "glue"), this tissue functions to bind together the nervous tissue proper. Some authors consider neuroglia to include all interstitial tissues, e.g., capsule cells of peripheral ganglia, but we shall restrict the term to a group of numerous scattered cells situated within the central nervous system. There are approximately ten neuroglial cells for each neuron in the central nervous system. The neurolemma, capsule, and satellite cells of the peripheral nervous system probably subserve functions in the peripheral nervous system similar to those of neuroglia in the central nervous system. The term neuroglia includes the *macroglia* (astrocytes and oligodendrocytes), the *ependyma*, and *microglia*, the last being of mesodermal origin, the others of ectodermal origin. The original concept of the neuroglia as a collection of non-nervous supporting cells and fibers with intercellular spaces, intercellular material, and capillaries arranged in an interwoven, tangled mass no longer is acceptable. These cells form myelin, are phagocytic under normal and pathological conditions, and provide a supporting framework for the neurons. Together, they should be regarded as a dynamic system of functional significance in fluid and respiratory interchange between the neurons of the central nervous system and their environment. In addition, some of the glial cells are mobile.

Neuroglial cells are not seen well in ordinary preparations, for their processes are not visible. In an H and E preparation, for example, only the nuclei are visible, and identification of neuroglial cells is dependent upon the size and shape of nuclei and the arrangement of chromatin granules within them.

Astrocytes

Astrocytes, as the name suggests, are star-shaped cells with numerous, branching, cytoplasmic processes. Nuclei are large, ovoid or spherical, and pale staining with fine, sparse chromatin granules distributed mainly at the periphery in close association with the nuclear membrane. Nucleoli are not obvious. The cytoplasm contains the usual organelles and a centrosome may be obvious. Lipochrome pigment often is present. Two types of astrocytes are distinguished by the character of the cytoplasmic processes.

Protoplasmic Astrocytes. Protoplasmic astrocytes, also called *mossy cells*, have many branching processes and are found mainly within the gray matter of the brain and spinal cord, often closely adjacent to the neuron cell bodies. In such sites, they are a type of satellite cell.

Fibrous Astrocytes. Fibrous astrocytes, or spider cells, have longer, more slender processes which contain numerous cytoplasmic fibrils and are located mainly in white matter.

In both types, one or more of the cytoplasmic processes terminates in a small, platelike swelling lying in the adventitia of a blood vessel. Such "perivascular feet" from many astrocytes may be so numerous as to constitute an outer sheath or perivascular limiting membrane to the blood vessel. The processes of astrocytes and other glial elements lying between nerve cell bodies and their axons and dendrites constitute the *neuropil*. This appears particularly dense at the surface of the central nervous system immediately beneath the pia mater (one of the covering membranes of the central nervous system; see page 204) and beneath the ependyma lining the cavities of the central nervous system. Thus, nervous tissue everywhere is separated from mesodermal structures (the membranes and blood vessels) by a concentration of glial cells and their processes.

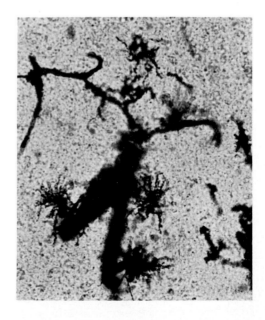

Figure 10-30. Photomicrograph of protoplasmic astrocytes. Note the end-feet attached to the wall of a capillary (solid black). Golgi method. × 300.

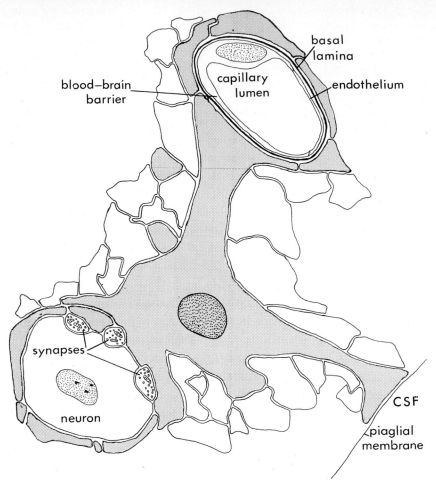

Figure 10-31.   Diagram of a protoplasmic astrocyte to illustrate the relationships between it and other components of the gray matter. Note that by its cytoplasmic processes it contacts a capillary (top), a nerve cell (bottom left), and the piaglial membrane (bottom right).

Oligodendroglia

Oligodendroglia have spherical or oval nuclei which are smaller than those of the astrocytes. They also are more numerous, being the most common of the neuroglial cells. The nuclei stain darkly owing to a high content of both coarse and fine chromatin granules, situated mainly adjacent to the nuclear membrane. Cytoplasm is scanty and nonfibrillar, and cytoplasmic processes are few and slender. In white matter, oligodendroglia are located in rows between myelinated fibers, and in gray matter, like protoplasmic astrocytes, they may be closely applied to nerve cell bodies as another type of satellite cell. In both gray and white matter, they may be associated closely with capillary blood vessels.

Astrocytes and oligodendroglia are derived from *spongioblasts*, a primitive ectodermal cell. Spongioblasts may be present in adult nervous tissue as a fourth type of neuroglial cell. Such cells have spherical nuclei, smaller than those of astrocytes and oligodendroglia, which contain much chromatin and thus are darkly staining. Cytoplasm is extremely scanty.

Microglia

Microglia, unlike the other two types, is of mesodermal origin and comprises fibroblast-like cells, presumably derived from the pia mater or from connective tissue which penetrated nervous tissue with ingrowing blood vessels. Nuclei are small and elongated with chromatin granules distributed throughout the karyoplasm. Cytoplasm is scanty and often appears as a slender thread at each pole of the elongated or kidney-shaped nucleus, but frequently shows numerous, small "spiny" processes. Microglial cells are distributed throughout gray and white matter, usually near blood vessels or as nerve satellites. They have no perivascular feet.

Ependyma

The entire central nervous system develops as a hollow cylinder—the neural tube—and cavities remain in the adult as the ventricles of the brain and the central canal of the spinal cord. The lining of these cavities is the ependyma, which retains the epithelial character present in the early embryo. In the embryo, the cells of the ependyma are ciliated, but in the adult the cells appear to be of the cuboidal epithelial type without cilia. By electron microscopy, it can be shown that on the luminal aspect ependymal cells have numerous microvilli and the cytoplasm contains fibrils which may extend into basal cytoplasmic processes.

Blood-Brain Barrier

Many substances are exchanged rapidly between the blood and brain tissue; others are not. In the adult human brain, nervous elements do not abut directly upon capillaries except in certain special situations, e.g., parts of the hypothalamus. Usually they are separated from capillaries by intervening neuroglial cells or their processes; the majority of these cells are astrocytes. The apposed plasma membranes of adjacent end bulbs of the neuroglial cells fit closely together by specialized "closed contacts" so that there are no extracellular diffusion channels. Nervous tissue is isolated from blood by neuroglial elements, which thus have an important function in the regulation of exchange of materials between the blood and the nervous tissue.

MEMBRANES AND VESSELS OF THE CENTRAL NERVOUS SYSTEM

Living nervous tissue of the central nervous system is soft and delicate and requires both adequate protection and nourishment. Protection is provided in the first place by a complete bony case covering brain and spinal cord in the form of the cranium (skull vault) and the vertebral column. Within the bony case are three membranous investments called the meninges. The outermost, the *dura mater* or *pachymeninx*, is fibrous, tough, and relatively inelastic and lines the cranium, being attached firmly to bone. At the foramen magnum, it continues as a tubular investment surrounding the spinal cord within the vertebral canal but is separated from bone by an *epidural* or extradural space. The middle membrane is the *arachnoid*, composed of fine, cobweb-like strands of interlacing reticular fibers. The most internal layer, which closely invests the brain and spinal cord, is the *pia mater*. In this layer are found the blood vessels supplying the central nervous system. Pia and arachnoid have a similar structure and sometimes are regarded as a single layer called the *leptomeninx* or *leptomeninges*.

Dura Mater

The cranial dura mater usually is described as consisting of two layers.

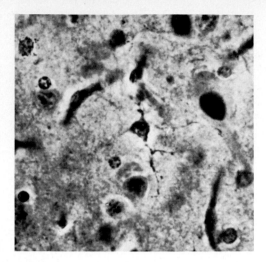

Figure 10-32. Photomicrograph of a microglial cell from the cerebral cortex. Golgi method. × 750.

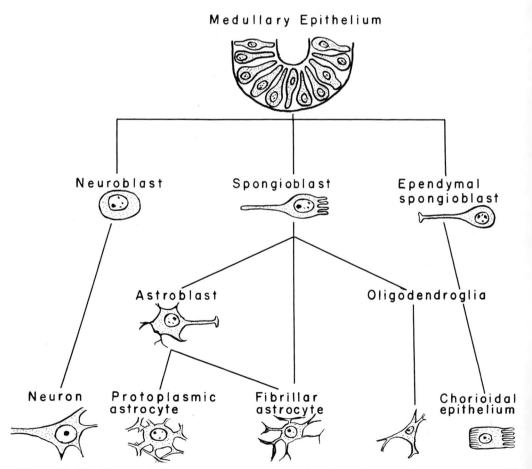

Figure 10-33. Diagram to illustrate the histogenesis of cells in the central nervous system. All are derived from the medullary epithelium of the neural tube. Microglial cells (not illustrated) are derived from mesenchymal cells which invade the developing nervous system.

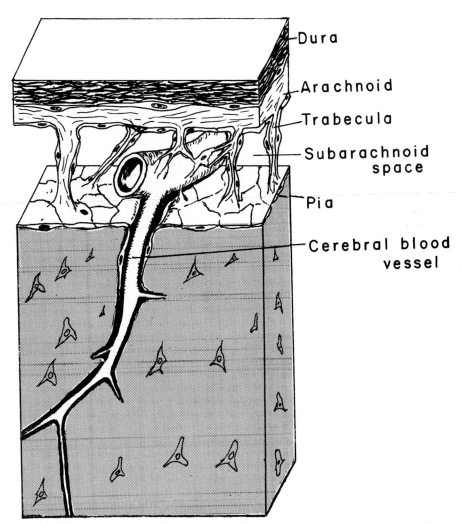

Dura

Arachnoid

Trabecula

Subarachnoid
space

Pia

Cerebral blood
vessel

Figure 10-34.   Diagram to illustrate the relationship of the meninges to the brain.

The first is an outer layer of dense connective tissue, containing numerous blood vessels and nerves. This layer is in. direct contact with the inner surface of bone. It is, quite simply, the periosteum on the inner surface of the cranial bones and is termed the *endosteal layer*. The second is an inner layer of dense fibrous tissue with a single layer of flat, mesothelial cells on its inner surface. This, the *fibrous layer*, is separated from the outer layer in regions to form the large venous sinuses of the brain and also is reflected inward to extend into large fissures of the brain as partitions. Such partitions occur in the midsagittal plane (the falx cerebri) between the two cerebral hemispheres, horizontally between the occipital lobes of the cerebrum and the upper surface of the cerebellum (the tentorium cerebelli), and between the two cerebellar hemispheres as the small falx cerebelli. In addition, there is an extension of dura forming the roof of the pituitary fossa (the diaphragma sellae). The spinal dura corresponds to the inner fibrous layer of the cranial dura, with which it is continuous at the foramen magnum. The vertebrae have their own periosteum. Both inner and outer surfaces of the spinal dura are covered by a single layer of flat cells, and dura is separated from periosteum by a slender *epidural space* in which are anastomosing venous channels lying in fatty, areolar tissue.

Between dura and arachnoid is a narrow capillary interval, the subdural space, containing lymphlike fluid.

Arachnoid

The arachnoid is a delicate nonvascular membrane lining the dura and covering the brain surface without passing into the sulci. It is separated from the pia by an interval of varying extent which is crossed by numerous trabeculae passing between arachnoid and pia, thus subdividing this space

into numerous interconnected *subarachnoid spaces*. Over the spinal cord the trabeculae are few and thus the subarachnoid space is continuous. The membrane lining the dura and the trabeculae is composed of fine collagenous fibers with some elastic fibers. Surfaces of the membrane lining the dura and trabeculae and the surface overlying the pia are covered with a continuous, single layer of flat cells with large, pale, oval nuclei. These cells can become phagocytic.

The subarachnoid spaces are filled with cerebrospinal fluid. In certain regions, arachnoid is separated from pia by a considerable distance, the spaces so formed containing large quantities of cerebrospinal fluid. Such spaces are termed *cisternae*.

Pia Mater

The pia mater is a delicate membrane closely investing the surface of the brain and, unlike the arachnoid, it extends into the depths of the cerebral sulci. It often is described in two layers. The inner, membranous layer (intima pia) is composed of a close network of fine reticular and elastic fibers. This layer is adherent to underlying nervous tissue and sends a fibrous, posterior median septum into the substance of the spinal cord. As blood vessels enter nervous tissue, they take with them a covering of the intima pia, with an intervening perivascular space containing cerebrospinal fluid in the case of the larger vessels. The more superficial layer of the pia, the epipial tissue, is composed of a network of collagenous fibers with, of course, a few fibroblasts. This layer is continuous with the tissue of the arachnoid. The external surface of the epipial layer is covered with a single layer of flattened mesothelial cells continuous with those covering arachnoid tissue. The epipial layer is more obvious over the spinal cord and contains the spinal blood vessels. That over the brain is less obvious, and vessels here appear to lie upon the intima pia within the subarachnoid space.

Branches of the internal carotid and vertebral arteries pass from the pia mater into the substance of the central nervous system. Capillary networks are richer in the gray matter than in the white. Venous return is to veins in the pia mater and thence to the dural venous sinuses. No lymphatics have been described in the central nervous system. Dura and pia contain a rich plexus of nerve fibers, mainly of the autonomic system to the blood vessels, but some sensory fibers are present also, these traveling from sensory receptors in the meninges.

CHORIOID PLEXUS AND CEREBROSPINAL FLUID

The central nervous system is made up of delicate tissue and, as stated previously, is protected by the bones of the cranium and spinal column, within which is the pia arachnoid containing fluid to function as a water cushion. This fluid is the cerebrospinal fluid, which also fills the ventricles of the brain and the central canal of the spinal cord. Fluid within the ventricular system of the brain freely communicates with fluid in the subarachnoid space and constantly is being replenished, for not only does it subserve a protective function but it also plays an important role in the metabolism of nervous tissue.

Cerebrospinal fluid is secreted by the *chorioid plexuses*, which are areas where brain tissue retains its embryonic character as a thin, nonnervous epithelium and is closely associated with pia mater which is extremely vascular. The plexuses are located in the roof of the third and fourth ventricles and in the medial walls of part of the lateral ventricles. In these sites the ventricular lining (ependyma) is composed of a regular layer of cuboidal cells with large,

central, spherical nuclei and a free, brushlike border. By electron microscopy, this surface shows many bulbous microvilli, and at both lateral and basal borders the plasma membrane is infolded into the cytoplasm. Both microvilli and membrane infoldings presumably are methods of increasing surface area. This epithelium rests upon a delicate connective tissue derived from pia-arachnoid and in which are numerous thin-walled blood vessels. The entire tissue of the chorioid protrudes into the ventricular cavities, and this is the site of secretion of the cerebrospinal fluid. In the roof of the fourth ventricle are three foramina—one central (the foramen of Magendie) and one lateral on each side (the foramina of Luschka)—and through these foramina cerebrospinal fluid can pass from the ventricles into the subarachnoid space. All the ventricles and the central canal of the spinal cord are continuous. Flow of cerebrospinal fluid usually is from the ventricles into the subarachnoid space.

Absorption of cerebrospinal fluid occurs mainly into the large venous sinuses inside the cranium. These are enclosed by the fibrous tissue of the dura, but in certain sites arachnoid protrudes into the lumina of the sinuses as finger-like projections termed the *arachnoid villi*. In these villi, cerebrospinal fluid is separated from blood within the sinuses only by arachnoid mesothelium and can diffuse back into the blood. Small amounts of cerebrospinal fluid return to the circulation via extracranial lymphatics which are in continuity with perineural spaces of the cranial nerves.

Thus, there is a constant secretion of cerebrospinal fluid by the chorioid plexuses and a consequent absorption back into the venous system.

Cerebrospinal fluid, a clear, colorless liquid similar to if not identical with the aqueous humor of the eye and tissue fluid, contains small amounts of protein and glucose, and some in-

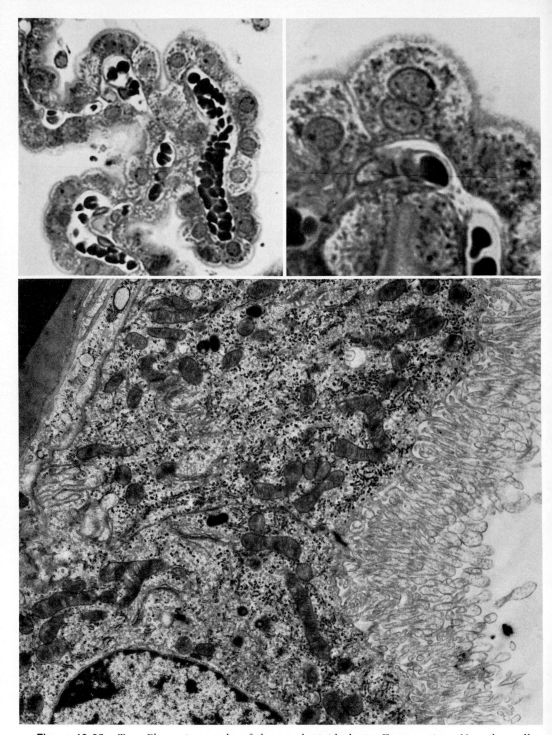

Figure 10-35. Top: Photomicrographs of the rat chorioid plexus, Epon sections. Note the well-defined brush border. Left, × 250; right, × 1250. Bottom: Electron micrograph of the chorioid plexus. Note the bulbous microvilli on the apical surface (right) and some basal infoldings of the basal plasma membrane (left center). There is a portion of a capillary containing a red blood corpuscle at top left. × 8500.

See filmstrip I, frame 40.

organic salts. It has a specific gravity of only 1.004 to 1.007. A few lymphocytes usually are present also.

CYTOARCHITECTURE OF THE CENTRAL NERVOUS SYSTEM

Although this subject is described fully in textbooks of neuroanatomy, a brief outline of the arrangement of nerve cells and their processes in the more important parts of the brain and spinal cord follows.

Spinal Cord

As shown in Figure 10-36, in cross section the spinal cord is oval in shape. Posteriorly, the cord is divided partially into right and left halves by the dorsal median septum while anteriorly

there is a deep longitudinal cleft called the anterior (ventral) median fissure. The entire cord is surrounded by pia mater which extends into the anterior median fissure.

Although there are variations in shape and structure at different levels—cervical, thoracic, lumbar, and sacral—the basic pattern of the cord is similar at all levels. Centrally in the cord in cross section is an H-shaped area of gray matter composed of nerve cells. On each side, the limbs of the H are called the anterior and posterior horns. In addition, extending throughout the thoracic and upper one or two lumbar segments, there is a lateral horn of gray matter. The central canal, lined by ependyma, is situated in the horizontal bar of the H. Nerve cell bodies lie in groups in the gray matter, the large motor neurons lying in the anterior horn.

The white matter, formed by nerve

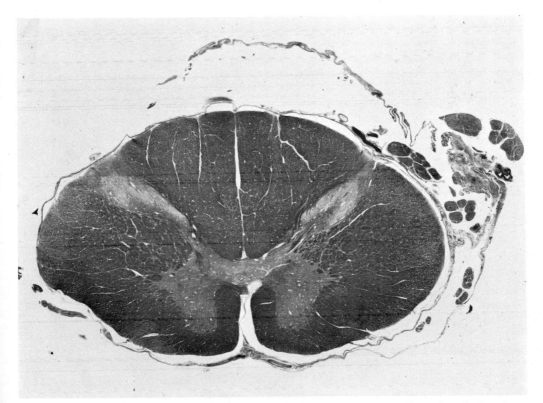

Figure 10-36.   Photomicrograph of a transverse section of the spinal cord. Weil method. × 3.

fibers, surrounds the gray matter and is divided into longitudinal columns or *funiculi*. Between the posterior horn of gray matter and the dorsal median septum is the posterior or dorsal funiculus. The remainder of the white matter is divided by the ventral horn and nerve roots and the anterior median fissure into lateral and ventral columns respectively. Between the tip of the posterior horn and the surface of the cord is a small area of white matter containing fine nerve fibers, called the *zone of Lissauer*.

Nerve cells in the gray matter are multipolar. The axons of some leave the cord as ventral root fibers, others send axons into the white matter of ipsilateral and contralateral sides, and still others have short axons which terminate on neurons near their origin, confined to the gray matter (Golgi type II). Generally the white matter contains no nerve cell bodies or dendrites and is formed by myelinated and nonmyelinated fibers. At the surface of the cord there is a narrow marginal area composed only of neuroglia.

Cerebellum

The cerebellum consists of right and left *hemispheres* and a central *vermis*, divided into lobules by transverse fissures. Each lobule comprises a part of the vermis with two lateral, winglike extensions into the hemispheres. The surface of the hemispheres shows numerous folds, or folia, arranged parallel to the main fissures so that in sagittal section there is the appearance of a central stem with numerous branches (the arbor vitae). Gray matter of the cerebellum is located on the surface as a thin cortex overlying the centrally placed white matter, but there are also small collections of nerve cells (nuclei) in the central parts of the cerebellum.

The cerebellar cortex on section shows three layers: an outer molecular layer of a few small nerve cells and many nonmyelinated fibers, a central

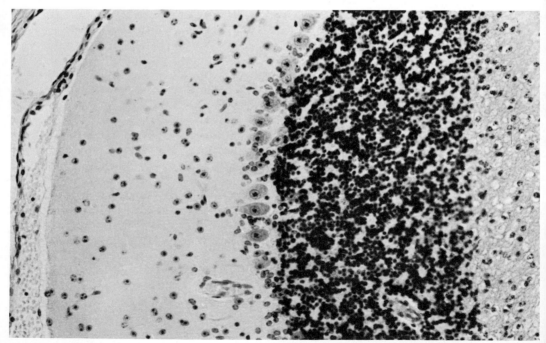

Figure 10-37. Photomicrograph of a section of the cerebellar cortex, cortical surface to the left. × 175.

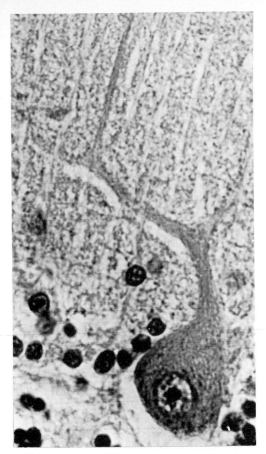

Figure 10-38. Photomicrograph of a Purkinje cell from the cerebellar cortex. Hematoxylin and eosin. × 750.

See filmstrip I, frame 41.

cell opposite to the dendrites, acquire myelin sheaths, and give off collaterals, and the main, myelinated axonal stem then traverses the granular layer to terminate in one of the deep cerebellar nuclei or to go to another part of the cortex. Cells of the molecular layer are small and stellate in form. Dendrites and axons of those situated near the surface are short, but those of the deeper layer, i.e., near Purkinje cells, have longer axons with collaterals in relation to several Purkinje cells.

In the cortex also are terminations of the *mossy* and *climbing* fibers, these passing into the cerebellar cortex from the white matter of the brain stem and spinal cord. The mossy fibers are thick and synapse on cells of the granular layer. Climbing fibers pass through the granular layer to terminate on Purkinje cells.

The cerebellum functionally is related to movements of striated muscle, being concerned with coordination, posture, and equilibrium.

Cerebrum

In the cerebral hemispheres, gray matter is located on the surface as *cerebral cortex* and centrally, surrounded by white matter, as ganglia or nuclei.

The surface of the hemispheres is convoluted, by which means the surface area is increased, the projecting folds being called the *gyri* with intervening depressions or *sulci*. The surface area of the cortex is about 200,000 sq. mm., and varies from 1.5 to 4 mm. in thickness, containing nerve cells, fibers, neuroglia, and blood vessels. Most of the cells are pyramidal, stellate (granule), and fusiform or spindle in type and they are arranged in a laminated manner so that six layers are recognizable in a section. These are, from superficial to deep: the molecular layer, composed mainly of fibers from cells in the deeper layers, these running parallel to the surface,

layer of a single row of large cells, called Purkinje cells, and an innermost granular layer of numerous small nerve cell bodies. Cells of the granular layer are small, with three to six short dendrites, and a nonmyelinated axon which ascends to the molecular layer where it divides into two lateral branches running along the length of a folium. The Purkinje cells are large and flask-shaped with several main dendrites which enter the molecular layer as a fan-shaped network of branching processes at right angles to the folium, and thus at right angles to the parallel terminal axonal branches of the granular cells. Axons from Purkinje cells arise from part of the

and a few small nerve cell bodies; the external granular layer of small, triangular nerve cell bodies; the pyramidal cell layer of large, pyramidal cells and many small granule cells; the internal granular layer of small stellate granule cells; the internal pyramidal or ganglionic layer of large and medium-sized pyramidal cells; and the multiform or polymorphic cell layer of cells of varying shape.

It should be emphasized that the layers blend with each other and that all layers contain neuroglia. Cells thus lie in the *neuropil*, a feltwork of naked nerve fibers and processes of neuroglia cells. The thickness of the different layers varies in different regions of the cerebral cortex, this being related to the particular functions of different regions.

The white matter underlying the gray cortex is composed of bundles of myelinated fibers passing in all directions. These fibers, of course, are supported by neuroglia, and, functionally, are of three main groups. Some fibers connect different parts of the cortex of one hemisphere and are called *association fibers*. Others connect areas of the cortex of one hemisphere with other areas of the opposite hemisphere and are termed *commissural fibers*. *Projection fibers* connect the cortex with lower centers.

DIFFERENTIATION AND PROLIFERATION

The details of development of the nervous system are given in textbooks of embryology and neurology. The *neural tube* is developed from an infolding of the ectoderm along the dorsum of the embryo, from which cells detach to form the *neural crests* on each side. From neural crests are developed the craniospinal ganglia and perhaps also the autonomic ganglia. The cells of the neural tube, the wall of which at first is composed of a single layer of epithelium, undergo rapid division and differentiate into

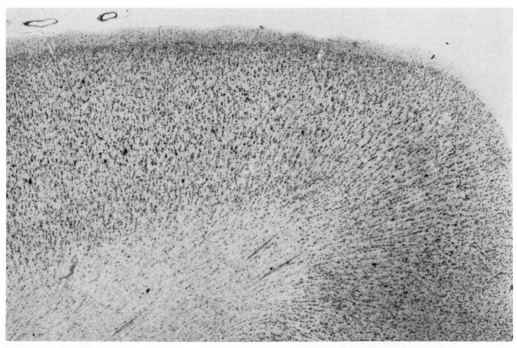

Figure 10-39.   Photomicrograph of cerebral cortex. Methylene blue. × 10.

neuroblasts, later forming neurons, and spongioblasts, which later form neuroglia. Ependyma develops from the primitive lining of the neural tube. In the neural crests, differentiation occurs and neurons, satellite cells, and neurolemma are formed. Microglia probably is formed by mesenchymal cells which enter the central nervous system with the blood vessels. A simplified scheme of development in the central nervous system is illustrated in Figure 10-33.

Throughout life, neuroglia, neurolemma, and capsule cells are capable of proliferation, but neurons become incapable of reproduction at about the time of birth. After destruction, they cannot be replaced.

DEGENERATION AND REGENERATION

Although neurons after birth cannot reproduce, they are capable of withstanding and recovering from a certain degree of injury. If a nerve fiber is crushed or severed, changes occur both in the central and peripheral portions of the neuron. As explained previously, the cell body undergoes chromatolysis, whereby the Nissl substance breaks down to a powderlike mass and becomes spread diffusely throughout the cell body. Reconstitution of Nissl substance after such an injury may occur rapidly in a few days or, depending on the nature of the injury, may take months. Peripherally, the axis cylinder swells and fragments within a period of days, and, in myelinated fibers, the myelin also is broken up. The degenerated and fragmented material of axis cylinder and myelin is removed by phagocytosis of macrophages which enter the neurolemmal tubes. These degenerative changes are accompanied by proliferation of neurolemma to form a band or cord of cells.

After an interval of about a week, the divided axon from its central end starts to grow peripherally at a rate of 1 to 2 mm. per day. It shows numerous fine branches or sprouts, and these grow across the scar tissue at the site of the injury and enter the cords of neurolemma, and thence follow them to reach the original site of termination. However, in such injuries usually many axons are divided and obviously may reach a termination which is functionally inappropriate. Others are lost in scar tissue. Myelin is re-formed but the process is slow. Unmyelinated fibers undergo a similar process but, of course, without a myelin sheath. In the central nervous system where a neurolemma sheath is lacking, regeneration is not possible.

SPECIAL STAINS

Ordinary staining methods show few details of nervous tissue, and it is necessary to employ special staining methods. However, no single stain shows more than a few features. Of the basic dyes, cresyl violet is useful as a stain for nuclei and Nissl substance and can be used to demonstrate chromatolysis. After mordanting in potassium bichromate, hematoxylin stains myelin, and methylene blue used supravitally is useful for demonstrating axons and nerve endings.

Various silver reduction methods, e.g., Golgi and Cajal, impregnate entire neurons (cell body and processes) with a silver deposit, but the results often are difficult to reproduce. Silver carbonate with gold toning is a good method for neuroglia. Osmium tetroxide blackens myelin and, when used with potassium bichromate (Marchi stain), demonstrates degenerating fibers.

REFERENCES

Adrian, E. D.: The Mechanism of Nervous Action. London, Oxford University Press, 1932.

Burkel, W. E.: The histological fine structure of perineurium. Anat. Rec., *158*:177, 1967.

Causey, G.: The Cell of Schwann. Edinburgh and London, E. & S. Livingstone, Ltd., 1960.

DeRobertis, E. D. P.: Histophysiology of Synapses and Neurosecretion. Oxford, Pergamon Press Ltd., 1964.

DeRobertis, E. D. P.: Ultrastructure and cytochemistry of the synaptic region. Science, *156*:907, 1967.

Geren, B. B.: The formation from the Schwann cell surface of myelin in peripheral nerves of chick embryos. Exp. Cell Res. 7:558, 1954.

Giese, A. C.: Cell Physiology, ed. 2. Philadelphia, W. B. Saunders Co., 1962.

Glees, P.: Neuroglia: Morphology and Function. Springfield, Ill., Charles C Thomas, 1955.

Gray, E. G.: Tissue of the central nervous system. *In* Electron Microscopic Anatomy, edited by S. M. Kurtz. New York, Academic Press, 1964, p. 369.

Hirano, A., and Dembitzer, H. M.: A structural analysis of the myelin sheath in the central nervous system. J. Cell Biol., *34*:555, 1967.

Hyden, H.: The neuron. *In* The Cell: Biochemistry, Physiology, Morphology, edited by J. Brachet and A. E. Mirsky. New York, Academic Press, 1960, Vol. 4, p. 215.

Kuntz, A.: The Autonomic Nervous System, ed. 4. Philadelphia, Lea & Febiger, 1953.

Millen, J. W.: Some aspects of the anatomy of the pia mater and choroid plexuses. Sci. Basis Med. Ann. Rev., 125, 1963.

Palay, S. L., and Palade, G. E.: The fine structure of neurons. J. Biophys. Biochem. Cytol., *1*:69, 1955.

Pease, D. C., and Schultz, R. L.: Circulation to the brain and spinal cord. Submicroscopic anatomy. *In* Blood Vessels and Lymphatics, edited by D. I. Abramson. New York, Academic Press, 1962, p. 233.

Peters, A.: Observations on the connections between myelin sheaths and glial cells in the optic nerves of young rats. J. Anat., *98*:125, 1964.

Ranson, S. W., and Clark, S. L.: The Anatomy of the Nervous System, ed. 10. Philadelphia, W. B. Saunders Co., 1959.

Robertson, J. D.: The ultrastructure of adult vertebrate peripheral myelinated nerve fibers in relation to myelinogenesis. J. Biophys. Biochem. Cytol., *1*:271, 1955.

Robertson, J. D.: The ultrastructure of Schmidt-Lanterman clefts and related shearing defects of the myelin sheath. J. Biophys. Biochem. Cytol., *4*:39, 1958.

Ross, L. L.: Peripheral nervous tissue. *In* Electron Microscopic Anatomy, edited by S. M. Kurtz, New York, Academic Press, 1964, p. 341.

Sandborn, E. B.: Electron microscopy of the neuron membrane systems and filaments. Can. J. Phys. Pharm., *44*:329, 1966.

Shanthaveerappa, T. R., and Bourne, G. H.: Perineural epithelium: a new concept of its role in the integrity of the peripheral nervous system. Science, *154*:1464, 1966.

Sherrington, C. S.: The Integrative Action of the Nervous System. New Haven, Yale University Press, 1906.

Truex, R. C., and Carpenter, M. B.: Strong and Elwyn's Human Neuroanatomy, ed. 5. Baltimore, The Williams & Wilkins Co., 1964.

Uzman, B. G., and Nogueira-Graf, G.: Electron microscope studies of the formation of nodes of Ranvier in mouse sciatic nerves. J. Biophys. Biochem. Cytol., *3*:589, 1957.

Van Harreveld, A., and Malhotra, S. K.: Extracellular space in the cerebral cortex of the mouse. J. Anat., *101*:197, 1967.

PART TWO

HISTOLOGY OF THE ORGAN SYSTEMS

CHAPTER 11

THE CIRCULATORY SYSTEM

The circulatory system comprises the blood vascular system and the lymph vascular system. The blood vascular system, which distributes nutritive materials, oxygen, and hormones to all parts of the body and removes the cellular products of metabolism, includes the heart and a series of tubular vessels, the *arteries, capillaries,* and *veins.* The heart is a modified blood vessel, specialized as an organ of propulsion. The arteries, which by branching constantly increase in number and decrease in caliber, conduct blood from the heart to the capillary bed. The capillaries, where the interchange of elements between the blood and the other tissues takes place, form a meshwork of anastomosing tubules. Veins return blood from the capillaries to the heart.

The lymph vascular system (commencing in the tissues as blind tubules) consists of lymphatic capillaries and various sized lymphatic vessels which return fluid (lymph) from tissue spaces to the blood stream via the large veins in the neck.

Frequently nerve fascicles lie in company with arteries and veins as they course through the various tissues. These are the so-called *neurovascular bundles.*

THE BLOOD VASCULAR SYSTEM

The blood vascular system has a continuous lining which consists of a single layer of endothelial cells. In the capillaries this single layer of cells forms the major component of the wall. Thereafter the addition of accessory coats can be traced progressively in larger vessels. Since the structure of the capillary is simpler than that of any of the other components of the vascular system, we shall describe the capillary first instead of following the system in its functional order of heart, arteries, capillaries, and veins.

Capillaries

The capillaries are simple, endothelial tubes which connect the arterial and venous sides of the circulation. They have an average diameter of about 7 to 9 microns (i.e., approximately the diameter of a single red

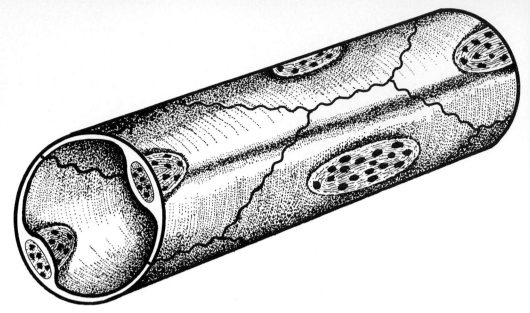

Figure 11-1.   Diagram to illustrate the arrangement of endothelial cells comprising the wall of a capillary. The boundaries of the endothelial cells may be outlined by silver impregnation.

blood corpuscle) and form a network of narrow canals. The meshes of the network vary in size and in shape in the different tissues and organs. The intensity of metabolism in a region determines the closeness of the mesh. There is a close network in the lungs, liver, kidneys, mucous membranes, glands, and skeletal muscle and in the gray matter of the brain. The network has a large mesh and is sparse in tendon, nerve, smooth muscle, and serous membranes. The network is best visualized in thick, cleared sections of material in which the capillaries have been injected with a colored gelatin or in living preparations such as the web of a frog's foot. Since capillaries pursue irregular courses, it is seldom that they are cut longitudinally in thin sections.

The wall of a capillary consists of a single layer of flat endothelial cells which is separated from a supporting bed of connective tissue by a basal lamina. Each endothelial cell is a curving, thin plate, with an ovoid or elongated nucleus. Usually the cells

are stretched along the axis of the capillary and have tapering ends. The cell borders, which can be made

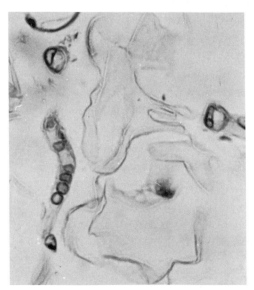

Figure 11-2.   Section of loose areolar connective tissue in which portions of three capillaries may be seen. Note the red blood cells occupying the lumen of the longitudinally cut capillary. × 400.

visible readily by the injection of silver nitrate, are serrated or wavy. The cytoplasm is clear or finely granular. Two or three cells, occasionally only one, line the circumference of a capillary at any level of section. Capillaries are surrounded by a thin sheath of delicate collagenous and reticular fibers and are accompanied by fixed macrophages and fibroblasts. Among the pericapillary elements, peculiar cells (*Rouget cells*) with long branching processes which surround the capillary wall have been described. Early studies indicated that these cells were contractile and were responsible for the contractility of capillaries. More recent work suggests that true capillaries in mammals do not possess Rouget cells and that capillary contractility is independent of them.

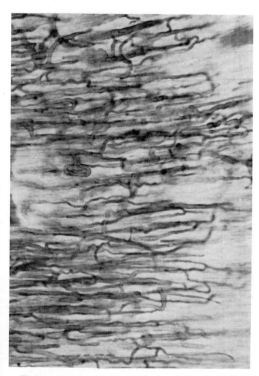

Figure 11-3. Unstained section of cardiac muscle in which the capillary network had been made visible by the injection of colored gelatin into the main arteries of supply. Note the close meshwork of capillaries between the individual cardiac muscle fibers. × 120.

Recently electron microscopic studies have added considerably to our knowledge of capillary structure. Practically all capillaries have numerous small vesicles (*pinocytotic vesicles* or *caveolae intracellulares*) along both the luminal and basal surfaces of the endothelial cells. The vesicles or caveolae appear to be formed by invagination of the cell membrane. Functionally, it appears that they represent sites of uptake of fluid for use by the endothelial cells and that they are involved in the transport of fluid across the capillary wall.

The ability to transfer substances through the wall of capillaries is referred to as permeability. Permeability varies regionally and, under changed conditions, locally. Whether the interchange occurs through the endothelial protoplasm or between adjacent endothelial cells is not known and at present it is the subject of considerable investigation. Most physiologists are of the opinion that changes in permeability can be accounted for by changes in the non-living component of the capillary wall (i.e., changes at the interphase between adjacent cells). In the capillaries of muscle, lungs, the central nervous system, and a number of other tissues, the endothelium forms a continuous layer around the lumen, and the margins of adjacent endothelial cells are closely opposed with little intervening "intercellular cement." Capillaries which exhibit such a complete endothelial lining have been referred to as *Type I (continuous) capillaries*. In the capillaries of many endocrine glands, the intestinal mucosa, and certain other organs, the endothelium is attenuated and contains "pores" ranging in diameter from 300 to 500Å. The pores, or circular fenestrations, may be covered by a diaphragm thinner than the cell membrane. Such capillaries are known as *Type II (fenestrated) capillaries*. Even more striking are the large pores found in the glomerular capillaries of the kidney. These pores

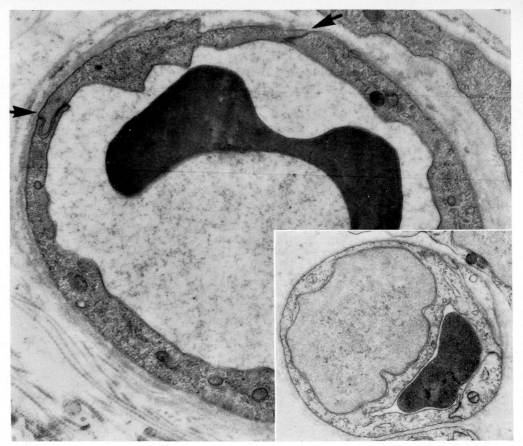

Figure 11-4. Electron micrograph of a capillary (Type I) in loose areolar connective tissue. The lumen contains a portion of a red blood corpuscle. Note the numerous pinocytotic vesicles in relation to the cell membrane of the endothelium and the two interphases between endothelial cells (arrows). × 18,500. Inset: A capillary, the wall of which is composed of two endothelial cells, one showing a prominent nuclear area. Present in the lumen is a red blood corpuscle. × 7500.

appear to be closed only by the continuous basal lamina which envelops the capillaries. The pores are thought to make an important contribution to the marked permeability of these capillaries in the production of the glomerular filtrate. *Sinusoids* and *sinusoidal capillaries* possess distinctive features not characteristic of ordinary capillaries. They are of relatively large caliber (up to 30 microns) and have irregular, tortuous walls. The walls are not formed by a continuous layer of endothelial cells, as in true capillaries, but they have an incomplete lining of phagocytic and nonphagocytic cells. The flat cells of the wall

belong to the reticuloendothelial (or macrophage) system. The lining of the sinusoids is separated from the parenchyma of the organs only by a fine network of reticular fibers.

Arterial (pre-) and *venous (post-) capillaries* are vessels intermediate between arteries and capillaries and capillaries and veins respectively. Arterial capillaries are a little wider than the capillary network (up to 40 microns in diameter) and may contain scattered smooth muscle cells in their walls. Venous capillaries not infrequently have a considerable diameter (up to 200 microns), may contain scattered smooth muscle cells in their

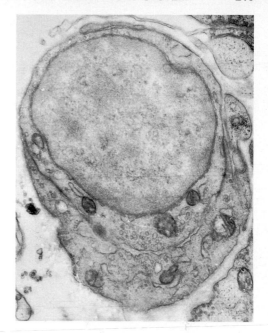

Figure 11-5. Electron micrograph of a closed-down capillary. The lumen of the vessel is represented by a narrow slit below the nuclear area. × 10,000.

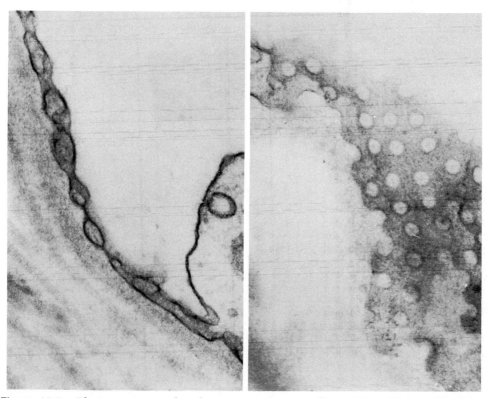

Figure 11-6. Electron micrographs of segments of two capillaries (Type II) from the chorioid plexus. In the left figure, the circular fenestrations (pores), each covered by a thin diaphragm, are cut transversely; in the right figure, the endothelium has been sectioned obliquely and the fenestrations are seen in surface view. Left, × 50,000. Right, × 40,000.

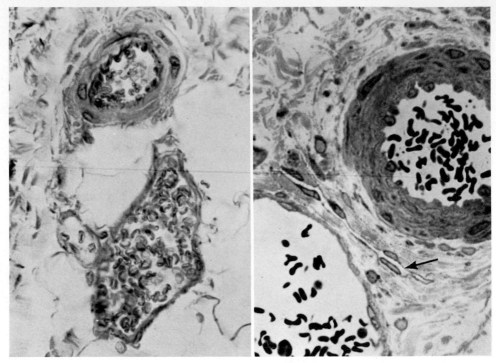

Figure 11-7.   Section of loose areolar connective tissue containing an arteriole and a venule. The prominent muscular wall and the internal elastic lamina of the arteriole distinguish it readily from the venule. Left: Paraffin section, × 300. Right: Epon section. Note the collapsed lymphatic capillary (arrow). × 450.   See filmstrip I, frame 42.

walls, and show denser concentrations of collagenous fibers than are found in the main capillary meshwork. The concept of arterial and venous capillaries, although rather indefinite, is helpful in understanding the transitions between capillaries and vessels with clearly defined coats. In such vessels, owing to the addition of connective tissue or smooth muscle or both, there is mechanical support, and control of vessel diameter becomes possible.

Arteries

All arteries show a common pattern of organization. The wall of a typical artery is composed of three tunics or coats. The innermost coat, the *tunica intima* (or *interna*), consists of an inner endothelial lining, a *subendothelial layer* of delicate fibroelastic connective tissue, and an external band of elastic fibers, the *internal elastic membrane*, which may be absent in many vessels. The middle coat, the *tunica media*, consists chiefly of smooth muscle cells, circularly arranged. The outer coat, the *tunica adventitia*, is composed principally of connective tissue, most of the elements of which run parallel to the long axis of the vessel. Closest to the media there may be a definite *external elastic membrane*. The structure and relative thickness of each of the tunics vary according to the type and size of the vessel.

Arterial blood vessels can be classified in three groups: *large arteries,* which contain a preponderance of elastic fibers; *small to medium-sized arteries,* containing numerous muscular elements; and *arterioles,* the smallest arterial vessels.

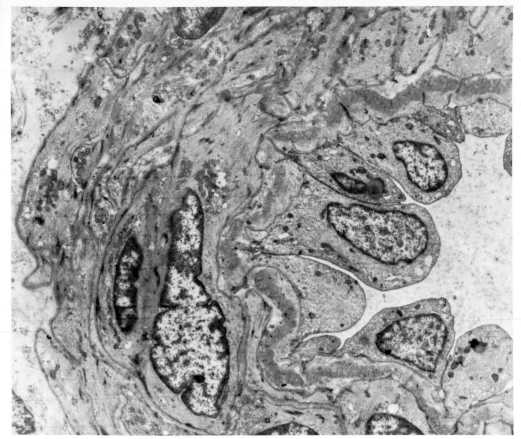

Figure 11-8. Electron micrograph of a segment of the wall of an arteriole. The internal elastic lamina may be identified between the endothelium and the tunica media. × 5000.

Arterioles. These vessels, with a diameter of 100 microns or less, have a tunica intima which consists only of endothelium and an internal elastic membrane. No subendothelial tissue is recognizable. The internal elastic membrane is really a network of fibers which by light microscopy appears as a thin, bright line just beneath the endothelium. The media is muscular and is composed of from one to five complete layers of muscle cells, among which are some scattered elastic fibrils. The adventitia, which usually is thinner than the media, is a layer of loose connective tissue with longitudinally oriented col-lagenous and elastic fibers. It merges into the surrounding connective tissue. No definite external elastic membrane is present.

The arterioles have relatively thick walls and narrow lumina. They are able to control the distribution of blood to different capillary beds by vasodilation and vasoconstriction in localized regions. They are the prime controllers of systemic blood pressure. Most of the fall in blood pressure occurs within the arterioles so that only a gentle stream passes into the delicate capillary beds.

Small and Medium-sized Arteries. This group comprises all arteries belonging to the *muscular type* and includes most of the arteries that bear names and all small unnamed ones. There is a gradual transition

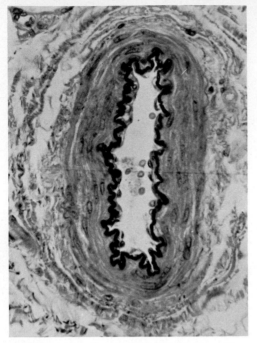

Figure 11-9. Section of a small artery. Note the prominent internal elastic lamina and the thickness of the tunica media. Aldehyde fuchsin stain. × 250.

between these vessels and the arterioles described above. The walls of the muscular arteries are relatively thick, owing principally to the large amount of muscle in the media. They also have been called *distributing arteries* because they distribute blood to different organs and regulate the supply of blood in response to different functional demands.

The tunica intima exhibits three definite layers. Beneath the endothelium there is the subendothelial layer comprising delicate elastic and collagenous fibers and a few fibroblasts. The internal elastic membrane, or lamina, is prominent and forms a thick fenestrated band composed of closely interwoven elastic fibers. In histological sections, it typically is thrown into folds because of postmortem contraction of the muscular elements of the media. In many arteries the membrane is split into two or more layers.

The media consists almost ex-clusively of circularly disposed smooth muscle cells. Between the layers of muscle (up to 40 in number) there are small amounts of connective tissue, the constituents of which are elastic, collagenous, and reticular fibers, and a few fibroblasts.

The adventitia is sometimes thicker than the media. It is composed of loose connective tissue containing collagenous and elastic fibers, most of which course longitudinally. The elastic fibers are concentrated in the inner layer of the coat, where they commonly form a definite external elastic membrane. The outer layer of the adventitia blends into the surrounding connective tissue without a sharp boundary between the two.

Large Arteries. The large arteries belong to the elastic type. The wall is relatively thin for the size of the vessel. The amount of elastic tissue present is sufficient to impart a yellow color to the freshly cut wall. This group includes the aorta and its largest main branches, the brachiocephalic, the common carotid, the subclavian, and common iliac.

The endothelial cells of the intima are polygonal in shape, not elongate, as in the smaller vessels. The subendothelial layer consists of collagenous and elastic fibers and scattered fibroblasts, and in the deeper portion of the intima small bundles of smooth muscle cells are present. Numerous elastic fibers, arranged mainly longitudinally, course in this deeper zone and pass into a fenestrated elastic membrane, which by its location corresponds with the internal elastic membrane.

The media is characterized by numerous distinct elastic membranes, 40 to 60 in number, which are arranged concentrically. They anastomose to form complex elastic nets. Interspaces between the concentric membranes contain fibroblasts, an amorphous ground substance, a fine elastic network, and smooth muscle cells which pursue a spiral course.

The adventitia is a thin coat and is

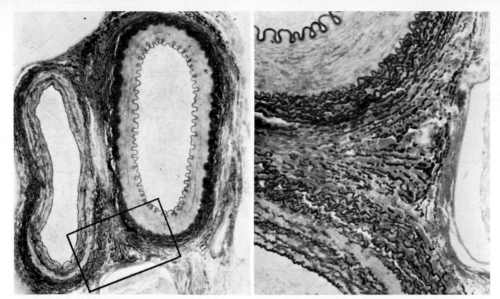

Figure 11-10.   Comparison of small artery and small vein. The artery is identified by the thickness of the tunica media. Elastic fibers are stained specifically by resorcin fuchsin. Left, × 40. Right (enlargement of blocked area of left figure), × 120.

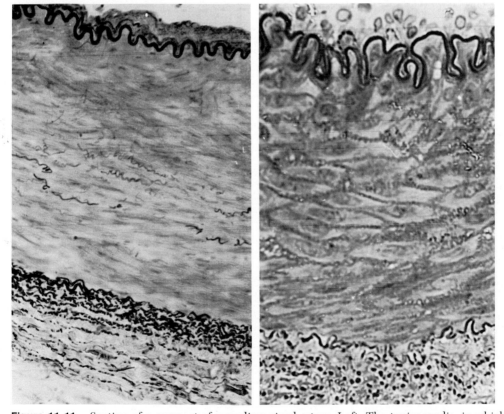

Figure 11-11.   Section of a segment of a medium-sized artery. Left: The tunica media, in which scattered elastic fibers may be seen, lies between the prominent internal and external elastic laminae. Resorcin fuchsin stain. × 120. Right: Individual smooth muscle cells may be identified clearly in the tunica media. Epon section. × 450.   See filmstrip I, frames 43 and 44.

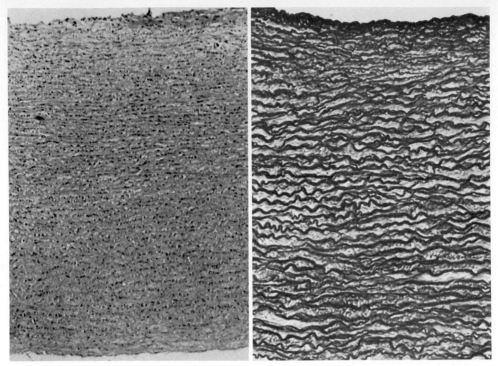

Figure 11-12.   Section of the aorta (large elastic artery). Left: Hematoxylin and eosin, ×50. Right: Resorcin fuchsin, × 80. In the latter micrograph, note the distinct elastic membranes, concentrically arranged.   See filmstrip I, frame 45.

not highly organized. It cannot be distinguished sharply from the surrounding connective tissue. There is no distinctive external elastic layer or membrane. The collagenous fibers present within the adventitia are oriented in an open spiral.

The elastic arteries absorb some of the pulse beat by the expansion of the elastic tissue within their walls and make the blood flow less intermittent than it would be if the vessels were rigid tubes. Often they are termed *conducting arteries*, emphasizing their function of conducting blood to the smaller ramifications of the vascular system.

Specialized Arteries. Certain arteries exhibit pronounced structural deviations from the generalized plan. These variations reflect adaptations to special locations and functional demands. Arteries protected within the skull have a thin wall and a well-

developed internal elastic membrane. Arteries of the lung have thin walls owing to a reduction of both muscle and elastic tissue. This is correlated with a lower blood pressure in the pulmonary circulation. The umbilical arteries possess a media composed of two thick, muscular layers, an inner longitudinal layer and an outer circular layer. These arteries lack an internal elastic membrane. In the penile arteries the intima is greatly thickened and contains many longitudinal muscle fibers. Cardiac muscle extends into the roots of the aorta and pulmonary artery.

Age Changes in Arteries. Arteries do not complete their differentiation until adult life. It is difficult to separate some of the final stages of differentiation from the retrogressive changes which develop gradually with age. Arteries of the elastic type show greater changes with age than do arteries of the muscular type. In the aging process the principal changes occur in the intima and media. The elastic tissue shows irregular thickenings, fat infiltrates the interstitial substance, and in the medium-sized arteries, calcification occurs within the media.

Veins

Blood in the venous system is under a pressure one-tenth of that in the arteries and hence must accommodate a volume of blood greater than that within the arterial system. The caliber of veins in general is larger than that of arteries, but their walls are much thinner, chiefly owing to a reduction of muscular and elastic components. Venous blood vessels are classified into three groups: venules, small to medium-sized veins, and large veins. This classification is somewhat unsatisfactory since the divisions are not rigid categories and there is greater individual variation within a group than occurs in arteries. The structure may be quite different in veins of the same caliber, and even the same vein may show great structural differences along its course. Thus a description of the venous wall is not so practical as that of arteries and can concern only the most general features.

Venules. The transition from capillary to venule is a very gradual one and involves the acquisition of connective tissue elements first and smooth muscle fibers later. The smallest venules possess an intima consisting of endothelium only and an outer sheath of collagenous fibers. When the vessel attains a diameter of about 50 microns, smooth muscle fibers appear between the endothelium and the connective tissue. In venules of 200 microns or more, the circular muscle fibers form a continuous layer (media), one to three cells thick, external to the endothelium. The adventitia is thick in comparison to the overall thinness of the wall and

consists of longitudinally oriented collagenous fibers and scattered elastic fibers and fibroblasts.

Small and Medium-sized Veins. These include practically all the named veins and their principal branches, excepting the main trunks. The diameter ranges from 1 to 9 mm. The tunica intima is thin. Endothelial cells are short and polygonal in shape. The subendothelial layer of connective tissue is inconspicuous. Sometimes it may be bounded externally by a network of fine elastic fibers.

The media is thin compared with that of arteries of the same size. It is composed of small bundles of circularly arranged muscle fibers separated by collagenous fibers and delicate networks of elastic fibers. The media is best developed in the veins of the lower limbs.

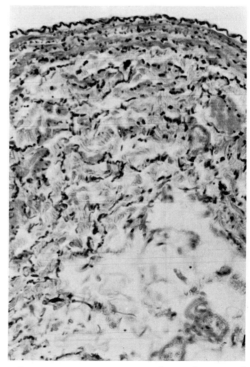

Figure 11-13. A segment of a medium-sized vein, lumen above. The tunica media is thin and the tunica adventitia, composed principally of collagenous fibers, comprises the bulk of the wall of the vein. Aldehyde fuchsin stain. × 135.
See filmstrip I, frame 46.

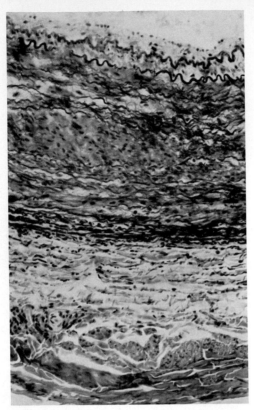

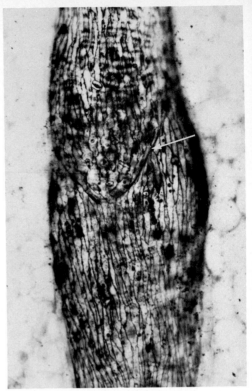

Figure 11-14. A segment of the inferior vena cava, a large vein, with the lumen above. Bundles of longitudinally arranged smooth muscle fibers, here sectioned transversely, are present in the tunica adventitia. Aldehyde fuchsin stain. × 120.

Figure 11-15. A spread preparation of mesentery, stained with silver nitrate. Shown is a segment of a small vein. The cell borders of endothelial cells and a valve (arrow) may be identified readily. × 120.

The adventitia is well developed and forms the bulk of the wall. It is composed of loose connective tissue with thick longitudinal collagenous bundles and frequently a few longitudinally arranged smooth muscle fibers.

Large Veins. This group includes the superior and inferior venae cavae, the portal vein, and the main tributaries of these trunks. The intima has the same structure as that of the smaller veins but may be a little thicker. The media is poorly developed and smooth muscle elements within it are much reduced or absent. The adventitia is the thickest of the three coats and contains prominent bundles of smooth muscle, longitudinally arranged.

Special Features of Certain Veins. Some veins lack smooth muscle and thus are without a media. In this group belong cerebral and meningeal veins, dural sinuses, and veins of the retina, bones, and the maternal component of the placenta. Veins which are rich in smooth muscle include those of the gravid uterus and of the limbs, the umbilical vein, some mesenteric veins, and certain other veins. Cardiac muscle extends for a distance into the adventitia of the venae cavae and pulmonary veins near their entrance into the heart.

Valves. Many small and medium-sized veins, particularly those of the lower limbs, are provided with valves which prevent the flow of blood away from the heart. The valves are semilunar folds or pockets produced by local folding of the intima. They usually are arranged in pairs and project into the lumen with their free margins directed toward the heart. Both surfaces of the valve are covered with endothelium, and on the side facing the current the subendothelial connective tissue contains a network of elastic fibers.

Arteriovenous Anastomoses

In addition to capillary and sinusoidal connections between arteries and veins, in certain regions arteries are connected directly to veins by *arteriovenous anastomoses*. In the anastomoses endothelium lies directly upon a specialized tunica media comprising a sphincter. These vascular shunts are especially numerous in the skin of exposed parts of the body, such as the palm, sole, lips, and nose, and in tissues where metabolic activity is intermittent, such as the thyroid gland and the digestive system. When the shunt is closed, arterial blood passes into the regular capillary bed. When the shunt is open, much of the blood is passed directly into the veins and thus by-passes the capillary bed.

In many regions the anastomosis is convoluted in outline and is surrounded by a definite connective tissue sheath, forming a *glomus*. Smooth muscle cells in the anastomosis are modified in shape and may be epithelioid in appearance.

Blood Vessels of Blood Vessels (Vasa Vasorum)

Arteries and veins with a diameter over 1 mm. are supplied with small, nutrient blood vessels, the *vasa vasorum*. These vessels enter the adventitia and terminate in a dense capillary network which penetrates as far as the deepest layers of the media. No capillaries are found in the intima. Networks of lymph vessels are found in the adventitia of many of the larger arteries and veins.

Nerves

The walls of blood vessels, particularly the arteries, have a rich nerve supply. Unmyelinated axons, which are vasomotor, arise from sympathetic ganglia, penetrate the adventitia, and end in relation to smooth muscle cells of the media. Myelinated nerve fibers, receptor or sensory in function, terminate in free sensory endings within the walls of the vessels.

The Heart

The heart, a highly specialized portion of the vascular system, propels blood through the blood vessels. It consists of four main chambers: a right and left *atrium* and a right and left *ventricle*. The superior and inferior venae cavae bring venous blood from the body to the right atrium, from whence blood passes to the right ventricle. Blood is forced from the right ventricle through the pulmonary arteries to the lungs, where gaseous exchange occurs, and is returned by the pulmonary veins to the left atrium. Blood passes from the left atrium to the left ventricle and then is circulated to the body by the aorta and its branches.

The wall of the heart consists of three layers: the inner layer, or *endocardium*; the middle layer, the *myocardium*, which forms the main mass of the heart; and the outer layer, or *epicardium*.

Endocardium. The endocardium is homologous to the tunica intima of blood vessels. It is lined by endothelium continuous with that of the blood vessels entering and leaving the heart. Beneath the endothelium there is a narrow zone of fine collagenous fibers forming a *subendothelial layer*. Still deeper there is a stouter layer containing numerous elastic fibers and some smooth muscle

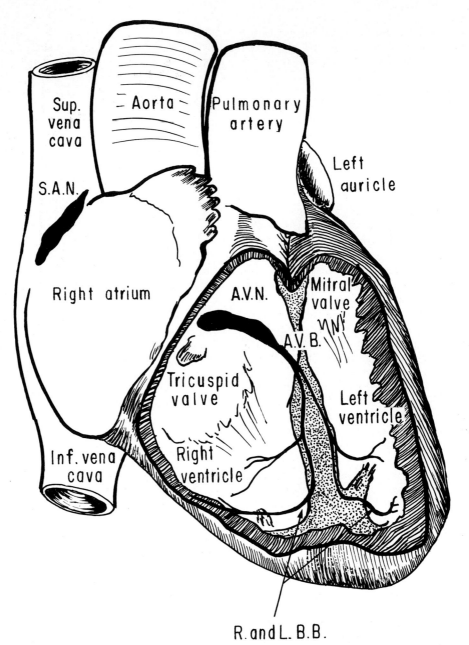

Figure 11-16.   Drawing of the heart, with the interior of the ventricles exposed, to show the main components of the conducting system. S.A.N., sinoatrial node; A.V.N., atrioventricular node; A.V.B., atrioventricular bundle (of His); R. and L.B.B., right and left branches of the bundle.

fibers. A *subendocardial layer* of loose connective tissue, which binds the endocardium proper to the underlying myocardium, lies farthest from the lumen. This layer contains numerous blood vessels and nerves and branches of the conduction system of the heart.

Myocardium. The myocardium, or middle coat, which corresponds to the tunica media, is composed of cardiac muscle, already described in Chapter 9. Its thickness varies in different parts of the heart, being thinnest in the atria and thickest in the left ventricle. In the atria the muscle fibers tend to be arranged in bundles which form a latticework. In the ventricles some bundles of muscle fibers are present in a more or less isolated fashion on the internal surface, covered by endocardium. These bundles are called *trabeculae carnae.* The spaces between muscle fibers and bundles contain reticular, collagenous, and elastic fibers.

The muscle is arranged in sheets which wind around the atria and ventricles in complex, spiraling courses. Most of the muscle fibers are attached to the central supporting structure of the heart, the *cardiac skeleton.*

Cardiac Skeleton. The central support of the heart is dense fibrous connective tissue on which cardiac muscle inserts and valves attach. Its main components are the *septum membranaceum,* the *trigona fibrosa,* and the *annuli fibrosi.* The annuli fibrosi, or fibrous rings, surround the origins of the aorta and pulmonary artery and the atrioventricular canals. The trigona fibrosa are masses of fibrous tissue between the arterial foramina and the atrioventricular canals. The septum membranaceum, the fibrous portion of the interventricular septum, also provides attachment for the free ends of some fibers of the cardiac musculature.

Epicardium. The external coat (also called the *visceral pericardium*) is a serous membrane. It is covered externally by a single layer of mesothelial cells. Beneath the mesothelium

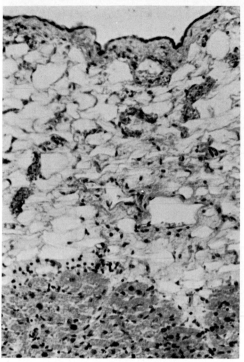

Figure 11-17. The epicardium of the heart. Above is the visceral pericardium (a mesothelium). The subepicardial layer, containing numerous fat cells and blood vessels, is prominent, and beneath it a portion of myocardium is shown. × 100.

is a thin layer of connective tissue containing numerous elastic fibers. A *subepicardial layer,* composed of areolar tissue containing blood vessels, many nervous elements, and fat, attaches the epicardium to the myocardium.

Cardiac Valves. The atrioventricular valves (*tricuspid* and *mitral*) are reduplications of endocardium containing a core of dense connective tissue continuous with that of the annuli fibrosi. The endocardium is thicker on the atrial than on the ventricular surface and contains more elastic tissue. The valves are connected to papillary muscles of the ventricles by fibrous cords, the *chordae tendineae,* which serve to restrain the valves and prevent eversion of the valves when the ventricles contract.

The *semilunar valves* of the aorta

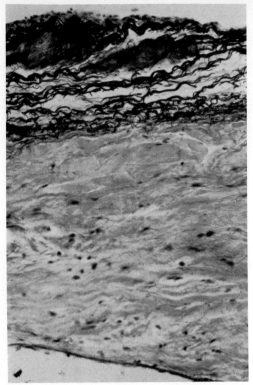

Figure 11-18. A portion of an atrioventricular valve, atrial surface above. Note the concentration of elastic fibers beneath the atrial surface. Resorcin fuchsin stain. × 120.

and pulmonary artery are similar in structure to the atrioventricular valves. Each valve has three cusps. The central, fibrous plate of each cusp forms a thickening (the *nodule of Arantius*) at the free border.

Impulse-conducting System. The heart possesses a system of specialized cardiac muscle fibers whose function is to coordinate the heart beat by regulating the contractions of the atria and ventricles. The modified fibers of this system (*Purkinje fibers*), which have a faster rate of conduction than ordinary cardiac muscle fibers, lie in the subendocardium. Purkinje fibers generally have a larger diameter than ordinary cardiac muscle fibers and contain relatively more sarcoplasm. The sarcoplasm often has a large amount of glycogen.

Myofibrils are reduced in number and usually are limited to the periphery of the fibers. Purkinje fibers ultimately lose their specific characteristics and pass by a gradual transition into ordinary cardiac fibers.

An impulse begins at the *sinoatrial node,* which lies at the junction of the superior vena cava with the right atrium. This node consists of a dense network of small Purkinje fibers. From here, since the modified fibers are in close association with typical cardiac muscle fibers, the impulse spreads to the *atrioventricular node,* which lies in the median wall of the right atrium. The atrioventricular node also consists of Purkinje fibers which form a dense tangled network whose meshes are filled with connective tissue. The node continues into a common stem, the *atrioventricular bundle (bundle of His)*, which lies in the membranous portion of the interventricular septum. This bundle divides into two trunks, one to each ventricle. Each trunk ultimately breaks up into a large number of branches which pass to all parts of the ventricle and terminate in the myocardium, where they connect with ordinary cardiac muscle fibers.

Blood Vessels of the Heart. Two *coronary arteries* supply blood to the heart, and the *cardiac veins* drain it. The arteries break up in the myocardium into a rich capillary plexus. The capillary plexus drains into cardiac veins, which empty into the right atrium via the *coronary sinus.* A small number of veins empty directly into the lumen of the heart.

The conducting system is abundantly supplied with special fine branches of the coronary arteries. The capillary network here is less dense than in the ordinary cardiac musculature.

Lymphatics of the Heart. Lymph channels are abundant within the heart and are intimately associated with muscle fibers. In addition to the network within the myocardium, there

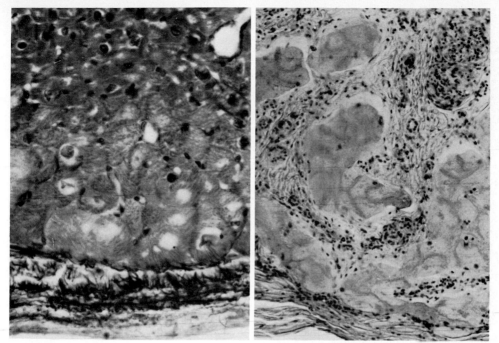

Figure 11-19. Endocardium of the right ventricle, containing Purkinje fibers. Left: Resorcin fuchsin stain, × 100. Right: Hematoxylin and eosin, × 60. In the left-hand figure, the larger Purkinje fibers, with distinct peripheral myofibrils, may be identified readily from the ordinary cardiac musculature above. In the right-hand figure, groups of Purkinje fibers are separated by connective tissue containing numerous nerve fibers.

are lymphatic networks in the subendocardial and subepicardial connective tissue.

Nerves of the Heart. The nerve supply is from the vagus and the sympathetic division of the autonomic system. The vagus and sympathetic fibers are antagonistic, the vagus fibers inhibiting and the sympathetic fibers accelerating the heart action. These fibers form extensive plexuses, often associated with small autonomic ganglia. Both sensory and motor endings are represented.

THE LYMPH VASCULAR SYSTEM

The lymphatic system is composed of lymphatic vessels and organs. The lymphatic vessels are tubes which collect tissue fluid and return it by a roundabout route to the blood stream. Lymph drainage is a one-way flow, not a circulation. The smallest lymphatic vessels, *lymph capillaries*, end blindly. Centrally the converging lymphatic vessels run into one of two main trunks, the large *thoracic duct* or the smaller *right lymphatic duct*, which empty into the great veins. Lymphatic nodes are located along the course of lymphatic vessels and add lymphocytes to the lymph passing through them.

Lymph capillaries and vessels are found in most tissues and organs. They are not found in the central nervous system, the bone marrow, the internal ear, and the coats of the eyeball.

Lymph Capillaries

Lymph capillaries, like blood capillaries, are delicate tubes but are

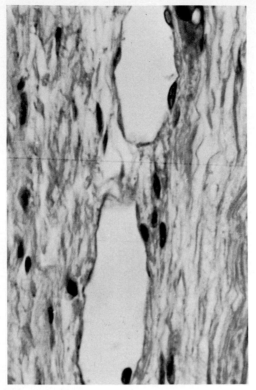

Figure 11-20. Lymph capillaries in the epicardium. Note the large lumen and the distinct endothelial wall. × 550.

somewhat broader and are not uniform in caliber. The wall is composed only of endothelium (see Figures 11-7 and 11-20), which rests upon a thin basal lamina. The capillaries form dense networks which often run in company with blood capillaries. Near surfaces they frequently end in loops or in blind, swollen projections.

Lymphatic Vessels (Collecting Vessels)

Lymph passes from capillaries into larger vessels which have thicker walls and valves. The endothelium is surrounded by collagenous and elastic fibers and a few smooth muscle cells. In the larger vessels three coats, intima, media, and adventitia, may be distinguished, but usually they are poorly demarcated. These vessels resemble the veins in structure, but their walls tend to be thinner than those of veins of equal caliber.

The tunica intima consists of endothelium and a thin layer of delicate elastic fibers. The media is composed of circularly arranged smooth muscle fibers, between which are a few elastic fibers. The adventitia is the thickest layer and consists of interlacing collagenous and elastic fibers and a few smooth muscle fibers.

Lymphatic vessels contain numerous valves which are more closely spaced than those found in veins. The valves occur in opposed pairs and their free margins are directed centrally. Each valve is a fold of the intima. Between valves the vessels are swollen; thus they have a beaded appearance.

Main Lymphatic Trunks

These are the thoracic and the right lymphatic ducts. In structure they are much like a vein of equal size except for the greater development of smooth muscle in the media. The intima consists of an endothelial lining, a subendothelial layer containing some longitudinal muscle, and a thin, inconstant, elastic membrane. The media is the thickest coat and consists of longitudinal and circular muscle bundles, separated by abundant connective tissue. The adventitia, which consists of coarse collagenous fibers and a few longitudinal muscle fibers, is poorly defined and blends into the surrounding connective tissue.

Blood vessels supply the wall of the main lymphatic trunks in much the same way as the vasa vasorum of the larger blood vessels. Nerve fibers, both motor and sensory, are found in the wall of the larger vessels.

DEVELOPMENT OF THE CIRCULATORY SYSTEM

The blood vessels and heart first appear as a collection of endothelial cells which differentiate from mesenchymal cells. The heart, main blood vessels, and peripheral vessels develop independently and later unite to establish a blood circulation.

Arteries and veins of all types first appear as ordinary capillaries, which later increase in size and acquire smooth muscle and connective tissue by differentiation from the surrounding mesenchyme. After the establishment of the circulation, new vessels arise by budding from pre-existing vessels.

The heart in the earliest human embryos is a tube with a double wall: the internal endothelium, from which the endocardium develops, and the external *myoepicardial* layer. From the myoepicardial layer are formed both myocardium and epicardium. The endocardium has important roles in the formation of partitions to separate the primary single cavity of the heart into chambers, and in the formation of the valves.

There are two opinions concerning the mode of development of the lymphatic vessels. According to one view the lymphatic vessels arise as evaginations or buds from veins. Most observers, however, believe that the lymphatics first arise independently of the veins as isolated intercellular clefts in the mesenchyme. The mesenchymal cells lining the clefts differentiate into endothelial cells, and the clefts enlarge and fuse to form the primary lymphatic vessels. These later establish communication with the veins. Later development of the lymphatic system occurs mainly by budding from the walls of pre-existing lymphatics in much the same way as in the blood vessels.

REFERENCES

Bennett, H. S., Luft, J. H., and Hampton, J. C.: Morphological classification of vertebrate blood capillaries. Amer. J. Physiol., 196:381, 1959.

Bruns, R. R., and Palade, G. E.: Studies on blood capillaries. I. General organization of blood capillaries in muscle. II. Transport of ferritin molecules across the wall of muscle capillaries. J. Cell Biol., 37:244, 277, 1968.

Chambers, R., and Zweifach, B. W.: Topography and function of the mesentine capillary circulation. Amer. J. Anat., 75:173, 1944.

Clark, E. R.: Arterio-venous anastomoses. Physiol. Rev., 18:229, 1938.

Davies, F.: The conducting system of the vertebrate heart. Brit. Heart. J., 4:66, 1942.

Fawcett, D. W.: The fine structure of capillaries, arterioles and small arteries. In The Microcirculation: A Symposium on Factors Influencing Exchange of Substances across Capillary Wall, edited by S. R. M. Reynolds and B. W. Zweifach. Urbana, University of Illinois Press, 1959, p. 1.

Florey, H.: The endothelial cell. Biol Med. J., 2:487, 1966.

Karnovsky, M. J.: The ultrastructural basis of capillary permeability studied with peroxidase as a tracer. J. Cell Biol., 35:213, 1967.

Krogh, A., and Vimtrup, B.: The capillaries. In Special Cytology, edited by E. V. Cowdry. New York, Paul B. Hoeber, 1932, Vol. 1, p. 477.

Leak, L. V., and Burke, J. F.: Fine structure of the lymphatic capillary and the adjoining connective tissue area. Am. J. Anat., 118:785, 1966.

Lewis, T.: The Mechanism and Graphic Registration of the Heart Beat. London, Shaw and Sons, 1925.

Majno, G.: Ultrastructure of the vascular membrane. In Handbook of Physiology, Section 2, Circulation, edited by W. F. Hamilton and P. Dow. Bethesda, Md., American Physiological Society, 1965, Vol. 3, p. 2293.

Muir, A. R.: Observations on the fine structure of the Purkinje fibers in the ventricles of the sheep's heart. J. Anat., 91:251, 1957.

Palade, G. E., and Bruns, R. R.: Structural modulations of plasmalemmal vesicles. J. Cell Biol., 37:633, 1968.

CHAPTER 12

LYMPHOID ORGANS

Several organs and structures within the body consist largely of *lymphoid (lymphatic)* tissue, which is not one of the primary tissue types but is merely a variety of connective tissue. It has two principal components: reticular tissue, comprising a framework of reticular cells and reticular fibers, and free cells, chiefly lymphocytes, which lie within the interstices of the reticular tissue. In many regions of the body the lymphoid tissue is not sharply delineated from the surrounding connective tissue and is known as *diffuse lymphoid tissue* in contrast to the more dense form (*lymph nodules*) in which the component cells are densely aggregated.

Diffuse lymphoid tissue occurs principally as an infiltration of the lamina propria of mucous membranes, particularly those of the digestive and respiratory systems. It shows no special organization. The reticular cells are arranged in an apparent syncytium in close relation to the reticular (argyrophil) fibers. Some cells have little cytoplasm and are relatively undifferentiated. Others possess more cytoplasm and have acquired phagocytic properties. These are fixed macrophages which, on detachment from the reticular network, become free macrophages. Small lymphocytes are the commonest of the free cells present.

In addition, hemocytoblasts (lymphoblasts), monocytes, and plasma cells are found within the meshes of the stroma.

Lymph, or *primary*, *nodules* are dense aggregations of lymphoid tissue arranged in spherical masses. They have been called the structural units of lymphoid tissue. Each nodule may be homogeneous or may consist of a darker *cortex* and a lighter central

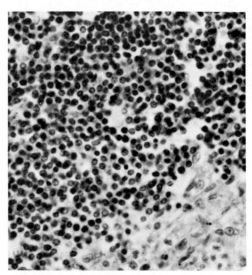

Figure 12-1. Section of a portion of the wall of the small intestine. Notice the accumulation of lymphocytes (diffuse lymphatic tissue) in the connective tissue. × 250.

234

area, the *germinal center*. The cortex comprises closely packed small lymphocytes, and the germinal center contains paler, larger cells, most of which are medium-sized lymphocytes. These are actively dividing elements. It should be emphasized that lymph nodules are not constant features, either in structure or in position. They appear, remain for a time, and then disappear. New nodules may arise in diffuse lymphatic tissue at any time since they are an expression of the cytogenetic and defense functions of the lymphatic tissue.

Lymph nodules may be isolated or may occur in aggregations in specific lymphoid organs such as lymph nodes, tonsils, and spleen. The *solitary nodules* or *follicles* of the digestive system are examples of isolated nodules. Nodules also may be aggregated into less highly organized structures than lymph nodes, forming the unencapsulated *Peyer's patches* of the intestine.

The lymph nodes are the only lymphoid organs which are interposed in the course of lymph vessels. Thus they possess both afferent and efferent lymphatic vessels. The tonsils, spleen, and thymus have efferent vessels draining from them, but they are not associated with afferent lymphatic vessels.

THE LYMPH NODES

Lymph nodes are variable in number but are found more or less constantly in certain definite regions of the body such as the prevertebral region, the mesentery, and the loose connective tissue of the axilla and groin. Frequently they occur in chains or groups. Each node is an oval or bean-shaped body, ranging from 1 to 25 mm. in diameter. It has a convex contour except at an indented region, the *hilum* (or *hilus*) on one side, where the blood vessels enter and leave the

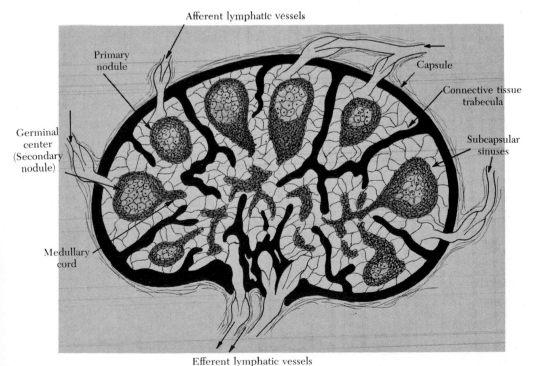

Figure 12-2.   Diagram to illustrate the general structure of a lymph node. The arrows indicate the direction of lymph flow.

node. Afferent lymphatic vessels enter at multiple points on the convex surface of the node. Efferent vessels leave only at the hilum.

Lymph nodes are covered by a definite *capsule* of connective tissue which is continuous with a number of *septa* or *trabeculae* extending into the substance of the organ. The latter, in turn, connect with a fine meshwork of reticular tissue. The parenchyma of each node is specialized into two regions, an outer *cortex*, characterized by the presence of lymph nodules, and an inner *medulla*, in which the lymphoid tissue is arranged chiefly in the form of irregular, anastomosing cords.

Framework

The capsule is a firm covering composed mostly of densely packed collagenous fibers. A loose network of elastic fibers, particularly on its inner surface, and a few smooth muscle fibers are found also in the capsule. At the hilum the capsule is greatly thickened. Trabeculae of dense collagenous fibers arise from the inner aspect of the capsule and project into the interior of each node, dividing the cortex into a number of incomplete compartments. In the medulla the trabeculae become highly branched and finally fuse with the connective tissue of the hilum. The capsule, the hilum, and the trabeculae constitute the collagenous framework. Within the framework there is a delicate meshwork of reticular connective tissue, comprising reticular fibers, reticular cells, and fixed macrophages. The spaces within this reticulum form the *lymph sinuses*, through which lymph percolates, and these sinuses contain the free cells.

Cortex

The degree of development of the trabeculae and the separation of the cortex into compartments vary in nodes

of different animals and in nodes taken from different regions of the body. In man the compartments are not so definite as in many lower mammals. Within the cortical compartments the lymphocytes are closely packed into nodules which are attached indirectly by reticulum to the nearby capsule and trabeculae. The nodules are separated from the capsule and trabeculae by spaces, the lymph sinuses, through which the lymph circulates. Although the cortex usually is found surrounding the medulla except at the hilum, it shows considerable variation in thickness.

The cortical nodules often contain lighter staining central areas, the germinal centers, but they are inconstant features. Component cells of each germinal center (also called a *secondary nodule*) are larger and possess more cytoplasm and paler nuclei than do the small lymphocytes. Hence the whole central area appears lighter in stained sections. Most of the cells are medium-sized lymphocytes. A few are large, undifferentiated lymphocytes (lymphoblasts) and plasma cells. During an active phase small lymphocytes are produced by the cells of the germinal center and are pushed outward into a peripheral zone, which becomes the *cortex of the nodule*. After a time mitotic activity diminishes, the former growth pressure subsides, and the sharp boundary between the germinal center and the cortex disappears. The center becomes inactive and the nodule returns to its homogeneous, resting appearance. Under certain pathological conditions some of the pale centers contain numerous free macrophages. These areas have been called *reaction centers*.

Medulla

The cellular components of the medulla and cortex are similar but there is a difference in arrangement. In the medulla the lymphoid tissue

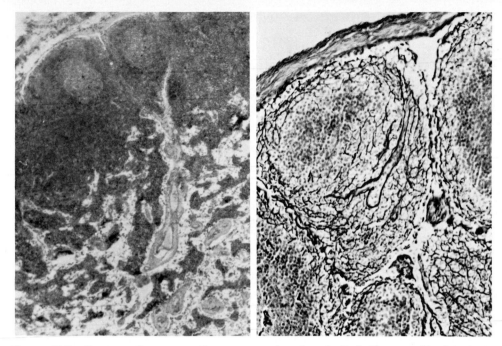

Figure 12-3.   Sections of a portion of a mesenteric lymph node. Left: Portions of both cortex and medulla are visible. × 25. Right: Section stained to visualize the reticular framework. A portion of the capsule is present above. Silver stain. × 75.   See filmstrip I, frames 47 and 48.

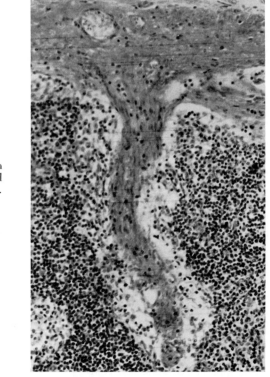

Figure 12-4.   Section of a portion of a lymph node, showing the capsule, a trabecula, cortical sinuses, and portions of two cortical nodules. × 100.

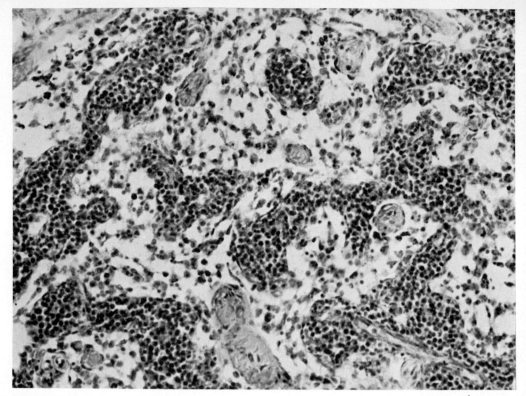

Figure 12-5.   Portion of the medulla of a lymph node, showing trabeculae, medullary cords, and medullary sinuses. × 175.   See filmstrip I, frame 49.

takes the form of dense lymphoid strands, or *lymph cords*, which run between the irregular branching and anastomosing trabeculae. Some lymph (*medullary*) cords are continuous with the deep surface of the cortical nodules. They are surrounded by medullary lymph sinuses. Reticulum, which bridges the sinuses, attaches the cords to adjacent trabeculae. This arrangement of dense lymph tissue, sinuses, and trabeculae is similar to that found in the cortex.

Lymphatic Vessels and Sinuses

The circulation of lymph through a lymph node involves afferent lymphatic vessels, a system of lymph sinuses within the node, and efferent lymphatic vessels. Several afferent vessels pierce the capsule on the con-

vex side of the node and open into the system of lymph sinuses. The afferent vessels are provided with valves which open toward the node. Each node contains a tortuous system of irregular channels, the *sinuses*, within the lymphoid tissue. Unlike the endothelial-lined blood vascular and lymphatic vessels, the sinuses have walls which are not continuous. They are incompletely lined by reticular cells and fixed macrophages, supported by reticular fibers. The sinus system comprises three parts. Afferent vessels enter the *marginal* or *subcapsular* sinus, which separates the capsule from the cortical parenchyma. From the marginal sinus lymph flows into the *cortical sinuses*, which lie between the cortical nodules and the trabeculae. Cortical sinuses are continuous with *medullary sinuses*, which are interposed between medullary trabeculae and medullary cords. The medullary sinuses pierce the thickened portion of the capsule at the hilum and continue into the efferent lymphatic vessels. The efferent vessels are fewer in number and wider than the afferent vessels and contain valves which open away from the nodes. The arrangement of valves in the afferent and efferent vessels allows a flow of lymph only in one direction through the node.

Blood Vessels and Nerves

Arteries enter the lymph node at the hilum and give branches to the medullary cords and to the trabeculae. The branches to the cords continue into the cortex to supply the cortical nodules. Branches to the trabeculae supply the connective tissue of the trabeculae and ultimately reach the capsule. Dense capillary plexuses are present within the medullary cords and the cortical nodules. From the capillaries blood is collected into veins which follow the same general route taken by the arteries and leave the node at the hilum.

Nerves, which are mostly vasomotor, enter the hilum with the blood vessels and follow them into the interior of the node.

Functions of Lymph Nodes

One of the primary functions of lymph nodes is the production of lymphocytes, which enter the sinuses partly by ameboid activity and partly by crowding pressure. Lymph is not markedly cellular until it has passed through a lymph node. The development of new lymphocytes from undifferentiated cells has been described previously (see Chapter 8). The actual stimuli for lymphopoiesis both in physiological and in pathological conditions are unknown. In certain pathological conditions extramedullary hemopoiesis occurs and the lymph nodes produce myeloid elements.

Lymph nodes filter lymph by means of the phagocytic activity of the fixed and detached reticular cells. They remove degenerating cells, including erythrocytes, and particulate matter from the lymph. A good example of the latter is provided by the bronchial lymph nodes. Inhaled carbon particles eventually reach the bronchial lymph nodes where they are taken up by the reticuloendothelial elements, often in such quantity that the entire nodes appear black.

The lymph nodes also play a role in the elaboration of antibodies and in the production of immunity. Any procedure which depletes the population of small lymphocytes of the body, such as thymectomy in neonatal life or treatment with lymphocytic agents, causes serious impairment of the production of humoral antibody. The mode of action of small lymphocytes in antibody production is unclear, but recent research indicates that in some

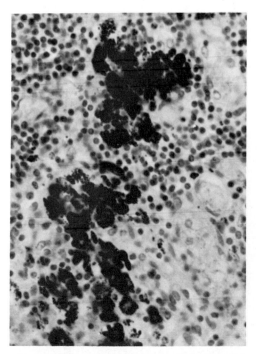

Figure 12-6. Portion of a bronchial lymph node from a 53-year-old man. Notice the accumulation of carbon particles in reticular cells. × 250.

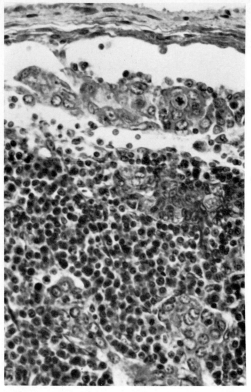

Figure 12-7. Portion of an axillary lymph node from a patient with carcinoma of the breast. Groups of cancer cells (metastatic growths) are present within the subcapsular sinus and the cortex. Notice that one cancer cell in the subcapsular sinus is in the process of dividing. × 250.

way they are transformed into large basophil cells which may be precursors of the plasma cell series. This transformation occurs in the germinal centers. The blast cells are thought to migrate from the centers into the medullary areas, where they complete their metamorphosis. In immune responses, lymphocytes exert their influence by transformation into large basophil blast cells either in the lymph nodes or in the grafted tissue itself.

Development of Lymph Nodes

Lymph nodes develop after the formation of the primary lymphatic vascu-

lar system. In connective tissue associated with plexuses of lymph vessels, condensations of mesenchymal cells occur which later infiltrate the vessels. Lymphocytes form *in situ* from the mesenchymal cells. Lymph sinuses develop as isolated lymph spaces within the mesenchyme. The spaces fuse to form a system of anastomosing sinuses throughout the developing node. Later this system comes into contact with the afferent and efferent lymphatic vessels. The connective tissue outside the marginal sinus becomes thickened to form the capsule and extends into the node as the trabeculae, which always remain separated from concentrations of lymphoid tissue by the sinuses.

Hemal (Hemolymph) Nodes

In certain animals, structures exist which are very similar to lymph nodes except that they contain large numbers of erythrocytes. These structures, the *hemal nodes*, are common in ruminants such as the sheep but probably do not occur in man. The general organization is similar to that of a lymph node in that the hemal node consists of a mass of lymphatic tissue covered by a connective tissue capsule. The sinuses, however, are purely blood sinuses. In the hog there are structures which are intermediate between a lymph node and a hemal node. Both blood vessels and lymphatics connect with the sinuses. In this instance the term *hemolymph node* is most appropriate.

Hemal nodes are lymphopoietic and also function to filter blood.

THE TONSILS

Three tonsillar groups, the *palatine tonsils*, the *lingual tonsil*, and the *pharyngeal tonsil*, form a ring of lymphoid tissue surrounding the pharynx, where nasal and oral passages unite. The tonsils are characterized

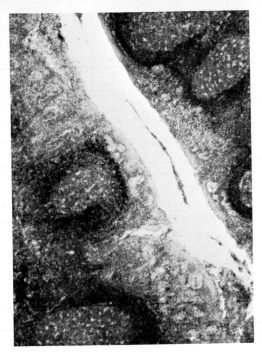

Figure 12-8. Portion of the palatine tonsil, showing the accumulation of lymph nodules covered by epithelium lining a tonsillar crypt. × 25.

those of lymph nodes, may contain germinal centers. In the deeper parts of the crypts there is no clear delineation between epithelium and lymphoid tissue because of an intense infiltration of the epithelium with lymphocytes. Adjacent to the deepest portions of the tonsil the fibrous tissue is condensed to form a thin capsule which covers the base and sides of the tonsil. The connective tissue septa extend into the interior of the tonsil and separate the various crypts, with their surrounding zones of lymphatic tissue, from one another. Small mucous glands lie in the connective tissue beneath the tonsil and its capsule. Their ducts open for the most part on the free surface; occasionally they may open into the tonsillar crypts.

The *lingual tonsil* is located in the root of the tongue, behind the circumvallate papillae. It consists of an aggregation of wide-mouthed epithelial pits, each surrounded by lymphoid tissue. Each simple pit or crypt is lined by a continuation of the surface by depressions of the surface epithelium around which aggregations of lymph nodules are grouped.

The palatine, or *faucal*, tonsils are paired, oval masses of lymphoid tissue which occupy the intervals between the glossopalatine and pharyngopalatine arches. They lie in the connective tissue of the mucosa and are covered on their free surface by a stratified squamous epithelium which is continuous with the lining of the mouth and pharynx. The epithelium rests upon a basal lamina, under which there is a thin layer of fibrous connective tissue. At various places on the surface of the tonsil, deep indentations, ten to twenty in number, occur. These indentations, or *tonsillar crypts*, penetrate into the interior of the tonsil and are lined by a continuation of the surface epithelium. Lymphoid tissue surrounds the crypts as a diffuse mass in which are embedded lymph nodules. The nodules, like

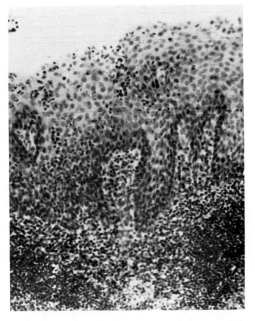

Figure 12-9. Portion of the palatine tonsil. Notice the invasion by lymphocytes of the epithelium lining a tonsillar crypt. × 100.

stratified squamous epithelium. The lymphoid tissue comprises a layer of lymph nodules, often with germinal centers. In most crypts there is marked infiltration of the epithelium with lymphocytes. Ducts of underlying mucous glands open onto the surface or into the crypts.

The *pharyngeal tonsil* is an accumulation of lymphoid tissue in the median posterior wall of the nasopharynx. The lymphatic tissue is similar to that of the palatine tonsils. The epithelium over the free surface is folded. In general it is pseudostratified, with cilia and goblet cells, but in the adult there may be islands of stratified squamous epithelium. The epithelium is extensively infiltrated with lymphocytes. A thin capsule surrounds the pharyngeal tonsil and sends septa into the core of the epithelial folds. Mixed seromucous glands occur in the connective tissue beneath the capsule, and their ducts open onto the free surface or into the furrows between the folds. Hypertrophy of the pharyngeal tonsil, with consequent obstruction to the nasal openings, is

common and is known clinically as *adenoids*.

The *tubal tonsils* sometimes are considered as a separate tonsillar group. Each tubal tonsil lies around the pharyngeal orifice of the pharyngotympanic (auditory) tube and constitutes a lateral extension of the pharyngeal tonsil. The tubal tonsil is covered with ciliated columnar epithelium.

Blood vessels course in the capsule and septa of the tonsils and supply the lymphoid tissue. The tonsils possess no afferent lymphatic vessels. Plexuses of lymph capillaries occur around the lymphoid tissue and drain into the efferent lymphatic vessels. The tonsils, which reach their maximum development in childhood and thereafter decline, constitute a discontinuous ring of lymphoid tissue around the pharynx. They participate in lymphocyte production. No other function has been established definitely. It is believed generally that they aid in the protection of the body against bacteria. On the other hand, epithelial erosion would seem to enhance an invasion by microorganisms, and the tonsils are known to be frequent portals of infection.

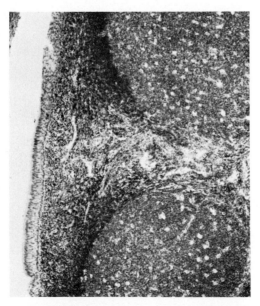

Figure 12-10. Portion of the pharyngeal tonsil. Pseudostratified columnar epithelium covers the masses of tonsillar tissue. × 40.

THE THYMUS

The thymus varies in size and development with the age of the individual. It attains its maximum development about puberty, after which it becomes inconspicuous. In the past it often has been grouped with the endocrine glands, but today it is considered to be predominantly a lymphoid organ.

It consists of two *lobes* closely applied and united by connective tissue, and it is situated in the anterior mediastinum behind the upper portion of the sternum. A lobe is composed of thousands of *lobules*, each containing *cortical* and *medullary* components. The lobules are not completely separate units since the medulla consti-

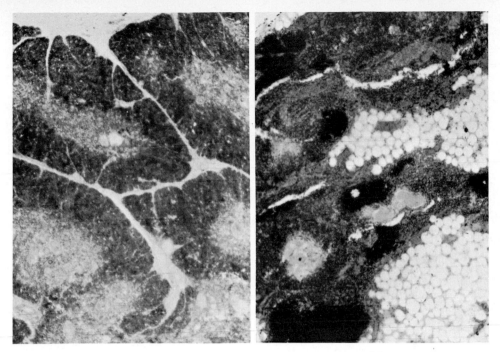

Figure 12-11. Left: Section through a part of the thymus of a 7-year-old child. The cortex of the lobules is dark, the medulla light. × 25. Right: Portion of the thymus from an adult. Notice the involution of the organ and the replacement with fat. × 40.   See filmstrip I, frame 50.

tutes a central core to each lobe and sends prolongations into each lobule. A capsule encloses each lobe and extensions from it (*septa*) delineate the lobules. The capsule consists of collagenous fibers together with a few elastic fibers, and interlobular septa extend from it as far as the medulla and partially separate the lobules from each other. In addition intralobular *trabeculae* arise from the capsule and pass into the cortex of the lobules. The reticular connective tissue of the thymus differs in some respects from that of other lymphoid organs. The reticular cells, which support the parenchyma, arise from entoderm rather than from mesenchyme and in tissue culture have been shown to possess epithelioid characteristics. They are stellate cells which do not phagocytose colloidal dyes, unlike true reticular cells of mesenchymal origin. Reticular fibers are sparse and are concentrated mainly around the blood vessels.

Cortex and Medulla

The cortex contains small lymphocytes, sometimes called *thymocytes*, that are densely and uniformly packed. They occupy the interstices of the sparse reticular meshwork and obscure the reticular cells. The lymphatic tissue, unlike that of lymph nodes, is not arranged in nodules. The medulla stains more lightly and is less compact than the cortex. The lymphocytes, or thymocytes, are less numerous in the medulla and consequently the reticular cells are prominent. The latter have an apparent syncytial arrangement. The medulla contains, in addition, a number of spherical or oval bodies composed of concentrically arranged epithelial cells. These are the *thymic corpuscles* (of Hassall) which are characteristic of the thymus. They are acidophil and vary in diameter from 20 to more than 100 microns. The central cells are large and often show

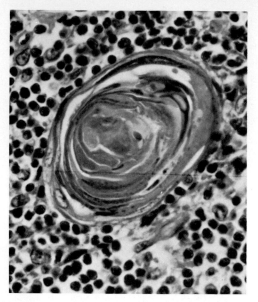

Figure 12-12. Portion of the medulla of thymus showing a Hassall's corpuscle. × 400.

evidence of hyalinization and degeneration. The surrounding cells are flattened and may retain connections with nearby reticular cells.

Blood Vessels

The arteries supplying the thymus are derived from the internal thoracic and the inferior thyroid arteries. They enter along the medullary core and are distributed first to the cortex. From capillary plexuses venules run in the medullary tissue and continue into larger veins which drain into the left brachiocephalic and thyroid veins.

Lymphatics

There are no afferent vessels and no lymph sinuses in the thymus. Lymphatics run mainly in the interlobular connective tissue.

Nerves

A few branches of the vagus and cervical sympathetic nerves reach the thymus. They are distributed mainly to the walls of the blood vessels.

Involution

The thymus reaches its maximum size at puberty, and then begins to involute, a process which continues into old age. Involution first involves a gradual loss of lymphocytes from the cortex with the result that the boundary between cortex and medulla becomes indistinct. The medulla also begins to atrophy at puberty. Adipose tissue replaces the thymocytes and reticular cells. The last elements to be replaced are the thymic corpuscles, which may be recognizable even in old age.

Functions

Lymphopoiesis is a known thymic activity and occurs principally during fetal and early postnatal life. Plasma cells and myelocytes also are formed in small numbers. In mice removal of the thymus shortly after birth results in lymphocyte deficiency and in some form of immunity lack. The mice grow for several months and then die, presumably owing to an inability to produce antibodies. In the meantime the mice do not resist bacterial infections and will not reject skin grafts from other strains of mice. Since these phenomena do not occur if thymectomy is delayed until a few days after birth, it is postulated that the thymus creates lymphocytes which are distributed by the blood stream to other lymphoid organs where they settle down and multiply. This process is known as *peripheralization*. In the adult the thymus continues to be an important source of small lymphocytes, particularly if the individual has suffered depletion of his lymphoid organs by irradiation. There is evidence that, in addition, the thymus exerts a humoral effect upon other lymphoid tissues, particularly with regard to immunological competence. Thus it can be considered as the pacemaker of the lymphoid tissues.

The thymus has some relations with the gonads, adrenals, and thyroid gland. Gonadal hormones induce involution and thyroidectomy hastens it.

There appears to be some relation between the thymus and *myasthenia gravis*, a clinical condition characterized by muscle weakness. Many individuals suffering from this disease have either a thymic tumor or an enlarged thymus, but the significance of the relationship remains obscure.

Development

In man the thymus arises as a paired ventral outgrowth from the third branchial pouch. Each outgrowth has a narrow lumen at first, but this quickly is obliterated by proliferation of the lining epithelial cells. The epithelial cells differentiate and some transform into reticular cells at about the end of the second month of pregnancy. Thymocytes (or lymphocytes) appear at this time also. Some authors believe that they arise from epithelial cells; others that they arise from mesenchymal cells which invade the developing thymus. The lymphocytes proliferate rapidly and the epithelium is converted into a reticular cell mass. Lobules form at this time and connective tissue invades the lobes to form septa and trabeculae. Hassall's corpuscles first appear during fetal life and continue to form until the time when involution is initiated. They are thought to arise from hypertrophied and degenerating epithelial cells.

THE SPLEEN

The spleen is the largest of the lymphoid organs and, with the possible exception of the hemal nodes, it is the only organ specialized for filtering blood. It has no afferent lymphatic vessels and its sinuses, as in the hemal nodes, are filled with blood instead of lymph.

The spleen, like the lymph nodes, has a collagenous framework within which is suspended a reticular network. It is surrounded by a capsule which itself is covered by a serous membrane, the peritoneum. Many trabeculae pass from the capsule into the interior of the organ. At one point on the surface of the spleen there is a deep indentation, the *hilum*, where blood vessels enter and leave. The parenchyma (*splenic pulp*) is of two distinct types. *White pulp* is typical lymphatic tissue which surrounds and follows the arteries. At intervals it is thickened into ovoid masses, the *splenic nodules* (or *malpighian bodies*). The *red pulp* is more abundant, often forms plates, the *pulp cords*, and is associated with numerous erythrocytes. The structure of the spleen and the relations between the red and white pulp depend upon the arrangement and distribution of blood vessels. Arteries are connected closely with the white pulp, and the terminal blood vessels (sinuses and veins) with the red pulp.

The trabeculae delineate many compartments, or *lobules*, within the spleen. A lobule is about 1 mm. in diameter and is bounded by several trabeculae. Each lobule is supplied by a central artery and is drained by veins which run in trabeculae to leave the lobule. The lobules are not distinct since they are not outlined completely by trabeculae.

Framework

The capsule and trabeculae of the spleen consist of dense collagenous connective tissue with a few elastic fibers and some smooth muscle fibers. The capsule is thickest at the hilum where it surrounds the major blood vessels. The external surface of the capsule is covered by a layer of flat-

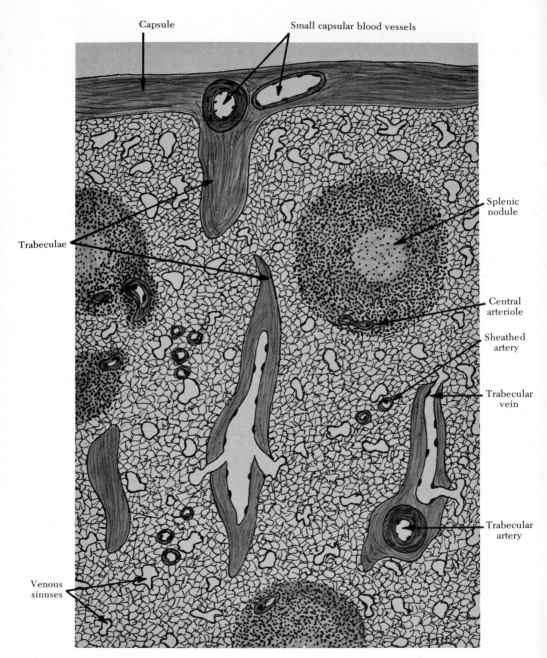

Figure 12-13. Diagram of a section of spleen. The white pulp consists of nodules and aggregations of lymphocytes, and the red pulp is an open mesh with sinusoids.

tened mesothelial cells, a component of the peritoneum. Trabeculae radiate inward from the hilum and from the internal surface of the capsule. They branch and anastomose repeatedly to produce a complex framework throughout the interior. Smooth muscle elements within the capsule and trabeculae are responsible for the slow, rhythmical changes in volume of the spleen. The splenic pulp is supported by a fine meshwork of reticular fibers which blends with the capsule, trabeculae, and walls of the blood vessels. The cells in relation to the reticulum are, as in other lymphoid organs, primitive reticular cells and fixed macrophages.

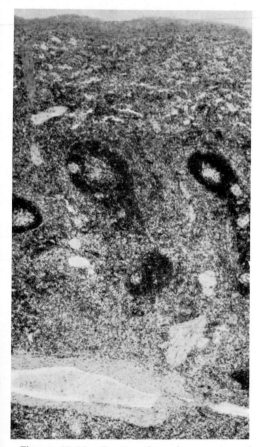

Figure 12-14. Section through a portion of spleen showing capsule (top), splenic nodules, and a trabecular vein (bottom). × 40.

White Pulp

White pulp appears on a cut surface as scattered gray areas of compact pulpal tissue. It forms a sheath about the arteries, the adventitia of which is largely replaced by reticular tissue. The reticular tissue is infiltrated with lymphocytes, which form areas of diffuse and nodular lymphatic tissue. The amount of lymphoid tissue is not constant but varies as it does in all lymphatic tissue in response to certain stimuli. *Splenic nodules* are denser accumulations of lymphocytes along the strands of white pulp. They are typical lymph nodules which may show germinal centers. In the spleen the nodules are arranged around a blood vessel, the so-called *central artery*, which in most instances is an arteriole, eccentric in position since it avoids the germinal center. The number of splenic nodules decreases with age.

Red Pulp

The red pulp is a pastelike, red mass which can be scraped from a freshly cut surface. It is looser in texture than white pulp and is infiltrated with all elements of circulating blood. It occupies all space not utilized by trabeculae and white pulp. It contains numerous venous sinuses. Between the sinuses the pulp appears as cellular cords (*splenic* or *Billroth cords*) which form a spongy network of modified lymphatic tissue that merges gradually into the white pulp.

The support of the pulp is a typical reticulum with its associated reticular cells, both primitive and phagocytic. Within the meshes of this framework are lymphocytes, free macrophages, and all the elements of circulating blood. Lymphocytes of large, medium, and small sizes are numerous in the white pulp but are less numerous and more loosely arranged in the red pulp. The various types of

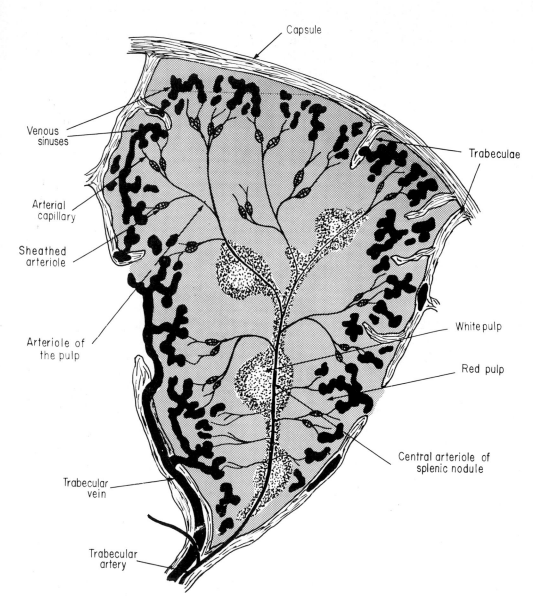

Figure 12-15.   Diagram of a splenic lobule. The principal vascular relations within a lobule are depicted diagrammatically.

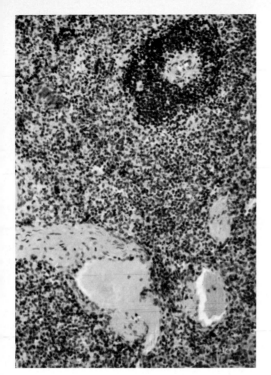

Figure 12-16. Section of a portion of spleen showing a splenic nodule (top) and a trabecular vein (bottom). × 100.

the vascular arrangement. An appreciation of this arrangement is necessary also to an understanding of the structure of the spleen as a whole.

The arteries enter the spleen at the hilum and divide into branches which pass along the trabeculae as *trabecular or interlobular arteries.* As the trabeculae branch, the arteries subdivide also. When reduced to a diameter of approximately 0.2 mm., they leave the trabeculae to enter the splenic parenchyma. As they do so, the tunica adventitia of the arteries loosens, takes on the character of reticular tissue, and becomes infiltrated with lymphocytes. At various points along the course of the vessels the lymphatic sheath is increased in amount to form the splenic nodules. These vessels, which are called "central arteries or arterioles" although they are eccentric with reference to the corpuscles, supply capillaries to all the white pulp. After numerous divisions, the arterioles become reduced in size, lose their investment of white pulp, and enter the red pulp. Here each

lymphocytes arise in the white pulp and spread to the red pulp by amebism. Monocytes also are fairly numerous. Some are brought by the blood stream; others arise within the spleen by proliferation of existing cells or by differentiation from hemocytoblasts. The red pulp also contains numerous plasma cells, granular leukocytes, and erythrocytes.

In many mammals and in mammalian embryos the red pulp of the spleen contains megakaryocytes, myelocytes, and erythroblasts. These myeloid elements are absent from the spleen in adult man except in certain pathological conditions when the spleen undergoes *myeloid metaplasia.*

Blood Vessels

The distribution and organization of the red and white pulp depend upon

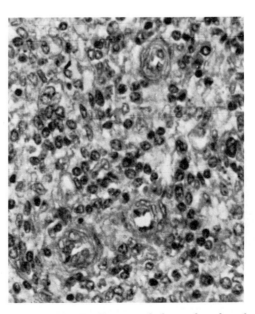

Figure 12-17. Portion of the red pulp of spleen showing three sheathed arterioles in cross section. × 350.

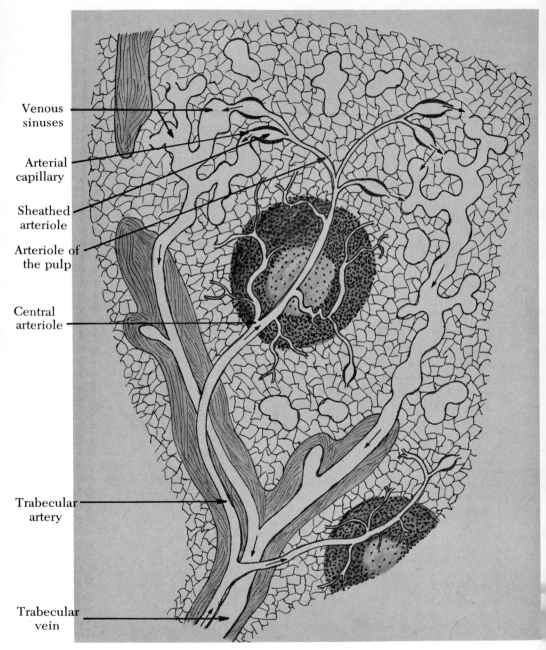

Venous
sinuses

Arterial
capillary

Sheathed
arteriole

Arteriole of
the pulp

Central
arteriole

Trabecular
artery

Trabecular
vein

Figure 12-18.   Diagram to show the route taken by blood through the spleen. At left, a closed circulation; at right, open circulation.

arteriole subdivides into several small branches that lie close together like a brush or *penicillus*. The *penicilli vessels* show three successive segments. The first portion, the longest segment, is the *pulp arteriole (artery of the pulp)*, which possesses a thin tunica of smooth muscle. This vessel becomes narrow and divides into the *sheathed arterioles*, or *ellipsoids*, which have markedly thickened walls, the *Schweigger-Seidel sheath*. The thickened sheath, which is not so well developed in man as in many lower mammals, is spindle-shaped and is composed of a mass of concentrically arranged cells and fibers continuous peripherally with the reticulum of the red pulp. Each sheathed arteriole divides into two or more *terminal arterial capillaries*, the terminations of which are the subject of considerable controversy. Some authors claim that the arterial capillaries open directly into the pulp reticulum and that the blood gradually filters into the venous sinuses (the "open" circulation theory). Other authors consider that the arterial capillaries empty directly into the venous sinuses (the "closed" circulation theory). Finally, some investigators hold a compromise view, that both types of circulation exist at the same time. The exact routing of the blood is, in a sense, a detail of academic interest only, since in any case there is an interchange of cells between the red pulp and the sinuses.

The *venous sinuses* constitute a system of irregular, anastomosing tunnels throughout the red pulp. They occupy more space than that occupied by the splenic cords which lie between them. These vessels are called *sinuses* since they have an irregular lumen and are highly distensible. The sinus wall is not endothelium but is composed of specialized reticular cells which are phagocytic and belong to the reticuloendothelial (macrophage) system. Component cells are rod-shaped and run longitudinally in the vessel wall. The cell bodies bulge into the lumen

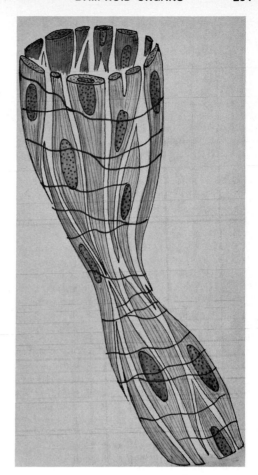

Figure 12-19. Diagrammatic reconstruction of a portion of a splenic (venous) sinus. Note the elongated reticuloendothelial cells and the circularly arranged, branching reticular fibers.

of the sinus. This bulging is most pronounced in the region of the nucleus. Outside these cells the wall of the sinus is supported by thick, anastomosing reticular fibers circularly arranged. There is some dispute concerning the integrity of the sinus wall. Some authors claim that a membrane exists between the cells which closes the meshes of the cellular framework. Other investigators believe that the sinuses open to the pulp by clefts between the lining cells.

The venous sinuses empty into the *pulp veins*, lined by endothelium. These veins leave the pulp and unite to form larger veins which pass into the trabeculae as *trabecular* or *interlobular* veins. The trabecular veins, which consist only of endothelium supported by the fibromuscular tissue of the trabeculae, travel to the hilum, where they drain into the splenic vein.

Lymphatics

Efferent vessels are present in the capsule and in the larger trabeculae. A few deep efferent lymphatic vessels, which follow the arteries, may be present also in the white pulp.

Nerves

Unmyelinated nerve fibers follow the arteries and terminate in the smooth muscle of their walls. A few branches enter both the red and white pulp but their endings here are unknown. Occasional myelinated fibers, which probably are sensory in function, are seen also.

Functions of the Spleen

Splenic functions are not understood completely. The spleen is said to be not essential for life. However, although in some cases it can be removed without harm to the individual, in others morbidity may follow the operation. Often the morbidity is related to an increase in the number of lymphocytes in the blood due to excessive compensation by the lymph nodes. After extirpation the spleen's functions are taken over by various organs, principally other lymphoid organs and the bone marrow.

The spleen is an important hemopoietic organ, producing both lymphocytes and monocytes. Lymphocytes are formed chiefly in the white pulp, in particular in its nodules. From the white pulp they pass to the red pulp, and so into the sinuses and splenic vein. Monocytes differentiate from hemocytoblasts in the red pulp. In

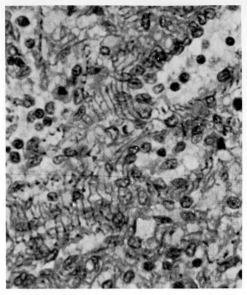

Figure 12-20. Section of red pulp of spleen stained by the periodic acid–Schiff (PAS) reaction to show reticular fibers in relation to splenic sinuses. × 425.

the embryo the spleen also produces myeloid elements. In certain pathological conditions it may undergo myeloid metaplasia, as mentioned previously, and produce all types of blood cells.

The spleen also acts as a store for red blood cells. It is an elastic, controllable reservoir that is important in adjusting the volume of the circulating blood. From time to time large numbers of red blood cells are retained in the spleen and then expelled when needed into the general circulation by contraction of the smooth muscle fibers and the stretched elastic fibers in the trabeculae and capsule.

The spleen filters the blood in much the same way as the lymph nodes filter lymph. The phagocytic cells of the spleen, both free and attached, remove foreign particles, bacteria, degenerating leukocytes, and erythrocytes. In the latter instance the spleen functions as an organ of blood destruction. Erythrocytes are engulfed by the phagocytic cells and iron recovered from the hemoglobin is stored in the cells. The iron is given up as needed and is utilized in the formation of new hemoglobin.

The production of antibodies is thought to be another important function of the spleen. Evidence indicates that young plasma cells, which are derived from reticular cells or hemocytoblasts, are the source of the antibodies.

Development

The primordium of the spleen in human embryos appears as a thickening of the mesenchyme in the dorsal mesentery of the stomach during the fifth week of embryonic development. At this time it consists of a mass of mesenchymal cells which later divide actively. The mass of the primordium is added to by apposition of cells from the covering mesothelium of the body cavity. The mesenchymal cells differentiate into cells of the reticulum and into primitive free cells resembling lymphocytes. Later the tissue becomes myeloid in type, containing all stages in the development of megakaryocytes, granulocytes, and erythrocytes. The development of lymphocytes and monocytes continues throughout life, but myeloid elements disappear shortly after birth.

In the early stages of development the spleen is supplied by a rich capillary plexus, but as a characteristic distribution of vessels is established, lymphocytes become compactly arranged around the arteries to form the white pulp. The venous sinuses develop as irregular spaces which later become connected with the established blood vessels.

REFERENCES

Burnet, F. M.: The thymus gland. Sci. Amer., 207:50, 1962.

Clark, S. L., Jr.: The reticulum of lymph nodes in mice studied with the electron microscope. Amer. J. Anat., 110:217, 1962.

Daniels, J. C., Ritzmann, S. E., and Levin, W. C.: Lymphocytes: Morphological, developmental, and functional characteristics in health, disease, and experimental study—an analytical review. Texas Rep. Biol. Med., 26:5, 1968.

Dependi, V., and Metcalf, D. (editors): The Thymus. The Wistar Institute Symposium, Monograph No. 2. Philadelphia, The Wistar Institute Press, 1964.

Elves, M. W.: The Lymphocytes. London, Lloyd-Luke, 1966.

Galindo, B., and Imaeda, T.: Electron microscope study of the white pulp of the mouse spleen. Anat. Rec., 143:399, 1962.

Good, R. A., and Gabrielsen, A. E. (editors): The Thymus in Immunobiology. New York, Hoeber Medical Division, Harper and Row, 1964.

Kohnen, P., and Weiss, L.: An electron microscopic study of thymic corpuscles in the guinea pig and the mouse. Anat. Rec., 148:29, 1964.

Lewis, O. J.: The blood vessels of the adult mammalian spleen. J. Anat., 91:245, 1957.

Maximow, A. A.: The lymphocytes and plasma cells. In Special Cytology, ed. 2, edited by E. V. Cowdry. New York, Paul B. Hoeber, 1932, vol. 2, p. 601.

Moe, R. E.: Electron microscopic appearance of the parenchyma of lymph nodes. Amer. J. Anat., 114:341, 1964.

Peck, H. M., and Hoerr, N. L.: The intermediary circulation in the red pulp of the mouse spleen. Anat. Rec., 109:447, 1951.

Roberts, D. K., and Latta, J. S.: Electron microscopic studies on the red pulp of the rabbit spleen. Anat. Rec., 148:81, 1964.

Snook, T.: The guinea-pig spleen. Studies on the structure and connections of the venous sinuses. Anat. Rec., 89:413, 1944.

Weiss, L.: A study of the structure of the splenic sinuses in man and in the albino rat, with the light microscope and the electron microscope. J. Biophys. Biochem. Cytol., 3:599, 1957.

Weiss, L.: The structure of fine splenic arterial vessels in relation to hemoconcentration and red cell destruction. Amer. J. Anat., 111:131, 1962.

Weiss, L.: An electron microscopic study of splenic white pulp. J. Cell Biol., 19:74A, 1963.

Yoffey, J. M., and Courtice, F. C.: Lymphatics, Lymph and Lymphoid Tissue. Cambridge, Harvard University Press, 1956.

Yoffey, J. M.: Lymphocytes—the fourth circulation. Discovery, 27:24, 1966.

CHAPTER 13

THE SKIN AND ITS APPENDAGES (THE INTEGUMENT)

The integument comprises the skin which covers the surface of the body together with certain specialized derivatives of the skin. These include nails, hair, and several kinds of glands.

The skin protects the organism from injurious substances and influences; it helps to regulate the temperature of the body; by sweating it excretes water and various waste products of catabolism; it is the most extensive sense organ of the body for the reception of tactile, thermal, and painful stimuli.

THE SKIN

The skin is composed of two layers: the *epidermis*, a specialized epithelium derived from the ectoderm, and beneath this, the *dermis* (or *corium*), of vascular dense connective tissue, a derivative of mesoderm; the dermis corresponds to the lamina propria of a mucous membrane. These two layers are firmly adherent to each other and form a membrane which varies in thickness from about 0.5 to 4 mm. or more in different parts of the

body. Beneath the dermis is a layer of loose connective tissue which varies from areolar to adipose in character. This is the superficial fascia of gross anatomy, sometimes referred to as the *hypodermis*, but it is not considered to be part of the skin. The dermis is connected to the underlying hypodermis by connective tissue fibers which pass from one layer to the other. The superficial fascia permits great mobility of skin over most regions of the body. It is only in local areas such as the palm and the sole, where there is considerable interlocking of fibers between dermis and hypodermis, that mobility is limited.

The free surface of the skin exhibits numerous ridges which can be seen with the naked eye. They run in various directions and are most apparent on the palms of the hands and the soles of the feet. The patterns are determined in the main by hereditary factors and correspond to similar patterns on the surface of the dermis, the *dermal ridges*. Thus, in sections, the boundary between epidermis and dermis appears uneven. However, varia-

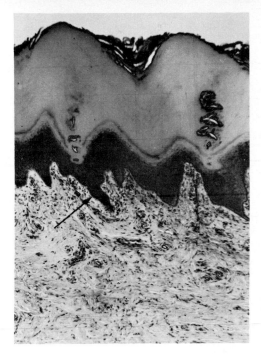

Figure 13-1. Low power photomicrograph of a section of thick skin of sole of foot. Note that the epidermis consists chiefly of keratin (stratum corneum), in which portions of two ducts of sweat glands can be seen as they pass through to the surface. The junction between the epidermis and the dermis (arrow) is irregular. × 100.

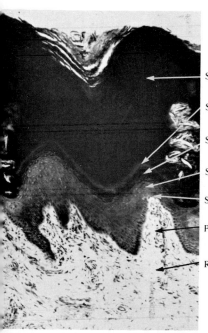

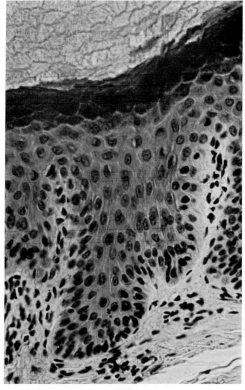

Stratum corneum

Stratum lucidum

Stratum granulosum

Stratum spinosum

Stratum germinativum

Papillary layer of dermis

Reticular layer of dermis

Figure 13-2. Sections of human sole, perpendicular to the surface, to illustrate the different layers of the skin. Left, × 165. Right, × 300.   See filmstrip II, frame 51.

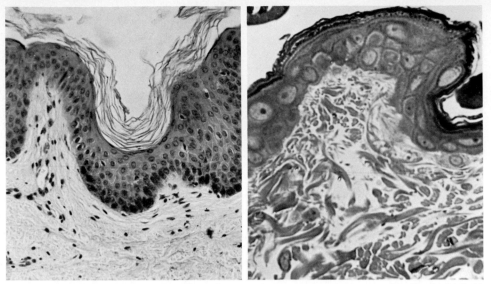

Figure 13-3. Left: Section of thin skin of a Negro. Compare with Figure 13-2 (thick skin). Note the scattered cells representative of the stratum granulosum and the thinness of the stratum corneum. There is marked deposition of pigment (melanin) in the lower layers of the epidermis, particularly in the stratum germinativum. × 180. Right: Section of thin skin of Caucasian. Epon section. × 550.

See filmstrip II, frame 52.

tions in the degree of development of ridges do occur, and ridges are absent on the forehead, external ear, perineum, and scrotum. The ridges seen on the skin of the palmar surface of the fingers constitute the basis for the prints used in criminal detection since they are subject to marked individual variation and never change (apart from enlargement) after they are formed during the third and fourth months of fetal life.

Skin is classified commonly as thick or thin, thick skin being found on the palms of the hands and soles of the feet, thin skin covering the remainder of the body. It should be emphasized that these terms, thick and thin, do not refer to the thickness of the skin as a whole, only to the epidermis. Thin skin itself varies greatly in thickness in different parts of the body and these variations are due, in actual fact, almost entirely to variations in the thickness of the dermis. The dermis of extensor surfaces is usually thicker than that of flexor surfaces. Both regions, however, have an epidermal component which is classified as thin.

The Epidermis

The epidermis, a stratified squamous epithelium, is composed of cells of two separate origins. The bulk of the epithelium, of ectodermal origin, undergoes a process of *keratinization* resulting in the formation of the dead superficial layers of skin. The second component comprises the melanocytes which produce melanin. The latter cells do not undergo keratinization. The superficial keratinized cells are continuously lost from the surface and must be replaced by cells that arise as a result of mitotic activity of cells of the basal layers of the epidermis. Cells which result from this proliferation are displaced to higher levels, and as they move upward they elaborate keratin. Keratin eventually replaces the majority of the cytoplasm, the cell dies and finally is shed. Thus it should be appreciated that the structural organization of the epidermis into layers reflects stages in the dynamic processes of cellular proliferation and differentiation.

Epidermis of the Palms and Soles. The epidermis here is particularly thick and exhibits maximal layering and cellular differentiation. It consists of five layers or strata: stratum germinativum or stratum basale, resting upon the dermis; stratum spinosum or prickle cell layer; stratum granulosum; stratum lucidum; and stratum corneum, the outermost horny layer.

The *stratum germinativum* consists of a single layer of columnar cells, each cell of which has short, thin, cytoplasmic processes on its basal surface. These toothlike processes fit into pockets of the basal lamina and appear to anchor the epithelium to the underlying dermis. Mitotic figures occur frequently in this layer, thus producing new cells which are displaced into the layer above.

The *stratum spinosum* is several layers thick and is composed of irregular, polyhedral cells, slightly separated from each other. Toward the surface the cells become flattened. The surface of these cells is covered with short cytoplasmic spines or projections which meet with similar projections of adjacent cells to form "intercellular bridges." It should be emphasized that these do not indicate cytoplasmic continuity between cells. Electron micrographs demonstrate that the short processes constituting a "bridge" make intimate contact at a desmosome. Hence the cells are independent entities. The cytoplasm of these cells is basophil, indicating a considerable content of RNA, in this case associated with protein synthesis for growth and division of cells. The cytoplasm also contains numerous bundles of filaments which form the tonofibrils. Many of these pass into cytoplasmic processes and terminate

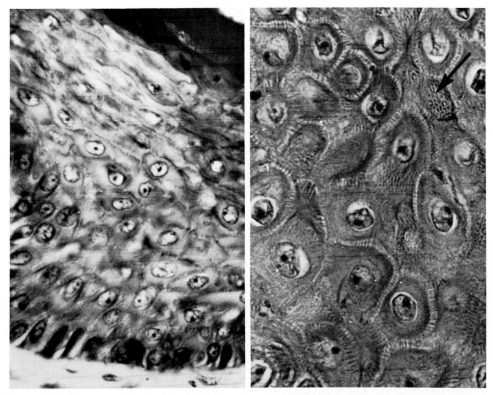

Figure 13-4.   Low power (left) and oil immersion (right) photomicrographs of a section of human palm, stained with iron hematoxylin, showing junctions between cells of the stratum spinosum. In one region (arrow), the contacts are seen in cross section. Left, × 560. Right, × 1200.

See filmstrip II, frame 53.

in the desmosome. They do not extend across cell membranes. It is thought that the tonofibrils are the principal precursor of keratin.

It should be mentioned at this point that the two layers just described, the stratum germinativum and stratum spinosum, are grouped together as the Malpighian layer (stratum [or rete] Malpighii) by many authors. This layer is responsible for proliferation and for initiation of the keratinization process.

The next layer, the *stratum granulosum*, consists of three to five layers of flattened cells whose long axis is parallel to the skin surface. The cytoplasm of these cells contains irregularly shaped granules of *keratohyalin*, which stain with some acid dyes and with certain basic dyes. The origin of these granules is obscure, but they appear to be involved in the process of formation of soft keratin. With increase in size and number of these granules, the nuclei become pale and indistinct, and show degenerative changes. At the same time, cell contacts and tonofibrils become indistinct. It is in this layer that the cells of the epidermis die.

The *stratum lucidum* is a clear translucent layer, three to five cells deep. Cells are not distinguishable clearly as separate entities. They are flattened and closely packed. Nuclei are indistinct or absent. The cytoplasm contains a semifluid substance, *keratohyalin*, which is presumed to be a product of the granules noted in subjacent layers.

The fifth and outermost layer, the *stratum corneum*, is composed of clear, dead, scalelike cells which become progressively flattened and fused. The nucleus is absent and the cytoplasm is replaced with keratin, thought to be derived principally from the tonofibrils of the deeper layers of the epidermis. This is "soft keratin," low in sulphur content, as distinct from "hard keratin" found in nails and the cortex of hairs. The most superficial layers of the stratum corneum are flat horny plates which are desquamated constantly. The stratum corneum stains pink with eosin and often is shredded during specimen preparation. Thus, from the surface of the epidermis, there is a constant loss of dead cells which are replaced by new cells formed as a result of mitoses in the deeper layers, principally in the stratum germinativum and the stratum spinosum, and pushed toward the surface during the process of keratinization.

Epidermis of the General Body Surface. The epidermis of the rest of the body is both thinner and simpler than that of the palms and soles. All layers of the epidermis are reduced and the stratum lucidum is usually absent. The stratum germinativum is similar to that of thick skin but the stratum spinosum is not so extensive. The granular layer may be present as one or two rows of cells or may be represented by scattered cells along the line where this layer might be expected. The reduction in thickness of the epidermis of thin skin is due probably to the fact that keratinization here is less marked and is not a continuous process.

Pigmentation. The color of the skin is dependent upon three factors. The color of skin itself is yellow, owing to the presence of carotene. Blood, showing through from the underlying vascular dermis, imparts a reddish hue. Finally, the presence of varying amounts of melanin pigment is responsible for shades of brown. Melanin is present mainly in the stratum germinativum and in the deeper layers of the stratum spinosum.

As cells move toward the surface, the granules of melanin become dustlike and cannot be identified as definite entities in the stratum corneum. In colored races, pigment is present in greater amounts in all layers of the epidermis. The pigment is not elaborated in the general cell population of the epidermis but in specialized cells derived from the neural crest, the *melanocytes*, which then distribute it to the epidermal cells.

Melanocytes are scattered just beneath the basal layer of the epidermis and send numerous cytoplasmic processes between epithelial cells. They also are present in the Malpighian layer of the epidermis. These cells contain an enzyme, *tyrosinase*, which is involved in synthesis of the pigment. Exposure to x-rays and to ultraviolet light increases the enzymic activity of these cells and thus leads to increased melanin production and deposition in the epidermis and to tanning. Melanocytes cannot be identified in normal preparations but can be made visible with a special reagent, "dopa," which they oxidize, coloring them black. The fate of the pigment in the epidermis is not clearly understood, but it is thought that it is probably broken down and eliminated with the epidermal scales. Characteristically, melanin granules in cells of the stratum germinativum are found related to the superficial aspect of the nucleus.

Dermis

It is difficult to define the exact limits to the dermis since it merges into the underlying subcutaneous layer (hypodermis). However, the average thickness varies from 0.5 mm. to 3 mm. or more It is composed of dense irregularly arranged connective tissue and is subdivided into two strata, the *papillary layer* superficially and the *reticular layer* beneath. The papillary layer includes the ridges and papillae which protrude into the epidermis. Papillae tend to occur in double rows and often are branched. Some papillae contain special nerve terminations (nervous papillae); others possess loops of capillary blood vessels (vascular papillae). The papillary layer is composed of thin collagenous, reticular, and elastic fibers arranged in an extensive network. Just beneath the epidermis, reticular fibers of the dermis form a close feltwork which in ordinary preparations appears as a homogeneous zone, into which the basal processes of cells of the stratum germinativum are anchored. This is the basal lamina.

The reticular layer is the main fibrous bed of the dermis. It consists of coarse, dense, and interlacing collagenous fibers, in which are intermingled a few reticular fibers and numerous elastic fibers. The predominant direction of all fibers is parallel to the surface. Owing to the direction of the fibers, lines of skin tension, *Langer's lines*, are formed. The direction of these lines is of surgical importance since incisions made parallel with the lines gape less and heal with less scar tissue than incisions made at right angles to or obliquely across the lines.

The predominant cellular elements of the dermis are fibroblasts and macrophages. In addition, fat cells may be present, either singly or, more commonly, in groups. Apart from the usual types of connective tissue cells, pigmented, branched, connective tissue cells, *chromatophores*, may be present. They are numerous only in areas where the overlying epidermis is heavily pigmented, for example, in the areola of the nipple and the circumanal region. They do not elaborate their pigment but obtain it apparently from melanocytes. True *dermal melanoblasts* are rare. These, like the melanocytes of the epidermis, are dopa-positive. They may accumulate in the sacral region, where they form the "mongolian spot," or in certain tumors of the dermis (blue nevi). Generally, the papillary layer contains more cells and smaller and finer connective tissue fibers than the reticular layer.

Smooth muscle fibers may be found in the dermis. They are arranged in small bundles in connection with hair follicles (*arrectores pilorum* muscles) and are scattered throughout the dermis in considerable numbers in the skin of the nipple, penis, scrotum, and parts of the perineum. Contraction of the fibers gives the skin of these regions a wrinkled appearance. In the face and neck, fibers of some skeletal muscles terminate in delicate elastic fiber networks of the dermis.

Hypodermis. The subcutaneous layer (superficial fascia) is not part of the skin, but appears as a deep extension of the dermis. The density and arrangement of the subcutaneous layer determines the mobility of the skin. Depending upon the region of the body and the general state of nutrition of the organism, varying numbers of fat cells are present in the hypodermis. On the abdomen this layer may reach a thickness of 3 cm. or more. In the eyelids, penis, and scrotum the subcutaneous layer is devoid of fat.

THE NAILS

The nails are horny plates which form a protective covering on the dorsal surface of the terminal phalanges of the fingers and toes. Their structure and relationship to the epidermis and dermis are understood best if consideration is given to their

early development. Toward the end of the third month of intrauterine life, the epidermis over the dorsal surface of the terminal phalanx of each finger and toe invades the underlying dermis. Unlike the early development of a gland, which is a tubular ingrowth of epithelial cells into the underlying connective tissue, in the case of the nail the invasion occurs along a transverse curved line and slants proximally with relation to the surface. The invading plate of epidermis later splits to form a *nail groove,* and the epidermal cells of the deep (distal) wall of the groove proliferate to form the matrix of the nail. With continuing proliferation and differentiation of cells in the lower part of the matrix, the forming *nail plate* is pushed out of the groove and slowly advances over the dorsal surface of the digit toward the distal end. The epidermis immediately beneath the nail plate constitutes the *nail bed.* The nail plate itself is contained within the nail groove, which becomes U-shaped as seen from the dorsum, flanked by a skin fold, the *nail wall.* The nail bed,

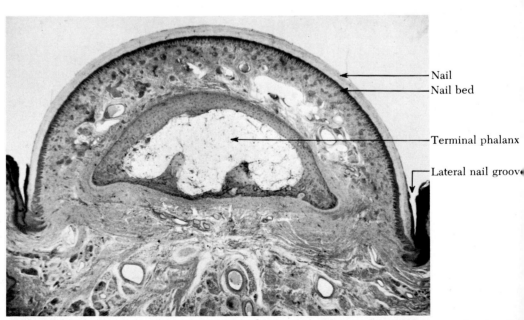

Figure 13-5. Low power photomicrograph of a cross section through a child's finger, showing the nail and nail bed. × 30.

which underlies both the exposed and concealed portions of the nail, consists only of the deeper layers of the epidermis and the underlying dermis, which is ridged longitudinally. It lacks sweat glands and hair follicles. The epidermis of the nail bed, the matrix, is thickest proximally, and it is here that nail growth chiefly occurs and the rate of cell division is rapid. Component cells contain numerous cytoplasmic fibrils which are lost at a later stage as the cells become homogeneous, cornify, and join the nail plate. At no time can keratohyalin granules be recognized in cells of the matrix, and the keratin of the nail is termed hard. The epidermis of the nail bed is continuous distally with the epidermis of the finger tip under the free edge of the nail. At the point of junction, the stratum corneum of the epidermis is thickened. This thickened epidermis is known as the *hyponychium*. The nail plate itself consists of intimately fused epidermal scales which do not desquamate. The body of the plate is translucent and transmits the pink color of blood vessels in the nail bed. The root is more opaque than the body since

cornification and drying are incomplete. The root becomes continuous with the body of the nail over a crescentic margin, a portion of which junction is visible distal to the nail groove. This is the *lunule*. The nail groove is lined by modified epidermis of the nail wall. Cells of the stratum corneum extend from the nail wall onto the free surface of the nail plate as the *eponychium*, or cuticle.

THE HAIR

Hairs are elastic keratinized threads which develop from the epidermis. They vary from 1 mm. or less to 1.5 meters in length and from 0.05 to 0.5 mm. in thickness. They are distributed over the entire skin except for the palms, soles, and region of the anal and urogenital apertures. Each hair has a free *shaft* and a *root* embedded in the skin. Enclosing the hair root is a tubular *hair follicle*, which consists of epidermal (epithelial) and dermal (connective tissue) portions. At its lower end the follicle expands into a *hair bulb*, which is indented at the basal end by a connec-

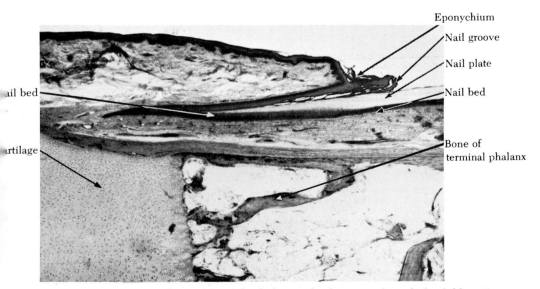

Figure 13-6.   Low power photomicrograph of a longitudinal section of a nail of a child. × 45.

tive tissue *papilla*. Associated with the hair follicle are one or more sebaceous glands and a bundle of smooth muscle. The muscle, the *arrector pili,* is attached at one end to the connective tissue sheath of the follicle and at the other to the papillary layer of the dermis. By its contraction it causes erection of the hair since the hair is not set perpendicularly to the skin surface but slopes at an obtuse angle.

Structure of the Hair

The hair consists of epidermal cells arranged in three concentric layers: the medulla, cortex, and cuticle. The medulla forms the loose central axis and consists of two or three layers of shrunken, cornified, cuboidal cells which are separated partially by air spaces. The medulla is absent in fine short hairs of the downy type and is missing also from some of the hairs of the scalp and from "blonde" hair. The cells often contain pigment. The keratin of medullary cells is of the "soft" type.

The cortex makes up the main bulk of the hair and is composed of several layers of long, flattened, spindle-shaped, cornified cells in which the keratin is of the "hard" type. Pigment granules are found in and between cells. Black hair contains pigment that is oxidized. Air also accumulates in the intercellular spaces of cortical cells and modifies the hair color. Superficially there is a single layer of thin clear cells, the cuticle. These are cornified cells which, except for those in the base of the root, have lost their nuclei. The cells overlap, like shingles on a roof, with their free edges directed upward. The appearance of hair in cross section varies from race to race. The straight hair of the Mongol races (Chinese, Eskimos, and American Indians) is round, whereas the wavy hair of many people, including Caucasians, is oval in cross section. The cross section of the wooly

hair of Negroes is elliptical or reniform.

The Hair Follicle

The hair follicle is a compound sheath which consists of an external connective tissue sheath (the *dermal root sheath*) derived from the dermis and an internal *epithelial root sheath* from the epidermis. The epithelial root sheath is subdivided into inner and outer components. Toward its deep end, the follicle is expanded into a hair bulb where the hair root and its sheath blend in a mass of primitive cells, the matrix. The base of the bulb is invaginated by a connective tissue papilla, and it is in relation to the papilla that the hair root and its sheaths merge. The hair papilla, although much larger, is similar in structure to other dermal papillae and contains delicate connective tissue fibers, cellular elements, and a rich plexus of blood vessels and nerves. All layers of the follicle are not found at all levels but are represented best in the portion of the follicle between the bulb and the entry of a sebaceous gland.

The dermal root sheath is composed of three layers, corresponding to similar strata of the dermis. The outer layer is poorly defined and consists of coarse bundles of collagen fibers running in a longitudinal direction. It corresponds to the reticular layer of the dermis. The middle layer is thicker and corresponds to the papillary layer of the dermis. It is cellular and contains fine connective tissue fibers, circularly arranged. The inner layer is a homogeneous narrow band, the *glassy membrane,* corresponding to the basal lamina beneath the epidermis. It consists of reticular fibers and amorphous ground substance.

The epidermal root sheath has an outer component, continuous with the deeper layers of the epidermis, and an inner component, which corresponds to the more specialized, super-

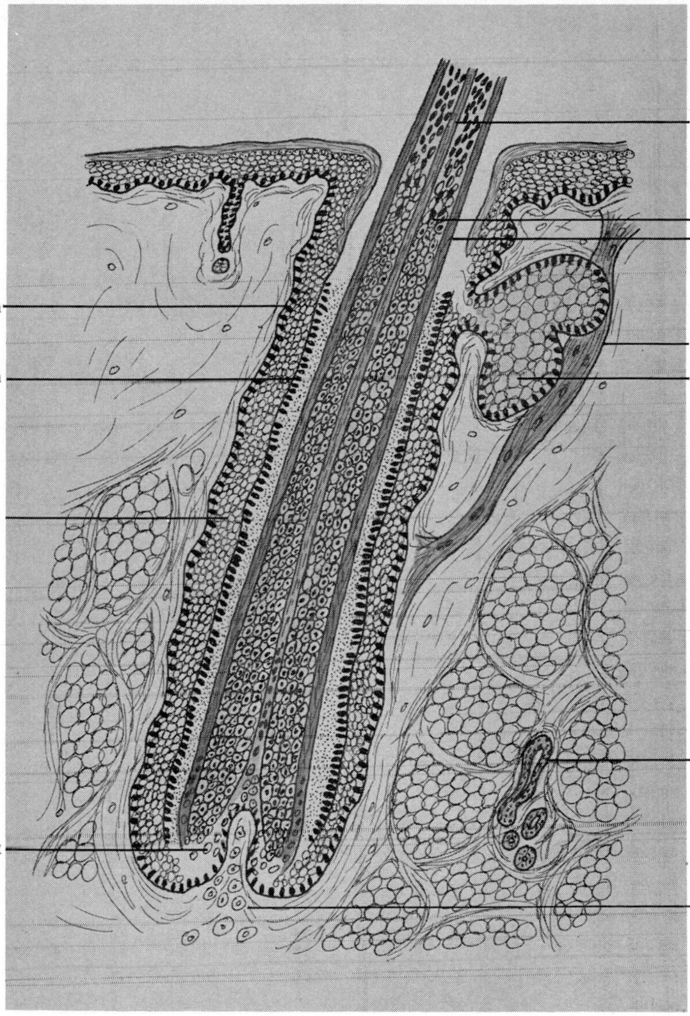
Medulla
Hair
Cortex
Cuticle
Connective tissue sheath
Internal root sheath
Arrector pili muscle
Sebaceous gland
External root sheath
Sweat gland
Matrix
Connective tissue papilla

Figure 13-7. Diagram of a hair follicle (length of follicle somewhat abbreviated) to show the general relationships.

See filmstrip II, frame 54.

ficial layers. The outer epithelial root sheath possesses a single row of tall cells directly in relation to the glassy membrane and an inner stratum of polygonal cells (with cell contacts) which resemble cells of the stratum spinosum of the epidermis. The inner epithelial root sheath is a keratinized sheath enveloping the growing hair root and, like the hair, it is pushed up by addition of cells from the bulb. It does not extend above the point of entry of the duct of the sebaceous gland into the follicle. It has three distinct strata: *Henle's layer, Huxley's layer,* and the *cuticle of the root sheath.* Henle's layer, directly in relation to the outer epithelial root sheath, is a single layer of flattened, clear cells which contain hyaline fibrils. Immediately internal to this is Huxley's layer, which consists of several rows of elongated cells whose cytoplasm contains *trichohyalin* granules, much like keratohyalin. The cuticle of the root sheath lies against the cuticle of the hair and is similar to the latter in structure. It is a single layer of transparent, horny scales, the free edges of which project downward

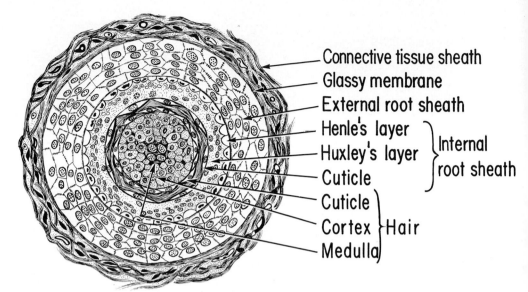

Figure 13-8. Diagram of a hair follicle in cross section beneath the level of entry of a sebaceous gland.

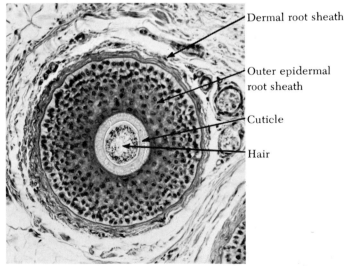

Figure 13-9. Cross section of human hair follicle above the level of entry of a sebaceous gland. × 180.

See filmstrip II, frame 55.

and interdigitate with the upward projecting scales of the hair cuticle. This interlocking explains why the inner root sheath is also removed when a hair is extracted.

Growth of the hair occurs following mitosis in cells of the undifferentiated matrix of epidermal cells above and around the dermal papilla of the follicle. Cells immediately above the apex of the papilla form the medulla; those above the slope and sides form the cortex and cuticle of the hair respectively. Cells immediately lateral to the papilla transform into the inner root sheath which, like the hair root, grows upward. Cells at the bottom of the follicle continue into the outer root sheath. The cells of the hair matrix are analogous to the Malpighian layer of the epidermis in that the life cycle of each terminates with the formation of cornified cells. In the case of the epidermis the product is soft keratinous material and the process is continuous. The product of matrix cells is a hard keratinous material and the process is intermittent and is dependent upon an inductive influence of a particular portion of the dermis. Hair has a definite period of growth. For the head it is about two to four years, for eyelashes only three to four months. Upon cessation of growth, multiplication of the undifferentiated cells at the base of the follicle ceases. The root of the hair then becomes detached from the matrix and the hair either falls out or is pulled out. After a resting phase, the remaining cord of epithelial cells of the follicle undergoes a period of growth and contacts either the old papilla or a new one. A new germinal matrix develops and a new hair begins to grow up the reforming follicle.

GLANDS OF THE SKIN

Glands of the skin include sebaceous, sweat, and mammary glands. Mammary glands, which are specialized sweat glands, are described with the female genital system (p. 439).

Sebaceous Glands

The sebaceous glands are, with a few exceptions, connected with hair follicles. Usually several drain into a single hair follicle but where they are independent of hairs, their ducts open directly upon the free surface of the skin, for example, in glans penis, labia minora, and tarsal (meibomian) glands of the eyelids. They are lacking entirely in the palms and the soles. Sebaceous glands are located in the dermis, where each gland is encapsulated by a thin layer of connective tissue. They are alveolar (saccular) glands which synthesize lipid. In most glands several alveoli open into a short wide duct, which itself empties into the neck of a hair follicle. The alveoli themselves are filled completely with a stratified epithelium. The epithelium of the secretory portion lies upon a delicate basal lamina, on the internal surface of which is a single row of small cuboidal cells, continuous with the basal cells of the epidermis at the neck of the hair follicle. Toward the center of the alveolus, cells become progressively larger and the cytoplasm is distended with fat droplets. Nuclei gradually shrink and then disappear and the cells break down into a fatty mass and cellular debris. This is the oily secretion (*sebum*) of the gland, which is of the holocrine type since it results from total destruction of epithelial cells. Cells lost in the secretory process are replaced by proliferation from the basal cells and from cells close to the wall of the excretory duct. The short, wide duct of sebaceous glands is lined by stratified squamous epithelium continuous with the external root sheath of the hair and with the Malpighian layer of the epidermis. Toward the alveolus, the layering decreases progressively until finally it

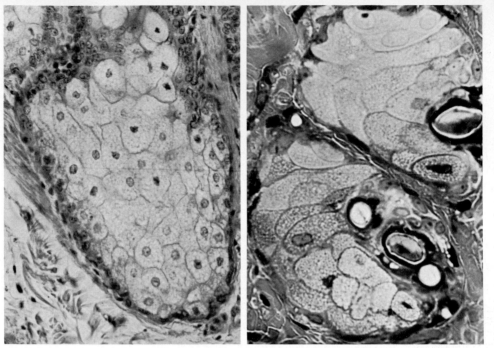

Figure 13-10. High power photomicrographs of human sebaceous glands. Left: Paraffin section. × 275. Right: Epon section. × 400.   See filmstrip II, frame 52.

merges with the row of low basal cells of the alveolus. Discharge of secretion is aided by contraction of the arrector pili muscle and by general pressure owing to an increase in the size of cells centrally within the alveolus.

Sweat Glands

The ordinary sweat glands (*eccrine* type) are unbranched, coiled, tubular glands distributed throughout the skin, except upon the nail bed, margins of the lips, glans penis, and eardrum. They are most numerous in the palms and soles. The secretory portion is situated deeply in the dermis, or in the hypodermis, and is coiled into a discrete mass. The excretory portion, or duct, rises to the epidermis by a slightly tortuous course, joins the epidermis, and spirals through it to reach the free surface where it opens by a minute pit, the *sweat pore.*

The coiled secretory portion of the gland is lined by a simple columnar or cuboidal epithelium supported by a distinct basal lamina. Three distinct cell types are present in the epithelium. The principal (clear) cells are serous and vary in height depending upon the activity of the gland. The nucleus is rounded and occupies a mid-position within the cell. The cytoplasm is vacuolated and contains fat droplets and, occasionally, pigment granules. Secretory capillaries (intercellular canaliculi) can be demonstrated between the cells. Scattered between serous cells are mucigenous cells, which contain small basophilic secretory granules. Between the bases of the cells and the bounding basal lamina, there is a zone occupied by spindle-shaped myoepithelial cells, which wind in longitudinal spirals around the tubule. The nucleus of such cells is elongated and the cytoplasm deeply acidophil. They are thought to be specialized smooth

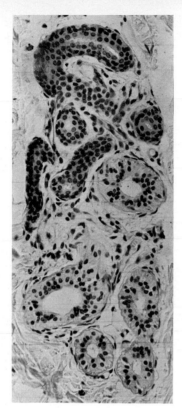

Figure 13-11. Medium power photomicrograph of a human (eccrine) sweat gland—duct portion above, secretory portion below. × 180. See filmstrip II, frame 56.

muscle cells which are contractile and aid in emptying the gland of secretion.

The secretory tubule narrows into a slender excretory duct which is lined with a double layer of darkly staining cuboidal cells. The cells which form the inner layer of the duct wall bear a specialized fibrous border along their free surface, where the cytoplasm appears homogeneous and stains intensely because of the concentration here of tonofilaments. The duct is surrounded by a basal lamina, but no myoepithelial elements are interposed between it and the lining epithelium. Where the duct joins the epidermis, it loses its own wall, becoming a specialized channel through the epithelium.

The ordinary sweat glands (eccrine type) are merocrine in their secretion, but there are certain large sweat glands found in the axilla, areola of the nipple, labia majora, and circumanal region which produce a thicker secretion than the sweat formed by the smaller glands. In these large glands, the apices of the gland cells frequently are broken off in the process of preparation, but this is an artifact and secretion is merocrine in type, although the glands traditionally still are called apocrine glands. These large sweat glands show less coiling than do ordinary sweat glands and the lumen of the secretory portion is much wider. Myoepithelial cells are larger and form a more complete layer between the epithelial cells and the basal lamina. The wax-secreting *ceruminous* glands of the external auditory canal and the *glands of Moll* in the margin of the eyelid also belong to this group of larger sweat glands.

BLOOD VESSELS, LYMPHATICS, AND NERVES OF THE SKIN

Blood Vessels

The blood supply to the skin is from large arteries in the subcutaneous layer. These vessels send branches superficially to form a horizontally orientated network (*rete cutaneum*) at the junctional zone between dermis and hypodermis. From this network, branches pass on one side to supply the subcutaneous tissue including sweat glands and the deeper portions of hair follicles, and on the other side to the dermis where they form a further network between the papillary and reticular layers (the *rete subpapillare*). From the latter plexus, small arteries are given off to the papillae, where they break up into capillary networks to supply the papillae, sebaceous glands, and the intermediate portion of the hair follicle.

Veins collecting blood from the area supplied by the rete subpapillare form a network immediately beneath the papillae. This network communicates

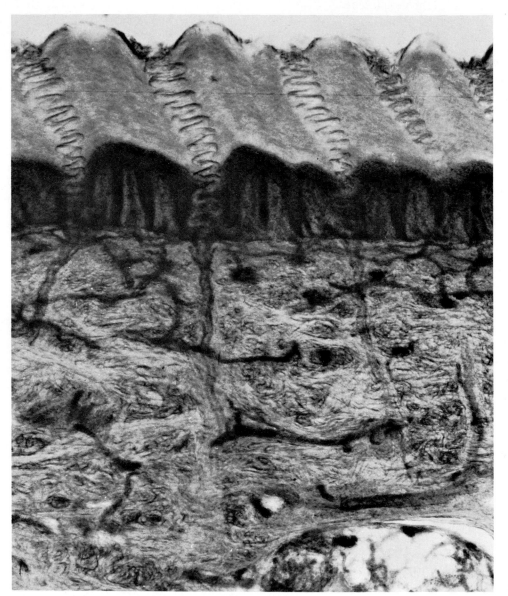

Figure 13-12.   Low power photomicrograph of a thick section of skin of human palm in which the blood vessels were injected with red gelatin. In this thick section, one also has a good demonstration of the spiral course taken through the epidermis by ducts of sweat glands. × 80.

with a second plexus just deeper than the first and via this with a third plexus at the junction of the dermis with the hypodermis. Into the latter plexus pass most of the veins from the fat lobules and sweat glands. From the third plexus, veins pass to a deeper network of large veins in the subcutaneous tissue which is drained by large veins accompanying the arteries.

Lymphatics

These begin as endothelial-lined clefts in the papillae, which pass to a horizontal network of lymph capillaries in the papillary layer. This network communicates with a network of larger lymph capillaries in the subcutaneous tissue. The latter also receives lymph from delicate plexuses surrounding sebaceous and sweat glands and hair follicles.

Nerves

The skin, together with its accessory organs, receives stimuli from the external environment and thus is abundantly supplied with sensory nerves. In the subcutaneous tissue, there are bundles of large nerves which send branches to several plexuses in the reticular, papillary, and subepithelial zones. In all layers of the skin and hypodermis there are numerous nerve endings of various kinds (see Chapter 20). Apart from free endings of unmyelinated sensory fibers in or close to the epidermis, there are numerous fibers supplying hair follicles. In addition to sensory nerves, there are efferent sympathetic fibers supplying the blood vessels, the arrectores pilorum, and the secretory cells of the sweat glands.

REFERENCES

Bertalanffy, F. D.: Mitotic activity and renewal rate of sebaceous gland cells in the rat. Anat. Rec., 129:231, 1957.

Birbeck, M. S. C., and Mercer, E. H.: Electron microscopy of the human hair follicle. J. Biophys. Biochem. Cytol., 3:203, 1957.

Bunting, H., Wislocki, G. B., and Dempsey, E. W.: The chemical histology of human eccrine and apocrine sweat glands. Anat. Rec., 100:61, 1948.

Chase, H. B.: Growth of the hair. Physiol. Rev., 34:113, 1954.

Ellis, R. A.: Fine structure of the myoepithelium of the eccrine sweat glands of man. J. Cell Biol., 27:551, 1965.

Giroud, A., and Leblond, C. P.: The keratinization of epidermis and its derivatives, especially the hair, as shown by x-ray diffraction and histochemical studies. Ann. N. Y. Acad. Sci., 53:613, 1951.

Hibbs, R. G., and Clark, W. H., Jr.: Electron microscope studies of the human epidermis. J. Biophys. Biochem. Cytol., 6:71, 1959.

Laidlaw, G. F.: The dopa reaction in normal histology. Anat. Rec., 53:339, 1932.

Montagna, W.: The Structure and Function of Skin. New York, Academic Press, 1962.

Montagna, W., and Lobitz, W. C. (editors): The Epidermis. New York, Academic Press, 1964.

Odland, G. F.: The fine structure of the interrelationship of cells in the human epidermis. J. Biophys. Biochem. Cytol., 4:529, 1958.

Rawles, M. E.: Origin of melanophores and their role in development of color patterns in vertebrates. Physiol. Rev., 28:383, 1948.

Rawles, M. E.: Skin and its derivations. In Analysis of Development, edited by B. J. Willier, P. A. Weiss, and V. Hamburger. Philadelphia, W. B. Saunders Co., 1955, p. 499.

Rogers, G. E.: Some aspects of the structure of the inner root sheath of hair follicles revealed by light and electron microscopy. Exp. Cell Res., 14:378, 1958.

Rothman, S.: Physiology and Biochemistry of the Skin. Chicago, University of Chicago Press, 1954.

Selby, C. C.: An electron microscope study of the epidermis of mammalian skin in thin section. J. Biophys. Biochem. Cytol., 1:429, 1955.

Zelickson, A. (editor): The Ultrastructure of Normal and Abnormal Skin. Philadelphia, Lea & Febiger, 1967.

CHAPTER 14

THE DIGESTIVE TRACT

GENERAL ORGANIZATION

The digestive tract is a long tube extending from the mouth to the anus, and basically each part of the tube has a similar structure. In addition to the digestive tube, there are associated glands situated outside the tube but delivering their secretions into it by duct systems. The process of digestion involves first the breaking down of food material to a small particulate size, accomplished primarily by the cutting and grinding action of the teeth and also by the action of hydrochloric acid and digestive enzymes. Digestive enzymes help to split or hydrolyze complex food materials (proteins, carbohydrates, and fat) into smaller residues and thus are to be classed as hydrolytic enzymes or hydrolases. Secondly, digestion involves the ab-sorption of such food materials into the circulation. It should be appreciated that any material within the lumen of the digestive tract virtually is outside the body and thus has to pass through the lining of the tract to enter the circulation. *Digestion, then, is the process whereby food material is converted into substances which can be absorbed into the circulation.* Materials which are useless, and some which even are toxic, are eliminated by fecal excretion.

The digestive tract will be described in three major parts: the oral cavity (including salivary glands and oropharynx), the tubular digestive tract (esophagus, stomach, small intestine, large intestine, rectum, and anal canal), and the major digestive glands (pancreas, liver, and biliary passages).

Part I — THE ORAL CAVITY

THE LIP

The oral cavity is closed anteriorly by apposition of upper and lower lips. The substance of each lip is composed of striated muscle fibers of the orbicularis oris muscle embedded in elastic fibroconnective tissue. Externally, the lip is covered by skin containing hair follicles, sebaceous glands, and sweat glands. At the free margin of the lip, the epithelium is modified by a high content of keratohyalin, which renders it more transparent, and the underlying dermis shows high papillae with a very rich plexus of blood capillaries.

It is blood in this plexus which is responsible for the red color of the free margin of the lip. In this region, there are no hairs, sweat glands, or sebaceous glands, and the surface epithelium can be kept moist only by licking with the tongue. On the internal aspect, the lip is covered by a mucous membrane consisting of a stratified squamous nonkeratinizing epithelium lying upon a connective tissue lamina propria with high papillae. Within the

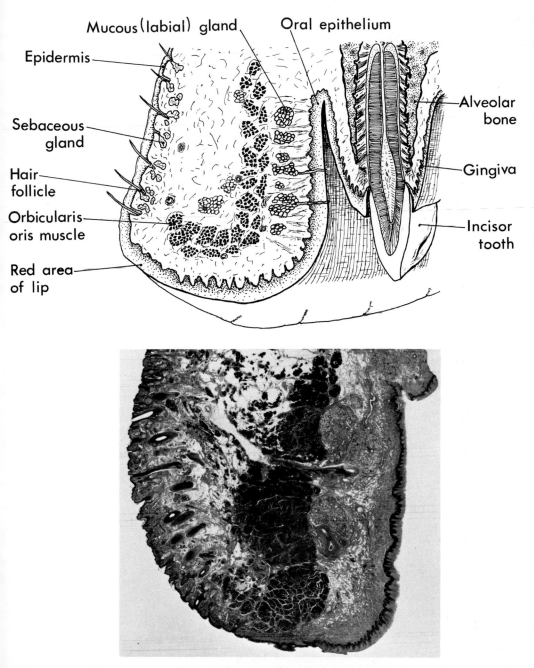

Figure 14-1. Top: Diagram of a vertical section through the upper lip and central incisor tooth. × 6. Bottom: Photomicrograph of a section through the upper lip, outer (skin) surface on the left. × 6.

connective tissue are numerous small mucous glands (the labial glands), the secretion of which passes to the surface via short ducts. In the epithelium, some keratohyalin granules can be found in the more superficial layers and the surface cells constantly are worn off and appear in the saliva. Numerous sensory nerve endings are found both in the dermis of the red lip margin and in the lamina propria of the oral mucous membrane.

THE CHEEK

The cheek has a similar structure to the lip with a core of striated muscle and elastic fibroconnective tissue lined internally by a mucous membrane covered by stratified squamous nonkeratinizing epithelium. A submucosa is present also, consisting of elastic connective tissue containing a rich vascular plexus. The elastic fibers are continuous externally with those around the striated muscle and internally with those of the lamina propria. They serve to bind the mucous mem-

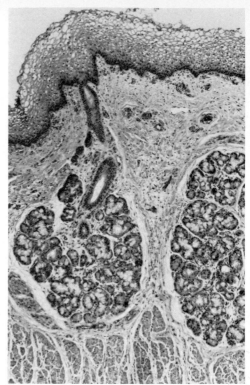

Figure 14-2. Photomicrograph of a section of the oral mucous membrane. Note the mucous glands in the submucosa. × 40.

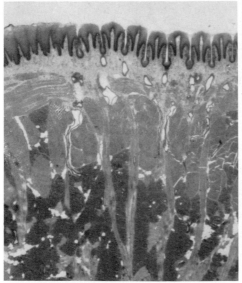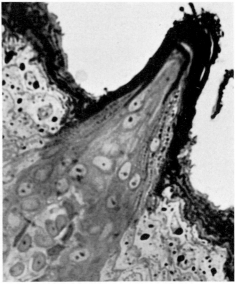

Figure 14-3. Left: Photomicrograph of a vertical section through the tongue. The surface mucosa shows filiform (left) and foliate (right) papillae, and deep to it are bundles of striated muscle, glands, and adipose tissue. Right: One filiform papilla from rabbit tongue, Epon section. Left, × 15. Right, × 450.

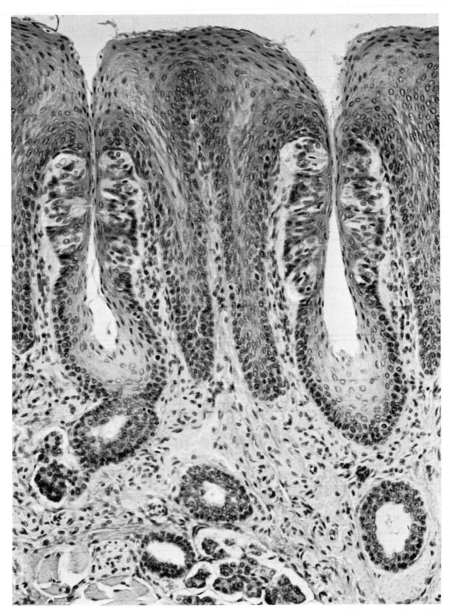

Figure 14-4. A higher magnification of part of Figure 14-3 to show a foliate papilla of the rabbit tongue with taste buds along its sides and parts of serous (Ebner's) glands and ducts below. × 175.

See filmstrip II, frame 57.

brane (mucosa) quite firmly to the muscle and prevent folds of the mucous membrane from being formed and bitten between the teeth when the jaws are closed. Mucous and mixed glands (mucous glands with serous demilunes) are present in the lamina propria of the cheek.

THE TONGUE

The tongue, which has been described as an epithelial covered bag of striated muscle and glands, is divided anatomically into anterior and posterior regions by a V-shaped groove, the apex of the V being directed posteriorly.

The mucous membrane on the under surface of the tongue is smooth and underlain by a submucosa, but on the upper surface the mucosa shows numerous small protuberances called *papillae*, which give the tongue a "furred" or roughened appearance. The papillae are of three main types in man: filiform, fungiform, and circumvallate. The *filiform papillae* are located mainly in rows parallel to the V-shaped sulcus and are 2 to 3 mm. in height; each has a primary, pointed, conical core of the connective tissue of the lamina propria with secondary papillae. The covering epithelium, although not keratinized, is quite hard. *Fungiform papillae* are disposed singly among the rows of filiform papillae and are more numerous toward the tip of the tongue. They are shaped like a mushroom (fungus) with a short stalk and a broader cap. The connective tissue core shows secondary papillae, over which the epithelium may be quite thin, so that the rich vascular plexus within the lamina propria imparts a pinkish or reddish tinge to the papillae. Taste buds may be present in the epithelium.

Circumvallate papillae (vallum, a wall), numbering only 10 to 14 in man, are located along the V-shaped sulcus. Each protrudes slightly from the surface and is surrounded by a moatlike, circular furrow. Secondary papillae are present but the surface epithelium is smooth. Taste buds are located on the lateral walls, viz., in the side of the circular furrow. Opening into the depths of the circular furrow are the ducts of specialized serous or albuminous glands (Ebner's glands), the glands themselves being located more deeply in the muscle tissue of the tongue.

The three types of papillae all contain numerous sensory nerve endings for touch, and in addition, taste buds are located on vallate and fungiform papillae.

The posterior third of the tongue has a nodular, irregular surface owing to the presence of lymphatic nodules (the *lingual tonsil*) (see page 241). Between the protrusions are cleftlike depressions of the surface epithelium termed *crypts*. Here the epithelium is infiltrated with numerous lymphocytes.

TASTE BUDS

The taste buds, responsible for the sense of taste, are located in the tongue epithelium of circumvallate papillae and fungiform papillae and in the surface epithelium between them. A few taste buds are found also in the palate and epiglottis. They are recognizable in sections under low power as pale, barrel-shaped bodies in the darkly staining epithelium. They have a laminated or layered appearance with a small external opening, the outer taste pore, and a small pit at the base, the inner taste pore.

By light microscopy, two cell types can be distinguished. The *supporting* or *sustentacular cells* are spindle-shaped with spherical, lightly staining nuclei, and they are arranged like the staves of a barrel around the inner taste pore. Between the sustentacular cells are the more darkly staining *neuroepithelial taste cells,* numbering only four to 16 in each taste bud. They are long and slender with a central, elongated nucleus, and each cell on the free apical surface has short *taste hairs* which

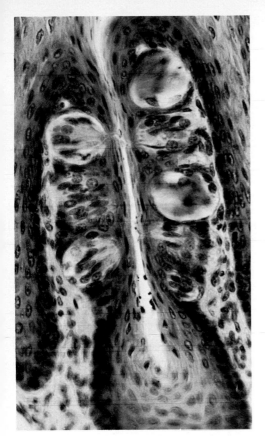

Figure 14-5. Photomicrograph to show taste buds in the walls of a foliate papilla. × 250. See filmstrip II, frame 58.

project into the cavity of the outer taste pore. By electron microscopy, dark and light cells are seen in a taste bud. In dark cells, which correspond to the neuroepithelial cells of light microscopy, apical microvilli that project into the outer taste pore contain prominent fibrillar or microtubular elements. The cytoplasm of these dark cells contains dense granules of 1000 to 3000 Å diameter and there is a dense, granular nucleus. Light cells differ in that their nuclei are more spherical and less granular, their apical microvilli are shorter, and they do not possess granules. Intermediate forms also are present. Radioautographic studies have demonstrated that there is a rapid turnover of cells within the taste bud. Surrounding epithelial cells divide and daughter cells enter the taste bud and move toward the center, perhaps first

becoming dark cells and then light cells. Although the darker, neuroepithelial cells formerly have been considered to be the cells which receive the sensation of taste, recent work has suggested that the light cells are the gustatory elements and that the dark cells are supporting elements, possibly also with an additional gustatory function.

Gustatory cells are stimulated only by substances in solution which enter the outer pore; i.e., the substances first are dissolved in saliva. Only four fundamental taste sensations can be detected: sweet, bitter, acid, and salty. The nerves from taste buds in the anterior two-thirds of the tongue pass by way of the chorda tympani branch of the seventh cranial nerve, those from the posterior third of the tongue by the glossopharyngeal nerve, and taste buds in the epiglottis and lower pharynx by the vagus nerve. All these nerve fibers are lightly myelinated but lose their myelin before reaching the taste buds, and then pass as fine terminal filaments both between taste buds and around taste buds. A few penetrate taste buds to end as terminal enlargements on taste cells.

The bulk of the tongue is composed of bundles of striated muscle fibers between which are numerous glands. The muscle fibers are both intrinsic and extrinsic, i.e., some are confined to the tongue, whereas others originate outside, principally on the mandible and hyoid bone, and pass into it. The glands in the base of the tongue are mainly mucous, whereas those nearer the tip are partially mixed with mucous acini and serous demilunes.

TEETH

Basically, teeth are derivatives of ectoderm and mesoderm. Each consists of a specially developed dermal papilla covered by calcified material originating chiefly in connective tissue but also in epithelium. Teeth, embedded in the bone of upper and lower jaws, are arranged in two arcs, the upper arc being larger than the lower with the result that the lower teeth are overlapped slightly by the upper. In man, two sets of teeth are distinguished. The *primary, milk,* or *deciduous* teeth of childhood number five in each half jaw (total 20), first erupt six to seven months after birth, and are a complete set by two years of age. They are shed between six and 12 to 13 years of age, being replaced gradually by the *permanent* set of adulthood. Permanent teeth number eight in each half jaw (total 32), the anterior five replacing milk teeth, the posterior three not being represented in the primary dentition.

Although individual teeth are modified for specific functions, eg., incisors for biting, molars for grinding, all show a similar histological structure. Each tooth has a *crown* projecting above the gum or gingiva, which thus is visible, and a *root* (or roots), which is buried in the alveolus of the maxilla or mandible. Crown and root meet at a region termed the *neck*. Each tooth is hollow containing a *pulp cavity* filled in life with connective tissue, and at the apex of the root this cavity communicates via one or more small pores or *apical foramina* with the connective tissue or *periodontal membrane* which holds the tooth in its socket or alveolus. This arrangement of a calcified tooth held in a bony socket by fibroconnective tissue is classified as a *gomphosis* or peg-and-socket type of fibrous joint.

The hard tissues of the tooth consist of *dentin,* which forms the bulk of the tooth and which surrounds the pulp cavity; *enamel,* which covers the dentin of the crown; and *cementum,* covering dentin of the root. The edge of the enamel thus contacts cementum at the neck of the tooth. The soft tissues include the pulp filling the pulp cavity, the periodontal membrane between bone of the alveolus and cementum covering the root, and the gingiva or gum. The last is continuous with the periodontal membrane and is that portion of the oral mucous membrane which surrounds a tooth at the neck and lower part of its crown. In a young person, gingiva is attached to enamel but gradually recedes from it in the adult so that the entire crown is exposed.

Dentin. Dentin, or dentine, is a substance harder than compact bone, but is of a similar chemical composition, being 72 per cent inorganic salts and 28 per cent organic material. In sections, dentin has a radially striated appearance owing to a multitude of fine canals or tubules termed the *dentinal tubules.* These run from the pulp cavity to the periphery of the dentin and are 3 to 4 microns in diameter at the bases and somewhat narrower near the periphery. Each pursues a wavy course through the dentin in the form of an open S. In the outer layers of dentin, the tubules may branch and anastomose. The dentinal tubules are occupied by processes of odontoblasts termed *Tomes's dentinal fibers.* The material between the dentinal fibers consists of a meshwork of collagenous fibers embedded in calcified ground substance. Immediately surrounding each dentinal tubule is a thin layer or sheath (of Neumann), which appears more dense and more highly refractile than the remainder of the intercellular substance between dentinal tubules. This sheath contains less collagen and is more highly calcified than the remainder of the dentin matrix. In addition, small areas of matrix remain incompletely calcified. These are termed the *interglobular spaces.*

The bundles of collagenous fibers of the dentin are 2 to 4 microns thick. In general they are orientated at right angles to the dentinal tubules and parallel to the long axis of the tooth, but in the crown of the tooth they run tangentially to the surface. The ground substance between the collagenous bundles is a mucopolysaccharide and is similar to that of bone but with a lower organic content. Dentin formation is cyclic and not regular, and in the fully developed tooth there are

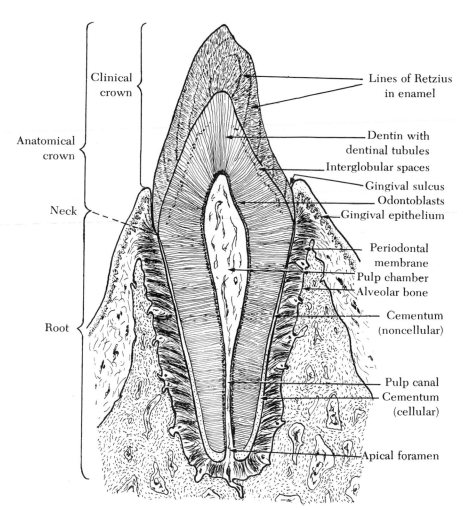

Figure 14-6.   Diagram of a longitudinal section through a lower lateral incisor tooth. × 6.

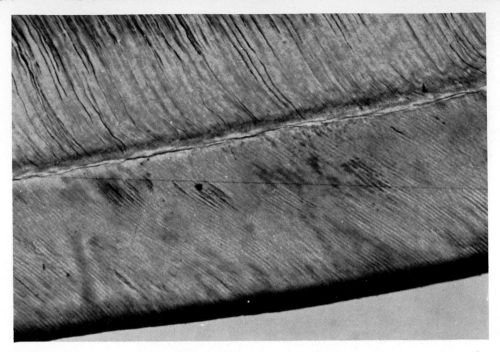

Figure 14-7. Photomicrograph of a ground section of a tooth, showing from above down, dentin with dentinal tubules, dentinoenamel junction, and enamel with enamel rods. × 100. (Courtesy of K. J. Paynter.)

growth or incremental lines (of Owen) which appear as growth rings in transverse section.

Dentin is sensitive to touch, cold, and hydrogen ion concentration, sensation being received by the Tomes fibers and not directly by nerve fibers.

Odontoblasts covering the pulp cavity remain viable throughout life and if stimulated, e.g., by excessive wear of the crown or irritation originating in the region of the periodontal membrane, new and excessive dentin or "secondary dentin" will be laid down at the periphery of the pulp cavity. This is irregular in structure and may be so excessive as to obliterate the pulp cavity.

Enamel. As mentioned previously, enamel is epithelial in origin and is extremely hard. Only 1 per cent of it is protein, the remainder (99 per cent) being inorganic salts of which more than 90 per cent is calcium phosphate in the form of apatite crystals. Enamel covers only the crown of the tooth.

The structural unit of enamel is the *enamel prism* and between the prisms is interprismatic substance. Both the prisms and the interprismatic substance are composed of apatite crystals in an organic matrix. Each prism, formed by a single ameloblast, is orientated perpendicularly to the surface of the dentin and traverses the entire thickness of the enamel, but does not run a straight course. Each is 6 to 8 microns in diameter, being thicker at the surface, and in cross section appears scalelike and basically hexagonal. The protein portion of enamel is perhaps a very primitive form of collagen and the matrix is in a state of low crystallinity; viz., it is not a highly ordered system. It may be in the form of a disordered protein gel with occasional crystalline regions. The crystals of enamel are particularly large when compared with hydroxyapatite specimens in other biological systems.

Like dentin, enamel is laid down rhythmically, and cross sections of the tooth crown show concentric, parallel, incremental lines (of Retzius). When

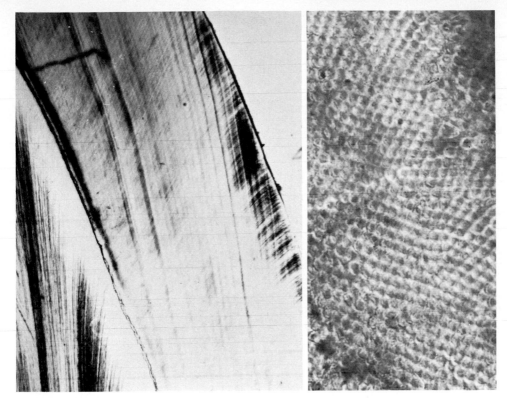

Figure 14-8.   Ground sections, left, in a longitudinal plane, of enamel to show the striae of Retzius (dentinal tubules also seen at lower left) and, right, in a transverse plane, to show enamel rods. Notice the scalelike appearance. Left, × 100. Right, × 550. (Courtesy of K. J. Paynter.)

the enamel is fully formed, the ameloblasts on its surface form a membrane about 1 micron thick and then disappear. Covering this membrane is a second membrane composed of a glycoprotein and derived from the enamel organ. Both membranes are worn off gradually after eruption. Unlike dentin, new enamel obviously cannot be added in the adult after the degeneration and disappearance of ameloblasts.

Cementum.   Cementum covers the dentin of the root of the tooth from the neck to the apex. Histologically, it is similar to bone with coarse bundles of collagen fibers in the calcified matrix. There are no cementocytes (osteocytes) in the upper one-third but bone cells are present in the lower portion, lying in lacunae. Haversian systems with blood vessels normally are not present but may appear if the cemen-

tum becomes increased in thickness, as may occur near the apex in old age. The coarse bundles of collagen fibers are continuous with bundles of fibers from the periodontal membrane which penetrate the cementum as Sharpey's fibers. These do not calcify and thus they appear as clear canals in ground sections.

Cementum under certain circumstances can undergo resorption and hyperplasia. Increase in thickness of cementum occurs by appositional growth, i.e., by addition of new layers on its surface. Destruction of cementum occurs rarely, e.g., in periodontal membrane disease.

Pulp.   The pulp of the tooth is derived from mesenchyme of the embryonic dental papilla, and it fills the pulp cavity consisting of both the main pulp chamber and the root canals. Being connective tissue, pulp consists of

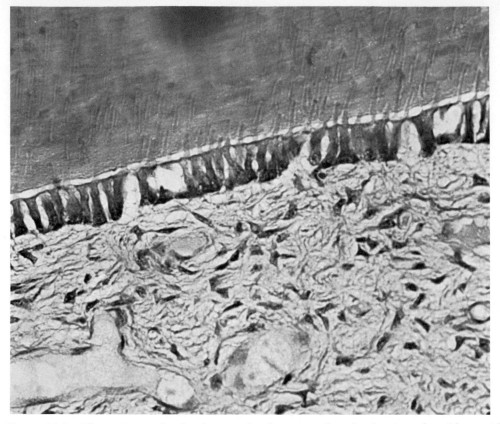

Figure 14-9. Photomicrograph of a demineralized section of tooth, showing odontoblasts with their processes entering dentinal tubules. The pulp chamber filled with mesenchymal-like tissue is below and contains a branching blood vessel (lower left). × 900. (Courtesy of K. J. Paynter.)

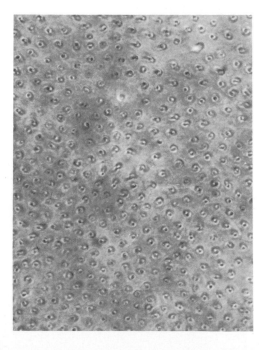

both cells and intercellular material. The cells of the pulp are fusiform or stellate, closely resembling mesenchymal cells in shape, but not in potentiality; in addition, there are extravascular lymphocytes and macrophages. Peripherally, underlying the dentin, is a single row of columnar, epithelium-like cells. These are the *odontoblasts*, of mesenchymal origin. Each odontoblast has one or more long, cytoplasmic processes extending into a dentinal tubule. The processes are the dentinal fibers (of Tomes). The cell body of the

Figure 14-10. Photomicrograph of a demineralized section of tooth, showing dentinal tubules in cross section. The black central dot in each hole is an odontoblast process; the dark area of modified matrix around the hole is the sheath of Neumann. × 900. (Courtesy of K. J. Paynter.)

odontoblast has a basally located nucleus, prominent mitochondria, and a Golgi apparatus. The odontoblasts are responsible for dentin formation.

Between the cells of the pulp are numerous, fine fibrils of collagen, not organized into bundles, and a basophil ground substance similar to mucoid connective tissue. The appearance of both cells and intercellular tissue in the pulp is similar to that of embryonic mesenchyme. However, the cells do not have the same potentialities for differentiation as do mesenchymal cells.

Contained within the pulp are vessels and nerves. Usually a single arteriole enters each root canal and breaks up in the pulp chamber into a dense capillary network with loops extending out to underlie the layer of odontoblasts. The capillaries drain into venules which leave via the root canal. Lymphatic capillaries have been described by some investigators. Myelinated nerve fibers, originating in the fifth cranial nerve ganglion, pass with the vessels into the pulp where they lose their sheaths and terminate as naked nerve endings between odontoblasts. Pain reception evidently occurs in the dentinal fibers, the stimulus being passed to the nerves. Unmyelinated nerve fibers of the sympathetic system also enter the pulp. These are vasomotor to the vessels of the pulp.

Periodontal Membrane. The periodontal membrane is a modified peri-

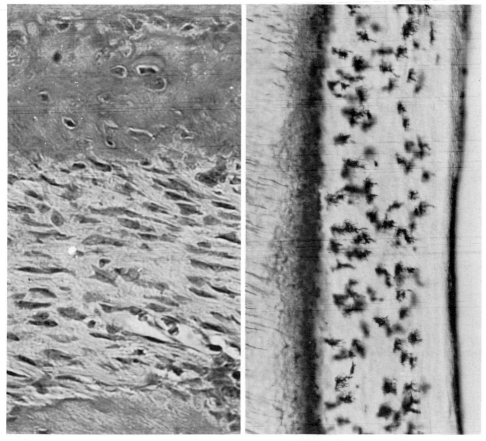

Figure 14-11. Left: Photomicrograph of a demineralized section of tooth, showing from above down, the dentin-cementum junction, cellular cementum with cementocytes, periodontal membrane with a blood vessel, and alveolar bone. × 900. Right: Ground section, showing cementocytes in cellular cementum. There is some dentin with dentinal tubules on the left of the photomicrograph. × 350. (Courtesy of K. J. Paynter.)

osteum of the alveolar bone and occupies all the space between the root of a tooth and its bony, alveolar socket. In addition to providing a firm connection between a tooth and its socket, it is continuous with, and supports, the gum. Unlike true periosteum, the periodontal membrane contains no elastic fibers but consists of strong, thick bundles of collagenous fibers running between alveolar bone and cementum. At the extremities of a bundle, collagen fibers extend into bone and cementum respectively as Sharpey's fibers. However, the fibers of each bundle are not taut and run a slightly wavy course, being attached somewhat deeper to the root of a tooth than to the

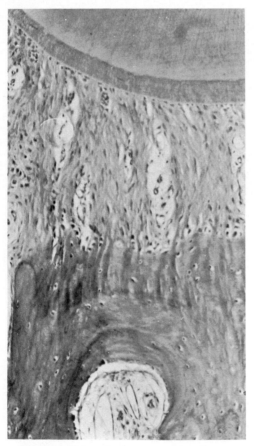

Figure 14-12. Photomicrograph of a transverse section through the root of a demineralized tooth, showing from above down, dentin, noncellular cementum, and periodontal membrane with Sharpey's fibers entering alveolar bone. × 500. (Courtesy of K. J. Paynter.)

alveolar bone. Thus, the tooth is "slung" in its socket and can move slightly in each direction, the periodontal membrane functioning as the suspensory ligament of the tooth. Between the fiber bundles are a few fibroblasts and some osteoblasts. Blood vessels and nerves pass through the membrane to reach the pulp cavity of a tooth but are not prominent in the membrane itself. However, the periodontal membrane has a relatively rich vascular supply, although the vessels are not seen readily in histological preparations. It also is highly sensitive to pressure changes and presumably, therefore, has a good nerve supply. There are lymph vessels and nerves in the membrane and small, scattered islands of epithelial cells derived from the embryonic root sheath. These may calcify to form small bodies termed cementicles.

Gingiva. The gingiva or gum surrounds each tooth like a collar and is the oral mucous membrane extending between and connected to the periosteum of alveolar bone at its crest and the tooth above its neck. Near the tooth, the gingiva extends around the tooth as the gingival crest, between the summit of which and the tooth is a narrow gingival crevice. More deeply at the bottom of the gingival crevice, the gingiva is attached around the circumference of the tooth crown. This attachment is to enamel cuticle and it extends deeply to the upper part of the cementum. The attachment to the enamel is not firm and with age the gingival sulcus deepens until the gingiva is attached only to cementum, thus exposing the entire crown.

The connective tissue papillae underlying the stratified squamous epithelium of the gingiva are high. The connective tissue itself consists of interlacing bundles of collagenous fibers with relatively few fibroblasts and numerous blood capillaries which form a rich vascular network immediately below the epithelium. It is blood in this network which is responsible for the pink color of the gums.

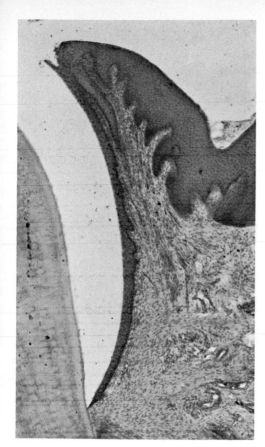

Figure 14-13. Photomicrograph of the gingiva and gingival sulcus. The sulcus is excessively wide owing to the loss of the enamel. × 150. (Courtesy of K. J. Paynter.)

Development of the Teeth. Each tooth has a mesodermal and an ectodermal component, the latter forming only the enamel. During the fifth week, ectoderm of the oral cavity develops horseshoe-shaped linear thickenings in the developing upper and lower jaws. Each thickening, a *labio-dental lamina,* is at first solid and bifid, extending deeply into underlying mesenchyme. The outer labial limb later splits to form the groove between the lip and the alveolar process of the jaw (i.e., the vestibule). The inner limb, the *dental lamina,* develops a series of budlike thickenings, or *tooth germs,* there being five in each half jaw or one for each deciduous tooth. Later, at 10 to 12 weeks, a second series of

tooth germs develops on the lingual side of each developing deciduous tooth (five) plus three more posteriorly for each adult molar (the molar is not preceded by a deciduous tooth). The tooth germs for the adult teeth do not appear until later (fourth month of intrauterine life for the first permanent molar, and first and fourth years after birth for the second and third molars). Each tooth germ, both deciduous and adult, develops further in identical fashion.

The epithelial tooth germ is invaginated from below by a papilla of mesenchymal connective tissue and thus becomes bell-shaped, still attached above by a cord of epithelial cells to the dental lamina. The bell-shaped epithelial bud, now termed the *enamel organ,* sits like a cap on the dental papilla. The whole is embedded in a layer of connective tissue, the dental sac, which soon completely invests the developing tooth when the connecting strand between the dental lamina and the enamel organ breaks down and disappears. The central cells of the enamel organ become separated by intercellular spaces, the cells remaining in contact only by long cytoplasmic processes to become reticulum-like in appearance. This is the stellate reticulum. Peripherally around the stellate reticulum, the epithelial cells are arranged in a regular sheet, one cell thick. The cells of the outer enamel epithelium remain small, but those of the inner enamel epithelium adjacent to the dental papilla become tall and columnar. These are the *ameloblasts,* responsible for enamel formation. Cells of the stellate reticulum which lie adjacent to the inner enamel epithelium (ameloblasts) form a single layer of cuboidal cells. This is termed the stratum intermedium and it plays an important role in attaching the epithelial tissues around the crown of the tooth to the oral mucous membrane during eruption of the tooth. By the time that ameloblasts have differentiated, the peripheral cells of the dental papilla in contact with ameloblasts

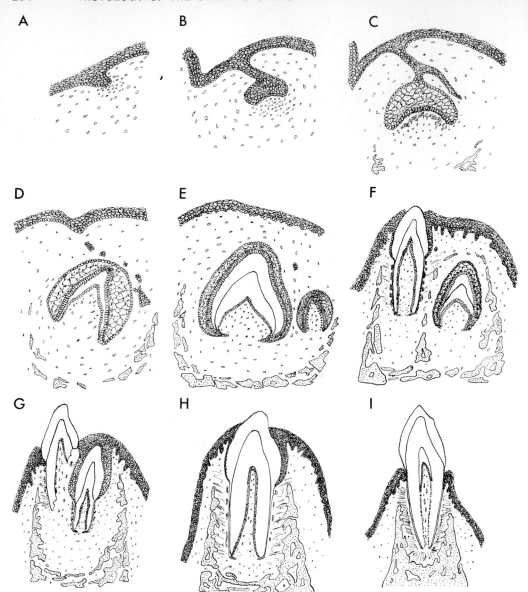

Figure 14-14. Diagram to illustrate stages in development of the lower central incisor. The approximate time is indicated in parentheses. *A*, Dental lamina formation from oral epithelium. (Six weeks intrauterine.) *B*, Early formation ("cap" stage) of the enamel organ of the deciduous tooth with condensation of underlying mesenchyme. (Seven to eight weeks intrauterine.) *C*, Early "bell" stage of the enamel organ with extension (to the right) of the dental lamina indicating formation of the permanent tooth. Alveolar bone is forming. (Ten weeks intrauterine.) *D*, Advanced "bell" stage with a cap of dentin now formed at the tip of the dental papilla. Connection between the tooth bud and the oral epithelium now is discontinuous. (Sixteen weeks intrauterine.) *E*, The crown of the deciduous tooth is complete with enamel formation, and the permanent tooth is in the bell stage. (Birth.) *F*, Early eruption of the deciduous tooth, the root of which now is formed, with the crown of the permanent tooth nearly completed, showing enamel and dentin. (Six months postnatal.) *G*, The deciduous tooth shows resorption of the root and the process of shedding is commencing. In the permanent tooth, root formation is complete. (Six to seven years.) *H*, The permanent tooth now is erupting. (Seven to eight years.) *I*, In the permanent tooth, early attrition is shown with some recession in the neck and formation of secondary dentin. (After 20 years.) Stages A to E drawn at higher magnification than stages F to I. (Based on diagrams supplied by J. G. Dale and K. J. Paynter.)

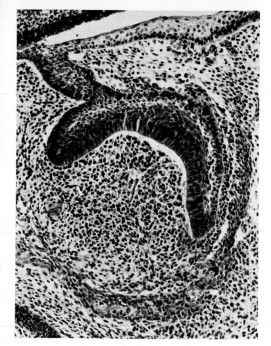

Figure 14-15. Photomicrograph of a developing tooth at the "bell" stage showing enamel organ attached to the dental lamina. Compare with Figure 14-14, *C.* × 100.

become arranged in a regular manner, one cell thick. These are the *odontoblasts* (dentinoblasts); they are separated from the ameloblasts only by basal lamina material.

By about 20 weeks of gestation, the hard tissues of the tooth begin to form. Dentin appears first between the two layers of cells (ameloblasts and odontoblasts) and at first is uncalcified and thus usually is called *predentin.* It gradually extends down toward the neck and increases in thickness by apposition on the internal surface. As it increases in thickness, cytoplasmic processes of the odontoblasts remain within the dentin as the dentinal fibers. Predentin thus is composed of odontoblast processes, collagen fibers, and ground substance. The collagen fibers originate in the pulp, and as mineralization occurs the fibers condense and thicken around odontoblast processes. Electron microscopy shows that odontoblasts form an acid muco-

polysaccharide which is concentrated in granules. These granules, situated mainly at the bases of odontoblast processes, are extruded later into the surrounding matrix where the polysaccharide lies on the surface of collagen fibers and in the interfibrillar spaces. Mineralization occurs in the patches of mucopolysaccharide and, later, upon the surface of fibers. Throughout dentin formation, collagen fibers invade the developing matrix and appear to be derived from fibroblasts within the pulp. Because mineralization occurs after the presence of fibers and ground substance, there is always a thin layer of predentin adjacent to the odontoblasts. As soon as dentin formation has been initiated, the ameloblasts commence to form enamel, layer by layer on the surface of the dentin. Ameloblasts, as seen by electron microscopy, contain abundant ergastoplasm, presumably associated with protein synthesis. It is believed that ameloblasts form enamel matrix which later is mineralized extracellularly. With the increase in thickness of the enamel, the ameloblasts recede from the dentin. It must be emphasized that enamel does not develop as a homogeneous mass but as enamel rods, each rod corresponding to a single ameloblast. Complete calcification in the enamel does not occur until late. Before the ameloblasts disappear, they elaborate the inner enamel cuticle which covers the bases of the enamel rods.

The development of the tooth as described above accounts only for the formation of the crown. At the periphery of the enamel organ in the future neck region, i.e., at the edge of the bell, where inner and outer enamel epithelia come together, a fold of epithelial cells develops and grows downward toward the root. This is the *epithelial root sheath* (of Hertwig). Root development occurs shortly before tooth eruption and gradually progresses as the crown emerges through the gingiva. Odontoblasts develop in relation to the epithelial sheath of Hertwig and form dentin. Cementum develops

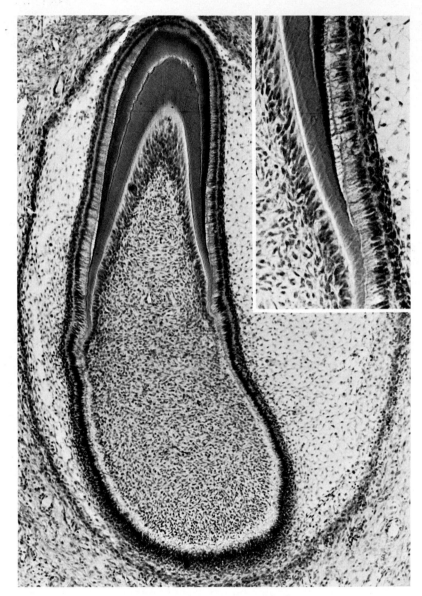

Figure 14-16.   Photomicrograph of a developing tooth at the stage in which crown formation is well advanced. (Compare with Figure 14-14, *E*.) Enamel and dentin are present with a thin layer of predentin in relation to odontoblasts. Note the connective tissue dental sac enveloping the entire developing tooth. × 75. Top right, inset: A higher magnification of part of the tooth showing, from left to right, pulp, odontoblasts, predentin, dentin, enamel (black), ameloblasts, stratum intermedium, and stellate reticulum. × 175.

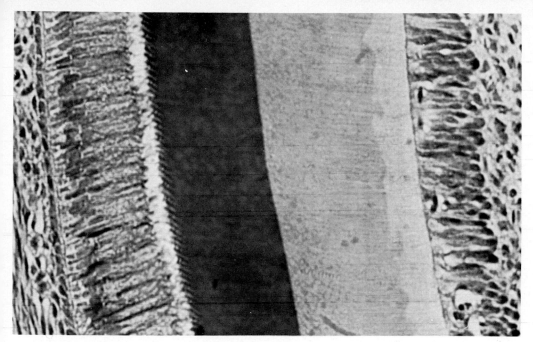

Figure 14-17. Photomicrograph of a developing monkey tooth, showing from left to right, stratum intermedium, ameloblasts, enamel (black), dentin, predentin, odontoblasts, and pulp. × 900. (Courtesy of K. J. Paynter.)

from mesenchyme of the periodontal membrane. The epithelial sheath of Hertwig disappears only when the root is formed completely.

During eruption of a permanent tooth, the deciduous tooth superficial to it gradually is resorbed by growth pressure, osteoclasts being prominent during the process. The deciduous tooth when finally shed consists only of the upper portion of the crown, the remainder having been resorbed.

THE MAJOR SALIVARY GLANDS

There are numerous small, intrinsic glands associated with the oral cavity which continuously secrete a liquid, *saliva*. This secretion moistens the mucous membrane of the oral cavity proper, the vestibule of the mouth, and the lips. In addition to these glands, there are three pairs of large, extrinsic glands, the ducts of which open into the oral cavity. These major salivary glands are the *parotid*, the *submandibular* or *submaxillary*, and the *sublingual*, and they secrete copious amounts of saliva intermittently on nervous stimulation. Such stimulations arise following mechanical, thermal, chemical, psychic, or olfactory stimuli owing to the presence or anticipated presence of food in the mouth cavity.

Saliva

Saliva, the mixed secretions of *all* the salivary glands, may amount to 1000 to 1500 ml. in 24 hours. Saliva is a viscid liquid containing water, mucin, proteins, salts, and two enzymes, *ptyalin* and *maltase*. Ptyalin splits starch, which is relatively insoluble in water, into less complex, soluble carbohydrates. Maltase splits the disaccharide maltose. Saliva also contains desquamated, degenerated, squamous epithelial cells from the oral epithelium and degenerated lymphocytes and granulocytes called "salivary corpuscles." These arise mainly from the tonsils. It should be noted that the quality as well as the quantity of saliva varies with different stimuli. The quality is affected by the varying contribution made by the different major salivary glands in response to different food materials.

The secretion of saliva subserves several functions. It constantly moistens the oral cavity and aids in cleaning the mouth of food debris which otherwise would provide a culture medium for bacterial growth, bacteria always being present in the oral cavity. Obviously, it moistens food and this permits both ease of swallowing and the appreciation of taste, for the chemical substances responsible for taste must be in solution to cause stimulation of the taste buds. Enzymatic digestion of carbohydrates by ptyalin and amylase commences in the mouth but ceases in the stomach where both enzymes are inactivated in an acid medium. The secretion of saliva is one important factor in the maintenance of fluid balance, a decreased secretion occurring when the body is dehydrated, giving rise to a sensation of thirst. Much of the fluid in saliva, of course, is returned to the circulation by absorption in the digestive tract. Finally, some heavy metals are secreted in the saliva.

The salivary glands are classified as merocrine and tubuloacinar in type. The student is referred to Chapter 5 for a general description of exocrine glands.

Parotid Gland

This, the largest of the major salivary glands, is situated below and anterior to the ear, being related to the mastoid process behind and the mandibular ramus in front. There is an anterior extension onto the face beneath the zygomatic arch and from this border the main duct (Stensen's duct) passes forward, through the cheek, and opens into the vestibule of the mouth opposite the second upper molar tooth. The gland is enclosed in a fascial sheet and contains serous acini composed of pyramidal-shaped cells, and intercalated and striated ducts.

From the fibrous capsule, relatively dense septa pass into the gland to divide it into lobes and lobules. The connective tissue of the septa often contains fat cells. Slips of fine connective tissue surround acini and ducts, and contained in this tissue are numerous blood capillaries.

Acini are elongated and enclosed in a basal lamina with some myoepithelial cells. All acinar cells have nuclei situated toward the base and show infranuclear cytoplasmic basophilia and apical secretion granules. By electron microscopy, two cell types have been described, one with widely dilated granular endoplasmic reticulum and homogeneous secretion granules which show a tendency to fuse into an irregular mass. The other type, probably merely a different secretory phase, has less dense, discrete secretion granules and a well-developed granular endoplasmic reticulum with flattened cisternae. Cell interfaces characteristically are complex and apical microvilli are present. By electron microscopy, two regions of the *intercalated duct* are identified. Cells in the proximal part are small, arranged in a tubular fashion from the lumen of an acinus, and show the presence of secretory granules. In the distal part, the cells contain no secretion granules, the lumen usually is of greater diameter, and myoepithelial cells may be present between the duct cells and the surrounding basal lamina. The intercalated duct continues into the *striated duct*. Cells here are tall and polygonal or columnar in shape and show basal striation, which by electron microscopy is resolved as basal invaginations of the plasma membrane with numerous elongated mitochondria in the pockets of cytoplasm so formed. The apical cytoplasm contains vesicles. The morphology of these cells is similar to that of cells in the distal convoluted tubules

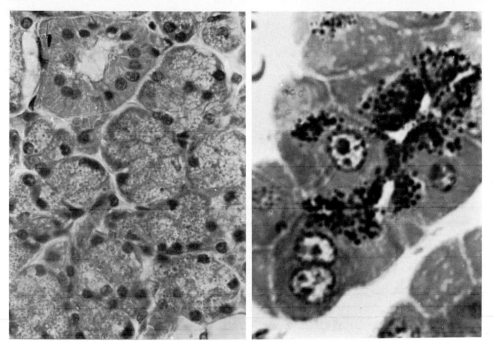

Figure 14-18. Left: Photomicrograph of human parotid gland, showing serous acini and a striated duct (top). × 375. Right: A single serous acinus, showing secretory droplets. Epon section, × 1250.

of the kidney, and it is suggested that they subserve a similar function of fluid resorption from the lumen to the interstitium. *Excretory ducts* commence with simple columnar epithelium which then becomes pseudostratified and finally stratified. Intralobular ducts particularly are prominent in this gland. (They are less so in, for example, the pancreas.)

Submandibular (Submaxillary) Gland

This gland is located in the floor of the mouth underlying the body of the mandible and extending beneath its lower border into the side of the neck. Its duct (Wharton's) opens into the floor of the mouth just behind the lower incisor teeth and beneath the tip of the tongue. It also is a tubuloacinar or compound acinar gland, the majority of the acini being serous. The remainder are mucous but usually with serous crescents, i.e., mixed acini. Like the parotid, the submandibular

gland has a capsule, septa, and a prominent duct system. Intercalated ducts are similar to those of the parotid, but with less secretion granules in the proximal part. By electron microscopy, striated ducts contain, in addition to the cell type described previously, a cell with masses of endoplasmic reticulum and some secretion granules. Striated ducts tend to be longer than those in the parotid and thus are more conspicuous in sections of this gland.

Sublingual Gland

The sublingual gland really is not a single gland but a collection of glands lying beneath the mucous membrane of the floor of the mouth in close relation to the duct of the submandibular gland, and each part has a duct opening separately. It is a mixed gland, the majority of the acini being mucous, but with some mixed units. Pure serous units are rare. There is no definite cap-

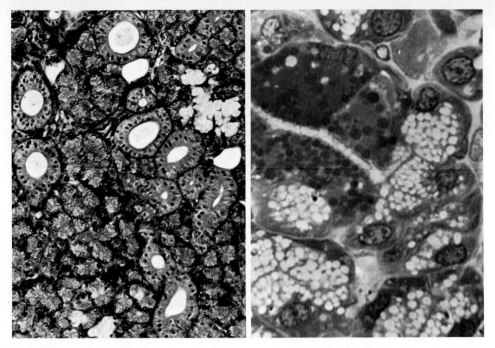

Figure 14-19.   Left: Photomicrograph of human submandibular gland showing serous, mucous, and mixed acini and striated ducts. × 100. Right: Submandibular gland showing a mixed acinus (center) with mucous and serous cells and mucous acini (below). Epon section, × 1250.

See filmstrip II, frame 59.

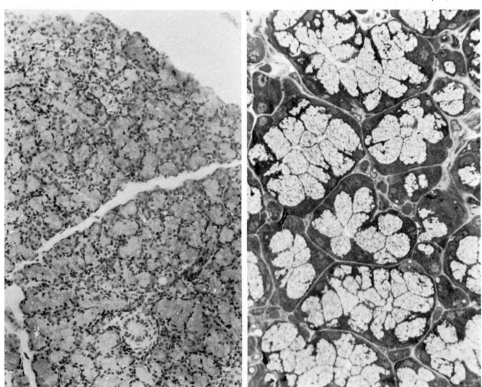

Figure 14-20.   Left: Photomicrograph of human sublingual gland, showing portions of two lobules, mucous acini, and an intralobular duct (lower center). × 100. Right: Mucous acini of sublingual gland. Epon section, × 750.

sule but septa are present. Myoepithelial cells usually are found in relation to acini. Intercalated ducts are short and not prominent, and the cells contain no secretory granules. The striated ducts are similar in appearance to those of the parotid and submandibular but are short and thus less commonly seen.

Each of the major salivary glands is provided with sensory nerve endings and motor nerves from both the sympathetic and parasympathetic nervous systems. The latter supply both secretory acini and blood vessels of the glands, the sympathetic being derived from the superior cervical ganglion and the parasympathetic from salivary nuclei located in the brain stem and associated with the seventh and ninth cranial nerves. There is some experimental evidence that stimulation of the glands by the sympathetic system causes secretion of a thick, mucous saliva and the parasympathetic causes a profuse watery secretion. The actual mechanism by which nervous stimulation causes acinar cell secretion is not well understood.

Palate

The roof of the mouth or palate is also the floor of the nasal cavity. The anterior part, termed the *hard palate,* contains bone (palatine processes of maxillae and palatine bones) and thus is rigid. The posterior portion, called the *soft palate,* has a core of strong fibroconnective tissue and thus is movable. The hard palate provides a rigid surface against which the tongue, a powerful muscular organ, can bring force to mix food material and expedite the swallowing mechanism. The oral surface of the hard palate correspondingly is covered by stratified squamous keratinizing epithelium, the lamina propria of which blends with the periosteum. Within the lamina propria are numerous small glands and some fatty tissue. In the midline, the lamina propria is thin and attached to a median ridge of bone. This linear region is called the *raphe.*

The soft palate functions to close off the nasopharynx from the oropharynx during swallowing, thus preventing aliment from entering the nasal cavity. It is covered inferiorly by stratified squamous nonkeratinizing epithelium, the lamina propria of which contains numerous glands. A layer of striated muscle (the musculus uvulus) lies between the lamina propria and the palatine aponeurosis, a sheet of fibroconnective tissue. On the nasal side, the soft palate is covered by the pseudostratified ciliated columnar epithelium of the nasal cavity, although posteriorly the oral type of epithelium extends around the posterior border of the soft palate and onto its superior, nasal surface. The lamina propria of this epithelium also contains a few glands.

Tonsils

The oral cavity is continuous with the oropharynx (see page 342) through a region termed the *fauces.* There are two mucosal folds, each containing a muscle, on each side between the palate and the side of the tongue and pharynx respectively. These are called the palatoglossal and palatopharyngeal folds and between them is a depression in which is located a mass of lymphoid tissue. This is the *palatine tonsil* (see page 241). Lymphoid tissue also is present in the nasopharynx (adenoids), around the openings of the pharyngotympanic (eustachian) tubes ("tubal tonsil"), and in the posterior part of the tongue ("lingual tonsil"). The parts of the pharynx are discussed on page 342.

Part II — THE TUBULAR DIGESTIVE TRACT

Each part of the digestive tube has four coats or layers, their nature and thickness varying with functional requirements in the different regions. These layers are as follows:

Mucous Membrane
(Tunica Mucosa)

This is a wet, surface epithelial membrane, lubricated by mucus, resting upon a basal lamina, in turn supported by a layer of connective tissue termed the lamina propria, and in many regions, with a thin, outer layer of smooth muscle, the muscularis mucosae. The last usually is arranged in two layers orientated as an inner circular layer and an outer longitudinal layer. In most regions, the mucous membrane is irregular and shows finger-like projections, the *villi*, which greatly increase surface area, and deep epithelial-lined invaginations, the *intestinal glands* or *crypts*. These glands extend deeply within the lamina propria to the muscularis mucosae in many regions and thus make the lamina propria difficult to identify as a separate entity. The lamina propria is classified as a loose, areolar, connective tissue but with lymphatic tendencies, the lymphoid material presumably functioning as a defense barrier against bacterial infection. Contained within the lamina propria are numerous blood and lymph capillaries into which absorbed food material passes.

Submucosa (Tunica Submucosa)

This extends from the mucosa to the muscularis externa and comprises coarse areolar connective tissue with some elastic fibers. It permits mobility of the mucosa. Contained in it are plexuses of larger blood vessels and nerves with some ganglion cells which are part of the autonomic nervous system, some being postganglionic fibers of the sympathetic system and others preganglionic fibers of the parasympathetic system. The ganglion cells are all parasympathetic. This is termed *Meissner's* or the *submucous plexus*. In some regions, e.g., the duodenum, there are submucosal glands.

Muscularis Externa
(Tunica Muscularis)

This characteristically consists of an inner layer of circularly orientated and an outer layer of longitudinally orientated smooth muscle fibers although there is striated muscle in the upper esophagus. Both layers actually are arranged in a spiral fashion, the inner following a tight helix and the outer a very open helix. Between the two layers is a vascular plexus and a nerve plexus associated with numerous small ganglia. This is *Auerbach's myenteric plexus* and is mainly parasympathetic with some postganglionic sympathetic fibers. The muscularis functions to propel onward food material in the lumen of the digestive tube, a process termed peristalsis, and by churning movements aids in mixing the food material with the digestive enzymes. It varies in thickness with the region of the tube; for example, a third layer is identified in the wall of the stomach.

Serosa or Adventitia (Tunica Serosa or Adventitia)

The outermost layer comprises a relatively dense areolar connective tissue, often blending with the connective tissue of surrounding structures. This is termed an adventitia. In many regions it is covered with peritoneum, i.e., by a single layer of mesothelial cells, and in these sites is termed a serosa rather than an adventitia. Blood

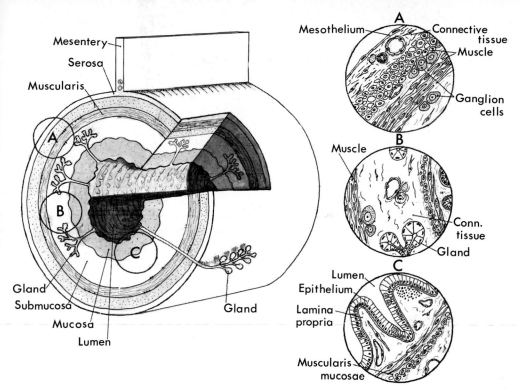

Figure 14-21. Diagram to illustrate the general plan of the gastrointestinal tract as seen in cross section.

vessels, lymphatics, and nerves are present and pass through it to the other layers.

Developmentally, the epithelial lining of the digestive tube is derived from endoderm with the exception of the external parts of the oral cavity and anal canal. These are ectodermal in origin. The connective and muscular tissues are derived from splanchnic or visceral mesoderm.

THE ESOPHAGUS

The esophagus, about 10 inches long, is a relatively straight, muscular tube, continuous with the lower extremity of the pharynx at the inferior border of the cricoid cartilage (see Figure 15-7) and extending through the lower neck and the mediastinum of the thorax to perforate the diaphragm and terminate by opening into the stomach. Its wall shows the four layers as described previously.

The mucous membrane consists of a stratified squamous nonkeratinizing epithelium continuous with that lining the pharynx, a lamina propria, and a muscularis mucosae. The epithelium is thick, and although cells in the superficial layers contain some keratohyalin granules, no true cornification occurs. At the lower end, there is an abrupt transition to the epithelium lining the stomach. Characteristically, the esophageal epithelium is indented by peglike protrusions of the underlying connective tissue lamina propria. This lamina is a loose areolar connective tissue, relatively acellular, containing some scattered lymphocytes and a few lymphatic nodules, and extending deeply to the muscularis mucosae. The muscularis mucosae, at the level of the cricoid cartilage, is continuous with the elastic layer of the pharynx and is

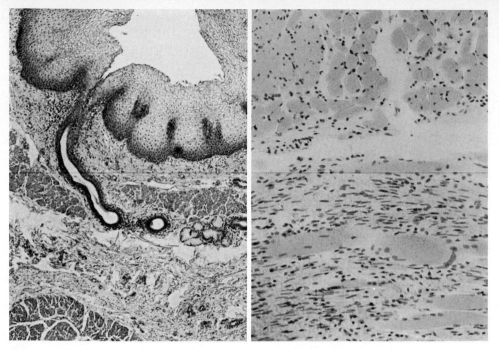

Figure 14-22.   Transverse sections of the esophagus. Left, through the lower third, showing mucosa, submucosa, and muscularis, and the duct of a submucosal gland. × 40. Right, through the muscularis of the middle third, showing a mixture of striated and smooth muscle fibers. × 325.

composed of longitudinal smooth muscle embedded in a fine, elastic meshwork.

The submucosa is a dense fibroconnective tissue, but in the empty esophagus is thrown into several folds which are longitudinally arranged. This gives the lumen a characteristic, easily recognizable, irregular outline in cross section. During passage of a food bolus the esophagus dilates and these longitudinal folds are "ironed out." The muscularis is composed of two layers of muscle, an inner circular and an outer longitudinal, but many bundles are arranged obliquely or in a spiral fashion. In the upper third of the esophagus, the muscle is entirely skeletal, striated muscle and the bundles of fibers are variable in orientation. In the second third, smooth muscle bundles are mixed with the striated and the proportion gradually increases until only smooth muscle is present in the lower third. Here the layers are more regular in arrange-

ment; i.e., they are in inner circular and outer longitudinal layers. External to the muscularis there is a layer of loose connective tissue, the adventitia, which blends with surrounding structures.

Since food passes rapidly down the esophagus and has been mixed previously with saliva, little additional lubrication is necessary. However, some glands are present. Throughout the length of the esophagus, there are in the submucosa some compound, tubuloacinar mucous glands, the ducts of which penetrate the mucosa to open on the surface. In addition, at the lower end of the esophagus and at its upper end there are glands in the lamina propria. These are compound, tubular glands, confined to the lamina propria, and they secrete mucin. Since they resemble the glands of the cardiac portion of the stomach they are termed *cardiac glands.*

Functionally, the esophageal epithelium is of a type to resist abrasion from

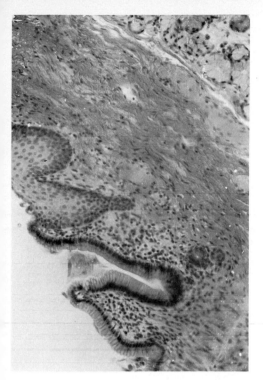

Figure 14-23. Longitudinal section through esophagogastric junction, showing abrupt change in epithelium from stratified squamous to simple columnar. Note the mucous glands in the submucosa. × 275. See filmstrip II, frame 60.

rough food material; some mucous glands aid its lubrication; the thick, loose submucosa permits great dilation during swallowing; and the thick muscularis, particularly in the upper portion where it is composed of striated muscle, provides the motive power for rapid propulsion of food material from the pharynx to the stomach. Indeed, swallowing is possible in the inverted position when the muscularis must work against gravity.

THE STOMACH

The stomach is capable of considerable distention and, although when empty it is only of slightly larger caliber than the large gut, it can accommodate two to three pints of material when distended. There is a sphincter at the entrance of the esophagus to pre-

vent regurgitation of material into the esophagus and a more powerful one at its junction with the small intestine. These are termed the *cardiac* and *pyloric sphincters*. To the left of and above the cardiac orifice (esophageal opening) is a dilatation or bulge termed the *fundus*. The main *body* of the stomach continues into a region called the *pyloric antrum*, in turn narrowing to the *pyloric canal*, which narrows to the *pylorus*, the opening into the duodenum. The stomach is flattened anteroposteriorly and has upper concave and lower convex edges called the *lesser* and *greater curvatures*. In the empty, contracted stomach, the lining mucosa is thrown into folds or *rugae*, orientated mainly longitudinally, but these disappear with distention.

Food enters the stomach as boli (bolus, a ball) of semisolid, masticated material, partially moistened by saliva, but leaves it intermittently after a period of three to four hours as a semifluid, pulplike mass termed *chyme*. The thick muscularis of the stomach functions to churn the contained material, mixing it thoroughly with the digestive juices secreted by the stomach. The *gastric juice* contains hydrochloric acid, enzymes, and mucus. One of the enzymes, *pepsin*, in an acid medium commences the digestion of proteins; *rennin* functions to curdle milk; and *lipase* starts fat digestion. In

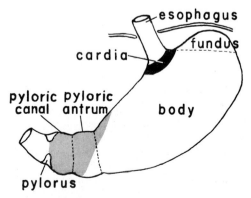

Figure 14-24. Diagram showing the anatomical and histological (shaded) areas of the stomach.

addition, the gastric mucosa secretes a factor necessary for the absorption of vitamin B_{12} (essential for hemopoiesis), and some absorption occurs, although this is limited to salts, water, glucose, alcohol, and some drugs.

The stomach wall is composed of four layers.

Mucosa

The mucous membrane of the living stomach is pale, grayish-pink, paler at the cardia and pylorus, and its entire thickness is occupied by a mass of *gastric glands* which open on the surface by *gastric pits* or *foveolae*. These pits usually are interpreted as tubular, but they also probably take the form of linear crevices. The gastric glands are simple tubular or branched tubular and extend deeply to reach the muscularis mucosae. Between them is the lamina propria, split up to such a degree to occupy the spaces between glands and pits that it is difficult to recognize it as a separate entity. On the basis of differences in the glands and pits, three zones are recognized: a narrow, ring-shaped area around the cardia containing *cardiac glands,* a main area comprising the fundus and body (the proximal two-thirds or more of the stomach) containing the *fundic* or *main glands,* and a distal area, the pyloric region, containing *pyloric glands,* this extending more proximally on the lesser than the greater curvature. The surface epithelium of the mucosa, however, is similar in form from cardia to pylorus.

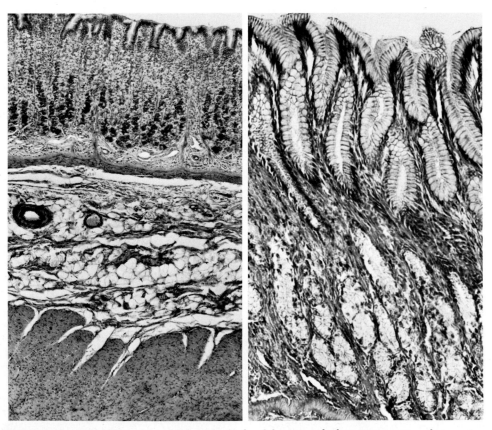

Figure 14-25.   Left: Photomicrograph of the body of the stomach showing mucosa, submucosa, and part of the muscularis. × 40. Right: Photomicrograph of the pyloric part of the stomach showing mucosa only. × 175.

Surface Epithelium

This is a tall, columnar epithelium (only one cell type being present) which distinguishes the stomach from all other regions of the digestive tract. At the cardia, it commences abruptly, adjoining the stratified squamous epithelium of the esophagus, and it is continuous at the pylorus with the intestinal epithelium. The columnar cells are mucin-secreting, the secreted material providing a protective coat for the epithelium. These mucin granules are peculiar in that they do not stain with some mucus-specific dyes. Nuclei are situated toward the bases of the cells, and the supranuclear region is occupied by round, discrete granules of mucin. As the epithelium extends into the mouths of foveolae, fewer mucin granules are present. Adjacent to the nucleus, but usually on the apical side, is a Golgi apparatus, and the subnuclear region is occupied by mitochondria. Terminal bars and apical microvilli are present. The mortality rate of the surface epithelial cells is high, and they are replaced by mitosis of less differentiated cells situated in the deeper parts of the foveolae and upper regions of the gastric glands.

Gastric Glands

As just outlined, these are branched tubular in type, are densely packed, and occupy the entire thickness of the mucosa, opening in small groups into the bottom of a gastric pit by which their secretions are carried to the surface. Each gland is surrounded by a basal lamina. They number some 35 million.

Cardiac Glands. These closely resemble the superficial mucosal glands of the lower esophagus; they are compound or simple tubular in type, extending over the deeper half of the mucosa, and several open into the base of a single gastric pit, the gastric pits occupying the superficial half of the depth of the mucosa. The cells of the cardiac glands are mucus-secreting, pale columnar cells interspersed with a few parietal cells. Their functional significance is not known.

Fundic Glands. These are the most important glands of the stomach and produce the majority of the enzymes and hydrochloric acid and some mucin. The pits are not as deep as those in the pylorus, extending for only a quarter to a third of the mucosal thickness. The glands thus are long and straight, although they may be slightly coiled in their upper extent. Usually in a section they are cut lengthwise. Each gland is said to have three parts: a base, a middle region or neck, and an upper isthmus which continues into a pit. Four cell types are present. In the isthmus, only surface epithelial cells and parietal cells are present. The main cell type in the neck is the mucous neck cell, between which are scattered parietal cells. The base is composed mainly of chief or zymogenic cells with some parietal and a few enterochromaffin cells.

CHIEF (ZYMOGENIC) CELL. Chief cells are situated in the lower portions of fundic glands, extend from the basal lamina to the lumen, and in a cross section of a gland, are pyramidal in shape and bear close similarities to pancreatic acinar and to salivary serous cells. The nucleus is spherical and situated toward the base of the cell, and the cytoplasm shows basal mitochondria and chromidial substance. The apical cytoplasm contains granules which do not preserve well and in a fixed preparation may be dissolved leaving a vacuolated appearance. By electron microscopy, the cells are cuboidal to pyramidal and show apical microvilli, a supranuclear Golgi complex, and numerous profiles of granular endoplasmic reticulum with some free ribosomes concentrated mainly at the base. Mitochondria are basally located also and in the apical cytoplasm are numerous, spherical, membrane-bound granules of low electron density. These appearances, of course, are consistent with a protein-secreting function, and this cell secretes enzymes, e.g., pepsin.

PARIETAL CELL. Parietal or oxyntic (i.e., acid-forming) cells are scattered singly and in small groups between the other cell types from the isthmus to the base of gastric glands, although they are most numerous in the neck and isthmus regions. They are characteristically spherical or pyramidal, of large size, and located peripherally in a gland so that their broad bases appear to bulge into the underlying lamina propria. Often their apices appear not to reach the lumen. The nucleus is spherical and central in position and the cytoplasm appears clear and stains readily with acidic dyes. An unusual feature is the presence of an intracellular canaliculus. This is a network of canals formed by infolding of the luminal surface which may be so extensive as to reach almost to the base of the cell. In ordinary preparations it appears as an irregular, unstained area. By electron microscopy it is obvious that these canaliculi are invaginations of the apical surface and not a true intracellular system. Numerous long microvilli project both into the glandular lumen and into the secretory canaliculi, where they may be so closely packed and interdigitated as to virtually occlude the lumen. The microvilli appear to lack the surface filamentous coat ("fuzz") of protein-polysaccharide found on other cells of the gastric mucosa. The cytoplasm of parietal cells contains numerous mitochondria and the Golgi apparatus is small and often located in an infranuclear posi-

tion. Free ribosomes are numerous; granular endoplasmic reticulum is sparse. A prominent component of the cytoplasm is agranular endoplasmic reticulum, usually of a tubular form. This organelle is considered important in hydrochloric acid secretion. Acid secretion may flow continuously through the tubular system into secretory canaliculi and so to the lumen of a gastric gland. Alternatively, as has been suggested by some authors, the tubules may contribute to the formation of long attenuated microvilli (by eversion, or turning inside out like the fingers of a glove), which then bring the secretory product, perhaps an ion exchanger, into contact with the luminal contents of a gastric gland. Certainly changes in the conformation of the agranular endoplasmic reticulum and of the microvilli do occur in the secretory cycle. No secretory granules are present in parietal cells. Recently radioautographic studies have shown that parietal cells are the site of intrinsic factor production (necessary for vitamin B_{12} absorption).

MUCOUS NECK CELL. These cells are relatively few in number and located only in the necks of fundic glands. They tend to be of irregular shape, as though deformed by the cells which surround them. The nuclei are ovoid, flattened, and basally located, and the apical cytoplasm contains pale, secretory granules which stain well with mucicarmine. Other staining reactions differentiate these cells from mucus-secreting cells of oral glands and from the gastric surface epithelial cells. By electron microscopy, these

---

Figure 14-26. A series of photomicrographs of the fundus of bear stomach. Epon sections, stained with toluidine blue and saffranin. A, Survey picture of the full thickness of the mucosa. The circled letters indicate regions from which following pictures were taken. × 125. B, Surface, showing surface epithelium (s) with mucin droplets, and parietal cells (p) in the isthmus of glands. × 450. C, The neck region, showing mucous neck cells (m) and parietal cells (p) with clear, unstained intracellular canaliculi. × 450. D, The bases of glands with parietal and chief or zymogenic (z) cells. Part of the muscularis mucosae is shown at the bottom. × 450. E, Surface epithelial cells with apical mucin droplets. × 750. F, Thin arrows indicate mucous neck cells, of irregular outline, seemingly squashed between parietal cells; the broad arrow shows a parietal cell with an extensive intracellular canaliculus. × 1250. G, Cross section through the base of a gland lined totally by chief cells with apical, unstained zymogen granules. × 750.   See filmstrip II, frames 61 and 62.

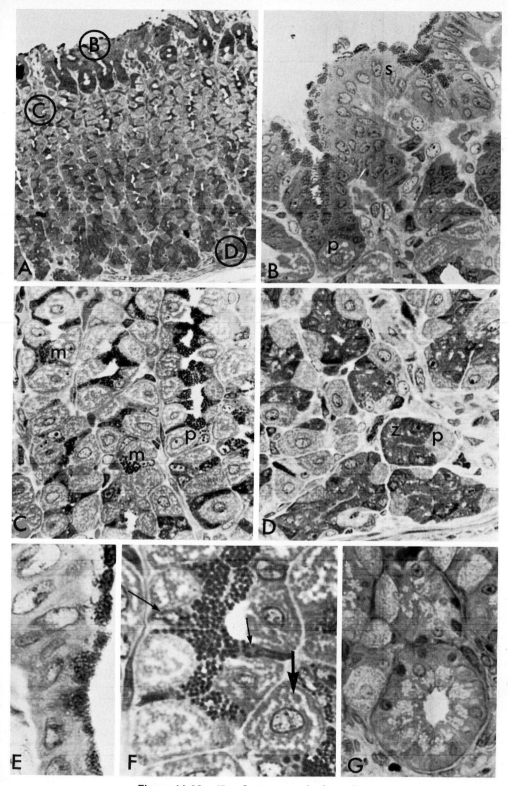

Figure 14-26. *(See facing page for legend.)*

cells show stubby, apical microvilli with a characteristic "fuzz" owing to the presence of very fine filaments attached to the surface. The secretory granules are dense and of varying shape.

ENTEROCHROMAFFIN CELL. Enterochromaffin, or argentaffin, cells are not numerous in the gastric mucosa and are most common in the small intestine. They are present, however, in the lining of the digestive tube from the esophagus to the anus. In gastric glands they are found, usually singly, in the bases and lying between chief cells. They appear not to reach the lumen but are situated between chief cells and the basal lamina of the gland. They are of a flattened, pyramidal shape and the cytoplasm is filled with small granules which can be stained with silver and chromium salts. At least two types of enterochromaffin cell are present. The granules of one type reduce silver salts without any pretreatment and the granules of the other first must be exposed to a reducing substance before they will react with silver. By electron microscopy, the granules are concentrated in the basal or infranuclear cytoplasm. Several types of cell can be distinguished on the basis of the morphology of the granules. In some there is a dense core with a loosely fitting limiting membrane and in others the granule is of a lower density with a closely applied membrane. The location of the granules in basal cytoplasm suggests that they are secreted into extracellular space and not into the lumen. The cells are known to be sites of synthesis and storage of 5-hydroxytryptamine (serotonin), a potent vasoconstrictor substance.

Pyloric Glands. Here the foveolae are deep, extending to half of the thickness of the mucosa. The pyloric glands thus are short and are simple or branched tubular, but they are of greater diameter than those of the fundus and coiled so that rarely are they sectioned along their lengths.

With the exception of a few argentaffin and parietal cells, only one cell type is present. This is very similar to the mucous neck cell, has a pale cytoplasm with indistinct granulation and a flattened basal nucleus, and produces mucin.

Lamina Propria

The lamina propria is scanty and consists of a delicate meshwork of collagenous and reticular fibers and a few fibroblast or reticular cells. Scattered in the meshes are some lymphocytes, plasma cells, mast cells, and white blood cells, the lymphocytes occasionally being present in small, local accumulations, these being more obvious at cardiac and pyloric regions. Occasionally single smooth muscle elements are present. The lamina propria, as explained earlier, owing to the masses of cardiac glands, is not extensive, being limited to the narrow, slitlike spaces between adjacent glands. The lamina is more obvious toward the surface of the mucosa where spaces are more extensive between foveolae.

Muscularis Mucosae

This is not thick and the smooth muscle of which it is composed is arranged into inner circular and outer longitudinal laminae. In some regions there is a third external coat which is circular or oblique. A few slips from the muscularis mucosae extend into the lamina propria between gastric glands.

Submucosa

This tunic or coat, of relatively dense fibroconnective tissue with collagenous, reticular, and elastic fibers, extends into the rugae or longitudinal

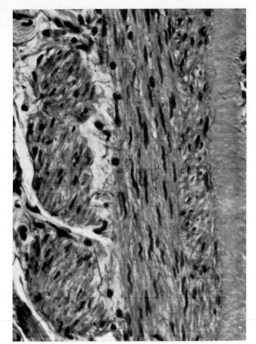

Figure 14-27. Photomicrograph of the muscularis mucosae of the cat stomach, showing three layers of smooth muscle. Aldehyde fuchsin, light green stain. × 250.

folds present in the contracted stomach. In addition to fibroblasts, macrophages, plasma cells, and lymphocytes, some fat cells usually are present. Contained in the layer are blood and lymph vessels and a few peripheral nerves.

Muscularis

There are three layers of smooth muscle, each orientated in a different plane. The outermost layer is longitudinal and continuous with that of the esophagus. The middle layer is circular, continuous with the inner layer of the esophagus, and greatly thickened at the pylorus to form the *pyloric sphincter*, where it is the thickest and most obvious layer. The innermost layer is oblique and takes the form of loops of muscle extending from the cardiac orifice around the fundus and corpus. It is not a complete layer.

Serosa

This consists of a layer of loose areolar tissue in which vessels and nerves are present, external to the muscularis and covered by a mesothelial layer, the peritoneum. At greater and lesser curvatures of the stomach, it is continuous with the greater and lesser mesenteries (omenta). The *greater omentum* hangs down from the greater curvature, is covered by peritoneum, and consists of areolar connective tissue which usually becomes increasingly adipose with age. The major blood vessels to and from the stomach course in the omenta.

THE SMALL INTESTINE

The small intestine extends from the pyloric orifice, where it is continuous with the stomach, to the ileocecal junction, where it continues into the large intestine. It is about 20 to 23 feet in length, is much coiled within the abdominal cavity, and is divided into three parts. The first part, the *duodenum*, is only 10 to 12 inches long and is relatively fixed to the posterior abdominal wall as it has no mesentery throughout the greater part of its length. The remainder of the small intestine is divided into the jejunum, the next two-fifths of the length, and the *ileum*, the remaining three-fifths. The jejunum and ileum are suspended from the posterior abdominal wall by the *mesentery* although the terminal ileum again is fixed to the posterior abdominal wall. The functions of the small intestine are to transport food material (chyme) from the stomach to the large intestine, to complete digestion by the secretion of enzymes from its wall and from accessory glands, to absorb the final products of digestion into blood and lymph vessels in its wall, and to secrete certain hormones.

To subserve these functions, particularly of absorption and digestive secretion, the small intestine shows cer-

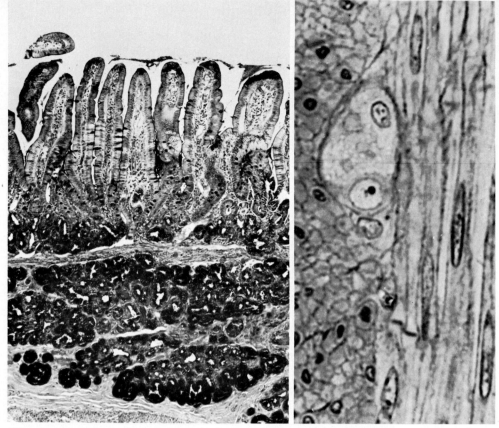

Figure 14-28. Photomicrographs of duodenum. Left: Longitudinal section showing mucosa with villi and intestinal glands, and submucosa with submucosal glands of Brunner. × 75. Right: Part of the muscularis showing a small collection of ganglion cells of Auerbach's plexus between the two layers of smooth muscle. × 1250.   See filmstrip II, frame 63.

tain specializations that increase the surface area of its mucosa.

Mucosal Surface Specializations

Plicae Circulares (Valves of Kerckring). These are permanent circular or spiral folds of the entire thickness of the mucosa with a core of submucosa. Any one fold may extend two-thirds or more around the circumference of the intestine, but rarely do the folds completely encircle the lumen. Branching of some plicae occurs. The plicae commence in the duodenum within one to two inches of the pylorus, reach their maximum development in terminal duodenum and proxi-

mal jejunum, and thereafter diminish, disappearing in the distal half of the ileum.

Villi and Crypts. Villi are small finger- or leaf-like projections of the mucous membrane, 0.5 to 1.5 mm. in length, found only in the small intestine. The length of villi varies and is reduced by distention of the intestine. They, of course, are covered by epithelium and have a core of lamina propria, but unlike plicae, the muscularis mucosae and submucosa do not extend into them. In the duodenum, they are broad, spatulate structures but become cylindrical or finger-like in the ileum. Crypts or intestinal glands (of Lieberkühn) are tubelike structures opening between the bases of villi, 0.3 to

0.5 mm. in depth, and extending deeply through the thickness of the mucous membrane nearly to reach the muscularis mucosae. They are not packed so closely as the gastric glands, the spaces between them being filled with connective tissue of the lamina propria. Crypts also are present in the large intestine although villi are not, and thus it is important for identification of sections that the student be able to recognize differences between villi and crypts when cut in cross section. Villi appear as circular or oval profiles with a core of connective tissue (lamina propria) covered by epithelium. A crypt in cross section appears as a central lumen lined by epithelium, the whole embedded in connective tissue of the lamina propria.

Microvilli. To further increase surface area, the columnar absorptive cells covering villi and lining crypts have a brush or striated border composed of numerous microvillous processes. Each microvillus is covered by an extension of the plasma membrane, the outer lamina of which is associated with a feltwork of fine filaments giving a fuzzy appearance. This filamentous coat, which occupies the spaces between microvilli and at their tips, forming a continuous surface layer, contains an acid mucopolysaccharide and is resistant to proteolytic and mucolytic agents. In the cores of microvilli are thin, longitudinally orientated filaments which at the bases are continuous with the filaments of the terminal web (see later).

To the food material in the lumen of the small intestine are added the secretions of many glands. These are of three main types: the intestinal glands,

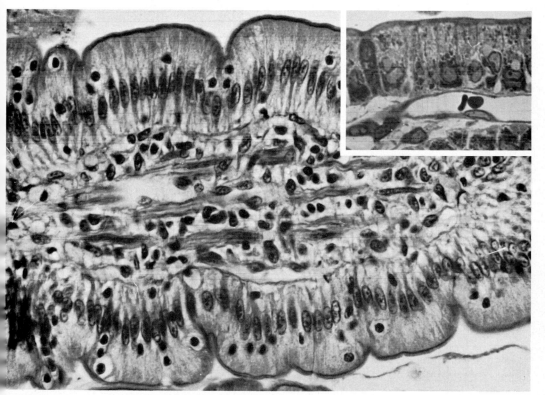

Figure 14-29. Photomicrograph of a longitudinal section of part of a duodenal villus showing surface epithelium with brush border and a core of lamina propria containing smooth muscle cells. × 375. Inset, top right, shows the close relationship between a blood capillary (containing two red blood corpuscles) and the surface epithelium of a duodenal villus. Epon section, × 300.

See filmstrip I, frame 14.

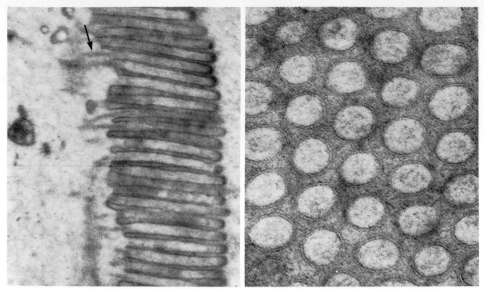

Figure 14-30. Electron micrographs of the human duodenum to show microvilli in longitudinal section (left) and in cross section (right). Note the associated surface "fuzz" of mucopolysaccharide, and longitudinal filaments in the cores of microvilli, continuous with the terminal web (left, arrow). Left, × 20,000; right, × 98,000.

the submucosal glands, and the glands situated outside the digestive tract but passing their secretions into its lumen by a duct system. Intestinal glands, as just explained, are found in both small and large intestines. Submucosal glands are located in the duodenum, are compound tubular in type, and are termed the *duodenal glands* (of Brunner). Usually, they are more extensive in the first part of the duodenum near the pylorus. Glands situated outside the digestive tract are the liver and pancreas, and both deliver their exocrine secretions into the duodenum.

Epithelium

The epithelium of the intestinal mucosa is simple columnar in type but differs from the surface epithelium of the stomach in that more than one cell type is present. There are columnar cells with a striated border, goblet cells, and enterochromaffin cells. The columnar cells show a relatively clear apical cytoplasm beneath the microvil-

lous border with elements of smooth endoplasmic reticulum and some mitochondria and a Golgi apparatus lying in a supranuclear position. The nucleus is situated toward the cell base with an infranuclear zone containing more mitochondria. The cells rest upon a basal lamina. With the electron microscope, the microvilli appear as tubular processes, tightly packed, and often with a relatively electron-dense core (see Figures 2-5 and 14-30). Beneath the microvilli, apical cytoplasm contains no organelles, but in it is a meshwork of very fine filaments, orientated parallel to the surface, and this *terminal web* converges at the cell surface into the *terminal bar*. By electron microscopy, these terminal bars are seen to correspond to the zonula adherens and zonula occludens of the junctional complex, as described in Chapter 5, the zonulae forming a complete corona around the cell. The zonula adherens, together with maculae adherentes present on cell interfaces, provides firm cohesion between cells, and the zonula occludens probably prevents passage of

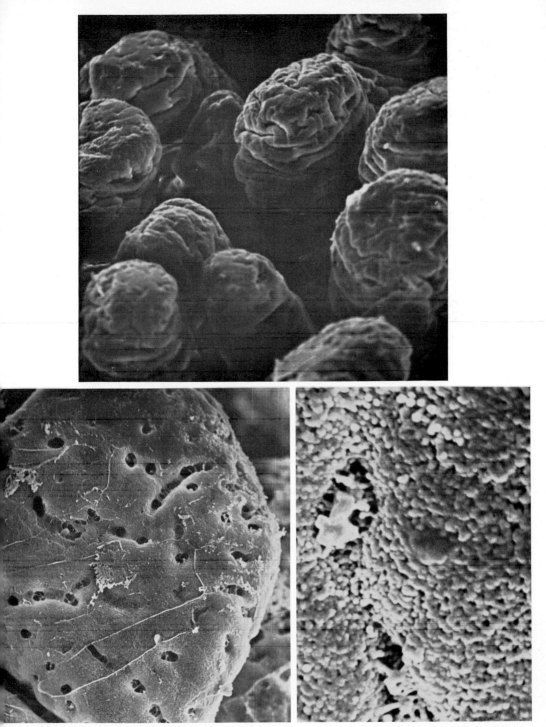

Figure 14-31. Scanning electron micrographs. Top: Low power showing finger-like villi. × 536. Botton left: A single fingerlike villus to show goblet-cell orifices with interconnecting troughs and strands of mucus (white) on the surface. × 1070. Bottom right: Cell surface showing microvilli and two goblet cells with mucus. × 10,300. (Courtesy of Doctors N. M. Marsh, J. A. Swift, and E. D. Williams.)

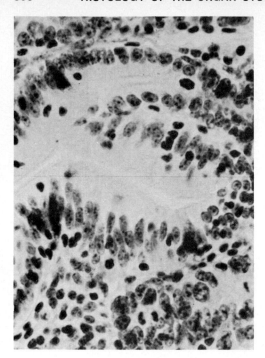

Figure 14-32. Photomicrograph of one (bifid) duodenal gland stained to show enterochromaffin cells (black). Silver stain. × 450.

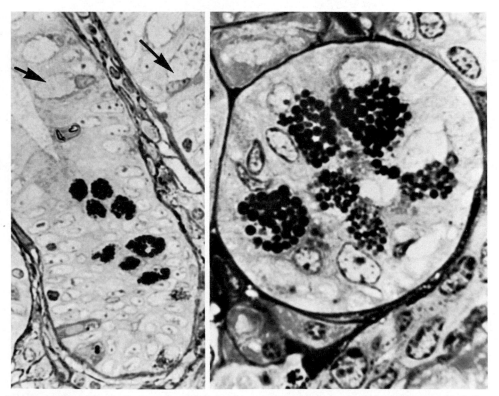

Figure 14-33. Photomicrographs of bases of intestinal glands in the human duodenum in longitudinal section (left) and transverse section (right) to show Paneth cells with discrete, dense granules. Goblet cells also are present, but unstained (arrows). Epon sections. Left, × 650. Right, × 1250.

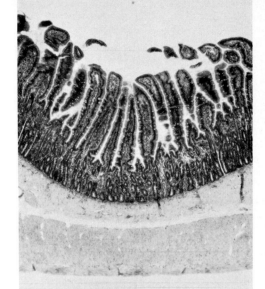

Figure 14-34. Photomicrograph of the jejunum, showing all layers. Note villi and intestinal glands. Goblet cells (clear dots) are visible in the epithelium. × 30.

See filmstrip II, frame 64.

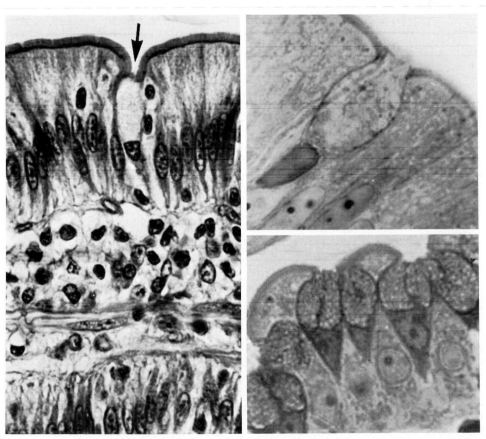

Figure 14-35. Photomicrographs particularly to illustrate goblet cells. Left: Part of a longitudinal section of a jejunal villus to show a goblet cell (arrow) between surface epithelial cells with a well defined striated border. × 600. Top right: A similar area. Epon section, unstained, phase contrast, × 1250. Bottom right: Goblet cells in the ileum. Epon section, toluidine blue and saffranin, × 650.

See filmstrip II, frame 65.

material from the lumen into the inter-cellular cleft.

Goblet cells are scattered between the columnar cells, whereas en-terochromaffin cells (see page 300) are scattered singly in the intestinal glands. Also present are migrating lymphocytes passing from the lamina propria ultimately to reach the lumen. Mitotic figures in columnar cells usu-ally are quite numerous in the intesti-nal glands, evidence for the rapid cell turnover. Epithelial cells of the small intestine undergo complete replace-ment every seven or eight days, arising by mitosis of relatively undifferenti-ated cells in the crypts and passing up the villi to be shed from their tips.

Cells at the bottom of the intestinal glands are pyramidal with a broad base and a narrow apex. Nuclei lie close to the basal lamina, the basal cytoplasm is occupied by chromophil substance, and the apical cytoplasm is filled with large, spherical acidophil granules. These are the *cells of Paneth*. Their function is not known, but their fine structure demonstrates an abundant content of granular endoplasmic reticu-lum, and while no digestive enzyme has been localized specifically to Paneth cells, it has been suggested that they may secrete peptidase. The granules are believed to contain lyso-zyme, an enzyme which breaks down bacteria.

Lamina Propria

The lamina propria extends between intestinal glands and into the cores of villi. Its character is quite distinctive with a network of reticular fibers and many features of loose lymphatic tis-sue. It is best described, perhaps, as a loose, areolar connective tissue with lymphoid tendencies. Present in the meshwork of reticular fibers are primi-tive reticular cells with large, oval, pale-staining nuclei, lymphocytes, macrophages and plasma cells. Eosin-ophil leukocytes, in particular, are evident, these having migrated from

blood vessels. Single smooth muscle cells orientated lengthwise in the cores of villi usually are related closely to lymphatic capillaries. These start blindly in villi, contain absorbed fat after a meal, and thus appear white in fresh or living tissue. They are called *lacteals*.

In addition to scattered lympho-cytes, there are present in the lamina propria large numbers of *solitary fol-licles* or isolated lymphatic nodules, more numerous distally in the intes-tine. If large, they may occupy the entire thickness of the mucosa and bulge the surface. There are no villi and may be no crypts on the surface of large follicles which are then separated from the lumen only by a simple columnar epithelium. In many re-gions, but mainly in the ileum, follicles may be so numerous and close to-gether as to aggregate into large masses of lymphoid tissue visible to the naked eye. They vary in size from 12 to 20

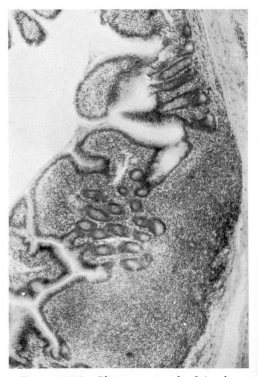

Figure 14-36. Photomicrograph of the ileum to show a small part of a Peyer's patch. × 60.

mm. long, and 8 to 12 mm. wide, the longer axis lying along the length of the intestine. Always they are situated on the antimesenteric border, i.e., on the side away from the attachment of the mesentery. These are the *Peyer's patches* or aggregated nodules.

The muscularis mucosae, submucosa, muscularis, and serosa do not merit a separate description, although it should be noted that the submucosa usually is infiltrated with lymphocytes in the region of Peyer's patches.

Duodenal Glands (of Brunner)

These submucosal glands of the duodenum are composed of tall cuboidal cells with dark, flattened, basal nuclei and a clear, vacuolated cytoplasm. They certainly are mucus-secreting but may also have other functions. The glandular portions continue into ducts lined by low cuboidal cells, and these penetrate the muscularis mucosae to open into intestinal glands. Often, the muscularis mucosae does not form a complete layer over the glands, and slips of smooth muscle extend in the connective tissue between the glandular units. Occasionally, Brunner's glands extend into the upper part of the jejunum, and, more commonly, may be found in the pyloric region of the stomach.

THE LARGE INTESTINE

The large intestine is about five feet in length and consists of the *cecum*, continuous with the ileum at the ileocecal valve, the *appendix*, a small diverticulum from the cecum, the *colon*, continuous with the cecum and divided into the ascending, transverse, and descending parts, and then the *rectum* and *anal canal*, terminating as the *anus* at the body surface. Food material enters the cecum in a semifluid state; it becomes semisolid, the consistency of feces, in the colon. Thus, one function of the large intes-

tine is absorption of fluid. Other functions are secretion of mucus (lubrication becomes more important as fluid is absorbed and the fecal mass becomes harder and thus more likely to damage the mucosa) and digestion, accomplished by enzymes present in the food material and by putrefaction by bacteria always present in the large intestine. No digestive enzymes are secreted by the large intestine.

The large intestine lacks plicae and villi and thus the surface epithelium is more obvious than it is in the small intestine. Intestinal glands or crypts are present and are longer than those of the small intestine and more closely packed. Epithelial cell types are identical to those of the small intestine but the goblet (mucus-secreting) cells are more numerous.

Ileocecal Junction

At the ileocecal junction there is an abrupt change in the character of the mucosa, which is thrown into anterior and posterior folds to form two *valves*. These folds consist of mucosa and submucosa supported by a mass of circular smooth muscle, a thickening of the inner layer of the muscularis, and because of their position the ileocecal orifice has the form of a vertical slit.

The ileocecal junction is located at the lower right side of the abdomen and is fixed to the posterior abdominal wall; i.e., the terminal ileum has no mesentery. The cecum is a small blind pouch hanging down from the ileocecal junction and has a structure identical to that of the colon.

Appendix

The appendix is a small, slender, blind diverticulum of the cecum arising about one inch below the ileocecal valve. In cross section, the lumen is small and usually of irregular outline, often contains cellular debris, and may be completely occluded. Villi are absent and intestinal glands are few and

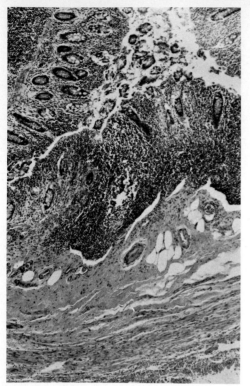

Figure 14-37. Photomicrograph of a cross section of the human appendix. Note the intestinal glands and the infiltration of the mucosa by lymphatic tissue. × 40.

of irregular length. The surface epithelium is composed of columnar, striated-border cells mainly, with only a few goblet cells. In the crypts there are a few Paneth cells, and enterochromaffin cells are numerous. The lamina propria is occupied by a mass of lymphoid tissue similar to that of the palatine tonsil. The muscularis mucosae usually is incomplete. The submucosa is thick and contains blood vessels and nerves, and the muscularis is thin but shows the usual two layers. The serous coat is identical to that covering the remainder of the intestine.

The appendix so commonly is the site of acute and chronic inflammation that it is difficult to obtain a completely normal appendix. Usually, some eosinophils and neutrophils are present in lamina propria and submucosa. If present in large numbers, they are

evidence of chronic and acute infection respectively.

Cecum, Colon, and Rectum

The intestinal glands are of greater depth in the large than in the small intestine and are packed more closely. They increase in depth to 0.75 mm. in the rectum, being 0.5 mm. in the colon. Goblet cells are numerous and enterochromaffin cells are occasional in the depths, but Paneth cells usually are not present. Most of the cells in the depths of the glands are undifferentiated epithelial cells which undergo rapid mitosis. The lamina propria between glands is similar in appearance to that of the small intestine and contains scattered lymphatic nodules which extend deeply into the submucosa. The muscularis mucosae is well developed but may be irregular or defi-

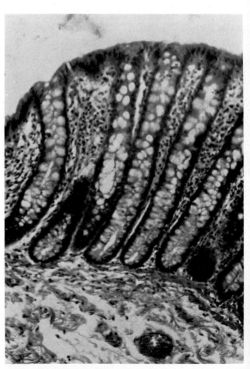

Figure 14-38. Photomicrograph of the rectum to show the mucosa. No villi are present. Intestinal glands are straight tubules. Goblet cells are abundant. × 125.

cient at the sites of lymphatic nodules. In the cecum and colon, the outer longitudinal coat of the muscularis is not a complete layer and is present as three longitudinal bands, the *taeniae coli*. In the rectum, it again becomes a complete layer. The serous coat shows, on the surface not attached to the posterior abdominal wall, small, taglike protuberances composed of adipose tissue, the *appendices epiploicae*. In the transverse colon there is a true mesentery.

Rectoanal Junction

In the lower end of the rectum, the intestinal glands become short and disappear in the anal canal. Here, the mucous membrane is thrown into a series of longitudinal folds termed the *rectal columns of Morgagni*. In this region, the muscularis mucosae becomes broken up into a series of bundles and finally disappears so that there is no distinction between lamina propria and submucosa. In this region there are numerous longitudinal, thin-walled veins which, if dilated and convoluted, cause protrusion of the mucous membrane over them. Such a condition constitutes *internal hemorrhoids* or *piles*. About one inch above the anal orifice, the columnar epithelium abruptly changes to a stratified squamous epithelium which extends downward for a short extent only as a transition zone between intestinal epithelium and skin. At the anus, the epithelium is keratinized and beneath it are branched tubular glands termed the *circumanal glands*.

The muscularis at the rectoanal junction shows certain modifications. In the lower rectum, the longitudinal layer appears to be shorter than the length of the rectum and thus causes the mucosa to bulge into the lumen as transverse shelves termed the *plicae transversae*, there being two such shelves on the right and one on the left. These may aid in the support of feces but also are thought to help the separation of feces from flatus. In the lower rectum and anal canal the internal layer of the muscularis is thickened as the *internal sphincter* of the anus. Surrounding the anal canal are bundles of striated muscle, the external sphincter of the anus.

Intestinal Absorption

The digestion of food material within the intestinal lumen involves the reduction of foodstuffs to molecular size. This is accomplished by the secretions of the major digestive glands (pancreas and liver) and by secretions of intestinal juice, produced mainly by the intestinal glands (of Lieberkühn). Bile from the liver reduces lipid to triglycerides, while pancreatic juice contains lipolytic, proteolytic, and carbohydrate-splitting enzymes. Intestinal juice contains lipase, maltase, and peptidase, possibly located in the microvillous border. In the adult, aminoacids resulting from the intraluminal digestion of proteins are absorbed by the intestinal epithelium. The majority of lipid is absorbed as micelles of fatty acids and monoglycerides which are re-esterified to triglyceride in the agranular reticulum of apical cytoplasm. The triglyceride then is combined with protein to form *chylomicrons*, which later enter the lacteals by an as yet unknown mechanism.

Blood Vessels

Generally throughout the digestive tract the arrangements of blood and lymph vessels are similar. Basically, arteries entering the tract pass through the muscularis to form an extensive submucous plexus. From this plexus, branches pass toward the lumen and supply capillaries to the muscularis mucosae and capillary networks throughout the mucosa and around the glands. Venous return commences superficially, from the mucosal capillary plexus, as large caliber vessels which form an extensive venous plexus just internal to the muscularis mucosae. From here, veins pass outward into the submucosa where there is a second extensive plexus which is drained by large veins passing through the muscularis to the serosa. These large veins run with the entering arteries.

In the small intestine, the arterial pattern is more extensive than that just described. In addition to capillary networks around the intestinal glands, other arteries originate in the submucous plexus and are destined specifically to supply villi, each villus receiving one or more such arteries. Having entered the base of a villus, these arteries break up into a dense capillary network situated adjacent to the basal lamina of the epithelium. Small veins arise from this superficial capillary network at the tip of a villus and pass outward to join the venous plexus internal to the muscularis mucosae.

Lymphatic capillaries form an extensive system surrounding glands in the superficial layers of the mucosa, and in the small intestine this plexus is joined by lacteals. Lacteals start blindly in the apices of villi, and run axially in the cores of villi. From the mucosal plexus, branches pierce the muscularis mucosae and form a plexus of lymphatics in the submucosa from which larger lymphatics pass outward through the muscularis and follow blood vessels to the retroperitoneal tissues. In the muscularis, lymphatics receive many tributaries from another lymphatic plexus located in the muscularis.

Part III — THE MAJOR DIGESTIVE GLANDS

There are two large abdominal organs which connect to the digestive tract by duct systems. These are the pancreas and the liver.

THE PANCREAS

The pancreas is a large, elongated organ lying in the concavity of the duodenum and extending behind the peritoneum of the posterior abdominal wall toward the left to reach the hilum of the spleen. It is both an exocrine and an endocrine organ, the two functions being performed by different cell types.

In the fresh condition, it is pale pink or white and has no definite fibrous capsule, but is covered by thin, areolar tissue from which thin septa extend into the gland to divide it into obvious lobules. Fine, delicate reticular tissue surrounds individual acini.

Exocrine Portion

The pancreas can be classified as a large, lobulated, compound, tubuloacinar gland.

Acini

Acini or alveoli are tubular or pear-shaped, surrounded by a basal lamina and composed of five to eight pyramidal cells arranged around a small central lumen. Myoepithelial cells are not present. Between acini is delicate connective tissue containing blood vessels, lymphatics, nerves, and excretory ducts. The acini are packed in an irregular fashion, and thus in any section, they will be cut in every possible plane. Obviously, the lumen of all will not be sectioned, and in addition, the caliber of the lumen varies with the secretory phase and may contain small cells. These, the *centroacinar cells*, belong to the duct system, which often commences not from the terminations but from the central parts of acini.

In an acinar cell, the nucleus is spherical, lies toward the base, and contains abundant chromatin and one to three large nucleoli. The basal cytoplasm is basophil and may show a longitudinal striation owing to the presence of numerous, elongated mitochondria. The apical cytoplasm con-

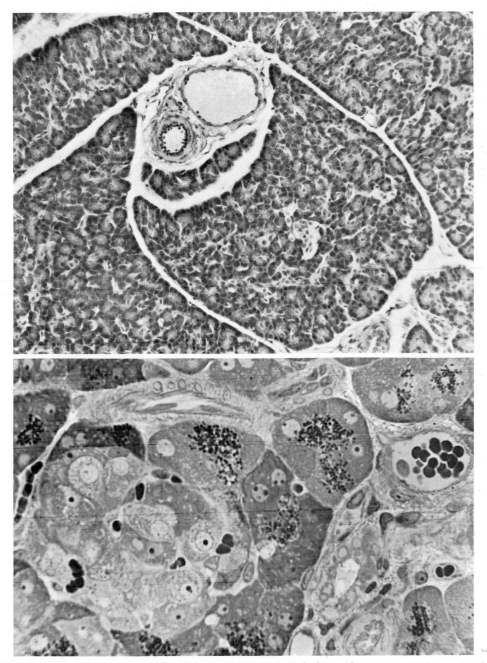

Figure 14-39. Photomicrographs of the pancreas. Top: Lobules with numerous serous acini. No islet tissue is obvious. × 100. Bottom: Parts of several serous acini with dense zymogen granules and an islet of Langerhans (left) are shown. Epon section, × 450.   See filmstrip II, frame 66.

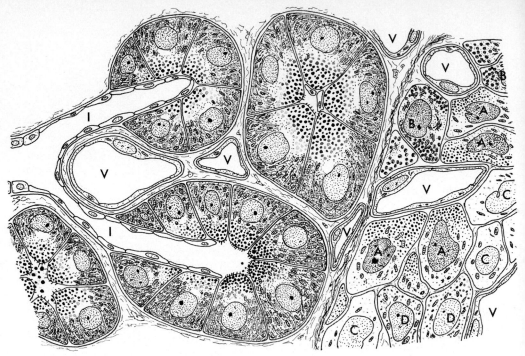

Figure 14-40.   Diagram of a small portion of the pancreas as seen by low power electron micros-copy. In the exocrine portion (left) parts of four acini are illustrated. Two are drained by intercalated ducts (I) and one (top center) shows two centroacinar cells. In a typical exocrine cell, identify the following features: nucleus with nucleolus, basal ergastoplasm and mitochondria, supranuclear Golgi zone (clear space) and apical zymogen and prozymogen droplets. In the endocrine islet of Langerhans (right), A, B, C, and D cells are labeled. Note the variation in type of secretory granules and their relation to capillary blood vessels (V). × 1500 approximately.

tains acidophil secretion (zymogenic) droplets or granules which are highly refractile. In a supranuclear position also is an extensive Golgi apparatus, sometimes visible as a clear area among the zymogen granules. By elec-tron microscopy, acini are seen to be enclosed by a thin basal lamina sup-ported by reticular fibers. The nucleus of each acinar cell is large and dense, and nucleoli commonly are seen. The main features of these cells are the specializations for protein secretion (see Chapter 2). The cytoplasm largely is filled with flattened sacs of granu-lar endoplasmic reticulum (ergasto-plasm), particularly prominent in the basal region but extending also into the supranuclear zone. Mitochondria are quite numerous, usually elongated, and mainly orientated perpendicularly in the basal cytoplasm. A well-devel-

oped Golgi zone is located in a supra-nuclear position, and the vacuoles of this zone have a content of varying density representing formative stages of zymogen granules. Zymogen granules are large, spherical, and homogeneously dense with a limiting membrane. Some with a less dense matrix have been termed prozymogen granules. A few short microvilli are present at the apex.

The formation and secretion of zy-mogen granules have been studied by radioautography after injection of triti-ated leucine, glycine, and methionine. Such studies confirm the theory of pro-tein secretion as explained in Chapter 2. Radioautographic label appears rap-idly in the endoplasmic reticulum (about five minutes after injection) and later appears in the Golgi zone (in about 10 to 12 minutes), where protein

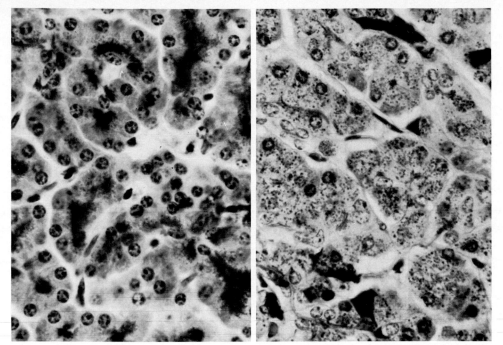

Figure 14-41. Photomicrographs of the pancreas stained to show secretion (zymogen) granules, left, before a meal, and, right, after a meal. Note that the majority of the granules have been secreted after feeding. Iron hematoxylin, osmic acid. × 350.

is built into prozymogen granules, and later in zymogen granules (in 30 to 40 minutes). The life span of a zymogen granule in an acinar cell is estimated at about 50 minutes only. These figures give some indication as to the extreme activity of the pancreatic acinar cells. Thus, in summary, it is believed that the digestive enzymes of the pancreas are synthesized in the basal region of the cytoplasm, and accumulate in the canals of the endoplasmic reticulum. From here, the enzymes pass to the Golgi region where they are segregated in membrane bound vesicles and concentrated into typical zymogen droplets, which later pass to the cell surface for release.

The pancreatic juice contains proteolytic enzymes, e.g., trypsin and chymotrypsin, which split proteins; carboxypeptidase, which cleaves peptides; ribonuclease and deoxyribonuclease, which break down RNP and DNP; amylase, which hydrolyzes starch and other carbohydrates; and li-

pase, which hydrolyzes neutral fat to glycerol and fatty acids.

Ducts

Three regions of the duct system are described, the cells of all three showing close similarities. They are, in order: centroacinar or centroductular, intercalated (intercalary) ductules, and intralobular to interlobular to main or accessory ducts. The transitions from one region to the next are gradual, the epithelium increasing in height from squamous through cuboidal to columnar. By light microscopy, in all regions cytoplasm is pale-staining and nuclei show little chromatin. Organelles are not prominent. Main features by electron microscopy are a thin basal lamina, lateral plasma membrane interdigitations with desmosomes and junctional complexes, indented nuclei, and apical microvilli. The interlobular and larger ducts lie in fibroconnective

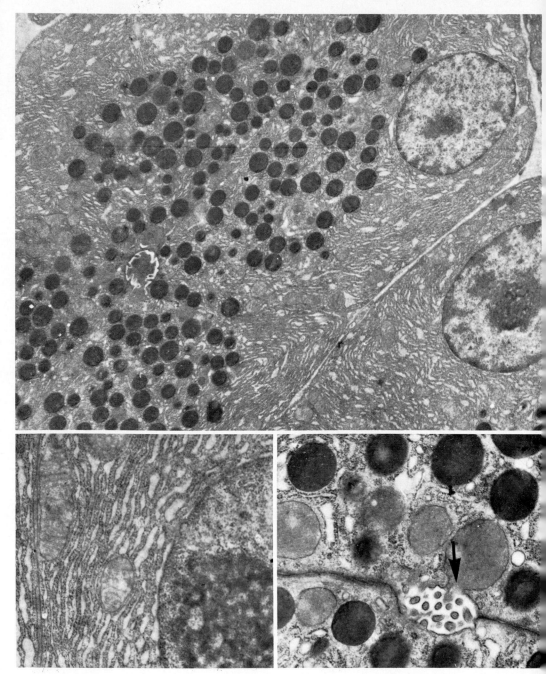

Figure 14-42. Electron micrographs of acinar pancreas. Top: The major portion of one acinus and part of another, showing nuclei, extensive basal ergastoplasm, apical zymogen droplets, and the lumen, containing electron dense material. × 5000. Lower left: Basal region of an acinar cell showing part of the nucleus and nucleolus, basal ergastoplasm, and mitochondria. × 13,500. Lower right: The lumen of an acinus between two acinar cells. Note apical microvilli and the variation in density of secretion droplets, one of which is in the process of discharging its contents into the lumen (arrow). × 13,500.

tissue, only fine reticular tissue surrounding intercalated and intralobular ducts. The relation of centroacinar cells and intercalated ducts is illustrated in Figure 14-40.

Endocrine Portion

The endocrine portion of the pancreas, the *islets of Langerhans,* are scattered throughout the pancreas and appear as irregular, spheroidal masses of pale-staining cells provided with a very rich blood supply. The endocrine pancreas thus can be termed a dispersed gland of internal secretion. The islets are delineated incompletely from surrounding acini by a thin "capsule" of reticular fibers. In the ordinary H and E preparation, the cells of the islets are seen to be polygonal, pale-staining, and arranged in cords between which are blood capillaries. Special staining methods are required to demonstrate secretion granules in

these cells, and such methods show that several cell types are present as distinguished by their granules. These are termed *alpha* or *A cells,* the granules of which are insoluble in alcohol, *beta* or *B cells,* with granules soluble in alcohol, *C cells,* deficient in granules, and *D cells,* which contain granules which stain blue with the Mallory-Azan method. (Alpha cell granules stain bright red, beta cell granules stain orange.) The function of C and D cells is unknown; A cells probably produce glucagon; and there is considerable evidence that B cells produce insulin. The Gomori aldehyde fuchsin and Ponceau technique stains the B cell granules a dark blue-purple and the A cell granules dark pink or red. In man, the B cells account for 60 to 80 per cent of the cells in each islet. A cells have been subdivided into two or more types by the presence or absence of cytoplasmic argyrophilia.

By light microscopy, all islet cells are of an irregular polygonal shape with central, spherical nuclei showing

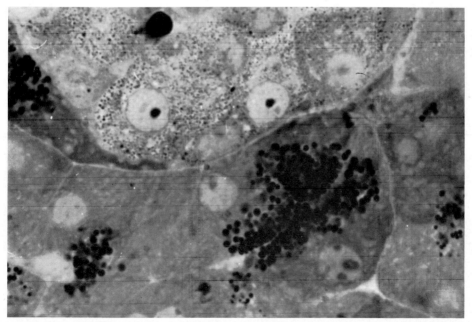

Figure 14-43.   Photomicrograph of a portion of an islet of Langerhans (above) and acinar tissue (below). Note that the cells in the islet are filled with small, discrete granules. Compare with Figure 14-40. × 1000.

well marked chromatin, small rodlike mitochondria, and a small Golgi apparatus. By electron microscopy, marked differences in the cell types are apparent, although there is considerable species difference. The A cells contain numerous granules of uniform size, each densely homogeneous and osmiophilic and surrounded by a membrane separated from the granule by a small interval. The remainder of the cytoplasm is of low density and contains the usual organelles. The number of granules varies from cell to cell and presumably is dependent upon the secretory phase. In B cells, the granules are spherical or oval, membrane bound, and of varying density, with a central more dense crystalline area of varying shape dependent on species. C cells have light cytoplasm and no granules and may represent a resting cell or a variant of A or B cells. D cells have granules which tend to be larger and less dense than those of A cells. They perhaps are not a distinct cell type but may represent altered alpha cells. The granules of all cell types usually are accumulated in the peripheral cytoplasm of a cell which abuts against a capillary. At the periphery of islets, cells are found which are intermediate between acinar and islet cells, containing both zymogen and A or B type granules.

Recent studies indicate that beta granules are formed in the ergastoplasm of the beta cell and released from

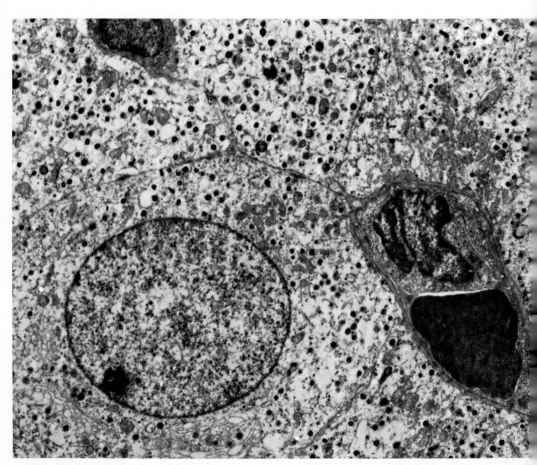

Figure 14-44.   Electron micrograph of a portion of an islet showing A cells (with cytoplasmic granules) around a capillary. × 7500.

the cell after stimulation of the cell by glucose.

Glucagon, secreted by A cells, is a polypeptide, has a molecular weight of 3485, and is released from A cells into the blood stream. In the liver, it produces gluconeogenesis with release of blood sugar to raise the blood sugar level. Insulin, having a molecular weight of about 6000, consists of two polypeptide chains, is secreted by the B cells, and promotes the transfer of glucose across certain cell membranes, particularly in muscle and liver, with a consequent lowering of the blood sugar level.

Blood Vessels and Nerves

The pancreas receives a very rich arterial supply from branches of the celiac and superior mesenteric arteries. Venous return is directly or indirectly to the portal system. Major vessels run in interlobular connective tissue with fine vessels passing into the lobules. As stated previously, capillaries in the islets of Langerhans are large and numerous. Nerves to the pancreas are from the sympathetic (celiac ganglion) and parasympathetic (vagus) parts of the autonomic nervous system. Some ganglion cells are present in interlobular connective tissue.

Development

The pancreas arises from two diverticula, ventral and dorsal, from the junction of fore- and mid-gut. The diverticula fuse, the epithelial lining branching to form acini connected to the primary outgrowths by a duct system. Some epithelial buds lose their connection to the duct system and differentiate into islet tissue. During development, the duct systems of the two diverticula become interconnected so that although the dorsal diverticulum forms the bulk of the pancreas, its secretion passes to the ventral outgrowth, the duct of which becomes the main pancreatic duct. The proximal part of the duct of the dorsal diverticulum remains as the accessory pancreatic duct, which opens into the duodenum at a higher level than the main duct. The latter has a common opening into the duodenum with the common bile duct from the liver.

THE LIVER

The liver is the heaviest gland in the body, weighing three or more pounds, is of soft consistency, and is situated beneath the diaphragm in the upper abdomen. It is dark red or reddish-brown in the fresh condition, the color being caused mainly by a very rich blood supply. Not only does it receive an arterial supply from the celiac artery, but it also receives blood from the intestinal tract via the portal vein. Its venous drainage returns to the inferior vena cava, and thus it lies interposed along the venous drainage of the intestinal tract. It receives all the material absorbed from the intestinal tract with the exception of lipid, most of which is transported in the lymphatic system. In addition to the digested and absorbed material which is assimilated and stored in the liver, the portal blood also carries to the liver various toxic materials which then are detoxicated in, or excreted by, the liver. Bile from the liver drains via a duct system into the duodenum and is partly a secretion in that it contains bile salts which are important in digestion and partly an excretion in that it contains waste and even harmful materials for ultimate evacuation in the feces. The portal vein and hepatic artery enter and the hepatic (bile) ducts leave the liver at a region called the *porta hepatis*, a transverse fissure on the inferior surface. The remainder of the liver is covered by a fibroconnective tissue capsule (of Glisson) from which thin connective tissue septa enter the substance of the liver at the porta hepatis to divide it into lobes and lobules. In some animals, e.g., the pig, the content

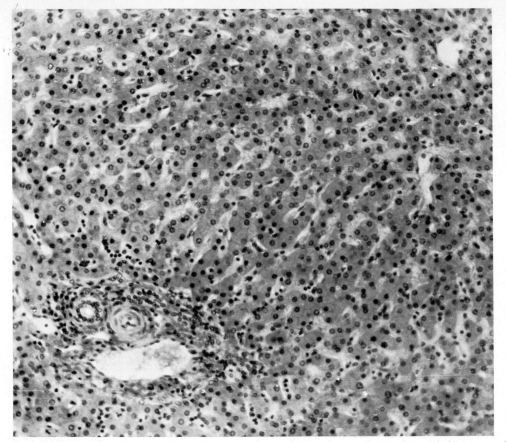

Figure 14-45.   Photomicrograph of the human liver, showing a portal area (lower left), a central vein (top right), and plates of liver parenchymal cells of part of a classical lobule extending between the two. × 175.

of connective tissue is much greater than it is in the human. Over a great area, the capsule is covered by peritoneum although there is an area (the "bare area") in direct contact with the diaphragm and viscera of the posterior abdominal wall.

General Histological Plan

In a section examined under low power, the liver is seen to be composed of masses of epithelial, parenchymal cells arranged in anastomosing and branching plates which form a three-dimensional lattice. Between plates are sinusoidal blood spaces. In this respect, the liver has the structure of

an endocrine gland. Also present are areas termed the *portal areas* or *portal canals,* each comprising branches of the portal vein, hepatic artery, and bile duct, often also with a lymphatic vessel, lying in a small amount of connective tissue. The portal areas are so arranged as to delineate lobules of liver tissue. Such a lobule, the *classical* or *hepatic lobule,* has several portal canals at its periphery, and in its center is a central vein, a tributary of the inferior vena cava, from which radiate plates of parenchymal cells like the spokes of a wheel from a central hub. This unit of structure is repeated thousands of times. With the afferent vessels (portal vein and hepatic artery) at the periphery of the lobule and the efferent

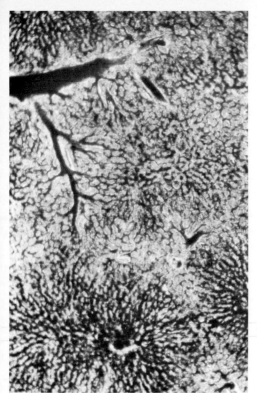

Figure 14-46. Photomicrograph to demonstrate blood vessels and sinusoids in the human liver. A large branch of the portal vein appears at top left and from it branches pass into sinusoids of classical liver lobules. Kull method. × 75.

cells in a liver lobule are either parenchymal (hepatic) cells, cells associated with the walls of hepatic sinusoids, or blood cells in the lumina of sinusoids.

Lobulation

The *classical* or *hepatic lobule* has just been outlined. It is a polygonal prism measuring about 1 by 2 mm., and usually appears hexagonal in cross section with a central vein at its center and portal canals peripherally at the corners. It is not delineated by connective tissue in man although it is in some mammals, e.g., the pig. Rarely in man are portal canals found at each of the six corners of the hexagon. It is obvious that such a lobule does not correspond to, for example, a lobule of an exocrine gland in which a lobule is that collection of tissue which drains into a duct, or that which clearly is demarcated by fibrous tissue. However, the classical liver lobule is of some functional significance in that it is a unit of structure from which the blood supply drains to a lobular (central) vein. In that its morphological determination is made by its vascular supply, it will be obvious to the student that the peripheral parts of a lobule, i.e., those nearest the portal vein and hepatic artery, will be supplied best with food materials and oxygen. The central area will not be supplied so well.

Other criteria have been used for demarcating functional units in the liver. A *portal lobule* has as its center a portal canal and consists of the tissue draining bile into the bile duct of that portal area. Such a unit is triangular in cross section, contains parts of three adjacent classical lobules, and has a central vein peripherally at each corner. Pathologically, however, liver damage usually is related to blood supply and a smaller unit of liver structure now is recognized on this basis. This is the *liver acinus* or the *functional unit*. Its dimensions are illustrated in Figure 14-47. As just explained, it is rare

vessels (the central vein) at the center of the lobule, it is obvious that blood flow is from the periphery through the sinusoidal channels between plates of liver cells to the central vein. Bile secretion, on the other hand, is from the liver cells to the small bile ducts at the periphery. Closer examination of a section at higher magnification reveals that each cord or plate of liver cells is so wide as to be composed of at least two rows of liver cells, between which are tiny channels, the bile canaliculi, which drain peripherally in a lobule to bile ducts. These bile canaliculi are simply spaces between adjacent liver cells and have no other lining epithelium. The sinusoidal spaces between liver plates are lined by reticuloendothelial cells, cells lying in a meshwork of fine reticular fibers. Thus,

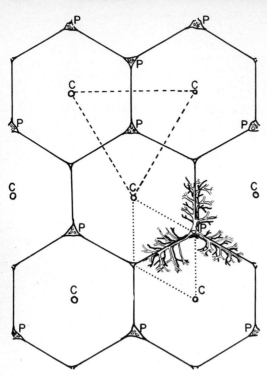

Figure 14-47. Diagram of hepatic lobules. The classical hepatic lobule is outlined with solid lines, the portal lobule with an interrupted line, and the liver acinus or functional unit with a dotted line. The branches of a portal vein and a hepatic artery (solid) from one portal area are shown at lower right. Portal areas are labeled "P," central veins "C." × 40.

to find a portal canal at each corner of the classical lobule. Such deficiencies are supplied by branches from an adjacent area which leave parent vessels at a right angle and course along the border between adjacent classical lobules. The vessels supply and the bile ductule drains an area of diamond shape in cross section with two central veins at two opposite corners and the portal canal branches coursing transversely between them.

Parenchyma (Hepatic Cells)

The parenchymal or hepatic cells are arranged in a series of branching and anastomosing perforated plates or laminae to form a spongework or labyrinth between which are the sinusoidal spaces. These plates extend from the periphery of the classical lobule to the central vein at its center in a radial fashion. Except at the sites of anastomosis and branching, the plates usually are only one cell thick, although

obviously any single parenchymal cell is bordered by several others within a plate. Around portal areas, the liver cells are arranged as a sheet, one cell thick, lying against the periportal connective tissue and termed the limiting plate. The limiting plate is composed of cells somewhat smaller than hepatic cells in the center of the lobule and is perforated by blood vessels (branches of the hepatic artery and the portal vein) and by branches of the bile ducts.

Hepatic cells are polygonal with six or more surfaces, usually 20 to 35 microns in size, and with a clearly defined cell membrane. The surfaces are either external and related to a sinusoidal space, closely applied to the surface of an adjacent liver cell, or partially separated from an adjacent cell to form a bile canaliculus. Nuclei are spherical or ovoid with a regular surface and show considerable variation in size from cell to cell, a variation associated with the condition of polyploidy. Occasionally, binucleate cells are pres-

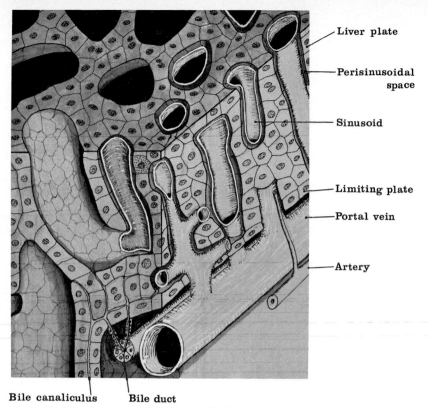

Liver plate

Perisinusoidal
space

Sinusoid

Limiting plate

Portal vein

Artery

Bile canaliculus   Bile duct

Figure 14-48. A three-dimensional diagram of the liver parenchyma in relation to its blood supply. On the front surface (center) one cell is shaded darkly. This cell appears at higher magnification as Figure 14-52.

ent. Each nucleus is vesicular in type with prominent, scattered chromatin granules and one or more nucleoli. Mitosis is rare in adult liver cells but numerous mitotic figures can be found during repair following injury.

The cytoplasm of hepatic cells shows considerable variation dependent upon functional activity, particularly in glycogen and fat storage. Both of these substances usually are removed during routine section preparation but are indicated by a lacelike appearance with spaces of irregular outline and by spherical vacuoles respectively. Present in all cells are clumps of basophil material, usually of such an extent as to give the cytoplasm a slightly basophil reaction. Mitochondria are small but numerous throughout the cytoplasm, and the

Golgi apparatus usually is demonstrable situated either near the nucleus or peripheral and adjacent to a bile canaliculus.

While all parenchymal cells show a similar structure, there are distinct variations in different regions and at different times in relation to feeding. This is dependent upon blood supply. The peripheral cells in a lobule have a good blood supply, but those near the central vein are farthest removed from their blood supply. After feeding, glycogen is deposited first in the peripheral zone. Only after a very heavy carbohydrate meal do the central cells show evidence of glycogen storage. Similarly, when glycogen is removed to increase a falling blood sugar level, glycogen first is removed from the central cells. Under certain conditions,

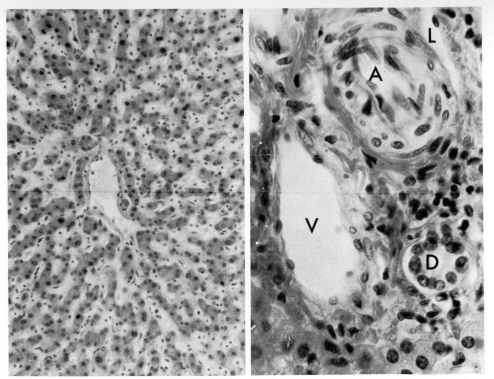

Figure 14-49. Photomicrographs of the human liver to show, left, the central area of a classical lobule with a central vein (× 250) and, right, the portal area with a branch of the hepatic artery (A), a branch of the portal vein (V), a small bile duct (D), and a lymphatic vessel (L). × 750.

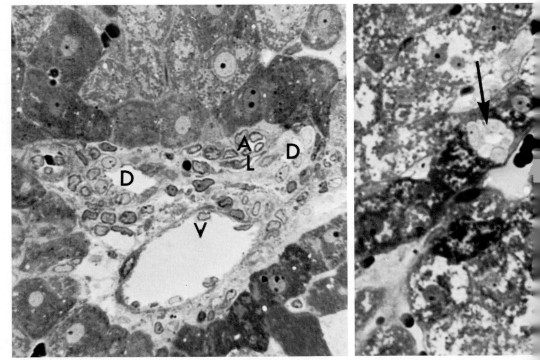

Figure 14-50. Left: Photomicrograph of an Epon section to show a portal area and associated parenchymal tissue. Labeling as in Figure 14-49 (right). × 550. Right: A small area of liver parenchyma in the region of the limiting plate to show a bile ductule or cholangiole (arrow, see page 328). Note that the parenchymal cells contain extensive unstained areas of glycogen. × 850.

324

fat too is deposited in parenchymal cells, and it always appears first in cells adjacent to central veins of lobules. These variations between cells in a lobule are not restricted to inclusions, for mitochondria show distinct morphological changes associated with glycogen storage, being small and spherical in peripheral cells and more slender and elongated in central cells.

Fine Structure

The hepatic parenchymal cell shows no special nuclear features although, as already noted, some binucleate cells are present. In the cytoplasm, both granular and agranular endoplasmic reticula are present, with areas of continuity between the two types. Granular reticulum usually occurs as groups of three to 15 parallel cisternae, the ends of which tend to expand. In addition to ribosomes attached to these membranes, groups of ribosomes or polysomes are present and are thought to be the sites of protein synthesis. The smooth reticulum appears as a meshwork of branching and anastomosing tubules. The Golgi apparatus usually is multiple, located near bile canaliculi, and consists of a few flat, closely packed lamellae, the ends of which may be dilated, containing dense granules 300 to 800 Å in diameter. Mi-

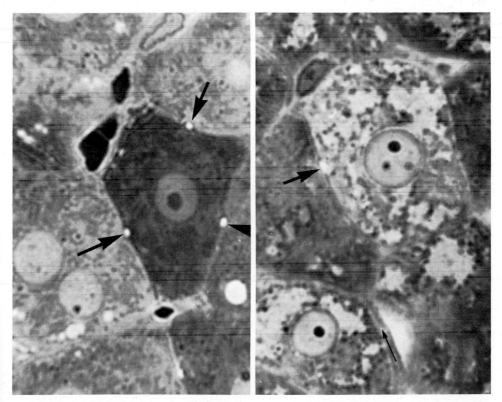

Figure 14-51. Photomicrographs of Epon sections of liver. Left: The dark parenchymal cell at center right shows five surfaces, two short ones adjacent to sinusoids containing red blood corpuscles, and three longer sides adjacent to surrounding parenchymal cells. On each of these three interfaces is a bile canaliculus (arrows). (Compare this cell with Figure 14-52 which has five similar surfaces.) Note also the binucleate cell (bottom left). × 1500. Right: The central parenchymal cell here shows extensive unstained areas of glycogen and one bile canaliculus (broad arrow). At bottom center, the perisinusoidal space between a parenchymal cell and a sinusoid lining is visible (narrow arrow). × 1500.   See filmstrip II, frame 67.

tochondria are numerous. Near bile canaliculi are membrane limited peribiliary bodies, about 0.2 to 0.5 micron in diameter, with an irregular dense internal material. They contain hydrolytic enzymes and are lysosomal in nature. Another body, called a microbody, has a crystalline content in a finely granular matrix and contains the enzyme uricase. The role of peribiliary bodies and microbodies in liver function remains obscure. Glycogen, usually present, appears as dense particles 300 to 400 Å in diameter. The glycogen particles may occur singly or in loose

aggregates 0.1 to 0.2 micron in diameter, usually in close association with areas of smooth reticulum.

The plasma membrane of the hepatic cell is of a typical unit membrane structure, about 75 Å thick, but shows specializations in certain regions. At the surface adjacent to a sinusoidal blood space, the hepatic cell is separated from the wall of the vascular channel by a narrow *perisinusoidal space* (the space of *Disse*) and at this surface the plasma membrane of the hepatic cell is covered by numerous, long microvilli, irregular in shape and size.

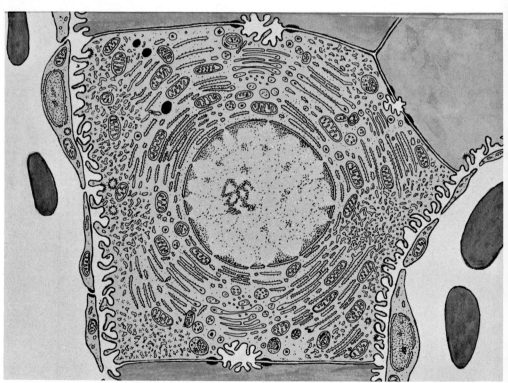

Figure 14-52. This diagram is of a single liver parenchymal cell (it is similar to the cell shaded darkly in Figure 14-48). On left and right sides are sinusoids, lined by reticuloendothelial cells. The parenchymal cell in this section shows five surfaces, two adjacent to sinusoids and separated from reticuloendothelium by the perisinusoidal space, and three opposed to other parenchymal cells. Irregular microvilli protrude into the perisinusoidal space, and on the other three surfaces, three bile canaliculi are illustrated, each limited laterally by desmosomes (maculae adherentes). In the parenchymal cell, the nucleus and its components are shown. In the cytoplasm, note the stacks of cisternae of granular endoplasmic reticulum (ergastoplasm). In some cisternae there are terminal dilatations containing granules in relation to the Golgi apparatus. This illustrates the mechanism of protein secretion in the endoplasmic reticulum and transport to the Golgi apparatus for packaging. In other areas granular endoplasmic reticulum is continuous with smooth endoplasmic reticulum, the latter being associated with particulate glycogen. Other organelles include mitochondria, lysosomes and microbodies.

Some of these microvilli branch. In some regions, however, where connective tissue fibers are present in the perisinusoidal space, microvilli are lacking. In the cytoplasm beneath microvilli, vacuoles and vesicles usually are present. The plasma membranes of adjacent hepatic cells at an interface show some irregularity with adjacent micropinocytotic vesicles in the cytoplasm, and an occasional desmosome near the perisinusoidal space. At the so-called "biliary pole," the two membranes of an interface separate to form an intercellular canal, the bile canaliculus, usually 1 to 2 microns across. Microvilli protrude from plasma membranes into the lumen of the canaliculus, and at each lateral border the interface usually is reinforced by a desmosome.

The union of bile canaliculi with the bile duct system is not easily demonstrated. At the periphery of a lobule, bile canaliculi drain into diverticula at the ends of the smallest bile ducts. These diverticula are located against parenchymal cells of the limiting plate, and then continue as small tubules with very thin walls. These short tubules, called bile ductules or *cholangioles*, pass in turn to bile ducts found in portal areas. The bile ducts have much more substantial walls and a wider lumen than the ductules.

Bile Canaliculi

Bile canaliculi can be seen occasionally in routine H and E preparations as tiny cavities between adjacent hepatic cells but can be better demonstrated by special staining methods, e.g., Gomori's reaction for alkaline phosphatase or silver impregnation. They form a three-dimensional network between liver cells, the walls of the canaliculi being adjacent parenchymal cells as just described. The junctions of bile

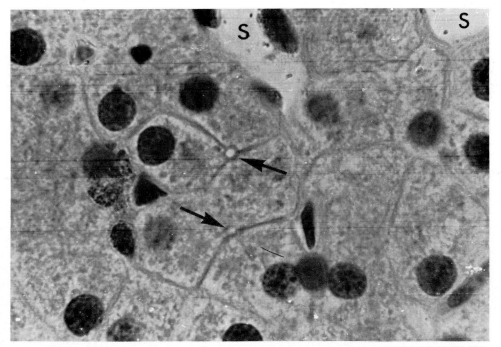

Figure 14-53. Photomicrograph of liver to demonstrate two bile canaliculi (arrows) between parenchymal cells. Two sinusoidal spaces (S) are visible. The spherical nuclei with chromatin granules are nuclei of parenchymal cells. The dark, irregular, or elongated nuclei are of cells associated with sinusoids. × 1500.

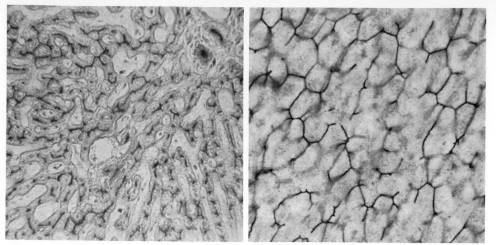

Figure 14-54. Photomicrographs to demonstrate bile canaliculi. Left: Alkaline phosphatase technique. A portal area is shown in the top right corner. (Courtesy of F. Jacoby.) × 200. Right: Silver injection. × 350.

canaliculi with bile ducts at the periphery of a lobule are not demonstrated easily. The junctions occur by means of an intermediate structure called the *ductule* or *canal of Hering.* At the periphery of a lobule, the parenchymal cells which form the wall of the bile canaliculus are replaced gradually by smaller, lighter-staining cells with dark nuclei and poorly developed organelles. These cells, the ductule cells, are underlain by a distinct basal lamina. The lumen of such a ductule eventually joins that of a bile duct in a portal area.

Blood Channels Within the Lobule

Sinusoidal Spaces. As previously explained, the blood supply of the liver lobule is via the sinusoids which form a very extensive spongework between the plates of hepatic cells. Blood enters the sinusoidal meshwork at the periphery of the lobule from interlobular branches of portal vein and hepatic artery and passes in a radial fashion through sinusoidal spaces to drain from the lobule by the central vein.

Sinusoidal spaces differ from capil-

laries in that they are of greater diameter (9 to 12 microns) and their lining cells are not typically of endothelium. The basal lamina around sinusoids is incomplete. Two main types of cell, with intermediate forms, are present in the sinusoidal lining of the adult liver.

"ENDOTHELIAL" TYPE. This cell has a small, elongated, darkly staining nucleus with greatly attenuated cytoplasm. The cytoplasm may interdigitate with, or even overlie, cytoplasmic processes of adjacent similar cells and cells of the second type. Organelles are few and small.

PHAGOCYTIC (STELLATE) CELL OF KUPFFER. This cell has a larger, paler nucleus and more obvious cytoplasm with processes which may extend into or even across a sinusoidal space. These cells are actively phagocytic and may contain pigment granules, engulfed and degenerating erythrocytes, and iron-containing granules. Because of this property of phagocytosis, the cells of Kupffer can be demonstrated by intravital injections of vital dyes, e.g., trypan blue, and particulate material, e.g., India ink.

Although not all sinusoid-lining cells are phagocytic, it is probable that all can become so and that the stellate cells of Kupffer are increased in number in time of need by differentiation

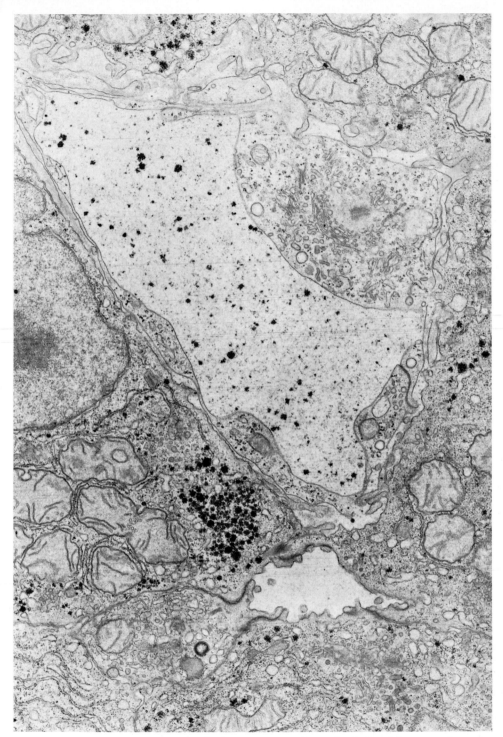

Figure 14-55. Electron micrograph of a hepatic sinusoid completely lined by parts of two sinus-lining cells. A narrow space (of Disse) separates it from surrounding parenchymal cells between which a bile canaliculus is shown below the sinusoid. The small, very dense particles are glycogen, some of which are present also in the lumen of the sinusoid. × 17,000. (Courtesy of J. Steiner and Anne-Marie Jezequel.)

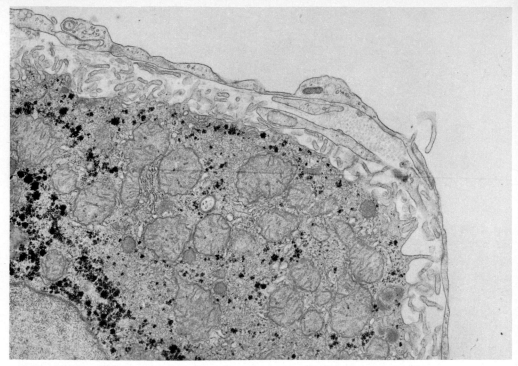

Figure 14-56.   Electron micrograph to show the perisinusoidal space of Disse. Note the irregular microvilli of a parenchymal cell protruding into the space which separates the parenchymal cell from reticuloendothelium lining sinusoids. There are a few collagen fibrils in the space. × 15,000. (Courtesy of J. Steiner and Anne-Marie Jezequel.)

of the more primitive, endothelial cells.

The sinusoids usually show some dilatation at their terminations into a central vein or a larger sublobular tributary of a hepatic vein, and there is some evidence that there are sphincteric mechanisms of smooth muscle at these sites.

One question concerning sinusoids is whether or not the lining is discontinuous. Discontinuities in the sinusoidal lining have been demonstrated by the electron microscope using a variety of preparative techniques, and particulate material of small diameter (following injection into the portal vein) rapidly passes into the perisinusoidal space. As just noted, the basal lamina around sinusoids is incomplete and thus there is no morphological barrier between sinusoids and the perisinusoidal space. There is direct access of plasma to the surface of the liver cell, a structural feature of great functional importance for active metabolic exchange between the liver and the blood. The perisinusoidal space itself is not a true lymph channel, for it is not lined by endothelium and is to be regarded as an interstitial space containing some formed reticular and collagenous fibers but in which fluid may circulate freely. Probably it plays an important role in lymph production (see page 332). Also contained in the perisinusoidal space are a few mesenchymal cells referred to as "pericytes," "fat storing cells," or "extravascular reticular cells." This cell in the adult liver is closely associated with reticular and collagenous fibers and probably is responsible for their formation. In fetal liver, this primitive mesenchymal cell probably is the stem cell for hemopoiesis. It differs from the two types of sinusoid lining cell not only in location but in that it does not be-

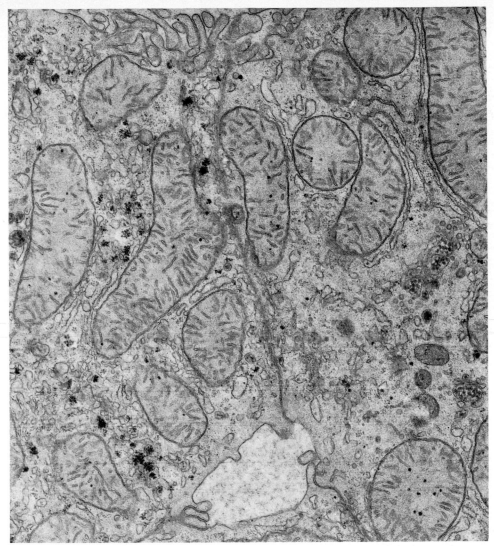

Figure 14-57. Electron micrograph to show a bile canaliculus (bottom) between three parenchymal hepatic cells. Microvilli at top center are in the space of Disse. × 28,000. (Courtesy of J. Steiner and Anne-Marie Jezequel.)

come phagocytic toward particulate material.

Central Veins. These are centrally located in the lobules and are the smallest radicles of the hepatic veins. They drain into larger sublobular veins which in turn join to form collecting veins, which themselves are tributaries of hepatic veins. The last drain directly into the inferior vena cava. Sinusoids normally drain into central veins although a few probably open directly into sublobular veins.

Portal Canals (Portal Areas). These are surrounded by small amounts of fibroconnective tissue and contain the "portal triad" of hepatic artery, portal vein, and bile duct, usually with a lymphatic vessel. The largest structure usually is the branch of the portal vein and is thin-walled; the smallest is the artery or arteriole, a branch of the hepatic artery; the bile duct is intermediate in size and recognized by its lining of cubical epithelial cells. In that a portal area is a region of

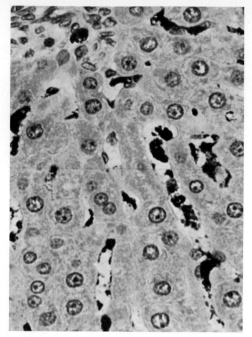

Figure 14-58. Photomicrograph of rat liver from an animal after intravital injection of India ink (carbon). The carbon particles (black) have been phagocytosed by the cells of Kupffer. × 450.

branching, commonly multiples of the triad are seen. Lymphatic vessels appear as slitlike spaces lined by endothelium. All components of a portal canal increase in size and are surrounded by stronger fibroconnective tissue nearer the hilum. The larger bile ducts are lined by a columnar epithelium.

In small portal areas, the portal vein gives off smaller venules with lateral branches lying between lobules. From these arise the terminal twigs which penetrate the limiting plate of hepatic cells and open directly into sinusoids. The terminal branchings of the hepatic artery are similar although some are said to penetrate deeply into a lobule before opening into a sinusoid. Direct communications between terminal branches of hepatic artery and portal vein also are said to exist but probably they are few in number and unimportant.

The lymphatic drainage of the liver via the large vessels in the porta hepatis is profuse but the origin of the lymph itself remains the subject of controversy. The fine lymphatic channels in small portal areas appear to terminate blindly in the connective tissue, and no direct communication with the perisinusoidal spaces has been established. However, the fluid of these spaces may be discharged into interstitial spaces of the connective tissue and thus pass indirectly into the lymphatic capillaries. Presumably, flow in the perisinusoidal spaces is toward the periphery of the lobule but this must be exceedingly sluggish and perhaps intermittent consequent upon variations in blood pressure in the sinusoidal spaces.

A few fine unmyelinated nerve fibers of the autonomic nervous system accompany the portal canals.

Stroma

Connective tissue of the liver, a large organ, is sparse. Over the liver surface, covered in most areas by the mesothelium of the peritoneum, is the relatively dense fibroconnective tissue of Glisson's capsule which at the porta hepatis is continuous with that around the portal canals. By this means, the entire organ is permeated by a fibroconnective tissue skeleton composed of collagenous fibers with relatively few cells, the majority of which are fibroblasts. Within the lobule, there is a fine meshwork of reticular and collagenous fibers around the sinusoids and within the perisinusoidal spaces, but no fibroblasts. The fibers here are elaborated and maintained by the sinus-lining cells and the pericytes of the perisinusoidal spaces. This fine meshwork is continuous at the periphery of the lobule with the connective tissue surrounding the terminal branches of the components of the portal canals.

Regeneration

After injury the liver shows quite a remarkable degree of regeneration.

The organization of the repair process depends upon the nature of the injury, but remaining hepatic cells are capable of both hypertrophy and hyperplasia. Bile ducts also actively proliferate, and it is possible that new hepatic cells may arise from this source also.

Functions

The liver is essential to life and, because of its unique position interposed in the venous drainage of the digestive tract, it is liable to damage from absorbed toxic materials. It subserves several functions. It is important in the maintenance of blood glucose concentration. Parenchymal cells take up blood glucose and store it as glycogen: glycogen also is formed from other compounds such as lactic and pyruvic acids. The liver also is important in lipid metabolism in that lipid is transported in the blood as lipoprotein, this substance being formed in the liver. It stores also vitamins A and B and heparin (originating in mast cells). It secretes bile salts into the biliary system and fibrinogen (an antianemic factor) and plasma albumins into the blood. Also, it synthesizes cholesterol, excretes bile pigments from the breakdown of hemoglobin of damaged erythrocytes, and produces urea (a byproduct of protein metabolism). Detoxication of various toxic materials circulating in the blood, phagocytosis of particulate material by the cells of Kupffer, and hemopoiesis in the fetus and newborn are additional functions.

Development

The liver develops as a ventral diverticulum (endoderm) of the fore- and

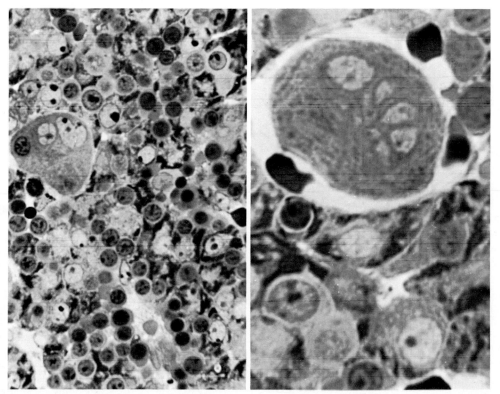

Figure 14-59. Photomicrographs of Epon sections of fetal liver to show hemopoiesis. Left: The normal liver structure is obscured by masses of cells of the red blood cell and granulocyte series. One megakaryocyte is shown. × 650. Right: A similar area showing a megakaryocyte. × 1250.

mid-gut junction and extends anteriorly into the mesenchyme of the septum transversum. Proliferation of the endodermal cells gives rise to the cords and plates of hepatic cells, which at first are tubular in arrangement with cells arranged around a central lumen. The sinusoids develop from vascular tissue associated with the vitelline veins, which themselves form the portal vein. Mesenchyme associated with the portal vein and that of the septum transversum develop into the connective tissue and capsule of the organ.

The original diverticulum of the gut and its main branches remain tubular as the bile and hepatic ducts. The gallbladder and cystic duct develop as a diverticulum from the main duct.

The liver, as stated before, is one of the main blood-forming organs in the fetus and retains this potentiality in the adult.

The Extrahepatic Biliary Passages

The arrangement of the major biliary passages is illustrated in Figure 14-60.

Extrahepatic Ducts. These all are lined by a tall columnar epithelium which is mucus-secreting. There is a

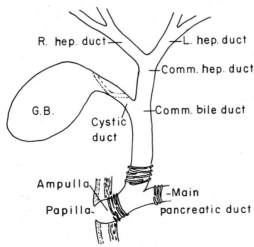

Figure 14-60. Diagram of the main bile duct system. The sphincter muscles and the spiral valve of the cystic duct are indicated.

layer of subepithelial connective tissue with a preponderance of elastic fibers and a marked lymphoid tendency. Many lymphocytes and occasional granulocytes are found migrating through the epithelium into the lumen. In the subepithelial layer there may be accumulations of tubuloacinar glands, mostly mucous in type, and blood vessels and nerves are prominent. In the common bile duct, there is in addition a layer of smooth muscle, at first composed of isolated bundles of smooth muscle fibers but near the duodenum forming a complete investment of oblique and transverse fibers. This layer, particularly the circular fibers, is thickened at the termination of the common bile duct (the sphincter of Boyden) and around the ampulla of the conjoined bile and pancreatic ducts just proximal to the ampullary opening into the duodenum (the sphincter of Oddi). Because the common bile duct traverses the lesser omentum, it is covered also by peritoneum.

THE GALLBLADDER

The gallbladder is a blind, pear-shaped diverticulum of the common hepatic duct to which it is connected by the *cystic duct.* The gallbladder is approximately 3 inches in length and 1½ inches in diameter but is capable of considerable distention. Its wall is composed of three layers:

Mucous Membrane

When empty, the mucosa is thrown into many folds or rugae and thus is irregular in section, often with the appearance of simple glands. All epithelial cells are similar, tall, columnar cells, with basally located nuclei. Electron microscopy demonstrates a fine, microvillous apical border. The cells are supported by a fine basal lamina and a lamina propria of delicate, reticular connective tissue with nu-

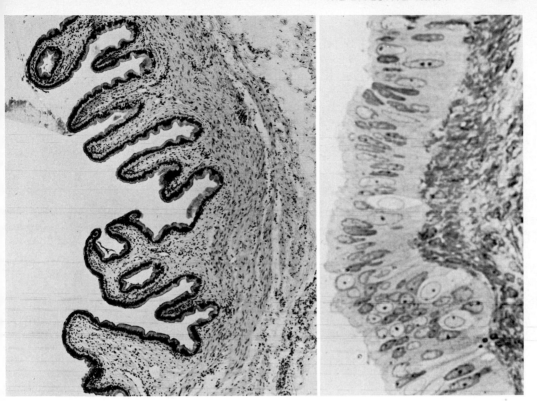

Figure 14-61. Left: Photomicrograph of the gallbladder. × 40. Right: Photomicrograph of the simple columnar epithelium lining the common bile duct. Epon section. × 550.

merous small blood vessels. Occasional small lymph nodules are present with a few mucous glands at the neck of the gallbladder.

Muscularis

There is no submucosa in the gallbladder and external to the mucosa is a layer of smooth muscle, irregular in thickness and orientation of its component bundles. In any section, smooth muscle will be cut in all possible planes, for the muscularis is a meshwork of interlacing bundles of smooth muscle fibers between which are collagenous, reticular, and some elastic fibers.

Adventitia or Serosa

The gallbladder lies on the inferior surface of the liver and its outer coat of dense fibroconnective tissue blends in

some regions with that of Glisson's capsule. Elsewhere the adventitia is covered by peritoneum.

The neck of the gallbladder continues into the cystic duct, and here the mucous membrane is thrown into a spiral fold with a core containing smooth muscle. This is termed the *spiral valve of Heister* and is believed to prevent sudden changes in capacity of the gallbladder following changes of pressure. The gallbladder itself functions as a reservoir for bile, secreted continuously by the liver but discharged intermittently into the intestine. In the gallbladder bile is concentrated by absorption of fluid by the epithelium.

REFERENCES

Beidler, L. M., and Smallman, R. L.: Renewal of cells within taste buds. J. Cell Biol., 27:263, 1965.
Bevelander, G.: Atlas of Oral Histology and

Embryology. Philadelphia, Lea & Febiger, 1967.

Bevelander, G., and Nakahara, H.: The formation and mineralization of dentin. Anat. Rec., 156:303, 1966.

Blackwood, H. J. J. (editor): Bone and Tooth, Proceedings of the First European Symposium. Oxford, Pergamon Press, 1964.

Boyden, E. A.: The sphincter of Oddi in man and certain representative mammals. Surgery, 1:25, 1937.

Burkel, W. E., and Low, F. N.: The fine structure of rat liver sinusoids, space of Disse and associated tissue space. Amer. J. Anat., 118:769, 1966.

Cardell, R. R., Jr., Badenhausen, S., and Porter, K. R.: Intestinal triglyceride absorption in the rat. An electron microscopical study. J. Cell Biol., 34:123, 1967.

Caro, L. G., and Palade, G. E.: Protein synthesis, storage, and discharge in the pancreatic exocrine cell. An autoradiographic study. J. Cell Biol., 20:473, 1964.

Daems, W. T.: The fine structure of mouse-liver microbodies. Microscop., 5:294, 1966.

Elias, H.: A re-examination of the structure of the mammalian liver: I, Parenchymal architecture. Amer. J. Anat., 84:311, 1949.

Elias, H., and Selkurt, E. E.: Hepatoportallienal circulation. In Blood Vessels and Lymphatics, edited by D. I. Abramson. New York, Academic Press, 1962.

Elwood, W. K., and Bernstein, M. H.: The ultrastructure of the enamel organ related to enamel formation. Amer. J. Anat., 122:73, 1968.

Hampton, J. C.: Liver. In Electron Microscopic Anatomy, edited by S. M. Kurtz. New York, Academic Press, 1964.

Herman, L., Sato, T., and Fitzgerald, P. J.: The pancreas. In Electron Microscopic Anatomy, edited by S. M. Kurtz. New York, Academic Press, 1964.

Ito, S.: The fine structure of the gastric mucosa. In Gastric Secretion Mechanisms and Control. Proceedings of the Symposium at The Faculty of Medicine, University of Alberta, Edmonton, Canada, September 13-15, 1965. Pergamon Press. Oxford and New York, 1967.

Ito, S.: Anatomic structure of the gastric mucosa. In Handbook of Physiology of the Alimentary Canal. Bethesda, Md., American Physiological Society, 1967, Vol. 2, pp. 705-741.

Jamieson, J. D., and Palade, G. E.: Intracellular transport of secretory proteins in the pancreatic exocrine cell. I. Role of the peripheral elements of the Golgi complex. J. Cell Biol., 34:577, 1967.

Jamieson, J. D., and Palade, G. E.: Intracellular transport of secretory proteins in the pancreatic exocrine cell. II. Transport to condensing vacuoles and zymogen granules. J. Cell Biol., 34:597, 1967.

Lacy, P. E.: The pancreatic beta cell. New Eng. J. Med., 276:187, 1967.

Leeson, C. R.: Structure of salivary glands. In Handbook of Physiology of the Alimentary Canal. Bethesda, Md., American Physiological Society, 1967, Vol. 2, pp. 463-495.

Mall, F. P.: A study of the structural unit of the liver. Amer. J. Anat., 5:227, 1906.

McMinn, R. M. H., and Kugler, J. H.: The glands of the bile and pancreatic ducts, autoradiographic and histochemical studies. J. Anat., 95:1, 1961.

Nylen, M. V.: Electron microscope and allied biophysical approaches to the study of enamel mineralization. J. Roy. Micr. Soc., 83:135, 1964.

Parks, H. F.: An experimental study of microscopic and submicroscopic lipid inclusions in hepatic cells of the mouse. Amer. J. Anat., 120:253, 1967.

Rappaport, A. M.: The structural and functional unit in the human liver (liver acinus). Anat. Rec., 130:673, 1958.

Rouiller, C.: The Liver. New York, Academic Press, 1964, Vol. 2.

Sedar, A. W.: Fine structure of the stimulated oxyntic cell. Fed. Proc. 24:1360, 1965.

Schour, I. (editor): Noyes' Oral Histology and Embryology, ed. 8. Philadelphia, Lea & Febiger, 1960.

Selkurt, E. E.: Gastrointestinal circulation. Microscopic anatomy. In Blood Vessels and Lymphatics, edited by D. I. Abramson, New York, Academic Press, 1962.

Sicher, H. (editor): Orban's Oral Histology and Embryology, ed. 5. St. Louis, C. V. Mosby, 1962.

Travis, D. F., and Glimcher, M. J.: The structure and organization of, and the relationship between the organic matrix and the inorganic crystals of, embryonic bovine enamel. J. Cell Biol., 23:447, 1964.

Walls, E. W.: Anorectal anatomy. Sci. Basis Med. Ann. Rev., 113, 1963.

Yamada, E.: The fine structure of the gall bladder epithelium of the mouse. J. Biophys. Biochem. Cytol., 1:445, 1955.

Zetterquist, H.: The ultrastructural organization of the columnar absorbing cells of the mouse jejunum. Stockholm, Karolinska Institutet, Aktiebolaget Godvil, 1956.

CHAPTER 15

RESPIRATORY SYSTEM

The main function of the respiratory system is to provide for an intake of oxygen by the blood and to eliminate carbon dioxide. *Respiratory tissue,* where these gaseous exchanges occur, is sited in the lungs, which lie within the thoracic cavity. This cavity virtually is a closed space. The lungs are connected to the exterior by a series of passages — the nose, the pharynx, the larynx, the trachea, and the bronchi. These passages are relatively rigid structures and are constantly patent, and together they comprise the *conducting* portion of the respiratory system. Thus, if the capacity of the thoracic cavity is increased, air will be drawn through the conducting tubes into the lung. Such inspiratory movements can be effective in drawing air into the lungs only if the passages to the exterior remain open, which explains why the conducting part of the respiratory system is rigid. This part also has other functions — it strains out particulate matter in the inspired air, washes and humidifies the air, and either warms or cools the air dependent upon the ambient temperature.

THE NOSE

The nose is a cavity divided by a midline septum into right and left nasal cavities. Each communicates an-

teriorly with the exterior by an *anterior naris,* or nostril, and posteriorly with the upper part of the pharynx, the nasopharynx, by a *posterior naris.* With the exception of the anterior naris, each nasal cavity has a rigid wall of bone and hyaline cartilage. The wall of the anterior naris is of fibroconnective tissue and cartilage and its dimensions can be varied by muscular action. Each nasal cavity is divided into a *vestibule,* the wider part immediately behind the anterior naris, and a *respiratory* part, which comprises the remainder.

The skin covering the external surface of the nose, which is characterized by some large sebaceous glands, extends into the anterior part of the vestibule where it contains some sebaceous and sweat glands and hair follicles with stiff, thick hairs. These hairs function to strain out coarse particles from the inspired air. Deeper in the vestibule, the stratified squamous epithelium becomes nonkeratinizing, and this type of epithelium gives way in the respiratory part of the nasal cavity to a pseudostratified ciliated columnar epithelium with goblet cells.

The epithelium which lines the respiratory passages lies upon a basal lamina which separates it from the underlying fibroconnective tissue, the lamina propria, in which are both

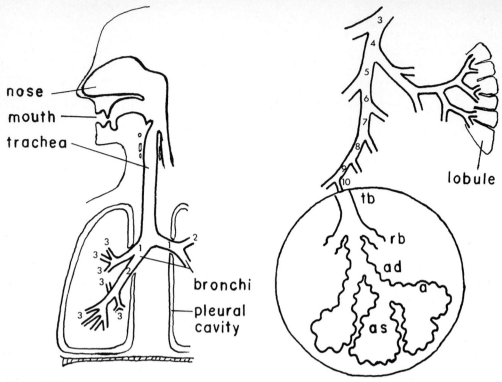

Figure 15-1. Diagram of the respiratory system. The numbers indicate the divisions of the bronchial tree; tb = terminal bronchiole; rb = respiratory bronchiole; ad = alveolar duct; as = alveolar sac; a = alveolus.

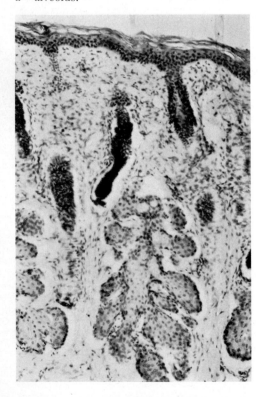

Figure 15-2. Section of the vestibule of the nose, showing large, lobulated sebaceous glands in the dermis. × 70.

mucous and serous glands. The deepest layer of the lamina propria blends into, and is continuous with, the periosteum or perichondrium of bone or cartilage in the wall of the nasal cavity. Accordingly, the mucous membrane of the nose often is termed a *mucoperiosteum* or a *mucoperichondrium* (the schneiderian membrane). The lamina propria contains both collagenous and elastic fibers, and fibroblasts, macrophages, lymphocytes, plasma cells, and granular leukocytes. Small collections of lymphatic tissue are characteristic, especially posteriorly near the nasopharynx.

In a frontal section, the nasal cavity is pear-shaped and is divided by the median nasal septum. Protruding into the cavity from the lateral wall are three curved plates of bone covered by the mucous membrane. These bones are the superior, middle, and inferior *conchae* (concha is a shell) or *turbinate* (scroll-like) bones. Of these, the inferior is the largest and it is covered by a thicker mucous membrane. In the lamina propria here, and elsewhere to a lesser degree, are numerous thin-walled, venous sinuses. This tissue has been termed *cavernous* or *erectile* tissue, but differs from the true erectile tissue of the penis in that it is venous in nature and that the smooth muscle which is present is located in the walls of the venous spaces and not in the septa between cavernous spaces.

The surface of the respiratory passage epithelium is covered with a layer of mucus produced by its goblet cells and by the glands in the lamina propria. The cilia of the ciliated cells in the epithelium constantly move this mucus backward to the nasopharynx whence it is either swallowed or expectorated. The mucous layer serves to pick up particulate matter in the air, which thus is eliminated from the inspired air. The fluid secretions from serous and mucous glands humidify the inspired air, which also is warmed by blood temperature in the dilated venous sinuses of the erectile tissue.

Organ of Smell

In the roof of each nasal cavity and extending down over the superior concha and the adjacent part of the septum is a region where the fresh mucous membrane is yellowish-brown in contrast to the pink color of the ordinary respiratory area. This specialized area contains the receptor organs for smell, and is called the *olfactory region* or *olfactory mucosa*.

The olfactory epithelium is pseudostratified columnar, lacks goblet cells, and has no distinct basal lamina. Three types of cell comprise the epithelium.

Supporting or Sustentacular Cells. These are tall, cylindrical cells, broad at their apices and narrow at their bases. The nuclei are oval and situated just above the center of the cells toward their apices. Near the nucleus is a small Golgi apparatus, and the apical surface shows a fine, striated border.

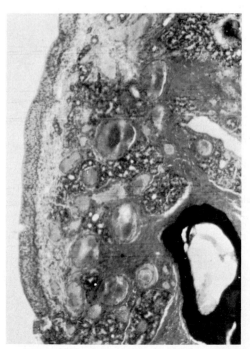

Figure 15-3. Section across the superior turbinate bone (black) with covering of olfactory epithelium and numerous glands and dilated venous channels in the connective tissue. × 40.   See filmstrip II, frame 68.

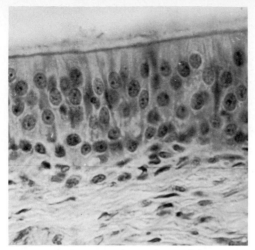

Figure 15-4. Section of the pseudostratified ciliated columnar epithelium (schneiderian membrane) of the nasal cavity. × 650.

This border is formed by long, slender microvilli which project into an overlying layer of mucus. The cells also contain a few pigment granules of a yellowish brown color.

Basal Cells. These are small, conical cells with dark, ovoid nuclei, and branching cytoplasmic processes.

Olfactory or Sensory Cells. These are evenly distributed between the supporting cells and are bipolar nerve cells. They are spindle-shaped with a central, nucleus-containing area and a peripheral (apical) slender process, a dendrite, which extends to the surface between supporting cells. This process terminates in a small, bulblike expansion called the *olfactory vesicle,* from which six to eight small, hairlike processes extend. These are the *olfactory hairs,* which are modified cilia and which function as the actual receptive elements. The proximal part of the cell narrows to a fine, cylindrical process about 1 micron in diameter, and this passes into the underlying lamina propria as the axon. Throughout the cytoplasm of the cell, neurofibrils can be demonstrated. In the lamina propria, the olfactory nerve fibers or axons are collected into small bundles, the *fila olfactoria,* which then pass superiorly through the fine canals of the cribriform plate of the ethmoid bone to enter the olfactory bulb of the brain. Also within the lamina propria are lymph and venous plexuses, the former communicating with the subarachnoid space via capillaries running with the fila olfactoria.

Within the lamina propria of the olfactory epithelium are branched, tubu-

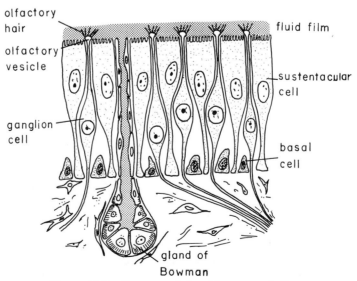

Figure 15-5. Diagram of the olfactory epithelium.

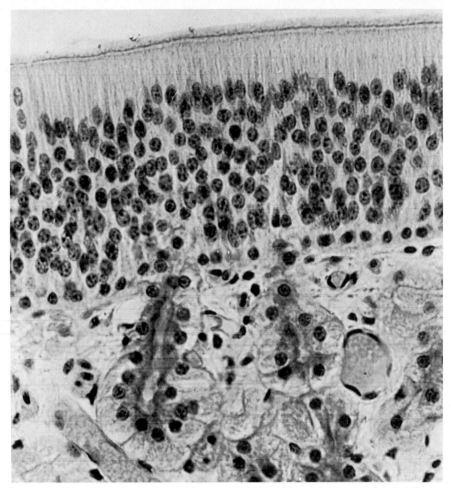

Figure 15-6. Photomicrograph of the olfactory epithelium. Note the serous glands (of Bowman) in the lamina propria. × 450.   See filmstrip II, frame 69.

loacinar serous glands (the *glands of Bowman*) from which a watery secretion is carried to the surface by narrow ducts. The secretion of Bowman's glands moistens the surface of the olfactory epithelium and serves as a solvent for odoriferous substances. Its continuous secretion serves to freshen the surface film of fluid and prevents repetition of stimulation of the olfactory hairs by a single odor. Repeated exposure of the sensory cells to trauma from infection and other causes results in frequent damage to, and loss of, some sensory cells. Consequently it is usual for the sense of smell to be diminished in the elderly, who show an atypical olfactory epithelium.

PARANASAL AIR SINUSES

The paranasal air sinuses are connected with the nasal cavities and are air-filled cavities within the bones of the skull. They are four in number and are termed the maxillary, frontal, ethmoidal, and sphenoidal sinuses. The epithelium lining them is continuous with that of the nose and also is of the pseudostratified ciliated columnar type. However, it is thinner and shows fewer goblet cells, and the basal lamina is poorly developed. The lamina propria too is thinner and contains fewer glands than that of the nose, and erectile tissue is not present. Like the mucosa of the nose, its deeper layers are continuous with periosteum, from which it cannot be separated.

THE NASOPHARYNX

The pharynx is a chamber, flattened anteroposteriorly, through which both food and air pass. It is subdivided into: the *nasopharynx*, situated below the base of the skull, behind the posterior nares of the nose, and above the soft palate; the *oropharynx*, behind the oral cavity and posterior surface of the tongue; and the *laryngopharynx*, behind the larynx.

The lateral and posterior walls of the pharynx are muscular, and thus the chamber can dilate or, by muscular contraction, be occluded. The nasopharynx, however, although its dimensions can change, cannot be closed completely. By apposition of the soft palate and the posterior wall of the pharynx, the nasopharynx can be isolated completely from the oropharynx. This movement occurs in swallowing, for normally no food material is permitted to enter the nasopharynx.

The epithelium lining the nasopharynx is either pseudostratified ciliated columnar or stratified squamous, the latter occurring in regions where the surface is subject to attrition, e.g., over the posterior edge of the soft palate and at the posterior wall of the pharynx where these two surfaces come into contact during the movement of swallowing. Elsewhere, a respiratory passage type of epithelium with some goblet cells is present. The lamina propria in this region contains much elastic tissue, especially externally where it is in contact with the striated pharyngeal constrictor muscles. A loose submucosa is present only in the lateral parts of the nasopharynx. In the lamina propria, glands are present, mainly of the mucous type, but serous and mixed glands also are found. Lymphatic tissue is abundant throughout the pharynx, and true lymphatic follicles are present posteriorly in the nasopharynx (the ad-enoids or pharyngeal tonsil), laterally on each side at the junction of oral cavity and oropharynx (the palatine tonsil), and in the root of the tongue (the lingual tonsil) (see Chapter 12). Collections of lymphoid tissue laterally in the nasopharynx around the openings of the pharyngotympanic (eustachian) tubes sometimes are of sufficient size to merit the term "tubal tonsil."

THE LARYNX

The larynx is that segment of the respiratory tract which connects the pharynx and the trachea. In addition to its function as part of the respiratory conducting system it plays an important role in phonation. In its wall there is a "skeleton" of hyaline and elastic cartilages, some connective tissue, striated muscle, and a mucous membrane containing serous and mucous glands. Figure 15-7 explains the relationship of these structures. The major cartilages of the larynx (the thyroid, cricoid, and arytenoids) are hyaline, the smaller (the corniculates, cuneiforms, and tips of the arytenoids) are elastic, as is the cartilage of the epiglottis. The cartilages, together with the hyoid bone, are connected by three large, flat membranes, the thyrohyoid, the quadrates, and the cricovocal. They are composed of dense fibroconnective tissue in which many elastic fibers are present, particularly in the cricovocal membrane. As illustrated in Figure 15-7, the true and false vocal cords (vocal and vestibular ligaments) are respectively the free upper borders of the cricovocal (cricothyroid) and the free lower borders of the quadrate (aryepiglottic) membranes. Extending laterally on each side between the true and false cords are the sinus and saccule of the larynx, a small slitlike diverticulum. The cricoid cartilage has the shape of a signet ring, broader posteriorly than anteriorly, and the cavity within it is continuous below with the lumen of the trachea. Behind the cricoid and arytenoid cartilages, the pos-

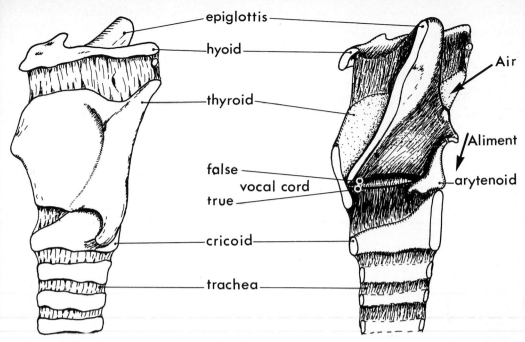

Figure 15-7.   Diagrams of the larynx. Left: External appearance, as seen from the left side. Right: A sagittal section, looking toward the right half of the specimen. The rima glottidis, the narrowest part of the larynx, lies between the two true vocal cords.

terior wall of the pharynx is formed by the striated muscle of the pharyngeal constrictor muscles, which is continuous at the lower border of the cricoid cartilage with the intrinsic musculature of the esophagus. Thus, from the larynx, the air passage extends between the vocal folds (the rima glottidis) through the cavity of the cricoid to the trachea, and aliment passes over the posterior surface of the cricoid into the lumen of the esophagus.

The epithelium of the mucous membrane lining the larynx varies with location. Over the anterior surface and upper one-third to one-half of the posterior surface of the epiglottis, the aryepiglottic folds (upper edges of the quadrate membranes), and the vocal cords, the epithelium is stratified, squamous, and nonkeratinizing. All these moist surfaces are subject to wear and tear. Over the remainder of the larynx, there is a pseudostratified ciliated columnar epithelium with

goblet cells, i.e., a typical respiratory tract epithelium. Although the epithelium above the vocal folds mainly is pseudostratified ciliated columnar in type, patches of stratified squamous epithelium are found commonly. Over the vocal folds, the lamina propria of the stratified squamous epithelium is dense and bound firmly to the underlying connective tissue of the vocal ligament. There is no true submucosa in the larynx, but the lamina propria of the mucous membrane is thick and contains numerous elastic fibers. Within it are tubuloacinar glands, of which the majority are mucous. Some acini possess serous crescents, and some purely serous secretory units also are present. In the epiglottis, mainly mixed salivary glands are present on both surfaces, predominantly on the posterior surface, and often they lie in irregular depressions in the elastic cartilage. On the posterior or laryngeal surface, there are a few taste buds

THE TRACHEA

The trachea is a rigid tube about 10 to 12 cm. long and 2 to 2.5 cm. in diameter, continuous above with the cricoid ring. It extends down through the lower part of the neck and superior mediastinum of the thorax where it terminates by dividing into the right and left main bronchi. It has a relatively thin wall and is pliable and capable of elongation with respiratory and postural movements.

The patency of the trachea is maintained by a series of about 20 horseshoe-shaped cartilages of irregular outline orientated one above the other with the deficiencies posteriorly. These cartilages on longitudinal section of the trachea are flat externally and convex internally. Between adjacent rings of hyaline cartilage, the relatively narrow gaps are filled by fibroconnective tissue which blends with the perichondrium of the rings. Numerous elastic fibers are present in this connective tissue and the bundles of collagenous fibers are so orientated as to give added elasticity to the tube. Posteriorly in the gaps between the ends of each horseshoe cartilage are interlacing bundles of smooth muscle fibers (the *musculus trachealis*), orientated mainly transversely and attached to the cartilages and elastic connective tissue so as to diminish the diameter of the trachea on contraction. External to the tube is loose fibroconnective tissue, termed the adventitia, containing small blood vessels and nerves (autonomic) which supply the trachea.

Internal to the cartilages is the submucosa, a layer of loose areolar fibroconnective tissue containing numerous small mixed glands and some serous secretory units. These glands lie mainly between adjacent cartilaginous rings and posteriorly, both within and external to, the smooth muscle. Their ducts pierce the lamina propria of the mucosa to open on the surface. Blood and lymph capillaries are prominent in this layer.

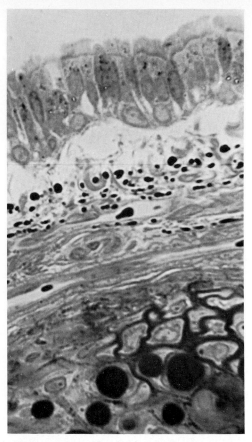

Figure 15-8. Photomicrograph of a section through part of the epiglottis to show the laryngeal surface. Note the typical respiratory tract type of epithelium (top), a loose lamina propria containing numerous elastic fibers (black), and elastic cartilage of the epiglottis (below). Epon section. × 550.

in the surface epithelium. Lymph nodules are scattered in the lamina propria.

Cilia of the laryngeal epithelium, as in all respiratory passages, beat toward the pharynx.

In any section of the larynx, striated muscle fibers will be found. In the posterior and posterolateral walls these are fibers of the constrictor muscles. In relation to the quadrate and cricovocal membranes they are fibers of the intrinsic musculature of the larynx, muscles associated with phonation, breathing, and swallowing.

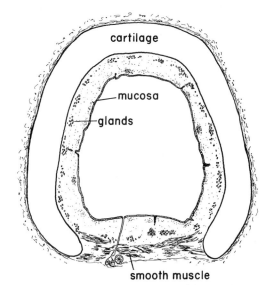

Figure 15-9. Diagram of a transverse section of the trachea.

cartilage

mucosa

glands

smooth muscle

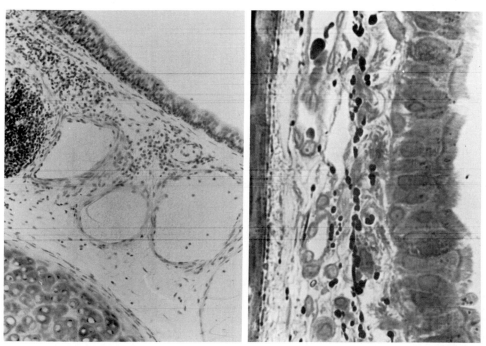

Figure 15-10. Transverse sections through the trachea. Left: Note the dilated venous channels and lymphatic tissue in the submucosa. × 140. Right: A higher magnification showing epithelium with cilia, lamina propria, submucosa, and the edge of a cartilage ring. Elastic tissue appears black and is concentrated in the lamina propria. Epon section. × 550.   See filmstrip II, frame 70.

The mucous membrane lining the trachea consists of a pseudostratified ciliated columnar epithelium with goblet cells which rests upon a thick basal lamina with a supporting lamina propria. Four cell types are distinguished in the epithelium: columnar ciliated cells, the cilia beating upward toward the pharynx; columnar cells with a microvillous or striated border; goblet mucus-secreting cells; and basal cells, some of which may represent lymphocytes or macrophages migrating through the epithelium. The lamina propria is relatively thin. There is a condensation of elastic fibers of the lamina propria to form a distinct elastic layer, the fibers of which are directed mainly longitudinally. Small accumulations of lymphocytes are common in the lamina propria. The lumen of the trachea characteristically is D-shaped in transverse section.

THE LUNGS

The lungs are paired organs situated one in each side of the thoracic cavity. The center of the thorax, the *mediastinum*, contains the heart and major blood vessels, the esophagus, the trachea, and the remnants of the thymus gland. On each side of this, the thoracic cavity is lined by a thin, mesothelial membrane, the *parietal pleura*, which at the *hilum* or root of the lung is reflected over the lung as *visceral pleura*. The potential space between parietal and visceral pleurae is occupied by a thin film of watery (serous) fluid; this space is the *pleural cavity*. Thus the lung is connected to the mediastinum by a relatively small area termed the *lung root* in which are located all structures passing to and from the lung. The right lung has three lobes and the left two lobes, each supplied by a branch (a secondary bronchus) of a primary bronchus, the two primary bronchi (right and left) being the terminal branches of the trachea. The right primary bronchus divides into upper and lower lobe bronchi before entering the lung, the right middle lobe bronchus arising from the latter within the lung. The left primary bronchus usually does not divide into upper and lower lobe bronchi until it has entered lung tissue. In turn, the major bronchus supplying a lobe of the lung divides further, the tertiary bronchi so formed supplying *bronchopulmonary segments*. Within each bronchopulmonary segment, further orders of dichotomous branchings occur, the cross-sectional areas of the two daughter branches exceeding that of the mother branch. This means, of course, that air travels more slowly in the smaller branches of the bronchial tree and fastest within the trachea. By branching, the air passage is reduced to a size at which the duct is termed a *bronchiole*. It is the bronchiole which supplies a *lobule* of the lung. A lobule, the basic unit of the lung, is pyramidal, but often highly irregular, with a base 1 to 2 cm. in diameter, a similar height, and an apex which points toward the hilum. In the human, the lobules are poorly delineated by incomplete interlobular septa of fibroconnective tissue, but these are dense and easily seen in the pig.

In summary, the basic organization of the conducting part of the respiratory system is: nasal cavity to pharynx, to larynx, to trachea, which divides into right and left primary bronchi (each supplying a lung), dividing into upper, middle (right only), and lower lobe or secondary bronchi (each supplying a lobe of a lung), dividing into tertiary bronchi (each supplying a bronchopulmonary segment, there being 10 in the right and 8 in the left lung), each continuing to divide into intrapulmonary bronchi of varying sizes, until finally a bronchiole supplies a lung lobule (about 30 to 60 lobules in each bronchopulmonary segment). Within each lobule, the terminal bronchiole continues into one to three *respiratory bronchioles*, each dividing into 2 to 11 *alveolar ducts*, from which *alveolar sacs* and *alveoli* arise. It has been estimated that there are 300 million to 500 million alveoli in the lung. From respiratory bronchiole to alveoli, gaseous exchange occurs.

The histology of each segment now will be described.

Bronchi

The extrapulmonary bronchi closely resemble the trachea in structure and differ from it only in being of smaller diameter. In the main bronchi, cartilage rings still are incomplete, the posterior deficiency being occupied by smooth muscle.

Intrapulmonary bronchi, however, differ from extrapulmonary bronchi in several basic features. First, the intrapulmonary bronchi are spherical in outline and so do not show a posterior flattening, as is seen in the trachea and extrapulmonary bronchi. This is due to the presence not of C-shaped cartilaginous rings but of irregular plates of hyaline cartilage, some of which completely encircle the lumen. These are

so irregular that on cross section the appearance of several small areas of cartilage around the circumference is common, each small piece of cartilage being a protuberance from a large plate. The hyaline cartilage plates are surrounded by dense fibroconnective tissue containing many elastic fibers. Internal to the ring of cartilage and connective tissue is a submucosa composed of loose connective tissue with some lymphoid tendencies and contained within it are mixed mucoserous and mucous glands. The ducts of these pass through the more superficial layers to open on the surface. At the junction of submucosa and mucosa, the condensation of elastic tissue seen in the trachea and extrapulmonary bronchi is reinforced by an outer sheet of smooth muscle fibers. These are not arranged in definite layers, as they are in the digestive tract, for example, but take the form of interlacing bundles of fibers arranged in open spirals around the bronchus, some with a left-handed and some with a right-handed twist.

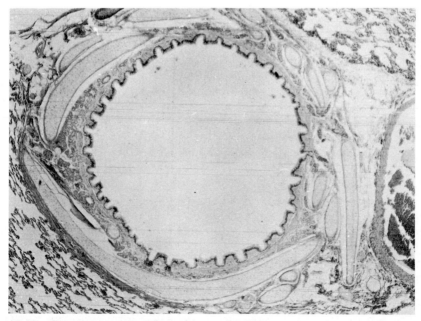

Figure 15-11. Transverse section through an intrapulmonary bronchus. The mucosa is thrown into longitudinal folds by the smooth muscle at the junction of mucosa and submucosa. Note the plates of hyaline cartilage, and mixed glands in the submucosa. × 25.

Intermingled with the bundles of smooth muscle fibers are numerous elastic fibers. The innermost layer is the mucosa, comprising an epithelium continuous with, and identical to, that of the trachea, and a well-defined basal lamina supported by a lamina propria of reticular and longitudinally oriented elastic fibers. Characteristically in sections, the mucosa shows numerous longitudinal folds owing to contraction of the smooth muscle.

Bronchi become smaller with successive divisions of the bronchial tree, but the basic structure as just described remains unchanged. However, the smallest bronchi contain less cartilage, which no longer forms complete rings, and the lining epithelium now is a ciliated columnar epithelium with goblet cells and is of less depth than the pseudostratified ciliated columnar epithelium lining the large bronchi. All bronchi are contained in connective tissue continuous with that of the hilum, and blood vessels are related closely to them and embedded in the same connective tissue.

Bronchioles

The term bronchiole in the past was applied to a conducting tube of less than 1 mm. in diameter. We regard a bronchiole as a small tube embedded in little or no connective tissue and surrounded by respiratory tissue. Thus a bronchiole may be compared with an intralobular duct of a gland. In larger bronchioles, the epithelium is ciliated columnar with some goblet cells, but with further divisions into smaller bronchioles (about 0.3 mm. in diameter) it becomes ciliated cuboidal with no goblet cells. Other characteristic features are the relative prominence of the smooth muscle, mingled with elastic fibers, and the absence of cartilage, glands, and lymph nodes. A thin adventitia of connective tissue is present. The smallest or *terminal bronchiole* is the finest part of the conducting system, its branches being within the respiratory tissue, and here the epithelium shows only patches of ciliated cells, the remainder being nonciliated.

Functional Correlations of the Conducting System. As explained previously, rigidity in the conducting tubes is essential to maintain patency, and this is achieved by the presence of cartilage from trachea to the smallest bronchi. The tubes, however, are capable of changes in length and diameter. Variation in diameter is achieved by the smooth muscle which is supplied by the autonomic nervous system. The abundance of elastic tissue in the walls of the bronchi and throughout lung tissue generally permits expansion of the lung with inspiration, and its elastic recoil aids contraction of the lung with expiration. As in the nose, mucus and cilia trap particulate matter and eliminate it from the system and secretions aid also in humidifying inspired air. It should be noted that cilia extend further down the respiratory tree than do goblet

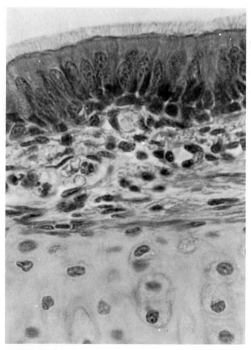

Figure 15-12. Section of a smaller bronchus showing respiratory passage epithelium with obvious cilia. Epon section. × 900.

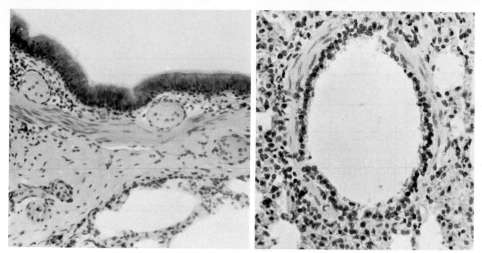

Figure 15-13. Left: Section through a large bronchiole. Note the band of smooth muscle and the ciliated columnar epithelium. × 90. Right: Section through a small bronchiole with cuboidal lining epithelium and smooth muscle. × 120.

cells and submucosal glands, thus preventing the respiratory tissue from becoming waterlogged or occluded by mucus. Cilia virtually constitute an internal drainage system for the respiratory tissue. In the smallest bronchioles, where cilia are absent, macrophages (by phagocytosis of material) take over the function of internal drainage.

Respiratory Bronchioles

Respiration, i.e., gaseous exchange, can occur only where blood in capillaries is separated from air by a very thin mass of material. Such an arrangement occurs from the respiratory bronchioles to the alveoli. Respiratory bronchioles are short, branching tubes, the diameter being less than 0.5 mm. Usually, two or more arise from each terminal bronchiole, and they themselves can branch. The lining epithelium is cuboidal or even low columnar with occasional cilia only in the larger respiratory bronchioles. Cilia are lost in the smaller ones and the epithelium becomes low cuboidal or squamous. No goblet cells are present. External to the cuboidal epithelium, the wall is formed by interlacing bundles of smooth muscle and elastic fibers em-

bedded in fibroconnective tissue. No cartilage is present. In that respiratory bronchioles are part of the respiratory tissue, a few alveoli are present and appear as small diverticula or outpouchings extending from the lumen of the bronchiole through deficiencies in its walls. The structure of these alveoli is identical to that of the main mass of alveoli in the lung (vide infra), and their number increases in the smaller bronchioles. Respiratory bronchioles terminate by branching into several alveolar ducts (2 to 11 in number).

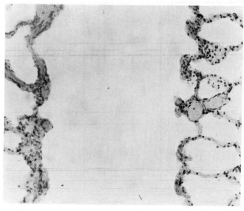

Figure 15-14. Longitudinal section through a respiratory bronchiole. × 75.

Alveolar Ducts

Alveolar ducts are cone-shaped, thin-walled tubes with a squamous epithelial lining which is so thin as to be difficult to resolve with the light microscope. External to the epithelium, the wall is formed by fibroelastic tissue. Opening from the alveolar duct around its circumference are numerous single alveoli and alveolar sacs (clusters of alveoli). Particularly at the orifices of alveoli and alveolar sacs, smooth muscle fibers are prominent. Indeed the openings of alveoli from alveolar ducts are so numerous that it is difficult to see the wall of the alveolar duct, although this is more obvious in thick sections where bundles of elastic, collagenous, and muscle fibers can be seen interweaving between the openings of alveoli along the wall of the alveolar duct.

Alveolar Sacs and Alveoli

The alveolar duct, the terminal part of which is of greater diameter than the proximal part, ends by branching into two to four chambers which, by some authorities, are termed *atria,* and which by others are regarded simply as the terminal alveolar ducts. From these arise single alveoli and alveolar sacs, the latter being a collection or cluster of alveoli opening into a central, slightly larger chamber.

Alveoli are polyhedral or hexagonal, with one wall lacking to permit diffusion of air from respiratory bronchiole, alveolar duct, atrium, or alveolar sac. Alveoli are packed so tightly that each does not have a separate wall. Rather, adjacent alveoli are separated by an *interalveolar septum.* However, each alveolus is lined by a squamous epithelium, which is greatly attenuated but complete. In thin sections, deficiencies in interalveolar septa can be seen, thus permitting communication between adjacent alveoli. These deficiencies are termed *alveolar pores.*

Contained within alveolar septa is an extremely rich capillary plexus. Thus an interalveolar septum is covered on each surface with attenuated epithelium lining alveoli, and contains blood capillaries in its supporting connective tissue framework.

The Interalveolar Septum

It is obvious that interalveolar septa must resist the pressures of air in the alveoli, a pressure which varies with the phase of respiration. The support of the septa is provided in the main by a framework of reticular and elastic fibers, only a little collagen being identifiable on light microscopy. By electron microscopy, the tissue space ("*zona diffusa*") of the septum is seen to contain unit fibrils of collagen, some fine elastic fibers, and small microfibrils. This space is limited by basal laminae underlying alveolar epithelium and covering blood capillaries. In many regions, the capillaries are related so closely to the alveolar epithelium that their respective basal laminae are separated by an interval of only 150 to 200 Å. These basal laminae virtually are complete but are traversed by alveolar or septal cells. Between the basal laminae is an amorphous type of ground substance in which the septal cells and fibers are embedded. Elastic fibers are randomly distributed throughout septa and show a concentration at the orifices of alveoli from alveolar ducts. Smooth muscle cells are seen only in these same regions at the openings of alveoli.

Several distinct cell types can be recognized in interalveolar septa.

Pulmonary Surface Epithelial Cells. They form a very thin, complete layer lining all alveolar spaces. By light microscopy, flattened nuclei of these cells can be recognized but the cytoplasm is so greatly attenuated as to be beyond resolution. By electron microscopy, it can be seen as a complete layer, only 0.2 micron thick or less. It is

(*Text continues on page 356.*)

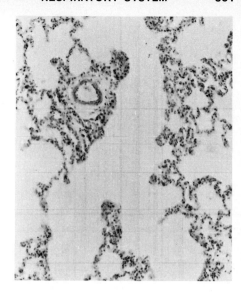

Figure 15-15. Longitudinal section through a single, trumpet-shaped alveolar duct which terminates by opening into two smaller terminal ducts or atria. × 75.

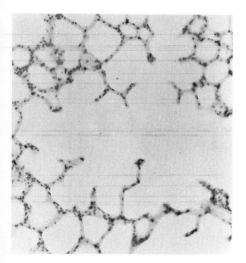

Figure 15-16. Section of alveolar sac and alveoli. × 60.

Figure 15-17. Terminal bronchiole and alveoli to show elastic tissue. Weigert's elastic stain. × 60.

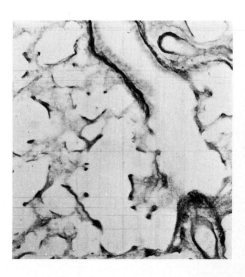

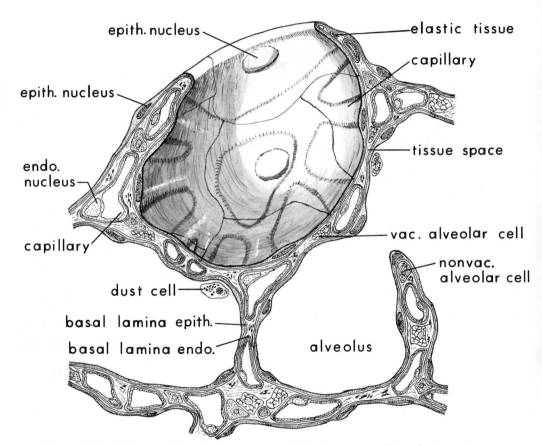

Figure 15-18.   Diagram of an alveolus as seen with the low power of the electron microscope.

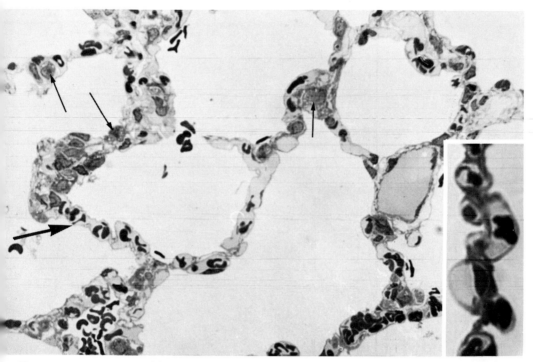

Figure 15-19. Section of lung showing alveoli and interalveolar septa. Thin arrows indicate alveolar phagocytes, and the thick arrow points to an interalveolar septum where blood capillaries are particularly prominent. Epon section, × 300. Insert, lower right: A single interalveolar septum, showing blood capillaries containing red blood corpuscles. × 800.   See filmstrip II, frame 71.

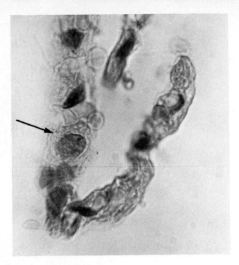

Figure 15-20. Section of an interalveolar septum containing a vacuolated septal cell (arrow). × 1200.

Figure 15-21. Interalveolar septum in which two interalveolar pores are present. Silver stain. × 370.

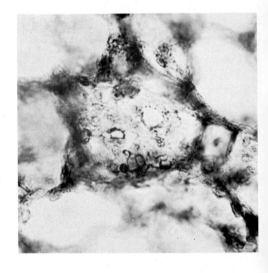

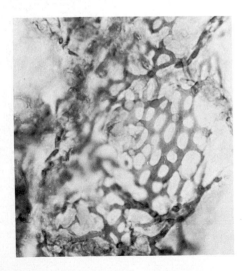

Figure 15-22. Capillary network in an interalveolar septum. Capillaries injected with colored gelatin. × 370.

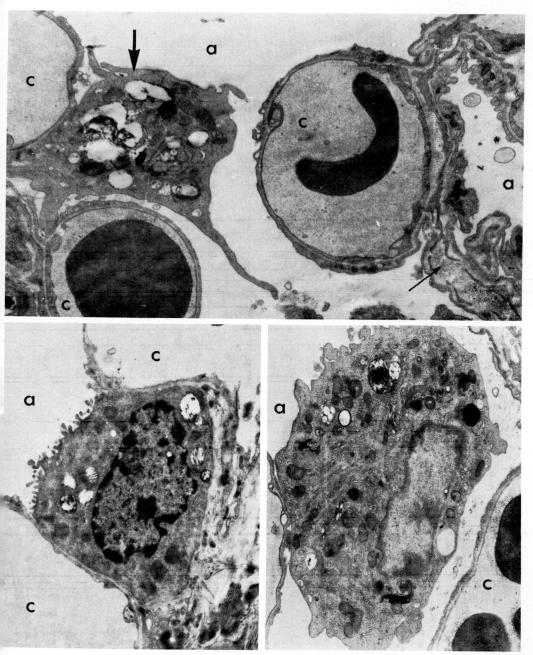

Figure 15-23. Electron micrographs of lung. Top: Part of an alveolus with interalveolar septa on right and left. Capillaries (c) are present in the septa, two containing red blood corpuscles; (a) indicates alveolus, the thin arrow points to collagen fibrils in a septum, the thick arrow to an alveolar or septal cell. × 6000. Lower left: An alveolar (septal) cell. × 5000. Lower right: A dust cell lying free in an alveolus. × 4200.

interrupted in places by migrating macrophages.

Endothelial Cells. These line the numerous blood capillaries. Their nuclei are distinguished from those of epithelial cells by being somewhat larger and, usually, less densely staining. The cytoplasm, as in capillaries elsewhere, is attenuated. The cells are more numerous than other elements in the interalveolar septum and are identified easily by their relationship to capillary blood spaces.

Blood Cells. Obviously, all formed blood elements—erythrocytes, granulocytes, lymphocytes, and monocytes—can be found in septa. When present in capillary lumina, they present no problem in identification, but several of the blood elements are migratory and may be found outside capillaries and in the tissue spaces ("zona diffusa") of the septa, from which they migrate further through epithelium into alveolar spaces.

Alveolar (Septal) Cells. These cells may lie deep to the surface epithelium or may bulge between surface cells into an alveolar lumen. They are cuboidal cells which usually occur singly or in small groups of three or four cells. By electron microscopy, they are seen to be located between surface epithelial cells and form junctional complexes with them as component cells of the alveolar lining. Characteristically, in addition to the usual organelles, the cytoplasm contains dense, osmiophilic bodies 0.2 to 1 micron in diameter. Internally these bodies show a multilamellated appearance and are rich in phospholipid. Occasionally they discharge their contents into the alveolar lumen and some investigators believe that they are concerned with the storage and release of a surface active agent (surfactant, see page 357).

Alveolar Phagocytes. Present in interalveolar septa are macrophages, many of which show evidence of phagocytosis. Generally they can be divided into *vacuolated* and *nonvacuolated*, or *granular*, cells. The vacuo-lated type, 7 to 14 microns in diameter, contain numerous cytoplasmic lipid droplets. Because lipid is removed by ordinary preparative techniques, the cytoplasm has a foamy or vacuolated appearance. It has been suggested that these cells remove blood lipids, particularly cholesterol, for they lie in close association with blood capillaries. The nonvacuolated, or granular, cell has a homogeneous, finely granular cytoplasm and perhaps is concerned with the elimination of inhaled particulate material. Both types migrate through the pulmonary epithelium, carrying their phagocytosed material, and are eliminated via the air passages, the cells finally appearing in the sputum. A few may be eliminated by lymphatic channels. These cells undergo a rapid turnover, being formed either by differentiation from fibroblast-like mesenchymal cells in the septa or by mitosis of other macrophages. However, once a macrophage has acquired a high content of phagocytosed lipid or particulate material, it probably is incapable of cell division.

In many alveoli free cells are present in the lumen. Many contain phagocytosed material, and if this material is inhaled dust, the cells are termed *"dust cells."* Others contain hemosiderin, the iron-containing pigment formed from disintegrating erythrocytes. They are found particularly in conditions in which there is stasis of pulmonary blood flow (e.g., congestive heart failure). These cells are called *siderophages* or *heart failure cells*. Occasionally such a cell may contain an entire erythrocyte as an inclusion.

Blood-Air Barrier

This comprises the structures interposed between air in alveoli and blood in pulmonary capillaries, i.e., the structures through which gaseous exchange occurs. They are the greatly attenuated cytoplasm of the pulmonary epithelial cells, the basal lamina of this epithelium, the capillary basal lamina,

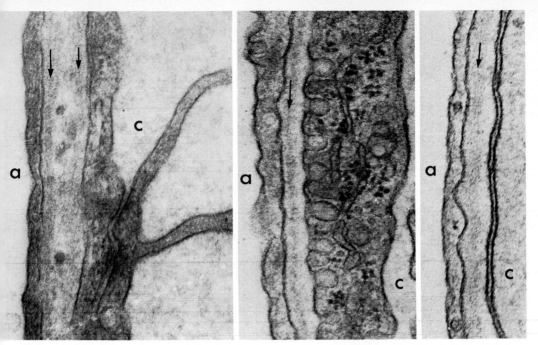

Figure 15-24. Electron micrographs that demonstrate the appearance of the blood-air barrier. In each micrograph the alveolar space (a) is to the left, lined by attenuated pulmonary surface epithelium, and the capillary blood space (c) is to the right, lined by endothelium. Basal laminae are indicated by arrows. Note that there is a fused (single) basal lamina in the center and right micrographs, and separate endothelial and epithelial basal laminae with an intervening zona diffusa or tissue space in the left micrograph. Extreme attenuation of epithelium and endothelium is shown in the right picture. The endothelium in the center picture shows extensive caveolae intracellulares. Each, × 68,000.

and the attenuated cytoplasm of the capillary endothelium.

Interposed between the basal laminae is the tissue space (zona diffusa) of varying extent. In some places it is practically nonexistent, and in other regions the two basal laminae may fuse into one. One further layer must be considered and that is a fluid film lining alveoli. This fluid, presumably secreted by either epithelial or alveolar cells, contains an agent which probably is a lipoprotein. Since this film must become thinner and "stretched" in inspiration, its surface tension may be a factor in aiding elastic expiratory recoil of the lungs. This fluid has the ability to change surface tension with surface area and to achieve a relatively low tension when surface area is reduced. It has been regarded as a type of anticollapse factor in alveoli.

The Lung Lobule

As explained previously, the lung lobule is the unit of structure of the lung, and is pyramidal, usually with the base at the pleural surface of the lung and the apex directed toward the hilum. At the apex, a terminal bronchiole, to be compared with an intralobular duct, enters the lobule accompanied by a branch of the pulmonary artery carrying venous blood to the respiratory tissue. In man, lobules are poorly and incompletely differentiated by connective tissue, continuous on the one hand with the deeper connective tissue layers of the pleura, and on the other with connective tissue around major vessels and bronchi and thus with connective tissue of the hilum. Branches of the pulmonary vein run alone in connective tissue of the poorly

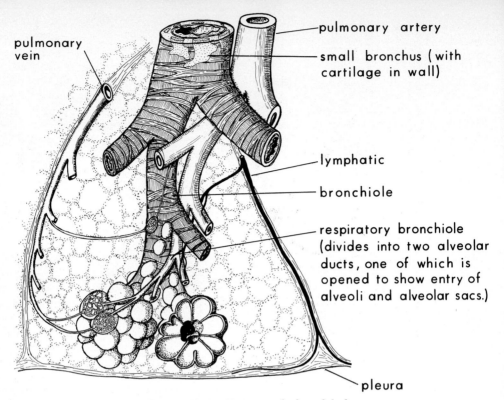

Figure 15-25.   Diagram of a lung lobule.

developed interlobular septa and, at the apex of the lobule, run in company with the bronchiole and branch of the pulmonary artery. Lymphatic capillaries also travel in interlobular septa and are continuous with vessels beneath the pleura and with others around major vessels at the hilum and its extensions. Lymphatics are important in the spread of carcinoma of the lung. Cancerous cells may break through from lymphatics in interlobular septa to adjoining pulmonary veins and thus into the systemic circulation, resulting in widespread metastases or secondary growths in, for example, bone.

Blood Vessels

There is a double blood supply to the lungs. Deoxygenated blood from the right ventricle enters the lungs by the pulmonary arteries, which are elastic arteries of large caliber. Their branches accompany those of the bronchial tree as far as respiratory bronchioles where terminal arterioles break up into a rich capillary network around alveoli, situated in interalveolar septa. Venules from these plexuses join with others draining the pleura and travel alone in the connective tissue of interlobular septa, finally running with branches of the companion artery at the apices of lobules. In addition to this system of pulmonary arteries and veins, there are bronchial arteries and veins. The former arise from the aorta and supply the tissues of the bronchi and the connective tissue of the lung with oxygenated blood. There are communications between the terminal branches of the bronchial arteries and the pulmonary arteries, and most of the blood in the former returns in the pulmonary veins. Some, however, is drained into bronchial veins which are tributaries of the azygos system.

Lymphatics

Two sets of lymphatic vessels, with interconnections, exist in the lung. The superficial or pleural set is situated in the pleura. Relatively large lymphatics demarcate the lung lobules on the surface of the lung. They often are blackened by inhaled carbon, particularly in city dwellers, and thus are visible to the naked eye. Smaller lymphatics form delicate meshworks within the outlines of the lobules. This set is drained around the periphery of the lung to the hilum. The deep or pulmonary set of lymphatics runs with the bronchus, pulmonary artery, and pulmonary vein. The latter start in interlobular septa; those with the pulmonary artery and the bronchi extend peripherally only to the alveolar ducts. All drain centrally to the hilum where they communicate with efferent channels of the superficial set. Lymphatic nodules are prominent at the hilum.

Nerves

Small nerve fibers can be found in the lung, particularly in the region of the hilum and related to major bronchi and large vessels. Those associated with the bronchial tree are from the pulmonary plexus, formed by branches of the vagus (bronchoconstrictor) and by branches of the thoracic sympathetic ganglia (bronchodilator). Both sympathetic and parasympathetic fibers run with the pulmonary vessels. In addition, small collections of nerve cells (parasympathetic ganglia) can be found in bronchial walls.

Pleura

This comprises a thin layer of fibroconnective tissue with collagenous and elastic fibers and few cells (principally fibroblasts and macrophages), covered by a layer of mesothelium. Contained within the connective tissue layer are numerous lymph and blood capillaries and a few small nerve fibers. The pleura is responsible for the secretion of the small quantity of pleural fluid which permits friction-free movement between the parietal layer lining the thoracic cavity and the visceral layer covering the lung surface.

DEVELOPMENTAL ORIGIN OF THE RESPIRATORY SYSTEM

In the embryo, the respiratory system originates as a ventral outgrowth from the floor of the primitive pharynx, the anterior part of the foregut. The outgrowth then extends inferiorly and divides into right and left bronchial buds, each of which undergoes repeated dichotomous branchings. The primary outgrowth becomes the trachea, each bronchial bud a main bronchus, and the orders of branchings the smaller bronchi, bronchioles, and terminal alveoli. Thus, the entire system

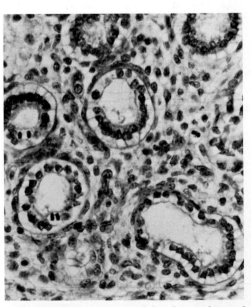

Figure 15-26.   Section of developing lung of the rat. Cross sections of epithelial (endodermal) tubules lie in a cellular mesenchyme. × 240.

has a lining which is of endodermal origin, being derived from the lining of the foregut. Respiratory tissue initially has a glandlike appearance of epithelial (endodermal)-lined alveoli embedded in mesoderm. The mesoderm forms the accessory coats of the system, e.g., connective tissue, muscle.

FUNCTION OF THE RESPIRATORY SYSTEM

As stated previously, the main function of the respiratory system is to provide for gaseous exchange. Oxygen in dissolved form passes from alveoli to blood capillaries through the blood-air barrier and carbon dioxide passes in the reverse direction. The functions of the conducting part of the system are to filter, wash, humidify, and warm or cool the inspired air. However, the lungs also function as an excretory organ in that water is lost in expired air.

REFERENCES

Amoore, J. E., Johnston, J. W., and Rubin, M.: The stereochemical theory of odor. Sci. Amer., *210*:43, 1964.

Avery, M. E.: The Lung and Its Disorders in the Newborn Infant. Philadelphia, W. B. Saunders Co., 1968.

Baradi, A. F., and Bourne, G. H.: Gustatory and olfactory epithelia. Int. Rev. Cytol., *2*:289, 1953.

Bertalanffy, F. D.: Respiratory tissue: Structure, histophysiology, cytodynamics. Part I. Review and basic cytomorphology. Int. Rev. Cytol., *16*:234, 1964.

Bertalanffy, F. D.: Part II. New approaches and interpretations. Int. Rev. Cytol., *17*:214, 1964.

Boyden, E. A.: Segmental Anatomy of the Lung: A Study of the Patterns of the Segmental Bronchi and Related Pulmonary Vessels. New York, Blakiston Division, McGraw-Hill Book Co., 1955.

Comroe, J. H.: Physiology of Respiration. Chicago, Year Book Medical Publishers, Inc., 1965.

De Reuck, A. V. S., and Porter, R. (editors): Development of the Lung. Ciba Foundation Symposium. London, J. & A. Churchill Ltd., 1967.

Leeson, T. S., and Leeson, C. R.: A light and electron microscope study of developing respiratory tissue in the rat. J. Anat., *98*:183, 1964.

Leeson, T. S., and Leeson, C. R.: Osmiophilic lamellated bodies and associated material in lung alveolar spaces. J. Cell Biol., *28*:577, 1966.

Low, F. N.: The pulmonary alveolar epithelium of laboratory animals and man. Anat. Rec., *117*:241, 1953.

Low, F. N.: The extracellular portion of the human blood-air barrier and its relation to tissue space. Anat. Rec., *139*:105, 1961.

Rhodin, J., and Dalhamn, T.: Electron microscopy of the tracheal ciliated mucosa in rat. Z. Zellforsch., *44*:345, 1956.

CHAPTER 16

URINARY SYSTEM

Metabolism of food by the body for the release of energy also involves the formation of waste materials, some of which are extremely toxic. In protein metabolism, especially, waste materials are formed. Such waste materials are eliminated by the urinary system which also subserves functions of fluid and salt balance by excreting these materials in varying quantity, dependent upon need. The urinary system comprises the two kidneys, where the *nephrons* or functional units are located, and a system of excretory passages to temporarily store and eventually conduct excreted materials to the exterior. Proper functioning of the system is, of course, essential to life. As might be expected, the kidneys have an extremely rich blood supply. Indeed, the blood supply is such that the total volume of circulating blood passes through the kidneys once every five minutes.

THE KIDNEY

The human kidneys are bean-shaped, about 10 to 12 cm. in length and 3.5 to 5 cm. thick, and are situated in the posterior part of the upper abdomen, one on each side of the upper lumbar vertebrae. Each is enclosed in a thin fibroconnective tissue capsule which may be stripped easily from the underlying parenchyma, an indication that no septa are present. On the medial aspect is a depression, the *hilum*, through which the blood vessels enter and leave, and from which the excretory duct, the *ureter*, leaves. The upper part of the ureter is expanded to fill the hilum of the kidney. This part, the *pelvis*, is subdivided into large and small cups, the major and minor *calyces*, there being usually two major and eight to 12 minor calyces. Each minor calyx envelops a conical protrusion of renal substance called a renal *papilla*, which is perforated by the openings of 10 to 25 *collecting ducts*. Vertical hemisection of the kidney shows that each papilla is the tip of a pyramidal area extending from the hilum toward the capsule and which in the fresh kidney is pale and striated. Such an area is a *medullary pyramid*, and its striated appearance is due to the presence of straight tubules and parallel blood vessels. The peripheral part or base of each pyramid does not show a clear demarcation from the dark, brownish, granular *cortex* of the kidney, since medullary material extends into the cortex as fine, radially orientated rays, the *medullary rays*. The student should not be confused by this term for although these medullary rays are composed of straight tubules and blood vessels, as is the medullary pyramid

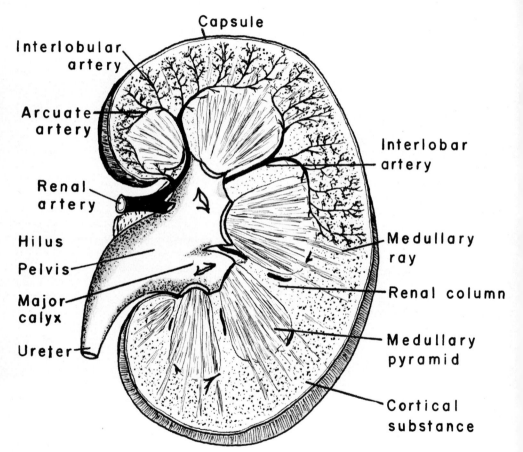

Figure 16-1.   Diagram of the human kidney, sectioned vertically. The arterial supply is indicated in the upper half of the kidney only.

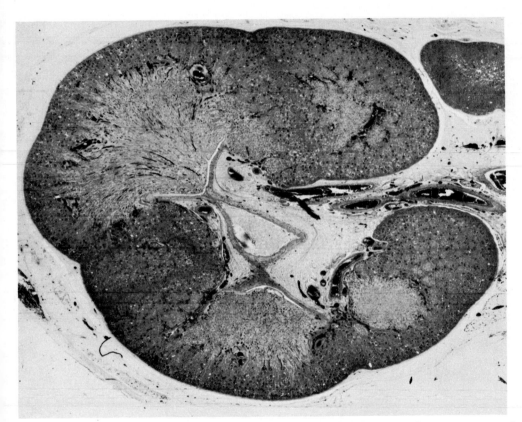

Figure 16-2. Transverse section of a human kidney. Notice the distinction between cortex and medulla, two minor calyces, and blood vessels in the hilum. Renal corpuscles are visible in the cortex as dark dots. A small portion of the adrenal gland is shown at the upper right corner. × 2.

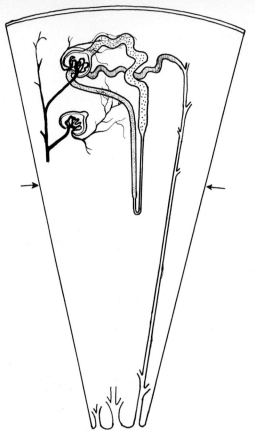

Figure 16-3. Diagram of approximately one-half of a renal lobule with an interlobular (cortical) artery (black, left) and a collecting duct (right) contained in a medullary ray and showing one nephron. Afferent and efferent arterioles and the glomerulus within the capsule of Bowman are shown. The proximal tubule (convoluted and straight parts) is dotted, the thin segment is white, and the distal tubule (straight and convoluted parts) is crosshatched and connected with a collecting duct. The arrows indicate the corticomedullary junction.

corpuscles, and convoluted uriniferous tubules. Thus, in section, the tubules will be cut in oblique or cross fashion.

Each pyramid with its associated overlying cortex is regarded as a lobe; hence the term *multipyramidal* or *multilobar* kidney. Some of the lower mammals, e.g., rat and rabbit, have a unilobar or unipyramidal kidney. In the adult human, the lobes of the kidney are not demarcated and the kidney surface is smooth. In the fetus and young child, the kidney surface is irregular and it is described as lobulated. This term is imprecise; the term lobated is preferable since lobes, not

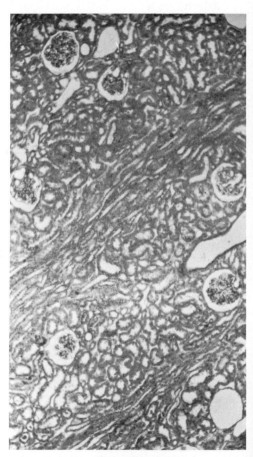

Figure 16-4. Photomicrograph of a portion of the renal cortex, showing two lobules, each with a medullary ray at its center and part of an interlobular artery (center right) between the lobules. × 40. **See filmstrip II, frame 72.**

itself, they are located in the cortex. The medulla can be divided grossly into inner and outer zones, this being a reflection of morphological variation of the walls of the tubules within the medulla. Between adjacent medullary pyramids, cortical material extends between the pyramids to separate them and forms the *renal columns* (of Bertin). The granular appearance of the cortex is accounted for by the presence of spherical bodies, the *renal*

lobules, are indicated. A *lobule* of the kidney is a smaller, functional unit comprising a medullary (cortical) ray, the *kidney units* or *nephrons* which drain into it, and the continuation of the ray in a medullary pyramid. In the cortex, lobules are outlined, but not clearly demarcated, by radially orientated interlobular or cortical blood vessels, but no demarcation exists in the medulla.

Uriniferous Tubule

The kidney can be considered as a compound tubular gland which secretes urine, each kidney containing a large number of uriniferous tubules. Each tubule consists of two parts, the *nephron*, which is about 30 to 40 mm. long, and the *collecting tubule*, approximately 20 mm. long. The two form a continuous tubule although they have different developmental origins. The nephron is responsible for urine secretion, and the collecting tubule is the excretory duct which conveys urine to the renal pelvis.

THE NEPHRON

There are a million or more nephrons in each kidney. Each is simply a long, epithelial-lined tube which starts blindly and terminates by joining an excretory duct, but the nephrons are so tortuous and so intermingled that histological sections of the kidney give no clear idea of their form. This can be achieved only by reconstructions from serial sections or by teasing out individual nephrons from kidneys after maceration. Each nephron consists of several segments of different structure and different function, and each segment is located in a definite position in the cortex or medulla.

The first part of the nephron, located in the cortex, is blind, dilated, and lined by a very thin epithelium. The expansion is invaginated into the form of a cup by a tuft of capillaries. This entire structure is called a *renal corpuscle* (of Malpighi); the expanded part is called *Bowman's capsule*, and the tuft of capillaries is known as the *glomerulus*. In the renal corpuscle an ultrafiltrate of plasma is formed from blood. This substance passes into the renal tubule, where later it is altered to form urine, both by secretions from tubule cells and by reabsorption of many of its filtered products. Connected to the renal corpuscle are convoluted and straight portions of the proximal tubule, a thin segment, and straight and convoluted portions of the distal tubule. The proximal convoluted tubule (convoluted part of the proximal tubule) and the distal convoluted tubule (convoluted part of the distal tubule) lie adjacent to the renal corpuscle in the cortex (see Figure 16-3). Between the tubules the remaining parts of the nephron form the *loop of Henle* which extends for a varying distance from the cortex into the medulla. The loop has descending and ascending limbs, running radially and parallel to each other and connected by a sharp bend. The descending limb comprises a thick portion (the straight part of the proximal tubule) and a thin portion, which continues round the loop as the thin part of the ascending limb. The thick remaining part of the ascending limb is the straight part of the distal tubule. The distal convoluted tubule continues into a collecting tubule or excretory duct.

Renal Corpuscle

Bowman's capsule, the epithelium-lined dilatation of the nephron, is invaginated by a tuft of capillaries, the glomerulus, thus acquiring a cup shape which is double walled. There is a narrow slitlike space, the capsular space, between the outer or parietal layer (capsular epithelium) and the inner or visceral layer (glomerular epithelium) which closely invests the capillary tuft. The entire renal corpuscle, i.e., Bowman's capsule plus the glomerulus of capillaries, is roughly spherical. It has a *vascular pole* where afferent and efferent arterioles enter and leave the glomerulus and where the parietal layer of the capsule is reflected onto the vessels as the visceral layer. The renal corpuscle also has a *urinary pole* at the opposite side of the corpuscle where capsular space is continuous with the lumen of the proximal convoluted tubule and where the parietal (squamous) epithelium is continuous with the cuboidal or low columnar epithelium of the proximal convoluted tubule.

In size, renal corpuscles vary from 150 to 250 microns in diameter; those in the deeper areas of the cortex adjacent to the medulla are larger than those situated peripherally beneath the capsule of the kidney. The larger,

juxtamedullary corpuscles are the first to differentiate during development.

The parietal layer of Bowman's capsule is composed of a simple squamous epithelium with nuclei which protrude slightly into the capsular space. Cytoplasmic organelles are poorly developed. At the urinary pole, these squamous cells increase in height over four or five cells to become continuous with the low columnar epithelium lining the proximal convoluted tubule. The visceral layer of epithelium closely invests the capillaries of the glomerulus and is difficult to delineate by light microscopy. Nuclei of these cells are located on the capsular side of the basal lamina covering glomerular capillaries and the cells do not form a complete sheet over the capillaries, i.e., there are discontinuities. By

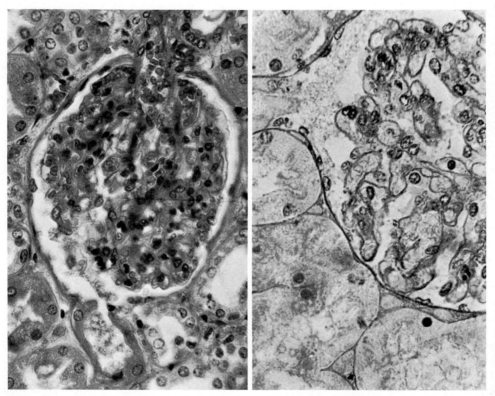

Figure 16-5.   Left: Photomicrograph of a single renal corpuscle, showing vascular pole (above) and urinary pole below. The macula densa is shown at upper right. × 700. Right: Part of a renal corpuscle with its urinary pole (upper left) and surrounding proximal convolutions to show basal laminae (black). PAS stain. × 900.   **See filmstrip II, frame 73**

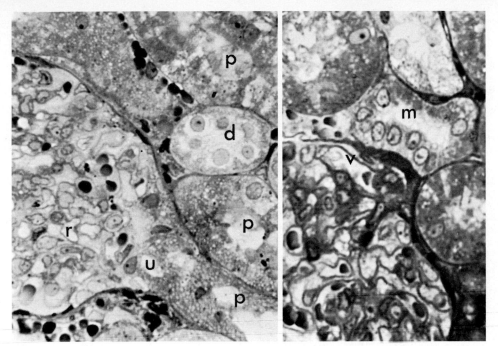

Figure 16-6.   Epon sections of rat kidney. Left: Renal corpuscle (r) and its urinary pole (u), proximal convoluted tubule (p), and distal convoluted tubule (d). × 700. Right: The vascular pole (v) of a renal corpuscle with macula densa (m) of a distal tubule. × 700.

electron microscopy, these cells show considerable morphological specialization. Nuclei are ovoid and surrounded by a small amount of cytoplasm or perikaryon which rarely is in close contact with the basal lamina of a glomerular capillary. Instead, the nucleus with its perikaryon usually lies apart from the capillaries but contacts one or more capillary loops by a series of cytoplasmic processes, the major processes, extending from the perikaryon in the manner of the tentacles of an octopus or the limbs of a starfish. A series of small footlike processes, the *pedicels*, extend from each major process and are attached to the outer (capsular) surface of the capillary basal lamina. The pedicels interdigitate in a complex manner with pedicels from other major processes of the same and other cells. This arrangement, illustrated in a simplified diagram, Figure 16-8, accounts for the name *podocytes*, a term now employed to describe the visceral epithelial cells.

Organelles are present in the major processes but do not extend into the small pedicels where the cytoplasm usually contains only a few RNP granules and some small vesicles.

Between pedicels as they extend to attach to the basal lamina are small slitlike spaces, about 250 Å wide, referred to as *filtration slits* or *slit pores*. These spaces are freely continuous with larger spaces beneath and between major processes. In turn, all drain into the capsular space and thus eventually into the lumen of the proximal convoluted tubule. However, near their attachment to the basal lamina, adjacent pedicels are connected by a thin membrane, *the slit membrane*, only 60 Å or less in thickness, extending between the outer leaflets of plasma membranes of adjacent pedicels at the surface of the basal lamina. These slit membranes perhaps can be compared to the diaphragms closing the pores of fenestrated (type II) capillary endothelium (see page 217),

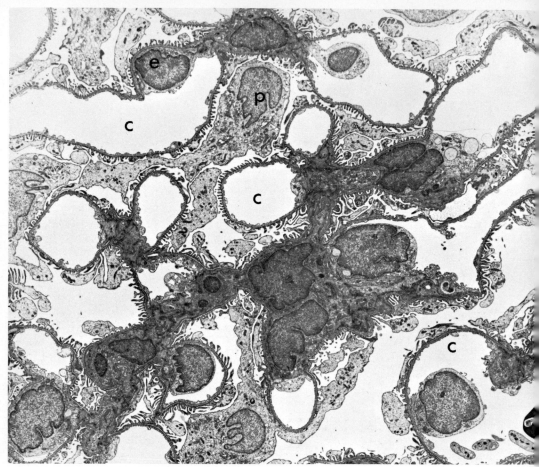

Figure 16-7. Survey electron micrograph of a portion of a renal corpuscle of the rat. Some of the capillary loops are labeled (c) and are lined by attenuated endothelium, one nucleus of which is indicated (e). Covering capillary loops are pedicels and cytoplasmic processes of the visceral epithelial cells or podocytes, one of which is labeled (p). × 3000. (Courtesy of Dr. Ruth Bulger, labeling added.)

and they close the filtration slits at their bases.

The endothelium lining glomerular capillaries is greatly attenuated and is perforated, the pores or fenestrae being spherical and some 500 to 1000 Å in diameter, i.e., somewhat larger than those in type II endothelium, and possibly unclosed by diaphragms. Between pedicels of podocytes and perforated capillary endothelium is a single, continuous basal lamina (basement membrane). High resolution electron microscopy demonstrates that the basal lamina contains fine filaments of at least two different thicknesses arranged in a feltwork.

Occasionally in the renal corpuscle, in addition to podocytes and endothelial cells, a third cell type is seen. These *mesangial* or *intercapillary cells* lie usually at the branchings of capillary loops between endothelium and basal lamina and do not contact the capillary lumen. They are stellate in shape and have numerous cytoplasmic filaments. They appear to be of mesodermal origin and resemble pericytes found elsewhere, although they may be modified smooth muscle cells. Their function remains obscure but in certain pathological conditions they proliferate and may become phagocytic. There is some evidence that they

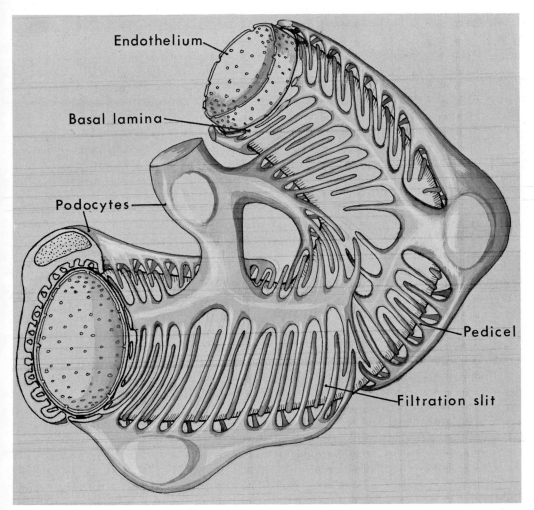

Figure 16-8. Diagram of a portion of a glomerular capillary loop as seen under the electron microscope. × approximately 10,000.

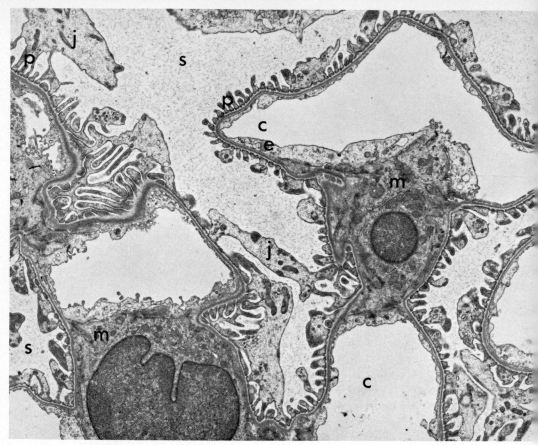

Figure 16-9. Electron micrograph of a portion of a renal corpuscle of the rat showing capillary lumen (c), endothelium (e), major processes (j) and pedicels (p) of visceral epithelial cells or podocytes and mesangial or intercapillary cells (m). Note the continuous basal lamina of the capillaries between endothelium and pedicels. Capsular space is indicated (s). × 7500. (Courtesy of Dr. Ruth Bulger, labeling added.)

are concerned in the maintenance of the basal lamina. Recently, these cells have been termed *stalk cells* and continuity between them and juxtaglomerular cells has been described. There are morphological similarities between the two cell types.

The glomerulus is a mass of tortuous capillaries located along the course of an arteriole; an afferent arteriole runs to the glomerulus and an efferent arteriole away from it. The afferent arteriole is of greater diameter than the efferent arteriole, and consequently the glomerulus is a relatively high pressure system. This aids the formation of tissue fluid in the capillary bed. Some of the smooth muscle cells in the wall

of the afferent arteriole are *"epithelioid"* in character, being large and pale-staining, and they contain conspicuous granules. These cells on one side contact the intima of the arteriole where the internal elastic lamina is absent or poorly developed. On the other side the cells are closely related to the *macula densa*, a specialized region in the wall of the distal convoluted tubule at its commencement. As shown by electron microscopy, the granules of these *juxtaglomerular (JG) cells* are of variable shape and membrane bounded, with an internal crystalline structure. There is considerable evidence that the JG cells are the source of the vasopressor sub-

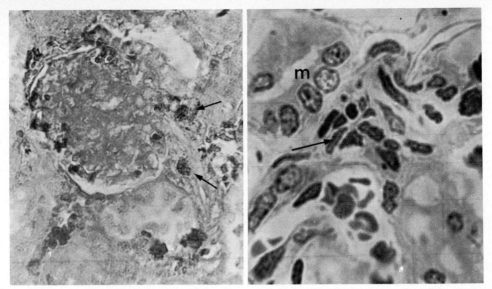

Figure 16-10. Left: Photomicrograph showing granules in juxtaglomerular cells (arrows). × 450. Right: Epon section of the vascular pole of a renal corpuscle showing macula densa (m) in close relation to epithelioid cells of the afferent arteriole (arrow). × 1200.

stance *renin*, which in the blood stream acts upon *angiotensin I* to convert it to *angiotensin II*, a hypertensive substance.

On entering the renal corpuscle, the afferent arteriole divides into three to five main branches, each entering a "lobule" to branch further into capillaries. The larger capillaries are interconnected, these channels probably functioning as by-passes to the main mass of capillaries in a lobule. The capillaries drain to larger channels which unite to form the efferent arteriole. The tunica media of circularly arranged smooth muscle fibers is thick in the efferent vessel, and by contraction it can regulate pressure in the glomerulus.

Filtration Barrier

The filtration barrier is a term applied to the structures which separate blood in the glomerular capillaries from the filtrate in the capsular space of the renal corpuscle. It comprises the fenestrated, attenuated endothelium, the basal lamina, and the pedi-cels of the podocytes. The basal lamina is the only continuous layer of the three and is regarded as the main filter preventing passage of large molecules. Experimentally, large particulate tracers, e.g., ferritin, pass through endothelial pores and are held up by the basal lamina for some time. Smaller particles, e.g., horseradish peroxidase (mol. wt. 40,000) pass through endothelial pores, basal lamina, and filtration slits to appear in capsular space. The larger myeloperoxidase (mol. wt. 160,000) is held up by the epithelial slit membranes after passing through endothelial pores and basal lamina. Presumably, therefore, the filtration slits constitute the barrier responsible for differential glomerular permeability.

It should be emphasized that the basal lamina is not static. There is experimental evidence that it is formed and added to by the epithelial podocytes and that the mesangial cells perhaps remove filtration residues and excess basal lamina material. Thus, while epithelial cells add new material externally, mesangial cells probably remove older material internally, and the overall thickness of the basal lamina remains constant. In addition, similarities in structure between the mesangial or stalk cells and juxtaglomerular cells suggest that there is a functional as well as a physical relationship between the two.

Functional Correlation

Physiologically, the renal corpuscle is regarded as an ultrafilter. The glomerulus is a high pressure system and tissue fluid leaves the contained blood along the entire extent of the capillary bed. The process probably is selective to some extent in that the endothelium and visceral epithelium may modify the filtrate by selective absorption, but the functional power mainly is that of hydrostatic (blood) pressure forcing a filtrate through the filtration barrier. In man, the total glomerular filtrate in 24 hours is from 170 to 200 liters, of which some 99 per cent will be resorbed by the uriniferous tubules, with only 1.5 to 2 liters remaining as urine. (The term "uriniferous tubule" encompasses the tubular part of the nephron and the collecting duct.)

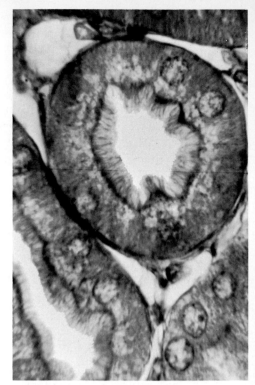

Figure 16-11. Photomicrograph of proximal convolution in cross and longitudinal sections, showing the brush or striated border. × 1400. (Courtesy of F. Jacoby.)

Proximal Convoluted Tubule

The proximal convoluted tubule, commencing at the urinary pole of a renal corpuscle, is approximately 14 mm. long with an outside diameter of 60 microns. As the name suggests, it follows a tortuous course and always takes one large loop toward the capsular surface of the kidney in addition to numerous minor twists and turns. It terminates by straightening out and passing into the nearest medullary ray where it becomes continuous with the loop of Henle. As the longest and widest part of the nephron, it constitutes the bulk of the cortex, appearing in sections as oblique and transverse profiles. In it, glomerular filtrate begins its transformation into urine by the absorption of some constituents and the addition of others.

At its commencement, there is a narrow zone termed the *neck* where there is a rapid transition from the squamous type of epithelium of the parietal cells of Bowman's capsule to the simple low columnar type of the proximal convolution. The cells are truncated pyramids, with cell interfaces which are defined poorly because cell membranes are irregular and cells interdigitate with their neighbors. The cytoplasm is abundant and usually intensely eosinophilic, the nucleus being large, spherical, and pale staining. Although there may be some six to twelve cells around the circumference of a proximal convoluted tubule, rarely are more than four or five nuclei seen, the cells being considerably greater in width

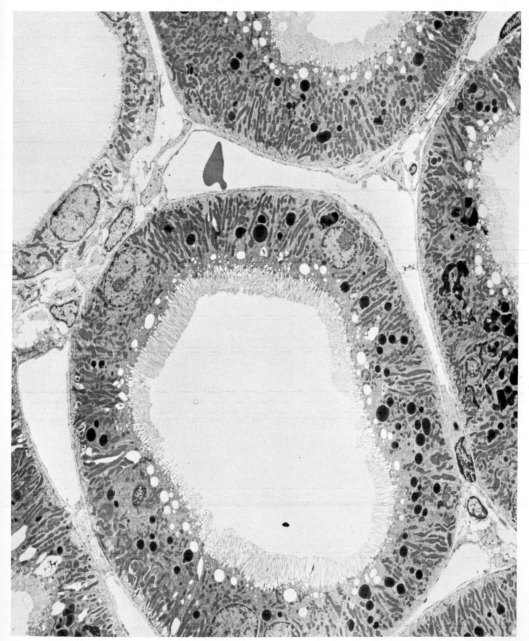

Figure 16-12. Electron micrograph of renal cortex showing proximal convoluted tubules and one distal convoluted tubule (top left). Note the elongated mitochondria and apical microvilli of the former, and the capillaries between the tubules. × 3300. (Courtesy of Dr. A. B. Maunsbach.)

than the thickness of the section. The height of the epithelial cells, and thus the diameter of the lumen, varies to some extent with functional activity although the lumen is never occluded completely in well fixed tissue.

In material well fixed immediately after death, the basal cytoplasm is striated by long, parallel mitochondria, and a brush border is obvious on the luminal surface. The brush border is alkaline phosphatase positive. A Golgi apparatus is located in a supranuclear position.

As evident by electron microscopy, the lumen is relatively wide, each cell having long, thin, closely-packed microvilli on its apical surface. The plasma membrane covering microvilli has a filamentous outer coat. Between the bases of microvilli are tubular pits or small apical canaliculi and the apical cytoplasm also contains numerous small vesicles, some of which appear to bud off from apical canaliculi. This may represent a mechanism for absorption of protein from the glomerular filtrate. The basal cytoplasm shows interesting specializations. The basal plasma membrane exhibits numerous infoldings, between which are elongated mitochondria. In addition, there is a complex interdigitation of adjacent cells, processes from one cell lying in basal pockets of adjacent cells. There also are complex intercellular interdigitations of lateral cell interfaces. Beneath the basal plasma membrane is a continuous basal lamina, separating the epithelial cells from surrounding capillaries, which are lined by a fenestrated (type II) endothelium.

The cytoplasm of proximal tubule cells contains a few, free RNP granules, a poorly developed granular endoplasmic reticulum, and a prominent Golgi zone in a supranuclear position.

The morphological appearance is similar in cells along the length of the proximal convoluted tubule although regional differences have been recognized in many species. In the straight portion of the proximal tubule (in the descending limb of the loop of Henle),

the cells are not as tall, and they show fewer basal infoldings and interdigitations, smaller mitochondria, and shorter and less numerous microvilli.

Functionally, the proximal tubule resorbs 85 per cent or more of the water and sodium chloride in the glomerular filtrate. The cells actively transport sodium, and the chloride and water follow passively to maintain osmotic equilibrium. Normally, all glucose also is resorbed but if the level of glucose in the blood is excessively high, the capacity for resorption is exceeded and glucose appears in the urine. This occurs, for example, in diabetes. Other substances also are resorbed, e.g., aminoacids, protein, vitamin C, and inorganic ions. In addition, cells of the proximal tubule pass materials into the lumen, a process of excretion. Some examples are creatinine and various dye materials, such as Diodrast and phenol red, which are used clinically to assess tubular function.

Loop of Henle

The loop of Henle consists of the straight part of the proximal tubule in the descending limb, a thin segment in descending and ascending limbs, and the straight part of the distal tubule in the ascending limb. The two limbs lie close together and are orientated radially in the kidney. There is some variation in loops of Henle in the human. Those of juxtamedullary nephrons are long with the loops formed by the thin limb (as shown in Figure 16-3) which may extend nearly to the apex of the medullary papilla. Loops of Henle of subcapsular nephrons are much shorter with the bend formed by the thick ascending limb, and the thin descending limb being very short. These loops extend only into the outer part of the medulla. This arrangement accounts for the zonation seen in the medulla.

The transition from straight portion of proximal tubule to descending thin

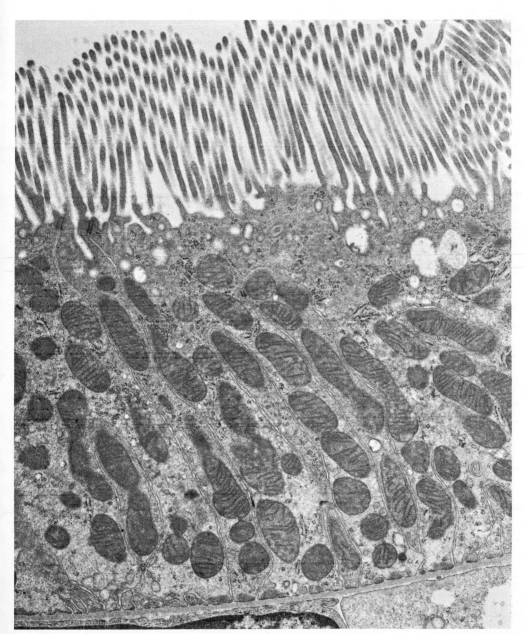

Figure 16-13.   Electron micrograph of part of a proximal convoluted tubule. Note the large number of mitochondria, the basal infoldings of plasma membrane and basal interlocking of cytoplasmic processes of adjacent cells, and the apical microvilli. × about 24,000. (Courtesy of Dr. Ruth Bulger.)

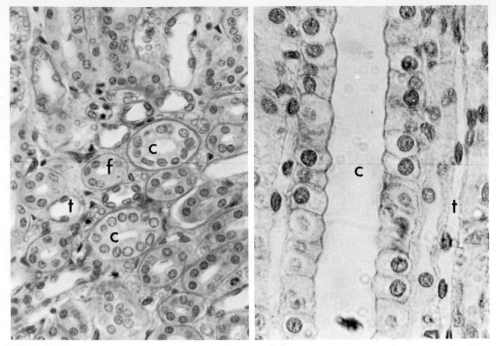

Figure 16-14. Photomicrographs of, left, cross sections through collecting ducts (c) and thin (t) and thick (f) segments of the loop of Henle, × 450, and, right, longitudinal sections through collecting ducts and the thin segment of the loop of Henle, × 750.

limb occurs abruptly over a few cells. The epithelium changes from low columnar or cuboidal to squamous, the thin limb having an outside diameter of only 14 to 22 microns. Nuclei of the squamous cells protrude into the lumen and only three to five are seen in a cross section of a thin limb. They resemble those of capillaries except that the nuclei protrude more and are closer together than those of endothelial cells. The cytoplasm is less eosinophilic than that of proximal tubule cells. By electron microscopy, the cells show only a few short apical microvilli and an occasional single cilium, small basal infoldings of the plasma membrane, and few organelles. Characteristically, there are numerous interdigitations of processes of adjacent cells with many lateral interfaces (extending from base to lumen). Thus, around the circumference of a thin segment in cross section there may be up to 20 or more portions of cells, only a few of which contain a nucleus.

The transition from thin segment to ascending thick limb (straight part of the distal tubule) also is abrupt with a rapid increase in height of the epithelium to cuboidal, this segment having an outside diameter of 30 to 50 microns. The straight part of the distal tubule ascends from medulla to cortex in a radial fashion to reach the glomerulus of origin at the vascular pole where it lies between afferent and efferent arterioles. This region is specialized and is termed the *macula densa* (dense spot).

Functionally, the loop of Henle is essential for the production of urine which is hypertonic to blood plasma. Fluid entering the loop already has been 80 per cent concentrated. In the descending limb, the wall is permeable to sodium and water but the ascending limb is impermeable to water. However, the cells of the ascending limb actively transport sodium from the urine to the interstitium (a "sodium pump"), thus increasing the osmotic

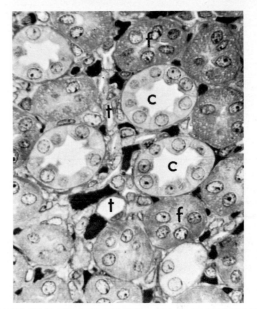

Figure 16-15. Epon section of the kidney medulla showing, in cross section, collecting ducts (c) and thick (f) and thin (t) segments of the loop of Henle. Vasa recta appear black. × 450.   See filmstrip II, frame 74.

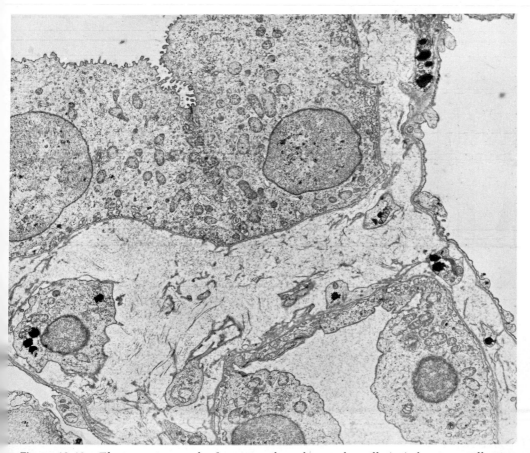

Figure 16-16. Electron micrograph of a section through a renal papilla (rat) showing a collecting duct (top left), a thin limb of the loop of Henle (bottom right), and a blood capillary (top right). × 4500. (Courtesy of Dr. Ruth Bulger.)

concentration of the interstitium. This rise in sodium concentration of the interstitium between and around descending and ascending limbs (which lie close together) results in water leaving the descending limb and sodium entering it by passive diffusion with consequent concentration of the urine. The straight blood vessels (vasa recta) of the medulla remove excess sodium and water but are arranged so that outgoing and ingoing vessels are connected by a sharp bend with outgoing fluid running in close proximity, but in the opposite direction, to inflowing fluid. This then is a countercurrent multiplier system allowing equilibration of concentration of blood in the descending and ascending limbs of the vasa recta. These vessels thus do not disturb the osmotic gradient in the medulla, i.e., there is a concentration of urine in a proximodistal direction in the loop of Henle. Presumably the thin segment functions mainly as a dialysing membrane for interchange between urine and the interstitium, i.e., mainly a passive loss of water and gain of sodium, while the sodium pump is located in the straight part of the distal tubule of the ascending limb of the loop of Henle.

Macula Densa. Where the ascending limb of the loop of Henle (straight part of the distal tubule) contacts the parent renal corpuscle between afferent and efferent arterioles, there is a specialized region of the distal tubule called the macula densa. The epithelial cells of the tubule, where they are immediately adjacent to an arteriole, show dense packing in a palisade manner. This is closely adjacent to the juxtaglomerular apparatus of the afferent arteriole, but a large macula densa also may be present in relation to the efferent arteriole. The tubule cells of the macula densa show less specialization and infolding of the basal plasma membrane, fewer mitochondria, and a Golgi zone which is subnuclear, i.e., near the arteriole. In addition, the basal lamina here is thin. The very close relation between the JG cells and the cells of the macula

densa suggests that there is an interchange of substances between them, perhaps related to the regulation of blood flow to the glomerulus.

Distal Convoluted Tubule

From the region of the macula densa, the nephron continues as the distal convoluted tubule, which follows a short, tortuous course in the cortex and terminates near a medullary ray by continuing into a collecting duct. The distal convoluted tubule is shorter than the proximal convoluted tubule, and thus in a section appears in smaller numbers, its overall diameter is less, and the cells are cuboidal, smaller, and have no brush border. Usually some six to eight nuclei are seen in a cross section. Generally the cells stain less intensely than those of the proximal convoluted tubule. As seen by electron microscopy, the cells are cuboidal with a clear cytoplasm and central, spherical nuclei. A few, short, apical microvilli are present. Mitochondria are small and elongated, and most of them are in basal cytoplasm between infoldings of the basal plasma membrane. These infoldings are developed more highly than in the proximal convoluted tubule.

When glomerular filtrate enters the distal convoluted tubule, some 85 per cent of its fluid has been resorbed and a further 14 per cent is resorbed in the distal convoluted tubule.

However, urine entering the distal convoluted tubule is hypotonic although reduced in volume. Under the influence of antidiuretic hormone from the posterior pituitary, the wall of the distal convoluted tubule and that of the collecting ducts become highly permeable to water. It is in the distal tubule also that urine becomes acidified—sodium is removed actively and replaced by potassium, hydrogen, and ammonia.

Each distal convoluted tubule drains by a short connecting duct into a small collecting tubule. Developmentally, the nephrons and the excretory or collecting ducts have different origins.

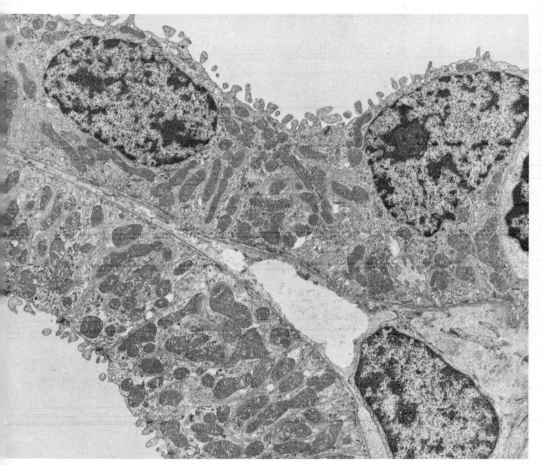

Figure 16-17.   Electron micrograph of distal convoluted tubules from the kidney of a spider monkey. × 4000. (Courtesy of Dr. Ruth Bulger.)

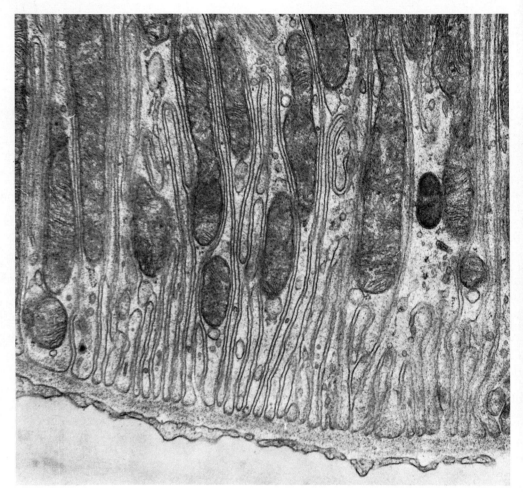

Figure 16-18.   Electron micrograph of the basal portion of a cell from the distal convoluted tubule. Note the invaginations of the basal plasma membrane, elongated mitochondria between the invaginations, and the underlying basal lamina. The cell is in close relationship to type II capillary endothelium lining a cortical capillary. × 26,000.

Collecting Tubules

The collecting tubules, or excretory ducts, are not considered parts of the nephron. Each distal convoluted tubule connects to a collecting tubule via a short side branch of the latter located in a medullary ray, there being several such branches. The collecting tubule passes in a medullary ray and down into the medulla. In the more central parts of the medulla, several collecting tubules join at acute angles to form large ducts which open onto the apex of a papilla. These are the *papillary ducts* of Bellini and have a diameter of 100 to 200 microns or more. Their openings onto the surface of a papilla are so large, so numerous, and so closely packed as to give the papilla the appearance of a sieve (the *area cribrosa*).

The cells lining these excretory ducts vary in size but all characteristically have a well-defined cell membrane, a darkly staining spherical or ovoid nucleus situated centrally in the cell, and a pale, watery, homogeneous cytoplasm with an apical bulge into the lumen. Cells of the smaller ducts are low cuboidal, those in the ducts of Bellini are tall columnar. As shown by electron microscopy, the cells contain few organelles, some clear apical vacuoles, a few microvilli, and some basal infoldings of the plasma membrane. Interspersed among these "clear" or "light" cells are occasional "dark" cells with more prominent organelles. These probably are functional variants of the light cells and not a different cell type. The collecting tubules conduct urine from the nephrons to the ureteric pelvis and under the influence of antidiuretic hormone, water passively leaves the urine.

Blood Supply of the Kidney

Each kidney receives a direct branch of the abdominal aorta, the renal artery, and in general blood passes through glomeruli before supplying the remainder of the kidney. At the hilum, the renal artery divides into three main branches, two passing anteriorly and one posteriorly to the renal pelvis, and each branch occasionally dividing further. There is little or no anastomosis between these major arteries, and each supplies three or four medullary pyramids and their corresponding cortical substance. This area of supply is termed a *renule*. In the adipose tissue around the hilum, each major branch divides into *interlobar* arteries which ascend between adjacent medullary pyramids in a column of Bertin, usually eccentrically placed to one side. There are also interlobar arteries at upper and lower poles of the kidney between the pyramids and the kidney surface.

At the corticomedullary junction, the interlobar arteries break up into several branches, the *arciform* or *arcuate* arteries, which leave the parent vessel almost at a right angle to arch over the bases of the medullary pyramids and run parallel to the surface of the kidney. From these, branches pass peripherally in the cortex in a radial fashion. These are located between medullary rays, viz., between lobules, and are termed the *interlobular* arteries. From the interlobular arteries, there are numerous side branches which enter cortical substance as *intralobular* arteries and branch into one or more afferent glomerular arterioles. The peripheral terminations of the interlobular arteries reach and supply the capillary bed of the renal capsule.

The efferent glomerular arteriole probably supplies the majority of the other parts of the same nephron. Efferent arterioles from juxtamedullary glomeruli pass into the medullary pyramids to supply them. These efferent arterioles run a straight, centripetal course and are called *arteriolae rectae spuriae* (false, straight arterioles) or vasa recta. These vessels

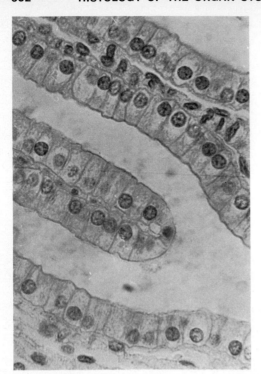

Figure 16-19. Photomicrograph of collecting ducts uniting to form ducts of Bellini. × 550.

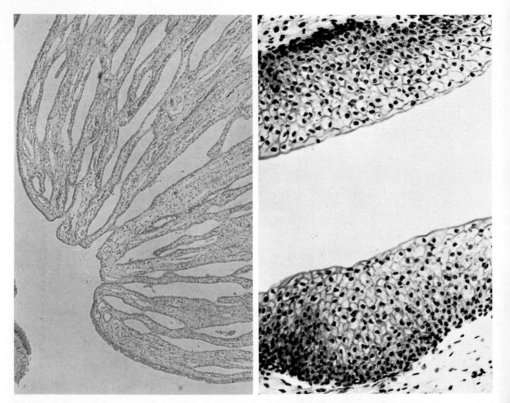

Figure 16-20. Photomicrographs of, left, the apex of a medullary pyramid to show the openings of ducts of Bellini through the area cribrosa and, right, the transitional epithelium covering a medullary pyramid. Note that in the left hand figure there is transitional epithelium visible on the outer (pelvic aspect of the pyramid. Left, × 125. Right, × 550.

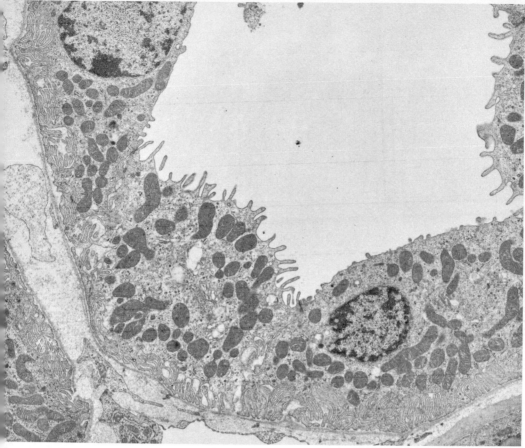

Figure 16-21. Electron micrograph of a portion of a collecting duct from the kidney of a spider monkey. × 4500. (Courtesy of Dr. Ruth Bulger.)

penetrate the medulla in a radial fashion, take sharp hairpin bends, and then return to the cortex to drain into arcuate veins. The endothelial walls of the vasa recta are very thin, the endothelium of the ascending (venous) limbs being perforated. This, together with the close proximity of the two limbs, permits rapid interchange of diffusible substances between the two limbs as a countercurrent exchange system. In the past, some investigators have claimed that the capillary networks of the medullary pyramids also are supplied by long, straight direct branches from arcuate and interlobular arteries *arteriolae rectae verae*—true, straight arterioles) but, if these do exist, they

probably are so few as to be of no functional significance.

Venous drainage has a similar arrangement to the arterial supply, except, of course, that there is no venous component in the glomerulus and its arterioles. In the cortex, capillaries collect into small venules (the *stellate* veins) which then join in a starlike pattern to form interlobular veins, which pass toward the medulla with interlobular arteries, receiving tributaries from all levels of the cortex. These join to form *arcuate* or *arciform* veins, which also receive straight vessels (the *venulae rectae*) ascending from medullary pyramids. Arcuate veins drain into interlobar veins,

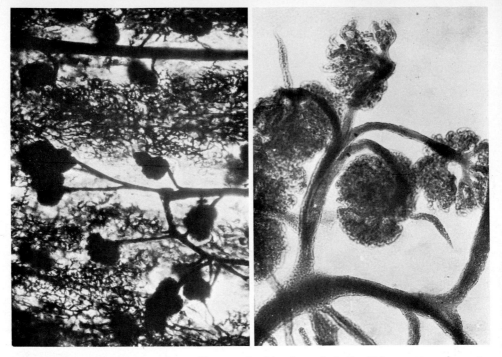

Figure 16-22. Photomicrographs to illustrate the blood supply to the kidney cortex, above, in an injection section, × 125, and, below, in isolated, microdissected whole glomeruli, × 350.

which pass toward the hilum and finally join to form the renal vein, which in turn drains to the inferior vena cava.

Lymphatics

There are networks of lymphatic capillaries in the capsule and in association with the renal vessels, and the two groups are connected by a few anastomotic channels. There is considerable disagreement on the extent of the lymphatic channels in cortical and medullary substance but certainly none is found in glomeruli. Small longitudinal channels are present in medullary pyramids. They commence blindly near apices and drain toward the cortex terminating in lymphatic vessels accompanying arcuate vessels. There are said to be extensive networks too between uriniferous tubules in the cortex. All vessels leave the kidney at the hilum.

Nerves

Nerves from the celiac sympathetic plexus enter the kidney with the arteries. They terminate in relation to large vessels and probably extend to glomeruli, and perhaps also between uriniferous tubules, although terminations between tubules have not been demonstrated satisfactorily.

Embryology

During development the kidney arises from intermediate mesoderm situated in the posterior abdominal wall. Primitive nephrons develop from the cords of mesenchymal cells and acquire a lumen, and the blind dilated end of the nephron (the future Bowman's capsule) is invaginated by a tuft of capillaries. The ureteric bud, a diverticulum arising from the mesonephric or wolffian duct, grows into the mass of developing kidney o metanephros. The mesonephric duct later becomes associated with the genital system, and by differential growth, the ureteric bud originating from it is taken up into the developing urinary bladder. When the growing end of the ureteric bud reaches the metanephros, it undergoes a series of divisions, each terminal branch becoming continuous with a developing nephron. The fine branches of the ureteric bud thus become the various orders of collecting or excretory ducts, and its main branches become the minor and major calyces of the renal pelvis; the ureteric bud itself becomes the ureter. As just indicated, the first nephrons to develop are those in the deeper layers of the cortex. At birth the kidney is irregular in outline (fetal lobulation), and the outer cortical region consists of undifferentiated

mesenchyme from which additional nephrons will develop for some months or even years after birth. When development is complete, the kidney outline becomes smooth.

Developmental abnormalities of the kidney and excretory passages are not uncommon. Early division of a ureteric bud before it reaches the metanephros can result in conditions such as bifid or double ureter, and double kidney. Failure of individual nephrons to connect with terminal divisions of the ureteric bud results in cysts, usually multiple (multicystic kidney).

EXCRETORY PASSAGES

The excretory passages convey urine from the kidney to the exterior. Essentially they are simple ducts, but they do add some mucus to the urine and may function to a limited extent to absorb a small amount of fluid. All parts have a relatively thick muscularis which on contraction aids the expulsion of urine.

Pelvis and Ureter

As noted, the upper expanded portion of the ureter, the pelvis, is situated in the hilum of the kidney and splits into major and minor calyces, each minor calyx fitting like a cup around a medullary papilla. The wall of the pelvis is thinner than that of the ureter itself, and, indeed, the thickness of the wall gradually increases from the start to the termination of the excretory ducts. The ureter is 10 to 12 inches in length, is situated in the posterior abdominal wall behind the peritoneum, and terminates by perforating obliquely the wall of the urinary bladder.

Mucosa. The lining mucosa of pelvis and ureter consists of transitional epithelium supported by a lamina propria. The epithelium consists of two to three layers of cells in the pelvis and four to five layers in the ureter. The

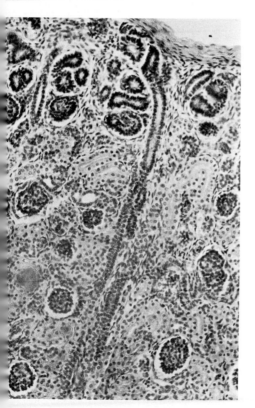

Figure 16-23. Photomicrograph of the cortex f developing human kidney of four months gestion. Note that the cortical renal corpuscles op) are less well developed than those near e medulla (bottom). × 125.

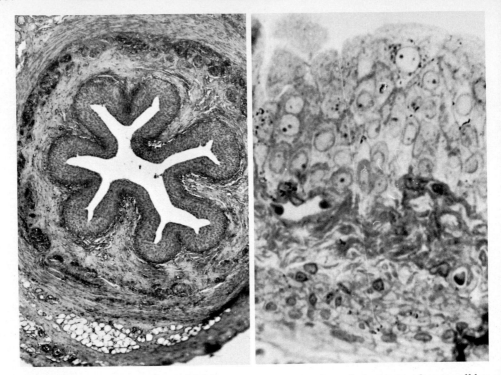

Figure 16-24.   Left, photomicrograph of a transverse section through the ureter, showing all layers, and, right, Epon section of the transitional epithelium lining the ureter. Left, × 35. Right, × 900.

See filmstrip II, frame 75

cells may be columnar if the tube is collapsed but become cuboidal if the lumen is distended. As described in Chapter 5, the cells of the surface layer present a convex border to the lumen and may be binucleate. By electron microscopy, the epithelium shows certain specializations. In cytoplasm immediately underlying the apical plasma membrane, there is a feltwork of fine filaments. The epithelium rests upon a fine basal lamina, usually not discernible by light microscopy, and this in turn is supported by relatively dense fibroconnective tissue of the lamina propria in which large numbers of elastic fibers are present. Some loose lymphatic tissue is present, and the deeper layers of the lamina propria have a much looser texture than the layer immediately subjacent to the epithelium. The elastic tissue in the lamina propria, the looseness of the outer layer, and the muscularis account for the presence of several longitudinal folds in the mucosa. The appearance in cross section is of a stellate, irregular lumen. No true submucosa is present but the outer, loose layer of the lamina propria has been so regarded by some investigators. No glands are present in pelvis and ureter, but small, solid clumps or knots of epithelial cells within the epithelium may be present.

Muscularis.   The muscularis is thick and consists of bundles of smooth muscle cells separated by strands of connective tissue. This smooth muscle is arranged as an inner longitudinal coat and an outer circular coat (the opposite orientation to that of smooth muscle in the intestine), but the layers are not clearly distinct and a third outer longitudinal or oblique layer is present at the lower end of the ureter. In the pelvis, the muscle mainly is orientated in a circular pattern around papillae and possibly has a sphincter action, perhaps squeezing or "milking" the papillae and thus expressing urine from the ducts of Bellini. At the lower end of the ureter, circularly arranged smooth muscle disappears but the two longitudinal layers, now not separated by the circular layer, are prominent and continue down to the ureteric orifice. Reflux of urine from the bladder up the ureter is prevented by a flap of bladder mucous membrane and by internal distention of the bladder. Urine does not flow continuously down the ureter but enters into the bladder in spurts, the longitudinal muscle fibers contracting to dilate the orifice.

Adventitia. External to the muscularis is a coat of fibroelastic connective tissue, which at the pelvis blends with the capsule of the kidney, and which is continuous with surrounding connective tissue of the posterior abdominal wall along the length of the ureter. The anterior surface of the pelvis and ureter is covered loosely by peritoneum.

The ureter has a rich arterial blood supply, with vascular and lymphatic plexuses in muscularis and lamina propria. Nerves, associated with some ganglion cells, are present and they supply motor fibers of the autonomic system to the muscularis. Sensory fibers extend through the muscularis to penetrate between the cells of the epithelium.

Bladder

The urinary bladder has a similar appearance to the ureter in sections. The transitional epithelium is thicker, consisting of six to eight layers of cells in the empty bladder, and only two to three layers in the distended bladder. The surface cells show, by electron microscopy, in their apical cytoplasm a collection of fusiform vesicles. These may represent a reservoir of surface membrane material which can be mobilized rapidly for expansion of the surface during distension of the bladder. A few small glands of clear mucus-secreting cells, with simple or branched ducts, are present in the lamina propria, particularly near the ureteric and internal urethral orifices. The lamina propria is thick with a loose external layer, sometimes called the submucosa, which permits the mucous membrane to become folded in the contracted bladder. The muscularis is of moderate thickness and consists of three layers, the middle circular layer being the most prominent and highly developed as a sphincter around the internal urethral orifice and, to a lesser extent, around the ureteric orifices. The adventitia is of fibroelastic tissue, with peritoneum covering only the superior surface of the bladder, where it is attached loosely.

The terminal urinary excretory passage connecting the bladder to the exterior is the urethra. That of the male differs markedly from that of the female.

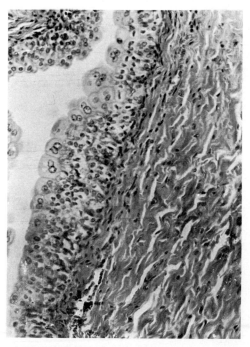

Figure 16-25. Photomicrograph of the transitional epithelium and lamina propria lining the contracted bladder. Note the surface cells, many of which are binucleate. × 275.

Male Urethra

This is 15 to 20 cm. in length and for descriptive purposes is divided into three regions. The first part passes inferiorly from the internal urethral orifice of the bladder to traverse the prostate gland. This is the *pars prostatica,* and opening into it are the two ejaculatory ducts and the ducts from prostatic glands. The second part, the *pars membranacea,* is short and passes from the apex of the prostate between striated muscles of the pelvis to perforate the perineal membrane and terminate in the bulb of the corpus cavernosa urethrae. The terminal urethra traverses the corpus spongiosum to open at the glans penis. This is called the *pars cavernosa* or *spongiosa,* or, simply, the penile portion of the urethra.

In the prostatic urethra, the lining epithelium is transitional in type but changes to a stratified or pseudostratified columnar epithelium in the remainder of the urethra, with patches of stratified squamous epithelium. The terminal dilatation of the penile urethra, the fossa navicularis, is lined by stratified squamous epithelium. A few mucus-secreting goblet cells are present. A loose, fibroelastic connective tissue lamina propria underlies the epithelium. The entire urethral mucous membrane is irregular with small depressions or pits extending deeply as branching tubular glands (of Littre). These are more numerous on the dorsal surface of the penile urethra, and are orientated obliquely with their bases situated proximal to their orifices. These glands are lined by epithelium similar to that lining the urethra and are mucus secreting.

Female Urethra

The female urethra is much shorter than that of the male, being only 1 to 2.5 to 4 cm. in length. It has a muscularis of two layers of smooth muscle orientated in a manner similar to those of the ureter, but reinforced by a striated muscle sphincter at its orifice. The lining epithelium is mainly stratified squamous in type, with patches of pseudostratified or stratified columnar epithelium. Glandular outpocketings, similar to the glands of Littre of the male, are present. The lamina propria is a loose fibroconnective tissue characterized by the presence of numerous venous sinuses resembling cavernous tissue.

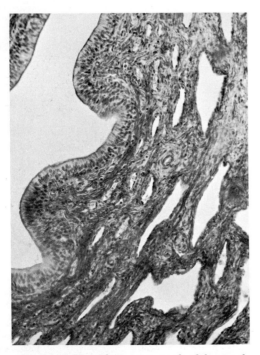

Figure 16-26. Photomicrograph of the penile portion of the male urethra. The lining epithelium here is stratified columnar. Note the surrounding cavernous tissue. × 125.

REFERENCES

Barajas, L.: The development and ultrastructure of the juxtaglomerular cell granule. J. Ultrastruct. Res., *15:*400, 1966.

Dalton, A. J., and Haguenau, F. (editors): Ultrastructure of the Kidney, Vol. 2. New York Academic Press, 1967.

Farquhar, M. G., and Palade, G. E.: Functional evidence for the existence of a third cell type in the renal glomerulus. J. Cell Biol., *13:*55, 1962.

Farquhar, M. G., Wissig, S. L., and Palade, G. E.: Glomerular permeability. I. Ferritin transfer across the normal glomerular capillary wall. J. Exp. Med., *113*:47, 1961.

Hall, B. V.: Further studies of the normal structure of the renal glomerulus. Proc. Sixth Ann. Conf. Nephrotic Syndrome. New York, National Nephrosis Foundation, *1*, 1954.

Hicks, R. M.: The function of the golgi complex in transitional epithelium. J. Cell Biol., *30*:623, 1966.

Kurtz, S. M.: The Kidney. *In* Electron Microscopic Anatomy, edited by S. M. Kurtz. New York, Academic Press, 1965, p. 239.

Latta, H., and Maunsbach, A. B.: The juxtaglomerular apparatus as studied electron microscopically. J. Ultrastruct. Res., *6*:547, 1962.

Latta, H., and Maunsbach, A. B.: Relations of the centrolobular region of the glomerulus to the juxtaglomerular apparatus. J. Ultrastruct. Res., *6*:562, 1962.

Leeson, T. S.: An electron microscope study of the postnatal development of the hamster kidney, with particular reference to the intertubular tissue. Lab. Invest., *10*:466, 1961.

Leeson, T. S., and Leeson, C. R.: The rat ureter. Fine structural changes during its development. Acta. Anat., *62*:60, 1965.

Maunsbach, A. B.: The influence of different fixatives and fixation methods on the ultrastructure of rat kidney proximal tubule cells. I. Comparison of different perfusion fixation methods and of glutaraldehyde and osmium tetroxide fixtures. II. Effects of varying osmolality, ionic strength, buffer system and fixative concentration of glutaraldehyde solutions. J. Ultrastruct. Res., *15*:242, 1966.

Pease, D. C.: Electron microscopy of the tubular cells of the kidney cortex. Anat. Rec., *121*:723, 1955.

Rhodin, J.: Correlation of ultrastructural organization and function in normal and experimentally changed proximal convoluted tubule cells of the mouse kidney. Stockholm, Aktiebolaget Godvil, 1954.

Symposium: Histochemistry and the elucidation of kidney structure and function. J. Histochem. Cytochem., *3*:243, 1955.

Vernier, R. L.: Ultrastructure of the glomerulus and changes in fine structure associated with increased permeability of the glomerulus to protein. *In* Ciba Foundation Symposium on Renal Biopsy, edited by G. E. W. Wolstenholme and M. P. Cameron. London, J. & A. Churchill, 1961.

Waugh, D., Prentice, R. S. A., and Yadav, E.: The structure of the proximal tubule: A morphological study of basement membrane cristae and their relationships in the renal tubule of the rat. Amer. J. Anat., *121*:775, 1967.

CHAPTER 17

THE ENDOCRINE SYSTEM

The endocrine system is composed mainly of glands which have lost connection with the parent epithelium. They possess no ducts and their secretions (hormones) are passed directly into the blood or lymph circulation; hence these glands are designated as *ductless glands* or *glands of internal secretion*. They have a rich and intimate blood supply which serves not only for the metabolic needs of the tissue but also for the transport of the secretory products. Most endocrine glands are separate entities, for example, hypophysis and thyroid. Some, however, are present as scattered masses within an exocrine gland, for instance, pancreatic islets, interstitial cells (of Leydig) of the testis, and corpora lutea of the ovary. These combined organs are called *mixed glands*. The liver also is a mixed gland, but here each hepatic cell exhibits both exocrine and endocrine functions. It secretes bile into the duct system and also passes internal secretions directly into the blood vessels.

Endocrine glands, as a group, have a very simple microscopic structure; they consist of either cords, plates, or clumps of cells separated by sinusoids or capillaries and supported by delicate connective tissue. The parenchyma is usually, although not invariably, composed of cells of epithelial or epithelioid character. The glands vary in their embryological derivation; as a group they are derived from all three germ layers in the embryo. The hypophysis, suprarenal medulla, and chromaffin bodies are of ectodermal origin. The ovaries, testes, and suprarenal cortex are derived from mesoderm. Parenchymal cells of thyroid, parathyroid, and islets of Langerhans arise from endoderm. The placenta possesses both maternal and fetal components.

Each endocrine gland secretes one or more specific substances called *hormones*. Hormones are discharged from cells of endocrine glands into the blood or lymph circulation and eventually are distributed to the tissue fluids everywhere. A hormone has an effect upon a particular tissue or organ or upon the body as a whole. Some hormones affect certain tissues and organs specifically; the organs affected are termed *target organs*. Only a minute quantity of hormone is required to produce an effect, usually an arousal or activation, occasionally an inhibitory type of response. Hormones differ greatly in their chemical composition; some are steroids, others polypeptide or proteins.

In some endocrine glands secretion accumulates within the cells of origin, e.g., pancreatic islets. In others the secretory product is stored in a central mass surrounded by secretory cells, thus forming a follicle, e.g., thyroid. In the suprarenal cortex, however, secretion is released almost as rapidly as it is formed.

This chapter deals with those endocrine glands which are separate organs. Other endocrine tissues, which are contained within organs of a wholly different type such as the pancreas and the gonads, will be described with the major organs of which they form a part.

HYPOPHYSIS

The hypophysis (pituitary gland) is the most complex of the endocrine glands. It is composed of two different tissues. The *adenohypophysis* (glandular portion) is derived from oral ectoderm which migrates dorsally as *Rathke's pouch* to surround partially the *neurohypophysis* (nervous portion), a ventral evagination from the floor of the diencephalon (forebrain). The hypophysis is buried in a bony fossa of the sphenoid bone, the sella turcica, and is covered by an extension of the dura mater, the *diaphragma sellae*. There is a small aperture in the diaphragm through which passes the hypophyseal stalk.

The hypophysis is about the size of a small, flattened grape. It is approximately 1 cm. in length, 1 to 1.3 cm. in width, and 0.5 cm. in height. It weighs

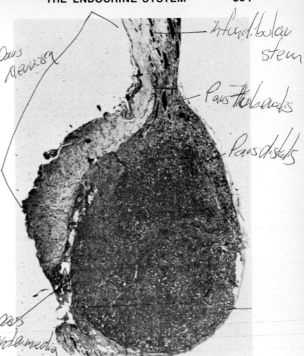

Figure 17-2. Low power microphotograph of a midsagittal section of human hypophysis. The pars nervosa, which lies to the left of the figure, is continuous above with the infundibular stem. The latter is in direct relationship anteriorly with the pars tuberalis. The pars distalis (darkly staining) is separated from the pars nervosa by the pars intermedia, represented here by a few large vesicles. Aldehyde fuchsin-trichrome stain. × 8.

about 0.5 to 0.6 gram in adults. It undergoes some enlargement during pregnancy and may weigh a gram or more in women who have borne children.

The adenohypophysis, which is pinkish in color in the fresh condition, is subdivided by the *residual lumen* of Rathke's pouch into two unequal portions. Anterior to the cleft is the *pars distalis*. An extension of this, the *pars tuberalis*, surrounds the neural stalk (see Figure 17-1). The third component of the adenohypophysis is the *pars intermedia*, which forms a thin cellular partition behind the cleft. The neurohypophysis, which appears white and fibrous in the fresh condition, consists of three parts. The major portion is the

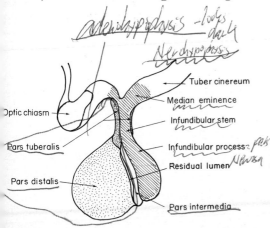

Figure 17-1. Diagram of midsagittal section of hypothalamus and hypophysis to show the various divisions.

Pars Distalis

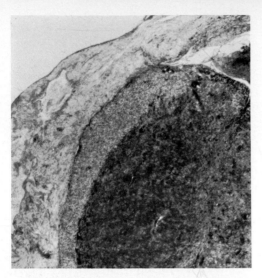

Figure 17-3. Midsagittal section of human hypophysis. The narrow pars intermedia is interposed between the pars nervosa (left) and the pars distalis (right). Aldehyde fuchsin-trichrome stain. × 20.

pars nervosa (infundibular process), which lies immediately posterior to the pars intermedia. Above, the pars nervosa is continuous with the *infundibular stem* and the *median eminence* of the tuber cinereum. The latter two together constitute the *infundibular (neural) stalk*. The *hypophyseal stalk* is composed of the infundibular stalk and the pars tuberalis.

The terms *anterior lobe* and *posterior lobe* are well established in the clinical and endocrinological literature; the anterior lobe refers to the portion anterior to the residual lumen, i.e., pars distalis and pars tuberalis, and the posterior lobe includes the parts posterior to the lumen, pars intermedia and pars nervosa.

The pars distalis constitutes about 75 per cent of the hypophysis, and is enclosed almost completely in a dense fibrous capsule. The parenchyma is in the form of anastomosing cords and clusters of epithelial cells supported by a network of reticular fibers continuous at the periphery with component fibers of the capsule. Between the parenchymal cells are sinusoidal capillaries.

The parenchyma is composed of two main categories of cells, *chromophils* and *chromophobes*. The former are subdivided into *acidophils* and *basophils* on the basis of the staining reactions of their cytoplasmic granules. However, the dyes used to distinguish these cells are acid dyes and do not distinguish acidic and basic properties of the cells. Recent workers have adopted the noncommittal terms *alpha* and *beta cells* for the two types of chromophils. The chromophobe cells, which have little affinity for dyes, sometimes are referred to as *chief* or *C cells*. The relative proportions of the cells vary markedly in man. Chromophobes constitute approximately 50 per cent of cells, acidophils 35 per cent, and basophils 15 per cent. The proportions may be altered considerably by castration, thyroidectomy, or other experimental procedures. Additional cell types may be demonstrated within the alpha and beta groups by special staining techniques and histochemical methods.

Chromophobes (C Cells). These faintly staining cells also are known as *reserve cells*. They are small, rounded or polygonal cells with relatively little

Terminology of the Pituitary Gland

Adenohypophysis (glandular lobe)	⎧ Pars distalis ⎫ ⎨ Pars tuberalis ⎬ ⎩ Pars intermedia ⎫	Anterior lobe
Neurohypophysis	⎧ Pars nervosa ⎫ ⎨ Infundibular stem ⎩ Median eminence	Posterior lobe

cytoplasm. The cell boundaries are not easily visible in ordinary preparations. The cytoplasm usually lacks specific granules. The chromophobes often appear in groups in the center of the cords. In Romeis's classification of pituitary cells the chromophobes are referred to as *gamma cells.*

Acidophils (Alpha Cells). The acidophils stain readily and are identified easily in ordinary preparations. They are larger than chromophobes and their cell boundaries are distinct. The cytoplasm is crowded with small specific granules which are stained by numerous dyes, such as eosin, acid fuchsin, orange G, and azocarmine. The affinity of the granules for the latter two dyes is used to differentiate two types of acidophils. Those whose granules take up the orange G of an azan stain are called *orangeophils* or *alpha acidophils;* those in which the granules

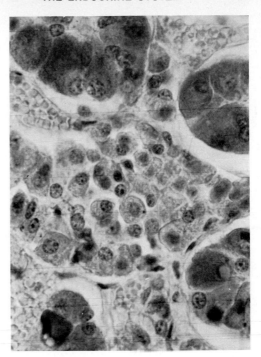

Figure 17-5. Human pars distalis. There is a large group of chromophobes (gamma cells) centrally. Note their small size relative to that of the chromophils (above). Hematoxylin and eosin. × 550.

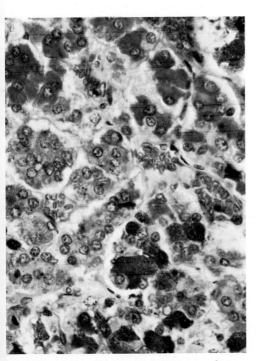

Figure 17-4. Representative area of pars distalis. Numerous acidophils occupy the upper part of the figure. The central region contains mainly chromophobes, and scattered basophils lie toward the lower portion of this micrograph. Aldehyde fuchsin-trichrome stain. × 250.

See filmstrip II, frame 76.

stain intensely with azocarmine are *carminophils* or *epsilon acidophils.* Electron micrographs appear to confirm the existence of two types of acidophils. In one kind, corresponding to the orangeophils, the granules are small (about 300 mμ in diameter) and are closely packed; in the other (carminophils), the granules are larger (up to 900 mμ in diameter) and are more scattered within the cytoplasm.

Basophils (Beta Cells). The basophils tend to be appreciably larger than the acidophils. The granules are less numerous than in acidophils and are smaller (about 150 to 200 mμ in diameter). They stain rather poorly with hematoxylin but are stained deeply with methylene blue. Basophils are best identified by the periodic acid–Schiff (PAS) technique where they are strongly positive owing to the concentration of glycoproteins in their secretory granules. In most

mammals at least two types of basophils can be distinguished. One type
stains with aldehyde fuchsin (*beta
basophil*), whereas the other (*delta
basophil*) does not.

In the chromophils, it is believed
that the granules are actual precursors
of the secretion. The degree of granularity is correlated with the physiological state of the cell when fixed. The
cells are thought to secrete cyclically
rather than continuously. Mitoses are
seen rarely in any of the cell types, and
it is certain that few if any of the cells
are destroyed when the secretory product is released. It appears that the
chromophobes represent reserve or inactive cells which give rise to the chromophils. As the chromophobes become active, granules form within
their cytoplasm. The granules are
specific for the different cell types. Engorged cells then secrete and the cells
revert to an inactive state.

Hormones Produced by the Pars Distalis

The pars distalis produces at least
six different hormones, most of which
are proteins of complex chemical
structure; some are polypeptides.

Growth Hormone. This hormone
(also called somatotrophic hormone or
STH) stimulates general body growth,
particularly growth at the epiphyses
of bones. Hypophysectomy causes a
cessation of growth which can be restored to normal by administration of
the hormone. Undersecretion leads
to dwarfism in certain animals, and
oversecretion, as in certain tumors of
the anterior lobe, causes *gigantism*
in children. If oversecretion occurs
after closure of epiphyseal discs, a
condition known as *acromegaly*, in
which the bones become thicker and
the hands and feet broader, results.

Thyrotrophic Hormone. This hormone (also called thyroid-stimulating
hormone or TSH), which has not been
as highly purified as most other hypophyseal hormones, maintains and stim-

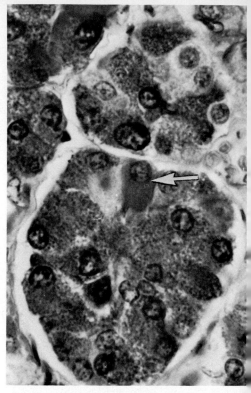

Figure 17-6. Human pars distalis. Basophils
are the principal cell type present on this micrograph. Note the discrete granulation of their
cytoplasm. One acidophil, in which discrete
granules are not apparent, occupies the center
of the field (arrow). Aldehyde fuchsin-trichrome
stain. × 625.

ulates the thyroid epithelium. Hypophysectomy results in atrophy of the
thyroid which may be restored to activity by administration of hormone ex-
tracts. Injections of TSH into normal
animals produce all the symptoms of
hyperthyroidism.

Adrenocorticotrophic   Hormone.
This hormone (also called ACTH)
causes growth of the suprarenal cortex and secretion of its hormones. The
atrophy of the suprarenal cortex which
follows hypophysectomy can be prevented by the administration of ACTH.

Follicle-stimulating   Hormone.
This hormone (also called FSH) promotes growth of ovarian follicles in the
female and activates the testes to produce spermatozoa in the male. In the

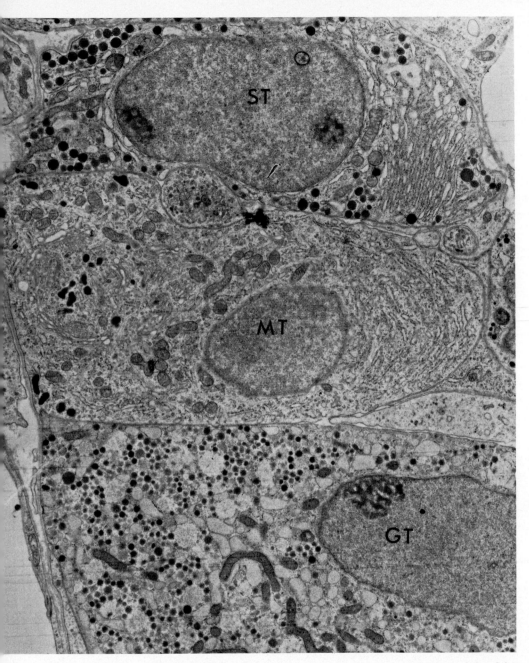

Figure 17-7. Electron micrograph of rat pars distalis. Note the varying appearance of the different cell types. In the anterior lobe of the rat pituitary, there are thought to be four morphologically distinct functional cell types: somatotrophs (ST), mammotrophs (MT), gonadotrophs (GT), and thyrotrophs (TT), so named to denote their association with the production of growth, mammotrophic (lactogenic), gonadotrophic (GT), and thyrotrophic hormones, respectively. With the light microscope, cell types are distinguished by differences in staining affinities of their secretion granules, somatotrophs and mammotrophs being acidophil, and gonadotrophs and thyrotrophs basophil. With the electron microscope, secretory granule size is the most useful criterion for identification of cell types. In the rat pituitary, maximum granule diameters are: ST, 350 mμ; MT, 600 to 900 mμ; GT, 200 mμ; TT, 150 mμ. × 7000. (Courtesy of M. G. Farquhar.)

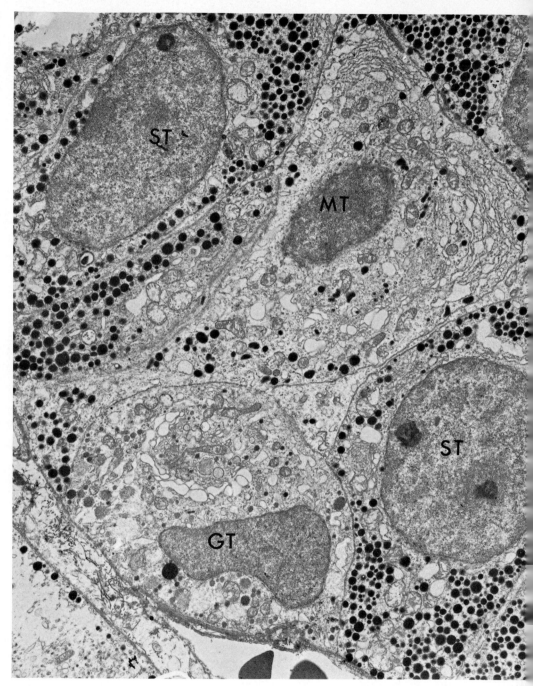

Figure 17-8.   Electron micrograph of rat pars distalis. For explanation, refer to Figure 17-7. A portion of a capillary is shown lower center. × 7000 (Courtesy of M. G. Farquhar.)

female, FSH acts usually in association with luteinizing hormone (LH), which ensures final maturation of the follicle, ovulation, and subsequent formation of the corpus luteum (*vide infra*). Atrophy of the sex organs occurs after hypophysectomy. They may be restored nearly to normal by administration of FSH, but complete recovery requires some LH in addition to FSH.

Luteinizing Hormone, Interstitial Cell-stimulating Hormone. Luteinizing hormone (LH) alone has no direct action on the ovary of a hypophysectomized animal. It acts only after prior stimulation of follicles by FSH. LH is necessary for the conversion of the ruptured follicle into a corpus luteum. In the male the luteinizing hormone (ICSH) stimulates the interstitial (Leydig) cells of the testes to produce an androgen, presumably testosterone, which in turn maintains the accessory reproductive organs and the secondary sex characteristics. The effect is augmented by the administration of FSH.

Prolactin. This hormone (also called lactogenic hormone, luteotrophic hormone, or LTH) causes secretion of milk following development of the ducts and secretory portions of the mammary gland in response to ovarian hormones during pregnancy. Another important function of this hormone is to stimulate the corpus luteum of the ovary to secrete progesterone in certain species (e.g., the rat).

Thus, although the pars distalis has only three principal cell types, it secretes at least six different hormones. Many attempts have been made to associate the secretion of the hormones with specific cell types. Much of the evidence as to the cell of origin is clinicopathological and is based upon the symptoms which result from tumors of specific cell types in the anterior lobe. In acromegaly and in gigantism, for instance, tumors of acidophils are present almost invariably. The suggestion that acidophils are responsible for the production of growth hormone is supported also by the finding that pituitaries in certain dwarfs have a deficiency of alpha cells. There is evidence that the acidophils also secrete prolactin (luteotrophic hormone). High titers of prolactin are found in areas of the pituitary which contain large concentrations of acidophils, and acidophils increase in size and in number during pregnancy. In most species in which two types of acidophils can be demonstrated, it appears that a separation can be made also as to the secretory product of each. The population of orangeophils (alpha acidophils) remains relatively constant during pregnancy in most species, whereas the carminophils (epsilon acidophils) show marked fluctuations. It appears, therefore, that orangeophils produce growth hormone and carminophils prolactin. Opposite conditions exist in the rat, in which the orangeophils react during pregnancy.

The follicle-stimulating hormone is thought to be produced by the basophils. After castration, the rat hypophysis contains increased amounts of gonadotrophic hormones and the basophils become enlarged and vacuolated (*castration cells*). Basophils are thought also to be responsible for the secretion of thyrotrophic hormone. Thyroidectomy, as well as castration, results in an increase in the percentage of basophils. There is further evidence that it is the beta basophils which are responsible for the production of the thyrotrophic hormone and that the follicle-stimulating hormone is elaborated in the delta basophils.

The present evidence as to the site of production of the adenocorticotrophic hormone is inconclusive, although most findings appear to indicate that it occurs in the basophils.

Chromophobes are believed to be inactive with regard to hormone production. Tumors of chromophobe cells usually cause symptoms of hypofunction of the pituitary.

Pars Intermedia

In man the pars intermedia is less well developed than in many other ani-

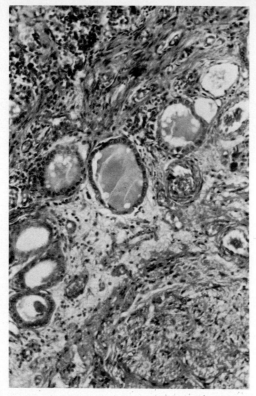

Figure 17-9. Pars intermedia. Follicles of the latter are interposed between the pars distalis (upper left) and the pars nervosa (lower right). × 100.

mals and usually is poorly defined. It forms only about 2 per cent of the hypophysis. It is composed of a thin layer of cells and of vesicles which contain colloid. It lies in close relation to the residual lumen, which virtually is obliterated in most adults. Some component cells, polygonal in shape, are small and pale staining; others are somewhat larger and granular, and stain deeply with basic dyes. The cells which are basophil frequently extend as cords for a short distance into the pars nervosa. The cells lining the colloid-containing vesicles commonly are ciliated, and some are mucus-secreting.

The function of the pars intermedia in man is not known. In certain species, e.g., amphibia, the pars intermedia is well developed and produces *intermedin,* a polypeptide hormone which causes expansion of the pigment-containing chromatophores in the skin. This expansion darkens the skin and enables the organism to blend better with its surroundings.

Pars Tuberalis

The pars tuberalis forms a collar of cells around the infundibular stalk. The cells, in close association with numerous blood vessels, are arranged in groups or short cords longitudinally oriented. They are cuboidal and the cytoplasm, which is weakly basophil, contains fine granules and some glycogen. Small vesicles, which contain colloid, are seen occasionally.

The function of the pars tuberalis, if any, is unknown.

Neurohypophysis

The neurohypophysis includes the median eminence of the tuber cinereum, the infundibular stem, and the infundibular process (pars nervosa). All three portions have the same characteristic cells and the same nerve and blood supply and contain the same ac-

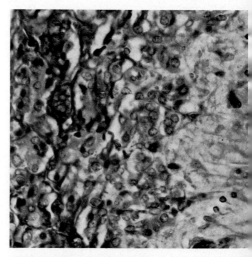

Figure 17-10. Pars tuberalis. A small portion of the infundibular stem lies to the right of the figure. × 200.

tive hormonal principle. Some 100,000 unmyelinated nerve fibers, constituting the *hypothalamo-hypophyseal tract*, pass into the neurohypophysis. Their cell bodies lie in the supraoptic and paraventricular nuclei of the hypothalamus.

The cells of the neurohypophysis, *pituicytes*, resemble neuroglia cells elsewhere in the central nervous system. Pituicytes are small cells with short branching processes which end in relation either to blood vessels or to connective tissue septa. Within the cytoplasm are fatty droplets, granules, and pigment. Pituicytes are present throughout the neurohypophysis and are especially abundant in the pars nervosa. The cells can be blackened by silver and, according to their morphological appearance in silvered preparations, four types are distinguished: *reticulopituicytes, micropituicytes, fibropituicytes,* and *adenopituicytes.*

A feature of the neurohypophysis is the presence within it of granules of varying size which stain deeply with chrome alum hematoxylin. These are the so-called *Herring bodies*, which

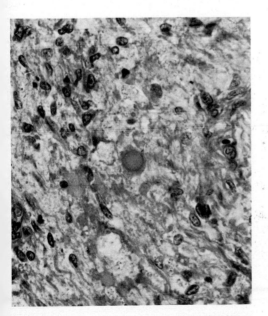

Figure 17-11. Pars nervosa. A distinct Herring body is present in the center of the field. × 250.

are particularly abundant in the pars nervosa. The earlier view that Herring bodies represented extracellular accumulations of secretory material has been disproved. Electron micrographs reveal granules in the cytoplasm of cells of the supraoptic and paraventricular nuclei, in the nerve fibers of the hypothalamo-hypophyseal tract, and in the nerve terminals. The secretory material is not elaborated in the pituicytes. Nerve cells of the supraoptic and paraventricular nuclei are neurosecretory and elaborate material which passes along the unmyelinated nerve fibers to the neurohypophysis where the secretion is stored. Herring bodies represent marked accumulations of neurosecretory material in the nerve terminals, which lie in close proximity to the capillary network. After sectioning of the hypophyseal stalk, there is a disappearance of neurosecretory material distal to the lesion and an accumulation of granules in relation to the severed nerve fibers in the stump.

The neurosecretory material is believed to be a protein which is associated with the actual hormones. The hormones of the neurohypophysis are *oxytocin* and *vasopressin*, both polypeptides. Oxytocin causes the smooth muscle of the uterus to contract. It also induces contraction of the myoepithelial (basket) cells of the alveoli and ducts of the mammary gland. Vasopressin is also known as antidiuretic hormone (ADH) and pharmacologically raises blood pressure by stimulating contraction of smooth muscle in the walls of blood vessels.

Blood and Nerve Supply of the Hypophysis

The blood supply of the hypophysis has unusual features and plays an important role in the secretory activity of the gland.

The anterior lobe is supplied by several *superior hypophyseal arteries* which arise from the internal carotids and the circle of Willis. Some arteries pass directly to the anterior lobe where they empty into sinusoidal capillaries. Others anastomose freely in the region of the median eminence and the infundibular stem and pass into a capillary network in the median eminence. The capillaries of this network drain into veins which run downward around the hypophyseal stalk to reach the sinusoidal capillaries of the anterior lobe. This system of venous connections between the capillaries of the median eminence and the sinusoidal capillaries of the adenohypophysis constitutes the *hypophyseal portal system*. The system appears to represent a connection by which neurohumoral substances ("hormone-releasing factors") from the median eminence may pass to the anterior lobe. It is an important pathway in the regulation of adenohypophyseal function.

The posterior lobe receives blood from the *inferior hypophyseal arteries*, branches of the internal carotids. Veins from anterior and posterior lobes drain into the cavernous sinuses.

The capillaries of the posterior lobe are smaller than the sinusoidal capillaries of the anterior lobe. Electron micrographs show an attenuated type of endothelium, with fenestrations, both in the capillaries and in the sinusoids. The deficiencies within the endothelial lining presumably facilitate passage of secretory material into the vessels.

The principal innervation of the neurohypophysis is the hypothalamo-hypophyseal tract, which originates mainly from the supraoptic and paraventricular nuclei. The unmyelinated nerve fibers of the tract course down the infundibular stalk to the infundibular process where they end in close relation to the fenestrated capillaries. It is questionable if any of the fibers extend into the anterior lobe.

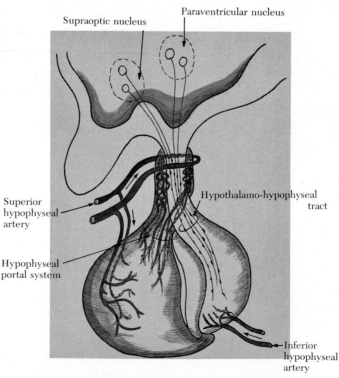

Supraoptic nucleus

Paraventricular nucleus

Superior hypophyseal artery

Hypophyseal portal system

Hypothalamo-hypophyseal tract

Inferior hypophyseal artery

Figure 17-12.   Diagram to illustrate the principal vascular and nervous relations of the hypophysis.

Histogenesis of the Hypophysis

The hypophysis arises from two separate sources. One portion arises as an evagination of the ectoderm of the primitive buccal cavity which extends as *Rathke's pouch* toward the floor of the diencephalon. The pouch comes in close relationship with a downgrowth, the *infundibulum*, from the floor of the diencephalon. The infundibulum gives rise to the neural stalk and the pars nervosa. Rathke's pouch loses its attachment to the pharyngeal roof by rupture of its original stalk and develops into the adenohypophysis. The cells of its anterior wall proliferate actively and reduce the lumen of the pouch to a narrow cleft. This proliferation forms the pars distalis and from its upper part cells extend around the neural stalk to form the pars tuberalis. The posterior wall of the original pouch, lying between the residual cleft and the pars nervosa, remains thin and becomes the pars intermedia.

THYROID GLAND

The thyroid gland, which is situated in the anterior region of the neck, consists of two *lateral lobes* connected by a narrow *isthmus*. The isthmus lies over the second to the fourth tracheal cartilages, and the lateral lobes lie in relation to the superior part of the trachea and to the inferior part of the larynx. Frequently a median *pyramidal lobe*, which extends upward anterior to the larynx, is present in addition.

The gland is enveloped externally by a connective tissue capsule which is continuous with the deep cervical fascia. Under this there is an inner, true capsule which is thinner and

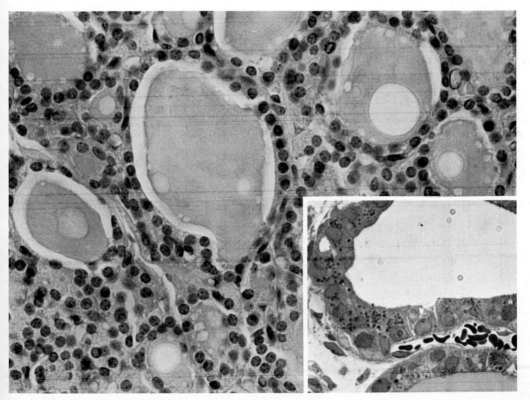

Figure 17-13. Thyroid gland. The lumen of each follicle is occupied by colloid. The interval between the colloid and the apical limit of the follicular epithelium is artifactual owing to shrinkage in preparation. × 375. Inset: Epon section. × 450.   **See filmstrip II, frame 77.**

which adheres closely to the gland. Delicate continuations of the inner capsule extend as septa into the gland, dividing it into indefinite *lobes* and *lobules.*

Follicles, the structural units of the gland, compose the lobules. They vary greatly in size, depending upon the degree of distention by secretion. They also vary in shape but usually are irregularly spheroidal. The follicles are embedded within a delicate meshwork of reticular fibers which also supports a close net of capillaries.

A follicle consists of a layer of simple epithelium enclosing a cavity which usually is filled with a stiff jelly called *colloid.* The shape of the component cells varies but commonly is cuboidal. The cells are low when the gland is hypoactive, high when the gland is hyperactive. Cell height in any one follicle is uniform and the arrangement is regular. The bases of the cells rest upon a delicate basal lamina. The

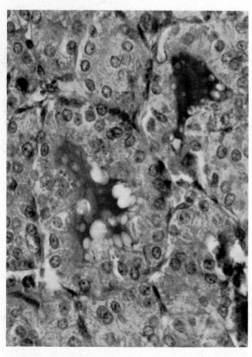

Figure 17-14. Thyroid follicles. Colloid stains deeply owing to the staining method used. Darkly staining granules are present in the apical cytoplasm of some follicular cells. PAS reaction. × 350.

large, vesicular nuclei lie centrally or toward the base. The cytoplasm is finely granular and basophil. The Golgi apparatus and centrioles are located above the nucleus. Lipid droplets and other inclusions, principally *colloid droplets,* are found in the cytoplasm of some cells. Junctional complexes are a feature of the interface between cells, and the free border is provided with small microvilli, visible only with the electron microscope. Some cells possess true cilia.

Colloid fills the follicular lumen. Fresh colloid is homogeneous, clear, and viscous. However, it undergoes shrinkage during the procedures employed in the preparation of microscopic sections and may show irregularities. Spaces often are present between the colloid and the epithelium and vacuoles may occur within the colloid. The irregularities are indications of the state of the colloid and are most common in activated glands. Colloid stains basophil in active follicles, whereas in inactive follicles it is weakly basophil or acidophil.

Colloid, which represents a reserve of secretion, is rich in nucleoproteins (hence its basophilia) and contains *thyroglobulin* and enzymes. Thyroglobulin is a glycoprotein containing several iodinated amino acids, the proportions of which vary from follicle to follicle. Thyroglobulin stains deeply with the PAS reaction.

The secretory process is complex and difficult to follow. It involves synthesis of the thyroid hormone, temporary storage, and release into the perifollicular capillaries. Both synthesis and release may occur at the same time. Thyroid cells remove iodine rapidly from the blood stream and concentrate it. The major part of the iodine is incorporated in follicles in an organic form. The incorporation of iodine in follicular cells and in colloid can be followed by the use of radioactive iodine (I^{131}). The iodine within the colloid is present in the form of *diiodothyronine,* *triiodothyronine,* and *tetraiodothyronine (thyroxine),* bound

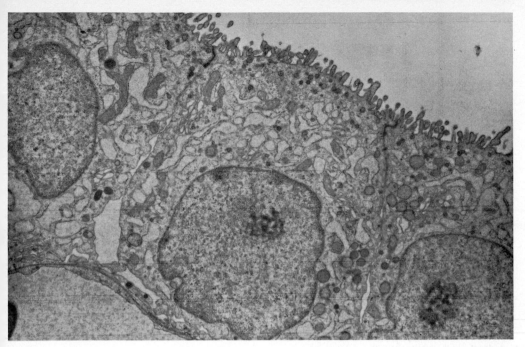

Figure 17-15. Electron micrograph of thyroid follicular cells. The cytoplasm contains dilated profiles of endoplasmic reticulum and scattered elements of the Golgi apparatus. The apical border is provided with small microvilli. A perifollicular capillary is present in the lower left corner of the figure. × 7200. (Courtesy of S. L. Wissig.)

to a globulin. These are components of thyroglobulin. The release of the active component also is difficult to follow. It may result from breakdown of the large thyroglobulin molecule by a proteolytic enzyme known to be present in the colloid. The smaller molecules resulting from the hydrolysis can be absorbed readily by the epithelium and discharged into adjoining capillaries.

Function of the Thyroid Gland

The most striking effect of the thyroid secretion is its regulation of the metabolic rate. Thyroxine increases cell metabolism and thus is concerned too with development, differentiation, and growth. *Hypothyroidism* in the infant leads to *cretinism*; hypofunction in the adult causes *myxedema*. Symp-

toms in both conditions are due to a reduction in the metabolic rate and may be removed by the administration of thyroid. *Hyperthyroidism* leads to overactivity and sometimes is complicated by the development of *exophthalmic goiter*. In hyperthyroidism some follicles become enlarged and follicular cells increase in height. Surgical removal of a part of the thyroid or the administration of antithyroid drugs or radioiodine reduces the metabolic rate.

Recent work has demonstrated that the thyroid gland elaborates, in addition to the thyroid hormone, a hormone called *thyrocalcitonin* (or *calcitonin*), a polypeptide which actively lowers the concentration of calcium in the plasma. The thyroid contains, in addition to the principal cells of the follicles, a smaller population of cells which have been known variously as "light cells," *parafollicular cells*, or C

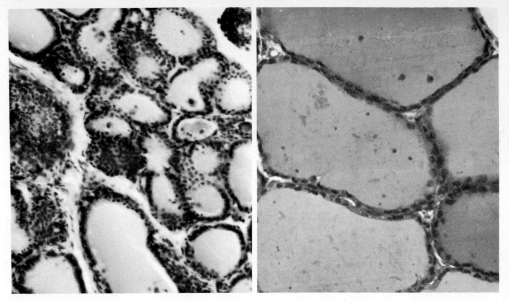

Figure 17-16. Rat thyroid gland: left, hyperactive; right, hypoactive. In the latter, follicles are large and the epithelial height is decreased. Left, × 100. Right, × 250.

cells. These cells, which lie adjacent to the follicles but within the basal lamina, possess distinct histological and histochemical features. From studies utilizing immunofluorescent techniques there can be little doubt that these cells are the site of production of thyrocalcitonin. The hormone lowers the calcium level in the plasma by a direct action on bone, inhibiting bone resorption. Hypercalcemia is the stimulus for secretion of the hormone and hypocalcemia inhibits secretion. It appears therefore that secretion is controlled by a feedback mechanism operating through the plasma calcium level in a manner similar to that of control of the secretion of the parathyroid hormone, but in the reverse direction.

The thyroid gland has certain interrelations with the anterior pituitary gland. Thyrotrophic hormone (TSH) stimulates release of thyroxine. Thyroidectomy results in hypertrophy of the anterior lobe with degranulation of alpha cells and the appearance of betacells which morphologically exhibit certain alterations (so-called *thyroidectomy cells*).

Blood Vessels and Nerves

Blood and lymph capillaries form intimate plexuses about thyroid follicles. Arteriovenous anastomoses are common. The architecture of the blood vessels indicates that there are fluctuations in the amount of blood supplied to different regions of the gland.

Numerous unmyelinated nerve fibers are present in the walls of the thyroid arteries. Most of these are vasomotor in function. A few fibers end in relation to the bases of some thyroid cells, but no definite secretory function has been ascribed to them.

Histogenesis of the Thyroid

The thyroid gland develops as a median downgrowth of the base of the tongue. The foramen cecum of the adult tongue is a vestige that indicates the site of origin. The thyroglossal duct, which connects the developing gland with the foramen cecum, usually becomes obliterated. Remnants of the duct may give rise to cysts or to the pyramidal lobe, a cranial extension of the isthmus. The thyroid gland may include also derivatives of the branchial pouches, such as the *ultimobranchial body*. Some authors consider this body to be the origin of parafollicular (C) cells.

The primordium of the gland initially is a compact mass of epithelial cells which later splits to form a network of solid cords or plates. These break up into small cellular groups, in each of which a lumen develops. As the lumen enlarges, the cells surrounding it become arranged into a single layer to form the definitive follicle.

PARATHYROID GLANDS

There are usually two pairs of parathyroid glands in man, but accessory glands occur frequently. The glands are small, brownish, oval bodies which lie in close relation to the thyroid gland. The upper parathyroids lie on the posterior surface of the thyroid about midway between the upper and lower poles of the lobes, whereas the lower ones are in relation to the lower poles of the thyroid lobes.

Each parathyroid gland is covered by a thin capsule which separates it from the thyroid. Delicate septa, which pass inward from the capsule, carry blood vessels and a few nerve fibers into the gland. A network of reticular fibers supports the parenchyma, which is composed of masses and cords of epithelial cells. The epithelial cells are of two types, *chief* or *principal cells* and *oxyphil cells*. Chief cells, which are more abundant than oxyphil cells, sometimes are divided into clear and dark forms. Clear chief cells have large vesicular nuclei and a clear, pale staining cytoplasm which contains no granules. Dark chief cells have smaller nuclei and a finely granular cytoplasm. Both forms are rich in glycogen.

Oxyphil cells are larger than chief cells and characteristically are present in small or large groups. They have small, darkly staining nuclei, and the cytoplasm is acidophil and contains

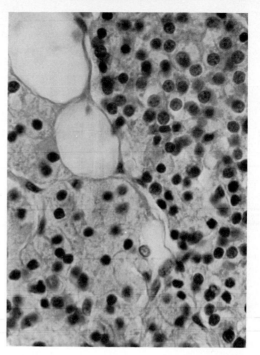

Figure 17-17. Parathyroid gland. There is a concentration of chief (principal) cells in the upper right hand corner of the figure and of oxyphil cells in the lower left hand corner. Two fat cells are present also. × 550.

fine granules and numerous mitochondria. They are not present in man until about five to seven years of age, and thereafter they increase in number, especially after puberty.

Small colloid follicles are seen occasionally and are more noticeable in old age. The material they contain has no functional relation to the colloid of the thyroid gland. Scattered fat cells are present within the parenchyma.

Function

The parathyroid glands elaborate the parathyroid hormone, a protein consisting of a single polypeptide chain. No association between the different cell types and the production of the hormone has been established. The hormone is important in the regulation of calcium metabolism. A lowering of the plasma concentration of calcium is followed by an increased output of the hormone, which in turn withdraws calcium from the bones. Atrophy or removal of the parathyroids causes a fall in blood calcium, which is accompanied by nervous hyperexcitability and muscular spasms, leading to death due to tetany. Administration of calcium or parathyroid extract relieves the symptoms. Hypertrophy of the glands occurs in conditions such as rickets, when there is a calcium deficiency. *Hyperparathyroidism* may result from tumor or hyperplasia and is associated with an elevated blood calcium level and extensive bone resorption.

Blood Vessels and Nerves

The parathyroids have a rich vascular supply, the larger vessels following the septa into the interior of the gland. A fine net of capillaries lies in relation to the parenchyma, and it is claimed that each parenchymal cell abuts directly against a capillary.

Unmyelinated nerve fibers, probably vasomotor, are scanty.

SUPRARENAL GLANDS

The suprarenal, or adrenal, glands are roughly pyramidal, flattened organs, one at the cranial pole of each kidney. The hilum is an indentation on the anterior surface. A sectioned, fresh gland shows two regions, an outer *cortex* which is yellow externally and reddish-brown internally and a thin inner *medulla* which is gray. These regions are distinct structurally, developmentally, and functionally. The cortex develops from epithelium (mesothelium) lining the primitive body cavity (coelom) and the medulla from the neural crest and presumptive autonomic ganglion (*sympathochromaffin*) tissue. In lower vertebrates the two tissues are not united into a single organ.

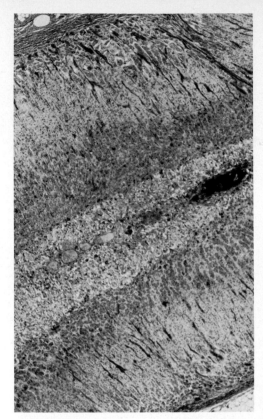

Figure 17-18. Low power micrograph of a section through the whole thickness of the suprarenal gland. Portions of the capsule are present in the upper left and lower right corners. The central region is occupied by the medulla. The darkly staining cortical cells in immediate relationship to the medulla constitute the inner portion of the zona fasciculata and the zona reticularis. × 25.

Each gland is surrounded by a tough connective tissue capsule which sends radial trabeculae, consisting principally of reticular fibers, into the cortex. Capillaries penetrate into the gland along the delicate trabeculae.

Cortex

The cortex, the major part of the gland, is divided into three ill-defined layers: a thin, outer zone, the *zona glomerulosa;* a thick, middle zone, the *zona fasciculata;* and an inner zone, the *zona reticularis*, directly in relation to the medulla.

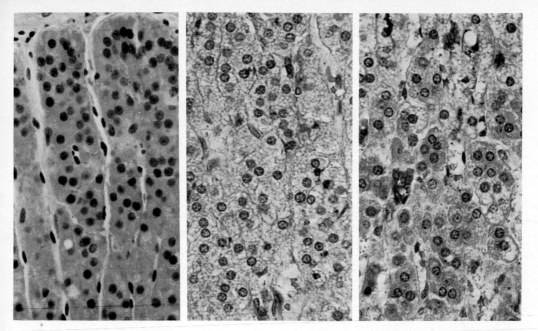

Figure 17-19. Representative areas of zona glomerulosa (left), zona fasciculata (center), and zona reticularis (right), Note the vacuolated appearance of the cytoplasm of component cells (spongiocytes) of the zona fasciculata. × 250.   See filmstrip II, frame 78.

The zona glomerulosa consists of columnar epithelial cells arranged in ovoid groups which normally show no central lumen. Nuclei stain deeply and the cytoplasm contains basophil material.

The zona fasciculata, the thickest layer, is composed of large, irregularly cuboidal cells arranged in long, radial cords, usually two cells wide. Nuclei are vesicular and frequently cells are binucleate. The cytoplasm is basophil and contains lipid droplets, composed of cholesterol, fatty acids, and neutral fat. Lipid droplets are most numerous in cells of the outer two-thirds of the zone. Since lipids are removed by the usual technical procedures, the cells here appear vacuolated and have a spongy appearance; hence sometimes they are called *spongiocytes*. The inner third of the zone is relatively free of lipid material and is more basophil.

In the zona reticularis, the cell cords form an anastomosing network. Near the zona fasciculata, component cells differ little from those of that zone; in general the cytoplasm contains fewer

lipid droplets. Near the medulla the cells appear "light" or "dark" depending upon their staining affinities. Many cells have shrunken nuclei and deeply staining cytoplasm and contain

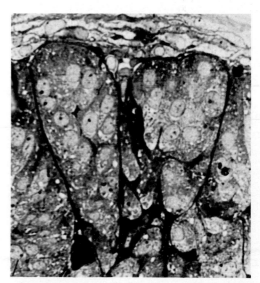

Figure 17-20. Zona glomerulosa of suprarenal gland. Note the ovoid groups of cells. Epon section. × 450.

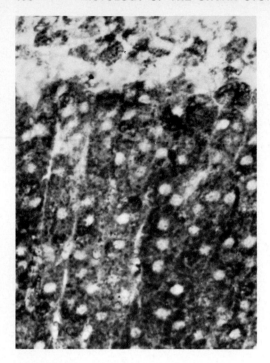

Figure 17-21. Zona fasciculata of suprarenal gland in a frozen section stained specifically to show lipid material, which appears as darkly staining droplets within the cytoplasm. The empty spaces represent the nuclear areas. A portion of the zona glomerulosa is present above. Sudan black B. × 375.

pigment granules. Both light and dark cells show evidences of degeneration.

The zonation just considered is based upon the general arrangement and organization of cells in the cortex. On the basis of cell structure, however, the cortex can be divided into four zones. The outer zone corresponds to the zona glomerulosa. The second zone is the outer two-thirds of the zona fasciculata, consisting of spongiocytes. The inner third of the zona fasciculata and the outer half of the zona reticularis comprise the third zone, a region poor in lipids. The fourth zone is the inner half of the zona reticularis (the juxtamedullary portion), in which many component cells are senescent and contain pigment. Previously it was thought that new cells were produced in the zona glomerulosa, migrated inward to the zona fasciculata, and finally degenerated in the zona reticularis. The observation of mitotic figures in all zones, particularly in the outer region of the zona fasciculata, and of degenerating cells in zones other than the reticularis has thrown doubt upon this hypothesis.

On electron microscopy, the most characteristic feature of component cells of the outer two zones is the well-developed, smooth-surfaced endoplasmic reticulum. In cells of the zona glomerulosa, this appears as an anastomosing network of tubules, and the extent of this network is even more marked in cells of the zona fasciculata. In the latter zone, the Golgi apparatus is large, and lysosomes and deposits of lipochrome pigment also are prominent features.

Medulla

The boundary between cortex and medulla usually is irregular in man, although in many other animals the boundary may be sharp. Cells of the medulla are ovoid and occur in groups or short, anastomosing cords, surrounded by venules and capillaries. Medullary cells have large, vesicular

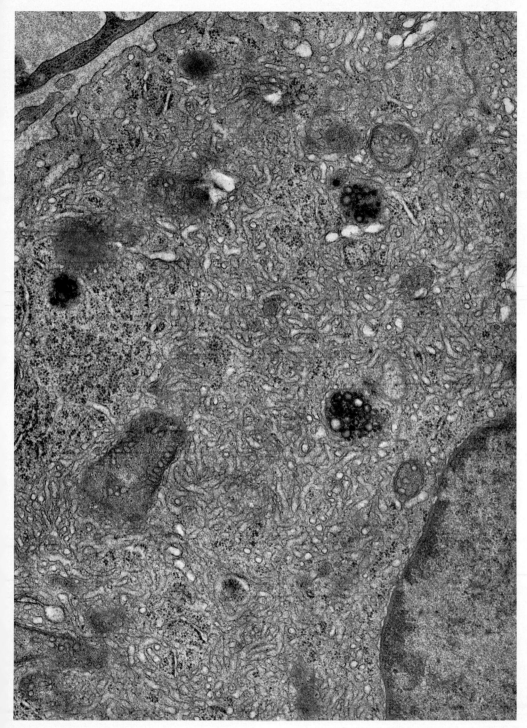

Figure 17-22.   Electron micrograph of a zona fasciculata cell of human adrenal cortex. Note the extensive development of smooth-surfaced endoplasmic reticulum (center). The dark masses are pigment granules. × 18,600. (Courtesy of J. A. Long.)

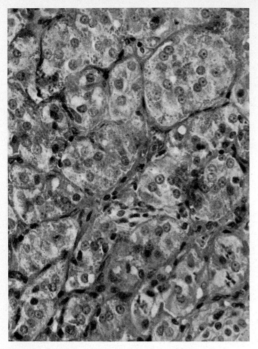

Figure 17-23. Suprarenal medulla. Component cells occur in groups, surrounded by capillaries and delicate connective tissue. Note the granularity of the cytoplasm. × 250.

nuclei, and their cytoplasm contains fine granules which become brown when oxidized by potassium bichromate. This is the *chromaffin reaction*, and the cells therefore are called *chromaffin* (or *pheochrome*) *cells*. The reaction is due in large part to the presence of the precursors of the hormone *epinephrine*. The granules also stain green with zinc chloride and brown with osmic acid. Each chromaffin cell is said to be orientated with one end abutting on a capillary, the other on a venule. In addition to chromaffin cells, the medulla contains a few autonomic ganglion cells.

Functions of the Suprarenal Glands

The cortex and medulla are functionally distinct. The cortex is essential to life. Cortical destruction by tuberculosis (Addison's disease) or

removal is fatal unless averted by administration of cortical extract. The cortex is necessary to man in a variety of essential factors. It maintains *water and electrolyte balance* in the body. After ablation of the cortex, there is concentration of the plasma, excessive excretion of sodium, and a shift of water from extracellular spaces to tissue cells. The cortex also maintains *carbohydrate balance*. If control is lost, glycogen stores in liver and muscle are depleted and *hypoglycemia* results. *Maintenance of the intercellular substances* of connective tissue is an additional function of the cortex.

More than forty steroid compounds have been isolated from the cortex, at least seven of which have been shown to possess physiological activity. In general, the active compounds can be divided into three categories as judged by their type of activity. Those of the first group are called *mineralocorticoids* (*aldosterone* and *deoxycorticosterone*), and they control electrolyte and water balance. Those of the second category participate in carbohydrate metabolism and are known as the *glucocorticoids* (*hydrocortisone* and *cortisone*). The latter compounds also affect connective tissues. Steroid hormones of the third category include both female sex hormones (estrogen and progesterone) and several androgenic hormones. Some tumors that arise in the cortex have a masculinizing or a feminizing effect.

There is some evidence pointing to a functional specialization of the various cortical zones. It appears that the mineralocorticoids are produced primarily in the zona glomerulosa, the glucocorticoids in the zona fasciculata, and, perhaps, the sex hormones in the zona reticularis.

The normal activity of the suprarenal cortex is partially under the control of the adrenocorticotrophic hormone (ACTH) of the adenohypophysis, which affects principally the zona fasciculata.

Marked changes occur in the human

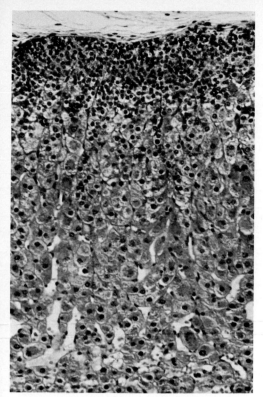

Figure 17-24. Fetal suprarenal cortex. Note the cellularity and lack of organization of the cortex immediately beneath the capsule. × 100.

suprarenal cortex after birth. Within two weeks after birth, most of the inner or *boundary zone* of the cortex (*fetal cortex*) has disappeared, leaving only *subcapsular (permanent) cortex*. The latter consists of zona glomerulosa and zona fasciculata. Zona reticularis becomes established by the end of the third year. The significance of the fetal cortex is poorly understood, but its development is thought to be dependent upon hormones elaborated by the placenta.

The suprarenal medulla is not essential to life. It produces *epinephrine* and *norepinephrine,* which are *catecholamines*. Their presence in the cytoplasmic granules can be detected by the chromaffin reaction. The number of chromaffin granules in a cell is an index of its secretory state. The two hor-

mones are closely related chemically and norepinephrine may be a precursor of epinephrine, but they have somewhat different effects. Epinephrine has a marked effect on metabolism, increasing oxygen consumption and mobilizing glucose from liver glycogen stores. It increases cardiac output and prepares the body to meet emergency situations. Norepinephrine has little general metabolic action, and its chief function is as the principal transmitter substance or mediator of adrenergic nerve impulses acting upon the heart and blood vessels to maintain blood pressure. Epinephrine has an additional effect upon the secretory activity of the anterior hypophysis, causing it to produce increased amounts of ACTH.

Blood Vessels and Nerves

The suprarenal glands receive a rich vascular supply. A variable number of arteries supplies each gland. As the arteries reach the gland, they branch into numerous arterioles which pierce the capsule. Some arterioles enter cortical sinusoids, which are lined by cells of the reticuloendothelial system. Other arterioles pass directly to the medulla where they empty into a capillary plexus. Venous blood both from the cortex and from the medulla drains into a system of venules which join to form a medullary vein.

Lymphatic vessels are found only in the capsule and in the connective tissue surrounding large veins.

Numerous unmyelinated nerve fibers from the splanchnic nerves enter the capsule in small bundles. A few fibers end in the cortex. Most fibers follow the trabeculae to the medulla and end as preganglionic fibers in relation to medullary cells. Every cell is said to be innervated. Stimulation of the splanchnic nerves causes a heavy discharge of epinephrine, whereas section of the splanchnic nerves inhibits secretory activity of medullary cells.

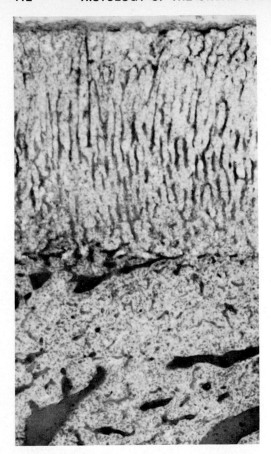

Figure 17-25. Section of suprarenal gland in which the blood vessels were injected with red gelatin. Note the longitudinally oriented cortical sinusoids and the large veins in the medulla. × 60.

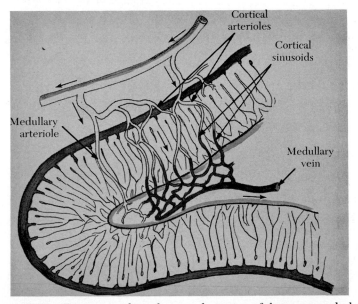

Figure 17-26. Diagram to show the vascularization of the suprarenal gland.

THE PARAGANGLIA
(CHROMAFFIN SYSTEM)

The term paraganglia embraces several widely scattered groups of cells which are similar in many ways to medullary cells of the suprarenal glands. The cell groups largely lie retroperitoneally, often in association with sympathetic ganglia. The largest groups are the paired or joined *para-aortic bodies of Zuckerkandl*.

Component cells of the paraganglia are chromaffin cells, and they stain positively with chromic and osmic acid. They lie in close association with capillaries. Because the cells are embryologically and morphologically similar to the chromaffin cells of the suprarenal medulla, it has been assumed that they secrete epinephrine, although this has not been established satisfactorily. The carotid and aortic bodies, which function as chemoreceptors, have associated with them small islands of chromaffin cells.

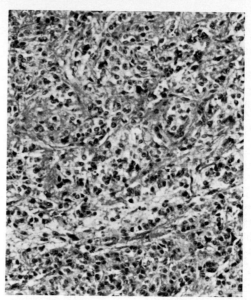

Figure 17-27. Low power micrograph of human pineal body. Component cells present no organized pattern on routine preparations. × 100.

THE PINEAL BODY

The pineal body, or *epiphysis cerebri*, is a small cone-shaped body attached by a stalk to the roof of the third ventricle. Pia mater covers the pineal body except at its attachment and forms a thin capsule which sends septa into the organ, dividing it incompletely into lobules. The lobules are composed of *epithelioid cells* and neuroglia. The epithelioid cells are difficult to define in routine preparations but can be seen well in silver preparations, when they appear as irregularly shaped cells with long, branching processes which terminate in bulbous endings. The cytoplasm is variable in amount and may contain granules and lipid droplets.

The neuroglial cells (astrocytes and microglia) serve as supporting elements.

The epiphysis attains its maximum development by about seven years of age and thereafter shows retrogressive

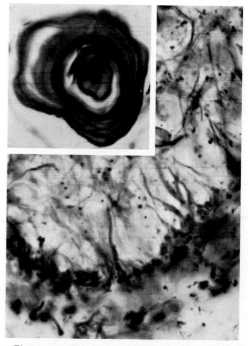

Figure 17-28. Human pineal body in which the epithelioid cells have been made visible with silver. Long branching processes of the cells terminate in bulbous endings. Del Rio-Hortega silver method. × 625. Inset: Acervulus ("brain sand"). × 250.

changes which involve principally the supporting elements. Connective tissue increases in amount and the lobules become well delineated. *Acervuli* (*brain sand* or *corpora arenacea*) are concretions which appear mainly in the capsule and septa. They are lamellated bodies which vary greatly in size and in number.

A few blood vessels and nerve fibers, both myelinated and unmyelinated, supply the gland. The nerve fibers are from the sympathetic portion of the autonomic nervous system. Electron microscope studies have shown that the nerve terminals end directly upon the pineal cells, instead of on blood vessels or smooth muscle cells, as in most other organs.

The epiphysis of mammals is a vestige of the photoreceptive pineal system of lower vertebrates. In mammals the epiphysis appears to have a secretory function. The pineals of many mammals, including human, have been shown to contain *melatonin* and *serotonin*, compounds which have a similar molecular structure. The content of both melatonin and serotonin in the rat pineal undergoes marked circadian rhythms. Melatonin, when injected into rats, slows the estrous cycle and causes the ovaries to lose weight. The ability of melatonin to modify gonadal function suggests that its secretion may be concerned with the timing of the estrous and menstrual cycles. Pineal tumors in children commonly are associated with delayed puberty as a result of increased pineal activity.

REFERENCES

Hypophysis

Bargmann, W.: Relationship between neurohypophysial structure and function. Proc. 8th Symp. Colston Res. Soc., 11, 1957.

Barnett, R. J., Ladman, A. J., McAllaster, N. J., and Siperstein, E. R.: The localization of glycoprotein hormones in the anterior pituitary glands of rats investigated by differential protein solubilities, histological stains and bio-assays. Endocrinology, 59:398, 1956.

Dawson, A. B.: The demonstration by differential staining of two types of acidophils in the anterior pituitary gland of the rat. Anat. Rec., 120:810, 1954.

Farquhar, M. G., and Rinehart, J. F.: Electron microscopic studies of the anterior pituitary gland of castrate rats. Endocrinology, 54:516, 1954.

Farquhar, M. G., and Wellings, S. R.: Electron microscopic evidence suggesting secretory granule formation within the Golgi apparatus. J. Biophys. Biochem. Cytol., 3:319, 1957.

Green, J. D.: The histology of the hypophyseal stalk and median eminence in man, with special reference to blood vessels, nerve fibers, and a peculiar neurovascular zone in this region. Anat. Rec., 100:273, 1948.

Green, J. D.: The comparative anatomy of the hypophysis, with special reference to its blood supply and innervation. Amer. J. Anat., 88:225, 1951.

Halmi, N. S.: Two types of basophils in the rat pituitary; "thyrotrophs" and "gonadotrophs" vs. beta and delta cells. Endocrinology, 50:140, 1952.

Harris, G. W.: Neural control of the pituitary glands. Physiol. Rev., 28:139, 1948.

Harris, G. W., and Donovan, B. T.: The Pituitary Gland (3 volumes). Berkeley and Los Angeles, University of California Press, 1966.

Kurosumi, K.: Functional classification of cell types of the anterior pituitary gland accomplished by electron microscopy. Arch. Histol. Jap., 29:329, 1968.

Scharrer, E., and Scharrer, B.: Neurosekretion. *In* Handb. Mikr. Anat. Menschen, edited by von Mollendorff. Berlin, Springer Verlag, 1954, Vol. 6, p. 953.

Sloper, J. C.: Hypothalamo-neurohypophysial neurosecretion. Int. Rev. Cytol., 7:337, 1958.

Turner, C. D.: General Endocrinology. 4th ed. Philadelphia, W. B. Saunders Company, 1966.

Thyroid

Anast, C. S.: Thyrocalcitonin—A review. Clin. Orthop., 47:179, 1966.

Bussolati, G., and Pearse, A. G. E.: Immunofluorescent localization of calcitonin in C cells of pig and dog thyroid. J. Endocrinol., 37:205, 1967.

De Robertis, E.: Cytological and cytochemical basis of thyroid function. Ann. N.Y. Acad. Sci., 50:317, 1949.

Ekholm, R., and Sjöstrand, F. S.: The ultrastructural organization of the mouse thyroid gland. J. Ultrastruct. Res., 1:178, 1957.

Grass, J.: The dynamic cytology of the thyroid gland. Int. Rev. Cytol., 6:265, 1957.

Leblond, C. P., and Gross, J.: Thyroglobulin formation in the thyroid follicle visualized by the "coated autograph" technique. Endocrinology, 43:306, 1948.

Leblond, C. P., and Gross, J.: The mechanism of the secretion of thyroid hormone. J. Clin. Endocr., 9:149, 1949.

Wissig, S. L.: The anatomy of secretion in the follicular cells of the thyroid gland. I. The fine structure of the gland in the normal rat. J. Biophys. Biochem. Cytol., 7:419, 1960.

Wissig, S. L.: The anatomy of secretion in the follicular cells of the thyroid gland. II. The effect of acute thyrotrophic hormone stimulation on the secretory apparatus. J. Cell Biol., 16:93, 1963.

Young, B. A., Care, A. D., and Duncan, T.: Some observations on the light cells of the thyroid gland of the pig in relation to thyrocalcitonin production. J. Anat., 102:275, 1968.

Parathyroid

Bensley, S. L.: The normal mode of secretion in the parathyroid gland of the dog. Anat. Rec., 98:361, 1947.

De Robertis, E.: The cytology of the parathyroid gland of rats injected with parathyroid extract. Anat. Rec., 78:473, 1940.

Munger, B. L., and Roth, S. I.: The cytology of the normal parathyroid glands of man and Virginia deer. J. Cell Biol., 16:379, 1963.

Suprarenal

Baxter, J. S.: The growth cycle of the cells of the adrenal cortex in the adult rat. J. Anat., 80:139, 1946.

Bennett, H. S.: The life history and secretion of the cells of the adrenal cortex of the cat. Amer. J. Anat., 67:151, 1940.

Bennett, H. S.: Cytological manifestations of secretion in the adrenal medulla of the cat. Amer. J. Anat., 69:333, 1941.

Brenner, R. M.: Fine structure of adrenocortical cells in adult male rhesus monkeys. Amer. J. Anat., 119:429, 1966.

Coupland, R. E.: Electron microscopic observations on the structure of the rat adrenal medulla. I. The ultrastructure and organization of chromaffin cells in the normal adrenal medulla. J. Anat., 99:231, 1965.

Coupland, R. E.: Electron microscopic observations on the structure of the rat adrenal medulla. II. Normal innervation. J. Anat., 99:255, 1965.

Deane, H. W., and Greep, R. O.: A morphological and histological study of the rat's adrenal cortex after hypophysectomy, with comments on the liver. Amer. J. Anat., 79:117, 1946.

Long, J. A., and Jones, A. L.: Observations on the fine structure of the adrenal cortex of man. Lab. Invest., 17:355, 1967.

Pineal

Anderson, E.: The anatomy of bovine and ovine pineals. J. Ultrastruct. Res., Suppl. 8, 1965.

Axelrod, J., Wurtman, R. J., and Snyder, S. H.: Control of hydroxyindole O-methyltransferase activity in the rat pineal gland by environmental lighting. J. Biol. Chem., 240:949, 1965.

Del Rio-Hortega, P.: Pineal gland. *In* Cytology and Cellular Pathology of the Nervous System, edited by Penfield. Baltimore, Williams & Wilkins Co., 1932, Vol. 1, p. 637.

Kelly, D. E.: Pineal organs: Photoreception, secretion, and development. Amer. Sci., 50:597, 1962.

Kitay, J. I., and Altschule, M. D.: The Pineal Gland: A Review of the Physiologic Literature. Cambridge, Harvard University Press, 1954.

Quay, W. B., and Harvey, A.: Experimental modification of the rat pineal's content of serotonin and related indole amines. Physiol. Zool., 35:1, 1962.

Wurtman, R. J., Axelrod, J., and Fischer, J. E.: Melatonin synthesis in the pineal gland: Effect of light mediated by the sympathetic nervous system. Science, 143:1328, 1964.

Wurtman, R. J., and Axelrod, J.: The pineal gland. Sci. Amer., 213:50, 1965.

CHAPTER 18

THE FEMALE

REPRODUCTIVE SYSTEM

The female reproductive system comprises the ovaries, a system of genital ducts (the uterine tubes, uterus, and vagina), and the external genitalia. The mammary glands, although not one of the genital organs, are included here since they are important glands of the female reproductive system.

THE OVARY

The ovaries are classified as double glands since they produce both exocrine (cytogenic) and endocrine secretions. They are slightly flattened, ovoid bodies, measuring about 4 cm. in length, 2 cm. in width, and 1 cm. in thickness. One lies on each side of the uterus on the lateral wall of the pelvic cavity. Each is attached at one of its margins, the *hilum*, by the *mesovarium*, a fold of peritoneum, to the broad ligament of the uterus. At the hilum the vascular connective tissue of the mesovarium becomes continuous with the ovarian stroma. The peritoneal covering of the mesovarium ceases abruptly at the hilum and is replaced by a layer of cuboidal cells, the *germinal epithelium*, which covers the free surface of the ovary. A basal

lamina is absent. Beneath the epithelium there is a layer of dense connective tissue which increases in density with advancing age.

In sections of the ovary two zones may be distinguished, an outer layer, the *cortex*, and an inner portion, the *medulla*, which merges with the vascular connective tissue of the mesovarium at the hilum. The medulla consists of loose fibroelastic connective tissue containing numerous large blood vessels, lymphatics, and nerves. The stroma contains scattered strands of smooth muscle fibers.

The cortex consists of a compact, cellular stroma that contains the *ovarian follicles*. The stroma is composed of networks of reticular fibers and spindle-shaped cells. Elastic tissue is sparse and occurs only in the walls of blood vessels. The follicles may be seen in all stages of development, and the appearance of the ovarian cortex depends upon the age of the individual and the stage of the ovarian cycle. Before puberty only *primary*, or *primitive, follicles* are seen. Sexual maturity is characterized by the presence of *growing follicles* and their end products (*corpora lutea, atretic follicles*). After the menopause follicles disappear and the senile cortex eventually

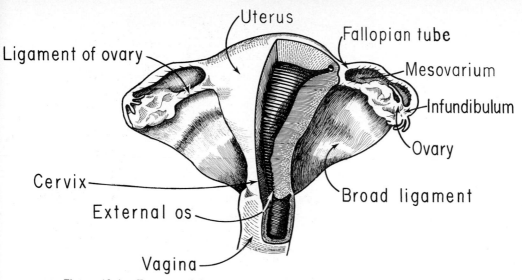

Figure 18-1. Diagram of the internal female genitalia as seen from behind.

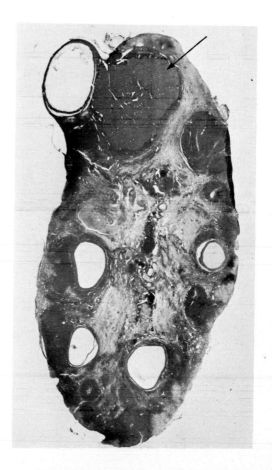

Figure 18-2. Section of the ovary from a 32 year old woman. Follicles in various stages of differentiation and a corpus luteum (arrow) are present in the cortex. Note the large blood vessels in the loose connective tissue of the medulla. × 5.

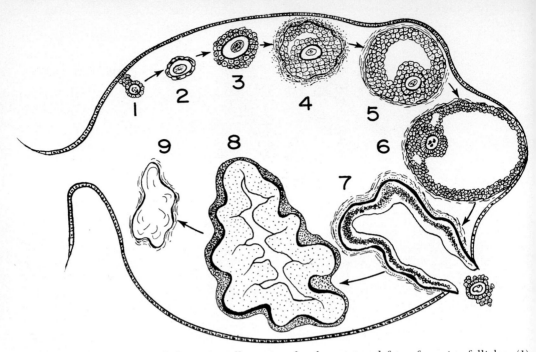

Figure 18-3. Diagram of the ovary, illustrating development and fate of ovarian follicles. (1) Oogonium, surrounded by follicular cells, the latter arising from germinal epithelium. (2) Primary follicle. (3-5) Maturing follicles. (6) Graafian follicle. (7) Ruptured follicle. (8) Corpus luteum. (9) Corpus albicans.

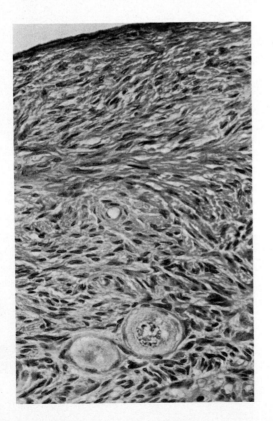

Figure 18-4. Portion of the cortex of an ovary from a 25 year old woman. The cortical stroma, which is markedly cellular, contains two primary follicles. × 250.

becomes a narrow zone of fibrous connective tissue.

Follicles

Each ovarian follicle consists of an immature ovum surrounded by epithelial cells. An immature ovum is a spheroidal cell with a large vesicular nucleus and a prominent nucleolus. The cytoplasm is opaque and finely granular.

In the newborn infant the follicles are believed to number about 400,000. Their number decreases progressively throughout life until virtually none is left soon after the menopause. Most follicles seen are *primary follicles*, which measure about 40 microns in diameter. A primary follicle consists of an immature ovum surrounded by a single layer of flattened *follicular cells*,

believed to be derived from the germinal epithelium.

Growing Follicles

The progressive development of follicles which occurs after puberty is characterized by growth and differentiation of the ovum, proliferation of follicular cells, and development of a connective tissue capsule from the surrounding stroma.

The ovum increases in size and a refractile, deeply staining membrane, the *zona pellucida*, is formed around it. The zona pellucida appears homogeneous in the fresh condition. It is elaborated probably by both the ovum and the surrounding follicular cells.

The flattened follicular cells become first cuboidal and then columnar in shape. They divide actively to produce

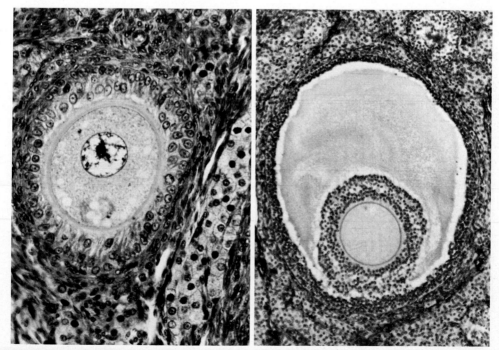

Figure 18-5. Left: Growing follicle, showing an immature ovum with a large vesicular nucleus and a prominent nucleolus, a zona pellucida, and a stratified layer of follicular cells. Also present is a group of large epithelioid cells, the so-called interstitial cells (right), derived from the theca interna of an atretic follicle. × 250. Right: A more mature follicle, showing a well-developed membrana granulosa, an antrum, and cumulus oophorus with an immature ovum. The ovum is sectioned tangentially and does not show a nucleus. × 100.   See filmstrip II, frame 79.

a stratified layer around the ovum. The proliferation occurs more rapidly on one side of the ovum so that the follicle becomes oval in shape and the ovum eccentric in position. Irregular small spaces filled with a clear fluid appear within the follicular mass. An increase in the amount of this fluid causes a further increase in the size of the follicle. The fluid-filled spaces fuse to form a single cavity, the *antrum*, within the follicular layer. The ovum, surrounded by a group of follicular cells, is pressed to one side and forms a definite projection into the antrum cavity. This eccentric mound is known as the *cumulus oophorus*. The follicular cells of the cumulus oophorus directly in relation to the ovum become radially arranged and form the *corona radiata*, separated from the ovum only by the zona pellucida. Elsewhere the stratified epithelium, composed of follicular cells, forms a continuous, regular layer around the antrum cavity.

As the follicle increases in size, the adjacent stroma organizes into a cap-sule, the *theca folliculi*, separated from the membrana granulosa by a basal lamina (the *glassy membrane*). The theca folliculi differentiates into two layers, an inner vascular layer, the *theca interna*, and an outer fibrous layer, the *theca externa*. The theca interna consists of enlarged (epithelioid) stromal cells between which are numerous capillaries. The theca externa, composed of closely packed collagenous fibers and fusiform cells, merges peripherally into the surrounding ovarian stroma.

Mature Graafian Follicles

It is believed that a follicle requires 10 to 14 days to reach maturity. A mature graafian follicle occupies the full breadth of the cortex and indents the medulla. It bulges on the free surface of the ovary. At this point, called the *stigma*, the tunica albuginea and the theca folliculi become attenuated. The large antrum, distended with fluid, is bound by the membrana gran-

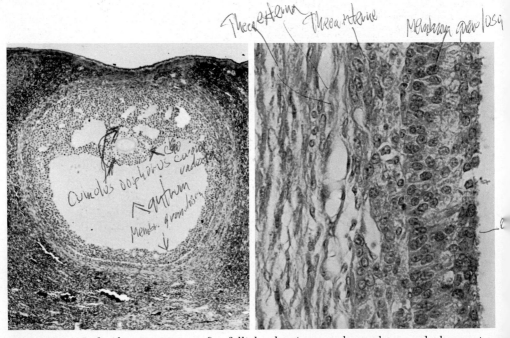

Figure 18-6.   Left: Almost mature graafian follicle, showing cumulus oophorus and a large antrum × 40. Right: High power micrograph of a portion of the wall of a mature graafian follicle. At the righ is the membrana granulosa lining the antrum and at the left of it are the theca interna and the theca externa, the latter merging into the surrounding ovarian stroma. × 250.

ulosa. The ovum has attained its full size, and it is surrounded by a thick zona pellucida and a conspicuous corona radiata. As follicular maturity is attained, small irregular spaces filled with fluid appear between the cells of the cumulus oophorus, thus weakening the connection of the ovum with the membrana granulosa.

Ovulation

As the follicle reaches maturity, there is increased secretion of liquor, more watery than that formed previously, which causes further expansion in diameter of the follicle. This is termed *preovulatory swelling*. The follicle, covered with thinned cortex, ruptures at the stigma and follicular fluid oozes out into the peritoneal cavity. The ovum, surrounded by cells of the corona radiata, is torn away from the cumulus and is discharged with the liquor. This process constitutes *ovulation*. Usually only one ovum is discharged at one time, but in some cases two or, rarely, more may be released. The free ovum retains the capacity to be fertilized only for 24 hours. In the human female ovulation occurs at intervals averaging 28 days.

Maturation of the Ovum: Oogenesis

The ovum which is released at ovulation is actually a *secondary oocyte* and technically is immature. In preparation for fertilization, the ovum passes through a series of nuclear changes similar to that described for spermatozoa (see Chapter 19). The end result is the same as with spermatogenesis, i.e., the reduction of the chromosomes to one-half the somatic (diploid) number.

Oogonia, or primitive ova, which contain the diploid number of chromosomes, divide mitotically to produce *primary oocytes* in the fetal ovary. During follicular development, the primary oocyte grows and then passes through a period of maturation in which it undergoes two maturation divisions, as a result of which the chromosomes are reduced to the haploid number. The first maturation division occurs shortly before ovulation. The chromatin is divided equally between the daughter cells, but the division of cytoplasm is extremely unequal. One of the daughter cells, the *secondary oocyte*, receives practically all the cytoplasm of the mother cell; the other becomes the *first polar body*, which soon degenerates. In each the chromosome assortment is reduced to a single set of 23 chromosomes. At about this time ovulation occurs and the secondary oocyte is released. It undergoes the second maturation division and again the cytoplasm is divided unequally. The majority of cytoplasm is retained in the mature *ovum*. The other daughter cell is the *second polar body*. Thus only one daughter cell of a primary oocyte becomes functional. The exact time of the second maturation division is unknown for the human ovum, but it is thought to occur at the time of fertilization.

The Corpus Luteum

After ovulation there is sometimes a little bleeding into the cavity of the follicle. The wall of the follicle collapses and is thrown into folds. The follicular wall becomes transformed into a temporary glandular structure, the *corpus luteum*. The granulosa cells of the follicle differentiate into large, pale-staining cells with large vesicular nuclei. The cytoplasm acquires an accumulation of fine lipid droplets and pigment granules. The transformed granulosa cells are called *granulosa lutein cells*, and they form a thick, folded layer about the remains of the follicular cavity.

Cells of the theca interna, which prior to ovulation have increased in size, form *theca lutein cells*. They are smaller in size than granulosa lutein

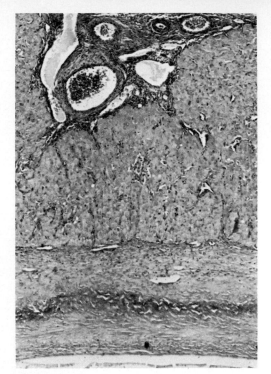

Figure 18-7. Portion of a corpus luteum from a woman 4 months pregnant. Note the folded outline and the large blood vessels in relation to the corpus luteum. × 40.

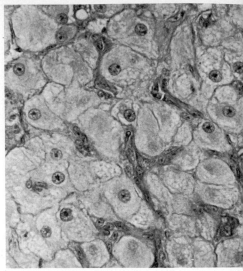

Figure 18-8. High power micrograph of a group of granulosa lutein cells from the corpus luteum depicted in Figure 18-7. The appearance is typical of a steroid-producing endocrine gland. Numerous capillaries lie between component cells. × 250.

cells and possess compact, dark-staining nuclei. They aggregate peripherally, especially in the recesses between the folds of granulosa lutein cells. The theca externa retains its regular ovoid outline, and component cells here do not undergo transformation.

Numerous capillaries and connective tissue from the theca invade the lutein mass. Fibroblasts organize a delicate reticulum throughout the corpus luteum and form a continuous lining on the inner surface of the lutein cells in relation to the reduced follicular cavity.

If the discharged ovum is not fertilized, the corpus luteum attains its greatest development about nine days after ovulation and then begins to degenerate. This is the *corpus luteum* of *menstruation*. The former rich vascularization declines, and component cells decrease in size and undergo a fatty degeneration. Connective tissue

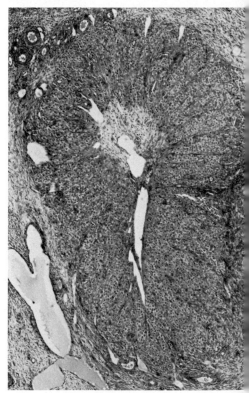

Figure 18-9. Early involution of a corpus luteum. Component cells are smaller than during the active phase, and connective tissue strands between lutein cells are prominent. × 35.

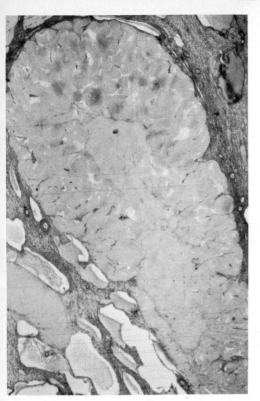

Figure 18-10. Corpus albicans. There has been complete replacement of the corpus luteum by connective tissue. × 20.

between lutein cells increases in amount and becomes hyalinized and gradually the corpus luteum is transformed into a white scar, the *corpus albicans*.

If the ovum is fertilized, the corpus luteum increases in size and is known as the *corpus luteum of pregnancy*. The cells continue to grow in size until the middle months of pregnancy, and thereafter a slow involution occurs. After delivery involution proceeds rapidly. The resulting corpus albicans is large and usually causes a retraction of the surface of the ovary following contraction of fibrous tissue formed as a result of involution.

Atresia of Follicles

Only about 400 follicles reach full maturity. The period of sexual activity in the human female is about thirty years, and during this time ordinarily only one ovum is discharged each month. All unsuccessful follicles undergo degeneration, either as primary follicles or after a varying period of growth. This involution of follicles is called *atresia*. Atresia appears to occur initially in the ovum. This is followed by degeneration of the follicular cells. In atresia of primary follicles the space resulting is filled with stromal tissue. Atresia of growing follicles is a more complicated process. As in primary follicles, the first degenerative signs occur in the ovum and follicular cells. The zona pellucida swells and may persist for some time after the disappearance of the ovum and follicular cells. Cells of the theca interna develop much like those in a corpus luteum. They increase in size and become arranged in vascularized, radial strands. The glassy membrane also increases in thickness and forms a hyalinized band. After resorption of follicular cells, the theca cells degenerate and are replaced by connective tissue. The resulting mass of scar tissue is similar in appearance to a corpus albicans, but is smaller.

Interstitial Cells

Large epithelioid cells are present in the ovarian stroma of some mammals, particularly rodents. These are the so-called *interstitial cells*, which are large spheroidal cells containing small lipid droplets. They are derived from the theca interna of follicles undergoing atresia. Thus they are most abundant when atresia is most marked. In the human this is in the first year of life. In the adult human ovary they either are absent or are present as small radiating cords of cells.

Hormones of the Ovary

The ovaries, in addition to producing sex cells (a cytogenic secretion), secrete the so-called female sex hormones, *estrogen* and *progesterone*. These are steroids. Estrogen (principally estradiol) is produced mainly by the growing follicles, progesterone primarily by the corpus luteum. Estrogen induces growth and development of the female reproductive tract and the mammary glands. Progesterone causes the uterine glands to secrete and renders the mucosa receptive to a nidating ovum.

Since the sequence of structural changes in the ovary is follicular growth, ovulation, and formation of a corpus luteum, the levels of the two hormones normally exhibit regular cyclic fluctuations. Estrogen secretion is high during the preovulatory period (follicular phase); progesterone production increases rapidly during luteinization of the ruptured follicle and remains at a high level until the corpus luteum regresses (luteal phase). These rhythmic changes in ovarian secretory activity are responsible for the cyclic changes which occur in the structure of the reproductive tract, notably in the mucosa of the uterus (see Figure 18-16).

The ovarian cycle in turn is activated and governed by the gonadotrophins secreted by the anterior lobe of the hypophysis. The gonadotrophins control the maturation of follicles and the formation of corpora lutea.

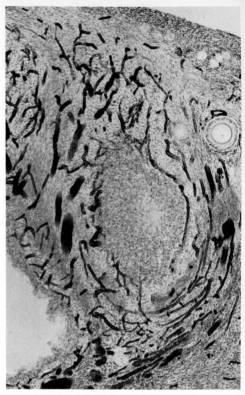

Figure 18-11. Section of a portion of an ovary in which the blood vessels had been injected with colored gelatin prior to sectioning. Note the abundant capillary networks in relation to the growing follicles. × 40.

Blood Vessels, Lymphatics, and Nerves

Large branches from the ovarian and uterine arteries enter the medulla and divide into a number of spiral vessels, often called *helicine arteries*. At the boundary zone between cortex and medulla these form a plexus from which smaller twigs pass into the cortex to ramify around follicles. Capillary networks are abundant in the theca interna of growing follicles. Veins, which arise from the capillary networks, accompany the arteries and leave the ovary at the hilum.

Lymph capillaries begin in the theca externa of follicles and unite to form larger vessels which pass to the medulla and leave at the hilum.

Nerve fibers, mostly unmyelinated, follow the blood vessels and supply their muscular coat. Some fibers penetrate into the cortex and form delicate plexuses around the follicles and beneath the germinal epithelium.

THE FALLOPIAN TUBES

The *fallopian (uterine) tubes*, or *oviducts*, are paired structures which extend from the ovary to the uterus in a fold of peritoneum, the upper free margin of the broad ligament. The tube is 12 to 15 cm. long and about 1

sists of a *mucous membrane*, a *muscular layer*, and a *serosa*.

Mucosa

The mucosal lining is thrown into characteristic longitudinal folds. In the ampulla the folds branch in a complex manner to divide the lumen into a labyrinth of spaces. In the isthmus the folds rarely branch and in the intramural portion of the tube the folds are low.

The epithelium consists of simple columnar cells, some of which are ciliated, whereas others are not. The nonciliated cells are narrow and peg-shaped and appear to be secretory in

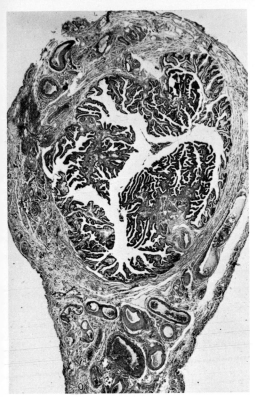

Figure 18-12. Section through the ampulla of the fallopian tube. The lumen appears markedly irregular owing to extensive folding of the mucosa. × 12.

cm. in diameter. The end of the tube in relation to the ovary opens into the peritoneal cavity; the other end opens into the uterine cavity. The uterine tube shows four regions. The *infundibulum* is the funnel-shaped opening into the peritoneal cavity. Its margins are drawn out into numerous fringed folds (*fimbriae*). The expanded intermediate segment, comprising two-thirds of the length of the tube, is the *ampulla*, which is thin-walled. It leads into the *isthmus*, slender and narrow, which connects with the uterus. The fourth part, the *intramural (interstitial) portion*, is the continuation of the canal through the uterine wall. The wall of the tube thickens progressively toward the uterus, whereas the lumen diminishes in size in this direction.

The wall of the fallopian tube con-

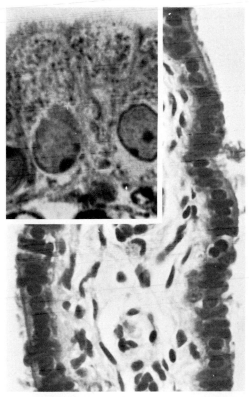

Figure 18-13. Portion of the mucosa lining the ampullary region of the fallopian tube. The specimen was removed from a woman four months pregnant. "Peg" cells are prominent between the groups of ciliated columnar cells. × 500. Inset.: Epon section, showing ciliated epithelial cells. × 1250.

nature. Ciliated cells occur in small groups, alternating with groups of cells that are nonciliated. The proportion of cells with cilia is greatest at the infundibulum and least at the isthmus. The cilia beat down toward the uterus. The height of the epithelium varies somewhat with the reproductive cycle, being greatest during the follicular phase and lowest during the latter part of the luteal phase. During pregnancy the epithelium is low and there is an increased number of "peg" cells.

The lamina propria of the mucosa is composed of an unusually cellular connective tissue containing a few scattered fusiform cells. There is no definite basal lamina. At the rim of the infundibulum the mucosal lining of the tube becomes continuous with the mesothelium of the serosa.

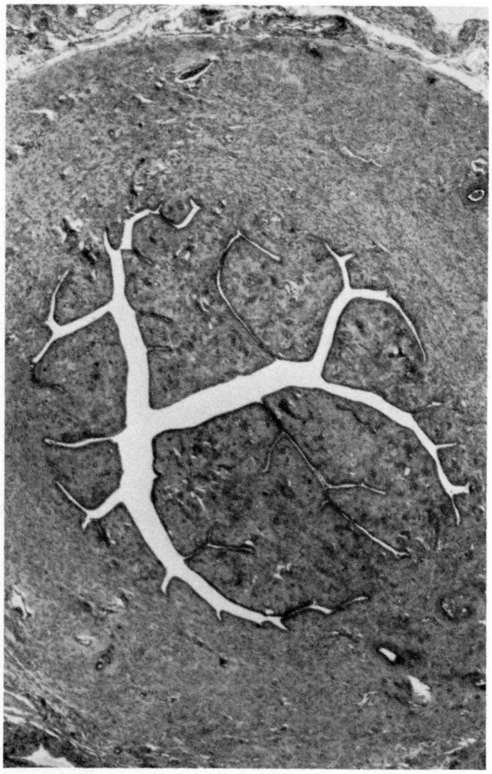

Muscularis

The mucosa rests directly upon the muscular coat, which consists of a broad inner circular layer and a thin outer layer. The outer layer is not continuous but consists of scattered bundles of fibers, orientated longitudinally. Toward the uterus the muscularis increases in thickness.

Serosa

The uterine tube is invested with a fold of reflected peritoneum, the serosa, consisting of loose connective tissue surfaced with mesothelium. The deeper layers of the connective tissue contain the longitudinal bundles of the muscularis.

Blood Vessels, Lymphatics, and Nerves

Numerous blood vessels and lymphatics are present in the lamina propria and the serosa. Nerves form a rich plexus in the serosa, from which nerve fibers pass to supply muscle fibers and the mucosa.

THE UTERUS

The uterus is the thick-walled segment of the tubular female reproductive system that is interposed between the fallopian tubes and the vagina. It is a pear-shaped organ, somewhat flattened in a dorsoventral direction, and averages 7 cm. in length, 5 cm. in width at its broadest part, and 2 to 3 cm. in thickness. Two major portions may be recognized: the expanded upper portion, the *body* or *corpus uteri,* and the lowermost, cylindrical portion, the *neck* or *cervix,* a part of which projects into the vagina as the *portio vaginalis.* The term *fundus* re-

Figure 18-14.   Isthmus of the fallopian tube. Folding of the mucosa is less marked than in the ampullary region, and the muscularis is increased in thickness. × 20.

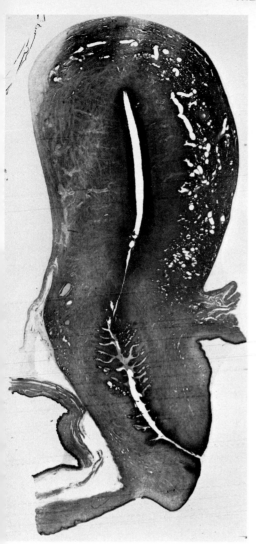

Figure 18-15. Median sagittal section through the uterus and upper portion of the vagina. Note the thickness of the uterine wall (principally myometrium), the prominent cervical glands, the portio vaginalis, and a portion of the bladder (anterior) to the left. × 2½.

fers to the rounded upper end of the body, from which the fallopian tubes extend. The *isthmus* is the narrow zone of transition between the body and the cervix.

The wall of the uterus consists of three layers: the outer—serosa or *perimetrium*; the middle—muscularis or *myometrium*; and the inner—mucosa or *endometrium*.

Perimetrium

The perimetrium is a typical serosa consisting of a single layer of mesothelial cells supported by a thin layer of connective tissue. It is continuous on each side of the organ with the peritoneum of the broad ligament and is deficient over the lower half of the anterior surface.

Myometrium

The myometrium is a massive coat of smooth muscle, about 12 to 15 mm. in thickness. The muscle fibers are arranged in bundles, separated by connective tissue. Individual fibers are large and their length varies from 40 to 90 microns. During pregnancy the fibers increase greatly in size and may attain a length of 600 microns or more. Three layers of muscle may be distinguished, although they are somewhat ill-defined owing to the presence of interconnecting bundles. There is an inner muscular layer consisting mostly of longitudinally orientated fibers, a thick middle layer of circular and oblique muscle fibers with numerous blood vessels, and an outer thin, longitudinal muscle layer immediately beneath the perimetrium.

Endometrium

The endometrium (mucosa), which is firmly adherent to the underlying myometrium, is subject to cyclic changes in response to ovarian secretory activity. These changes culminate in partial destruction of the mucosa leading to tissue necrosis and hemorrhage, an event known as *menstruation*. Menstruation occurs typically at intervals of about 28 days and lasts for three to five days. The first day of menstruation is counted as the first day of the menstrual cycle.

The body of the uterus is lined by a simple columnar epithelium which possesses scattered groups of ciliated

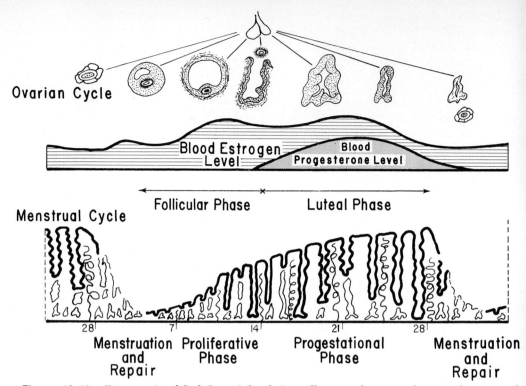

Figure 18-16.   Diagram (modified from Schroder) to illustrate the interrelations of ovary and endometrium during a menstrual cycle.

cells. From the surface epithelium, uterine glands extend through the full thickness of the mucosa. These are simple tubules which may branch toward their basal ends. They are separated from each other by connective tissue, the *stroma*. Stromal cells are irregular, stellate cells which have large, ovoid nuclei. They lie in a framework of reticular fibers which are condensed beneath the epithelium to form a basal lamina. Wandering lymphoid cells and granular leukocytes also are present in the stroma.

Blood Vessels, Lymphatics, and Nerves

Branches from the uterine arteries penetrate to the middle layer of the myometrium and from these vessels two systems of branches arise. One system supplies the superficial layers of the myometrium. The other system supplies the remainder of the myometrium and sends two sets of vessels to the endometrium. One set of arterial extensions supplies the basal part of the endometrium. Another set spreads out into a rich capillary bed superficially. Vessels of the latter set are more or less contorted and are termed *coiled arteries*. Thus the endometrium is supplied by a basal and a superficial set of vessels. The basal set does not undergo changes during the menstrual cycle, but the coiled arteries show pronounced modifications.

Veins in the endometrium are thin-walled and form an extensive network. A plexus of large vessels is present in the middle (vascular) layer of the myometrium.

Lymph vessels are abundant and form plexuses throughout the layers of the uterus with the exception of the superficial zone of the mucosa.

Myelinated nerve fibers enter the mucosa and form a plexus beneath the epithelium. Unmyelinated nerve fibers supply blood vessels and muscle bundles.

Cyclic Changes in the Endometrium

Beginning with puberty and ending at the menopause, the endometrium undergoes periodic changes. Four stages can be recognized in a continuous cycle of events, and each stage passes gradually into the next: the *menstrual stage*, during which there is external menstrual discharge; the *proliferative (follicular) stage*, which is concurrent with follicular growth and estrogen secretion; the *progestational (luteal) stage*, usually associated with an active corpus luteum; and the *ischemic (premenstrual) stage*, when there is interruption of blood flow in the coiled arteries.

The Proliferative (Follicular) Stage. This stage begins at the end of a menstrual flow and is characterized by rapid regeneration of the endometrium from the narrow zone remaining after menstruation. Epithelial cells from the remnants of torn glands glide over the denuded surface of the mucosa. Numerous mitoses occur in cells of the glands and of the endometrial stroma. The mucosa increases in thickness from 1 mm. or less to 2 mm. or more. This increase coincides with growth of ovarian follicles and secretion of estrogen. The glands proliferate, lengthen rapidly, and become closely packed. Rebuilding of the lamina propria occurs as a result of the mitotic activity of stromal cells. Toward the end of the proliferative phase the lumina of the glands widen and they become wavy. Glycogen accumulates in the basal region of the cells, but only a thin mucoid secretion is released at this stage. Coiled arteries grow into the regenerating tissue but are not found in the superficial third of the endometrium, which possesses only capillaries and venules.

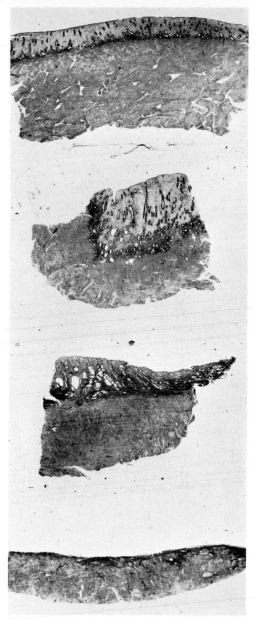

Figure 18-17. Series of sections through the uterus at various stages during the menstrual cycle. From top to bottom, early proliferative stage, late proliferative stage, late secretory stage, and late menstrual stage. Note the varying height of the endometrium and the character of the uterine glands. × 4.

The Progestational (Secretory) Stage. The endometrium increases in thickness and becomes 4 mm. or more in depth. The increase is due

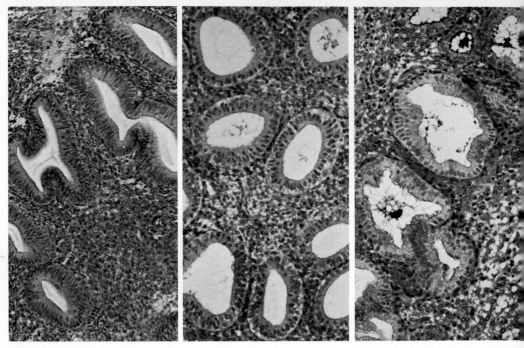

Figure 18-18. Portions of three endometrial biopsy samples taken during various stages of the menstrual cycle. Left, proliferative stage; center, early secretory phase; right, late secretory phase. Note the varying character of the glands and of the stroma. In the early secretory phase, vacuolation of the basal cytoplasm of glandular cells is indicative of glycogen accumulation; in the late secretory phase, secretion is present in the apical zone of cytoplasm and in the lumina of glands, which become irregular in outline. The stroma becomes less dense in the secretory phase owing to fluid accumulation. × 100. See filmstrip II, frame 80.

largely to hypertrophy of gland cells and to an increase of edema fluid. The glands swell and secrete profusely. Secretory material at first is localized in the basal portions of the cells. During the latter half of the stage the secretion moves to the apical zone of the cells. The secretion is thick and rich in glycogen. The glands become serrated and their lumina become wider. Coiled arteries grow nearly to the surface.

Once the structural changes associated with this stage become apparent, three zones of the endometrium can be distinguished. Nearest the surface is the *compact layer,* which is a relatively narrow zone. It contains the straight necks of the glands and shows little edema. Under this layer is a thick *spongy layer,* in which are the tortuous portions of glands, sepa-

rated by a lamina propria which is grossly edematous. The compact and spongy layers together are termed the *functional layer,* which is lost at menstruation and at parturition. Deepest of all is the thin *basal layer,* containing the blind ends of glands. This layer participates little in the cyclic changes and is not lost at menstruation or at parturition.

The Ischemic (Premenstrual) Stage. This occurs 13 to 14 days after ovulation and is characterized by extensive vascular changes. The coiled arteries constrict intermittently. The functional layer becomes pale and shrinks as a result of anemia and anoxia. The stroma increases in density and becomes infiltrated with leukocytes.

The Menstrual Stage. The functional layer undergoes necrosis and is shed. After a number of hours the coiled arteries relax, the walls of the vessels near the surface break, and blood is added to the secretion of the glands and the necrotic endometrial tissue. Patches of tissue separate and are lost. Blood oozes from veins exposed by the shedding process. The menstrual discharge thus contains altered arterial and venous blood, disintegrated epithelial and stromal cells, and glandular secretions. Finally the whole functional layer of the endometrium is lost, leaving a raw surface. The surviving basal layer remains intact, epithelial cells glide out of the torn ends of glands, and the surface epithelium is quickly restored once the menstrual discharge ceases.

As stated previously, the uterine changes are related closely to the ovarian cyclic changes. The proliferative stage corresponds to the preovulatory period of follicular maturation. The progestational stage is associated with the formation and activity of the

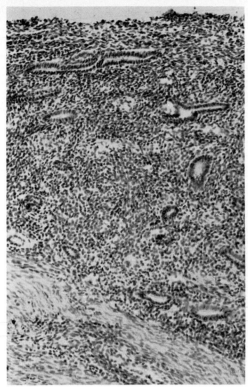

Figure 18-20. Section of the endometrium at the termination of the menstrual stage. Only the basal layer, consisting of the torn ends of uterine glands and a dense stroma, remains. Beneath is a portion of myometrium. × 100.

corpus luteum. The time lapse between its start and the onset of bleeding is quite uniform, regardless of the length of the cycle. The onset of bleeding corresponds to the beginning involution of the corpus luteum.

In certain instances the ovary may not produce a ripe follicle in the course of a cycle. Nevertheless bleeding will occur, but from a proliferative endometrium at the expected time. Such a cycle is known as an *anovulatory cycle.*

The Uterus During Pregnancy

The fertilized ovum undergoes segmentation as it moves down the fallopian tube and enters the uterus. By this time several cell divisions have

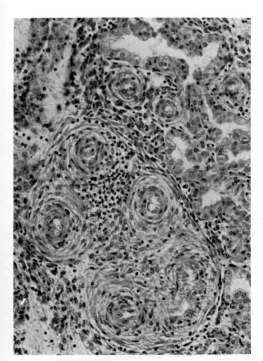

Figure 18-19. Horizontal section through the endometrium during the secretory phase of the cycle. Note the prominent coiled arteries in the stroma. × 100.

occurred, and it consists of a mass of cells. A cavity appears within the cellular mass, after which it is called a *blastocyst*. The blastocyst becomes implanted within the endometrium six or seven days after ovulation. At this time, the endometrium is in the progestational phase. It is thick and edematous and the glands are large and swollen with secretion. The site of implantation may be anywhere on the wall of the uterus but usually it is high up toward the fundus.

The blastocyst wall is composed of a single layer of cells, called the *tropho-blast*, with, in the cavity of the blasto-cyst, an *inner cell mass*. The inner cell mass will not be considered further here since it is from this mass that the embryo is destined to form. As the blastocyst attaches to the endome-trium, trophoblast cells proliferate and the trophoblast becomes several cells thick. The uterine epithelium breaks down at the point of attachment, and

the blastocyst sinks into the endome-trial stroma. The defect in the endo-metrium is closed temporarily by a plug of fibrin, but later the endometrial epithelium grows over the embedded blastocyst to restore continuity of the uterine lining.

Once the blastocyst becomes em-bedded within the endometrium, the trophoblast over the entire surface proliferates and by the eleventh day after ovulation it consists of two layers of cells. The inner layer of cells, the *cytotrophoblast*, is composed of cells with clearly defined cell boundaries. The outer layer is thicker and con-sists of a multinucleated protoplasmic mass, the *syncytial trophoblast*. From the surface of the syncytial tropho-blast epithelial cords extend out into the surrounding space. These are the *primary (primitive) villi*. Later primi-tive embryonic connective tissue comes into relation with the tropho-blast, and the two layers together con-

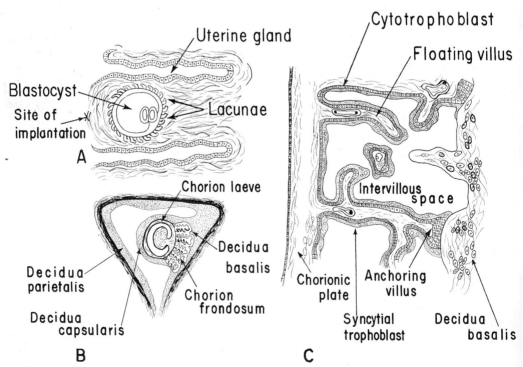

Figure 18-21. Series of diagrams, illustrating the relationships of the blastocyst to the uterus. A, Newly implanted blastocyst within the endometrium. B, Components of the decidua. C, Small segment of the early placenta, showing fetal and maternal contributions.

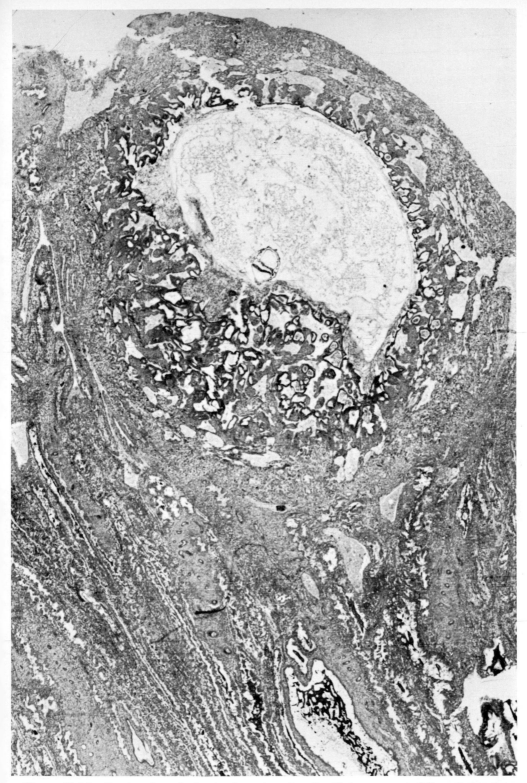

Figure 18-22. Section through the implantation site of a 15 day ovum. A differentiating inner cell mass lies within a large trophoblast cavity. The trophoblast, which is invading the endometrium, already shows more extensive development toward the decidua basalis (chorion frondosum) than toward the decidua capsularis (chorion laeve). × 15.

stitute the *chorion*. Connective tissue, containing fetal blood vessels, extends into the villi, which now are termed *secondary (chorionic) villi*.

Villi on the deeply embedded surface of the blastocyst grow rapidly and form the fetal component of the placenta, the *chorion frondosum*. Villi of the chorion frondosum are attached to a firm portion of the chorion, the *chorionic plate*. Villi on the surface of the chorion facing the uterine cavity do not grow as rapidly as on the deeply embedded surface, and they degenerate by the end of the third month of pregnancy. This portion of the chorion is known as the *chorion laeve*.

The endometrium also shows important structural changes during pregnancy. Since all the endometrium,

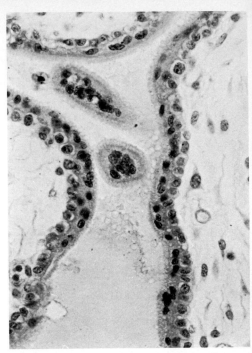

Figure 18-24. Portions of three chorionic villi during the third week of pregnancy. The trophoblast covering each villus consists of a complete layer of cytotrophoblast (cells with pale nuclei) and a layer of syncytial trophoblast, the cytoplasm of which contains numerous dark nuclei. The irregularity at the surface of the syncytial trophoblast is artifactual but is indicative of a microvillous border. × 250.

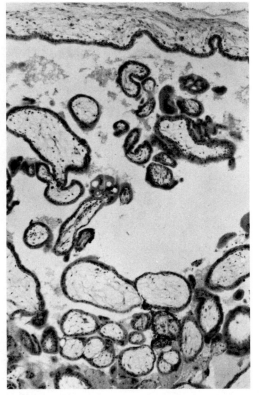

Figure 18-23. Section through the chorion frondosum during the third week of pregnancy. Above is a portion of the chorionic plate; below are sections through numerous villi, each containing a core of primitive mesenchyme. × 40.

except the deepest layer, is destined to be shed at parturition, the endometrium in a pregnant uterus is referred to as *decidua*. Three regions of the decidua are distinguished: overlying the blastocyst is the *decidua capsularis*; underlying it is the *decidua basalis*; all the remaining mucosa of the body of the uterus is the *decidua parietalis*. It is the decidua basalis which becomes the maternal component of the placenta. In the early part of pregnancy the endometrium increases in thickness. A characteristic feature is the presence of *decidual cells*, which are enlarged stromal cells. The cytoplasm is vesicular or finely granular and contains large amounts of glycogen. The function of these cells is obscure.

As chorionic villi grow into the decidua basalis, they destroy and erode endometrium, leaving spaces or *lacunae*. With further enlargement of villi, lacunae become interconnecting and contain blood liberated by penetration of the maternal vessels by the trophoblast. Diffusion of dissolved substances now can occur between the maternal blood in the lacunae and fetal blood in the capillaries of the villi.

The Placenta

By 16 weeks, the chorion frondosum is well developed and the placenta is discoid in shape. It continues to increase in size throughout most of the gestational period owing mainly to growth of the villi. It consists of two components, a fetal and a maternal. The fetal component consists of the chorionic plate and the villi which arise from the plate. The villi lie in lacunae through which maternal blood circulates. Villi usually are classified into two types, *anchoring villi* and *free villi*. Anchoring villi pass from the chorionic plate to the decidua basalis. They give rise to branches which float in the lacunae.

Villi are alike histologically. In the loose connective tissue core of each villus there is a fetal capillary lined with typical endothelium. Large cells with large spherical nuclei (*cells of Hofbauer*) also are present in the cores; possibly they are phagocytic cells. The trophoblast covering each villus consists of two layers until approximately the tenth week of pregnancy, after which time the cytotrophoblast progressively disappears until at parturition only isolated clumps of its cells remain.

The cytotrophoblast, also called *Langhans' layer*, rests upon a basal lamina and consists of large, discrete, pale cells. The cytoplasm contains vacuoles and some glycogen. The syncytial trophoblast is a dark layer of variable thickness in which numerous small dark nuclei are present. No

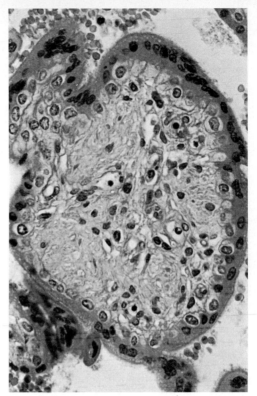

Figure 18-25. Section of a villus during the third month of pregnancy. The dense nuclei and dense (acidophil) cytoplasm of the syncytial trophoblast are prominent. Beneath this layer the pale cells with distinct cell boundaries comprise the cytotrophoblast, which already shows evidence of discontinuity.

See filmstrip II, frame 81.

intercellular boundaries can be distinguished. In some places the outer surface possesses microvilli. In the latter half of pregnancy the syncytial trophoblast thins out over the fetal capillaries to form a narrow layer. In other regions it often becomes aggregated into protuberances called *syncytial knots* or *sprouts*. On the surface of the villi irregular masses of an eosinophil, homogeneous substance called *fibrinoid* are present. This becomes increasingly abundant in older placentae.

The maternal component of the placenta is the decidua basalis. The enlarged endometrial stromal cells are known as decidual cells. Epithelial cells lining the glands are rich in glycogen and lipid droplets. By the third month, the glands of the decidua basalis become stretched and appear as horizontal clefts. Passing through the decidua basalis are spiral arteries which open into the intervillous space. The decidua is eroded more deeply opposite the anchoring villi than elsewhere, and this leaves projections of decidual tissue between the main villi. Such projections are termed *placental septa,* and they divide the placenta into lobules or *cotyledons.* From the fourth month on, the decidua basalis becomes loose in texture owing to the development of a dense venous plexus within it.

Functions of the Placenta. The placenta transfers from the maternal to the fetal circulation the nutritive and other substances necessary for the growth of the embryo. It also transfers waste products of fetal metabolism to the maternal circulation. The maternal circulation is separated from the fetal circulation only by the syncytial trophoblast, the cytotrophoblast (in the first trimester of pregnancy only), the basal lamina of the trophoblast, fetal connective tissue, the basal lamina of the fetal capillaries, and the fetal endothelium. These structures comprise the so-called *placental barrier,* which is selective against particulate matter, such as microorganisms, and against chemical substances over a certain molecular size.

The placenta elaborates hormones: it secretes estrogen and progesterone. Part of the fetal component of the placenta (cytotrophoblast) also produces *chorionic gonadotrophin.*

The Cervix

The cervix is the lowest segment of the uterus. The mucous membrane of the cervical canal, which shows branching folds on its surface, comprises an epithelium and a lamina propria. The epithelium consists of tall, mucus-secreting columnar cells. The oval nuclei lie at the bases of the cells and the cytoplasm above is pale. Some of the cells are ciliated. Numerous large, branching glands extend into the lamina propria. The glands sometimes become transformed into large cysts, the *nabothian follicles.* The lamina propria is a cellular connective tissue which contains no coiled arteries.

The portion of the cervix which projects into the vagina is covered by stratified squamous nonkeratinizing epithelium. The transition between the simple columnar epithelium of the cervical canal and the stratified squamous epithelium of the portio vaginalis is abrupt and occurs usually just inside the cervical canal.

The mucosa rests upon a myometrium which is composed chiefly of

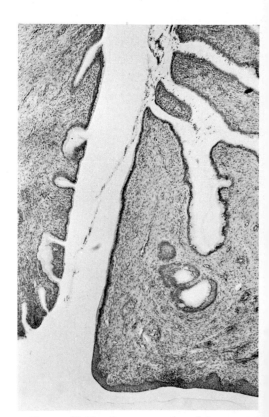

Figure 18-26. Lower portion of the cervix, including the portio vaginalis. Note the cervical glands and the transition between the simple columnar epithelium of the cervical canal and the stratified squamous epithelium of the portio vaginalis. × 35.

dense collagenous connective tissue. Smooth muscle present is arranged mainly in irregular bundles. The thin outer longitudinal layer continues into the vagina.

THE VAGINA

The vagina is a fibromuscular sheath lined with a mucous membrane. Under ordinary conditions it is collapsed and the anterior and posterior walls are in contact. The walls of the vagina consist of three coats: mucosa, muscularis, and adventitia.

The mucosa exhibits transverse folds, or *rugae*. It is lined with thick, stratified squamous epithelium which is nonkeratinizing. Component cells

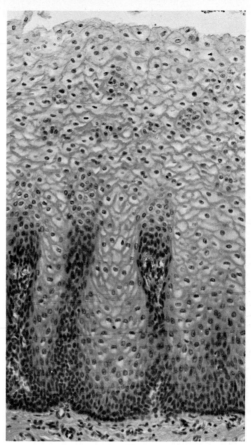

Figure 18-28. Portion of the vaginal mucosa. Note the depth of the epithelium, many component cells of which appear vacuolated, and the well-developed papillae of the lamina propria. × 100.   See filmstrip II, frame 82.

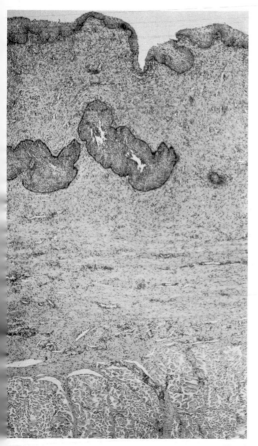

Figure 18-27. Section through the wall of the vagina, showing mucosa and a portion of the muscularis. × 25.

are loaded with glycogen and thus they appear vacuolated in most histological sections. The epithelium, which lacks glands, is lubricated by mucus which originates from the cervix. Beneath the epithelium there is a lamina propria which is a dense connective tissue containing numerous elastic fibers, lymphocytes, and occasional lymph nodules. Many lymphocytes invade the epithelium.

The surface cells of the vaginal epithelium are desquamated continuously and may be studied by the smear method. In subhuman primates and many other mammals, the vaginal epithelium undergoes cyclic changes correlated with other events of the reproductive cycle. In the human, the epithelium varies little during the cycle, although the study of desquamated vaginal cells is useful in the diagnosis of atrophic conditions and in evaluation of the effectiveness of estrogen therapy.

The muscularis of the vagina is composed of smooth muscle fibers which are arranged in interlacing bundles. The inner portion, where most muscle bundles are circularly arranged, is thin. The thick outer portion contains longitudinal bundles which are continuous above with the myometrium of the uterus. At the introitus there is a sphincter of skeletal muscle.

The adventitia is a thin layer of dense connective tissue which blends with that of surrounding organs.

The *hymen,* a transverse fold of the mucosa, partially occludes the opening of the vagina into the vestibule.

Blood Vessels, Lymphatics, and Nerves

Blood vessels and lymphatic vessels are abundant in the wall of the vagina. Veins are particularly numerous and give the lamina propria the appearance of erectile tissue.

The vagina receives both myelinated and unmyelinated nerve fibers. The latter form a ganglionated plexus in the adventitia and supply the muscularis and the walls of blood vessels. Myelinated nerve fibers terminate in special sensory endings in the mucosa.

THE EXTERNAL GENITALIA

The external genitalia, known collectively as the *vulva,* comprise the clitoris, the labia majora and minora, and certain glands which open into the vestibule.

The *clitoris* is a rudimentary and incomplete counterpart of the penis. It consists of two cavernous, erectile bodies which end in a rudimentary

glans clitoridis. It is covered with a thin, stratified squamous epithelium that is associated with specialized sensory nerve endings.

The *labia minora* are folds of mucous membrane which form the lateral walls of the vestibule. They are covered with a stratified squamous epithelium and have a core of richly vascularized connective tissue. Tall papillae of connective tissue penetrate far into the epithelium. Sebaceous glands occur on both surfaces of the fold, which is devoid of hair follicles.

The *labia majora* are folds of skin that cover the labia minor externally. The inner surface is smooth and hairless. The outer surface is covered with cornified epidermis which contains numerous hairs, sweat glands and

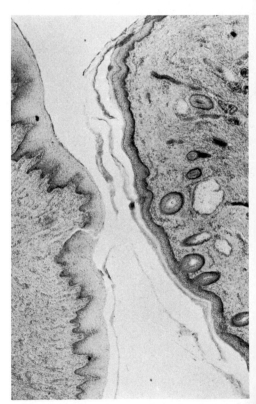

Figure 18-29. Section through portions of the labium minus (left) and the labium majus (right). The former is covered with nonkeratinized stratified squamous epithelium, the latter with cornified epidermis containing sweat and sebaceous glands. × 25.

sebaceous glands. The core of each fold contains a considerable amount of adipose tissue and some smooth muscle fibers.

The *vestibule,* into which the vagina and urethra open, is lined by a typical stratified squamous epithelium and contains numerous small glands, the *minor vestibular glands.* These are located mainly around the urethral opening and near the clitoris. They resemble the urethral glands (of Littre). The *major vestibular glands (glands of Bartholin),* analogous to the bulbourethral glands in the male, are located in the lateral walls of the vestibule. They are tubuloalveolar glands which secrete lubricating mucus.

THE MAMMARY GLAND

The mammary gland is a specialized, cutaneous gland located within the subcutaneous tissue. It is a modified sweat gland and is said to have an apocrine type of secretion. Mammary glands are present in both sexes and they develop only slightly during childhood. At puberty the glands enlarge rapidly in the female, principally as a result of development of adipose and other connective tissue, but very slowly in the male. The glands remain incompletely developed in the female until pregnancy occurs. After puberty there is no further development of the gland in the male.

The gland consists of 15 to 20 lobes, each of which actually is an independent gland with a duct opening at the apex of the nipple. A lobe is surrounded by interlobar connective tissue containing many fat cells. The fat and connective tissue also divide each lobe into numerous lobules. The intralobular connective tissue is loose, delicate, and cellular. Intralobular ducts drain into interlobular ducts, which join to form a single excretory duct from each lobe, the *lactiferous duct.* The lactiferous duct courses through the nipple and dilates near

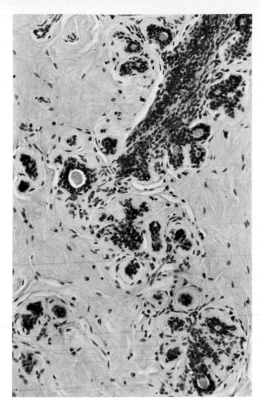

Figure 18-30.   Section of inactive mammary gland. The lobules, which are composed principally of ducts, are separated by abundant interlobular connective tissue. × 100.

its termination at the summit of the nipple into a *lactiferous sinus.*

Areola and Nipple

The nipple is traversed by lactiferous ducts which open by a pore on the surface. There are fewer pores than main ducts, owing to terminal fusions. The skin of the nipple is pigmented, and the underlying dermis is characterized by the presence of tall papillae and smooth muscle fibers. Contraction of the muscle hardens and elevates the nipple. The *areola,* an area of skin extending outward from the nipple, is pigmented and contains special *areolar glands (glands of Montgomery),* which are large, branched glands of the apocrine type. Sweat and sebaceous glands and a number of coarse hairs are present also.

(See filmstrip II, frame 83.)

Parenchyma

The parenchyma of the mammary gland shows extensive structural changes which are dependent upon the functional condition.

The Inactive Mammary Gland

The ducts are the principal epithelial tissue seen. Intralobular ducts are grouped together into lobules. The lining of the ducts changes from a simple cuboidal to a two-layered epithelium from the small to the main ducts. Alveoli, if present, are small buds. Between the epithelium and the basal lamina there is a layer of myoepithelial cells. Intralobular connective tissue is dense and abundant and contains varying amounts of adipose tissue.

The Mammary Gland During Pregnancy

The gland exhibits extensive changes in preparation for lactation. In the first half of pregnancy, intralobular ducts undergo rapid proliferation and form buds which enlarge into alveoli. Owing to the expansion of lobules, interlobular fat and connective tissue decrease in amount and the 15 to 20 lobes become distinct entities. Intralobular connective tissue also decreases in amount and becomes infiltrated with lymphocytes. During the second half of pregnancy, alveoli enlarge and begin to elaborate some secretory material. At the end of pregnancy some cloudy, watery fluid, colostrum, is secreted.

During pregnancy increased pigmentation occurs in the skin of the nipple and areola.

The Mammary Gland During Lactation

Soon after parturition, the mammary gland begins active secretion of milk. Many alveoli become dilated and appear as saccules. They are distended by milk and have a low epithelial wall. Other alveoli are resting; they have a relatively tall epithelial lining and small lumina. Individual alveolar cells undergo a cyclic process of secretion. Within the cytoplasm small fat droplets appear, which later coalesce in the region of the Golgi apparatus. The lipid droplets migrate toward the apical ends of the cells where they coalesce further to form large fat globules. Secretion appears to be, at least in part, of the apocrine type and contains, in addition to the fat, considerable quantities of protein. The apical cell membrane ruptures and the droplets escape together with some cytoplasm. The secretory cycle is then repeated. The alveolar cytoplasm is quite basophil during lactation, and electron microscopic studies suggest that secretory material arises in association with granular endoplasmic reticulum.

The alveolar epithelium rests upon a basal lamina. Between the alveolar cells and the basal lamina are stellate *basket* (myoepithelial) *cells*. These are thought to be contractile.

Intralobular ducts histologically appear similar to alveoli. Functionally they are true secretory ducts which also possess myoepithelial elements.

Regression of the Mammary Gland

After cessation of lactation, the gland undergoes retrogressive changes and returns to a resting state. Alveoli decrease in size and some cells degenerate. Connective tissue and fat again become abundant. However, the gland usually does not return to the nulliparous state; many alveoli remain recognizable as such and remnants of

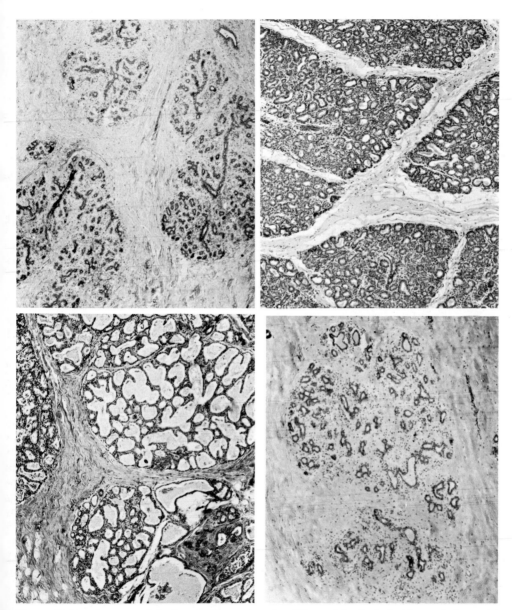

Figure 18-31. Sections of the breast, illustrating the different histological pictures during varying functional conditions. Top left: During the fourth month of pregnancy. Top right: Immediately after parturition. Bottom left: During lactation. Bottom right: After cessation of lactation. Note the degree of development of the lobules during these functional states. After cessation of lactation (bottom right) the breast does not return completely to the nulliparous state (compare with Figure 18-30). × 25.

See filmstrip II, frames 84 and 85.

secretory material may be retained within the ducts for a considerable time.

Involution of the Mammary Gland

After the menopause, the mammary gland undergoes involution. The secretory epithelium atrophies and only a few remnants of the duct system persist. Cystic dilatation of the remaining ducts occurs frequently. The connective tissue becomes increasingly dense and homogeneous.

Hormonal Control of the Mammary Gland

Growth of the duct system which occurs at puberty is influenced by estrogen and progesterone secreted cyclically by the ovaries. Further growth of the gland in pregnancy is due to continuous and prolonged production of both estrogen and progesterone by the ovaries and placenta. The initiation of secretion seems to be induced by the lactogenic hormone (prolactin) of the pars distalis of the hypophysis. Maintenance of lactation appears to depend upon a number of hormones.

Blood Vessels, Lymphatics, and Nerves

Blood vessels enter the gland from several sources, ramify in the stroma, and terminate in rich capillary plexuses around the ducts and alveoli. The vascular supply becomes much richer in the active gland. From the capillaries, veins arise which accompany the arteries.

Lymph vessels are found in the areola, around the ducts, and in the interlobular connective tissue. Collecting lymphatics pass to the axillary nodes; a few penetrate the intercostal spaces and follow the branches of the internal mammary artery.

Afferent nerve fibers supply the tactile organs of the nipple. Some nerve fibers follow the interlobular connective tissue and form delicate plexuses around the alveoli.

EMBRYOLOGY OF THE MALE AND FEMALE REPRODUCTIVE SYSTEMS

The primordia of the gonads arise as thickenings of mesodermal epithelium, the *genital ridges,* on the mesial surface of the mesonephros. The epithelial cells of the ridge proliferate and form a band of tissue composed of two types of cells. Most cells are small, cuboidal elements and scattered between them are large, spheroidal cells, the *primitive sex cells.* The epithelial cells penetrate the underlying mesenchyme and form *sex cords.*

In the male human embryo the testis becomes recognizable at about seven weeks. The sex cords become more distinct and elongate to form the seminiferous tubules. Their peripheral ends anastomose and unite with a number of mesonephric tubules to form the rete testis. At the onset of puberty component cells of the seminiferous tubules differentiate into spermatogonia and Sertoli cells.

Differentiation of the ovary does not commence until about the eighth week of gestation. The sex cords formed during the indifferent stage gradually disappear. The covering (germinal) epithelium continues to proliferate and produces the primitive cortex of the ovary. This mass of cortical cells is subdivided by strands of mesenchyme into clusters containing oogonia, probably derived from the primitive sex cells. Proliferation of cortical tissue continues into the latter half of fetal life.

Genital ducts develop in close connection with the embryonic urinary system. They are laid down initially as two paired longitudinal ducts, the *ducts of Wolff* and *of Müller,* the latter from mesoderm lining the coelomic cavity. In the male the wolffian duct is transformed into ductus epididymidis and ductus deferens. Connection of the ductus epididymidis with the rete testis is established by a number of mesonephric tubules, which become the ductuli efferentes. The müllerian duct involutes, leaving only small rudiments. In the female, the wolffian ducts regress and the müllerian ducts transform into the female genital ducts. Caudally the two müllerian ducts fuse to form a single tube which opens into the urogenital sinus (cloaca). The paired upper portions form the fallopian tubes and the unpaired terminal portion becomes the uterus and vagina.

Vestigial Structures

Certain vestigial structures occur in relation to the ovary.

The *epoophoron* consists of several blind tubules situated in the broad ligament between the ovary and the fallopian tube. The tubules fuse into a longitudinal canal, the *duct of Gartner*, which passes along the lateral wall of the uterus.

The *paroophoron*, consisting of a few blind tubules, lies in the connective tissue of the broad ligament close to the hilum.

Both epoophoron and paroophoron are remnants of mesonephric tubules. Gartner's duct represents a remnant of the mesonephric duct.

REFERENCES

Boyd, J. D., and Hamilton, W. J.: Development of the human placenta in the first three months of gestation. J. Anat., 94:297, 1960.

Boyd, J. D., Hamilton, W. J., and Boyd, C. A. R.: The surface of the syncytium of the human chorionic villus. J. Anat., 102:553, 1968.

Corner, G. W.: Cytology of the ovum, ovary and fallopian tube. In Special Cytology, edited by E. V. Cowdry. New York, Paul B. Hoeber, 1932, Vol. 3, p. 1565.

Dempsey, E. W., Bunting, H., and Wislocki, G. B.: Observations on the chemical cytology of the mammary gland. Amer. J. Anat., 81:309, 1947.

Dempsey, E. W., and Wislocki, G. B.: Histochemical reactions associated with baso-

philia and acidophilia in the placenta and pituitary gland. Amer. J. Anat., 76:277, 1945.

Enders, A. C., and Schlafke, S.: A morphological analysis of the early implantation stages in the rat. Amer. J. Anat., 120:185, 1967.

Gruenwald, P.: The development of the sex cords in the gonads of man and mammals. Amer. J. Anat., 70:359, 1942.

Hertig, A. T., and Adams, E. C.: Studies on the human oocyte and its follicle. I. Ultrastructural and histochemical observations on the primordial follicle stage. J. Cell Biol., 34:647, 1967.

Hertig, A. T., and Rock, J.: Two human ova of the previllous stage, having a developmental age of about seven and nine days respectively. Contributions to Embryology No. 200, Carnegie Institution of Washington Publ. No. 557, 31:67, 1945.

Hertig, A. T., Rock, J., and Adams, E. G.: A description of 34 human ova within the first 17 days of development. Amer. J. Anat., 98:435, 1956.

Kon, S. K., and Cowie, A. T.: Milk: The Mammary Gland and Its Secretion. New York, Academic Press, 1961.

Kurosumi, K., Kobayashi, Y., and Baba, N.: The fine structure of mammary glands of lactating rats, with special reference to the apocrine secretion. Exp. Cell Res., 50:117, 1968.

Linzell, J. L.: The silver staining of myoepithelial cells, particularly in the mammary gland, and their relation to the ejection of milk. J. Anat., 86:49, 1952.

Nilsson, O.: Electron microscopy of the glandular epithelium in the human uterus. I. Follicular phase. J. Ultrastruct. Res., 6:413, 1962.

Nilsson, W.: Electron microscopy of the glandular epithelium in the human uterus. II. Early and late luteal phase. J. Ultrastruct. Res., 6:422, 1962.

Papanicolaou, G. N.: The sexual cycle in the human female as revealed by vaginal smears. Amer. J. Anat., 52:519, 1933.

Papanicolaou, G. N.: Atlas of Exfoliative Cytology. Cambridge, Mass., Harvard University Press, 1954.

Ramsey, E. M.: Circulation in the maternal placenta of the Rhesus monkey and man, with observations on the marginal lakes. Amer. J. Anat., 98:159, 1956.

Rock, J., and Hertig, A. T.: The human conceptus during the first two weeks of gestation. Amer. J. Obstet. Gynec., 55:6, 1948.

Wislocki, G. B., and Bennett, H. S.: The histology and cytology of the human and monkey placenta, with special reference to the trophoblast. Amer. J. Anat., 73:335, 1943.

Wislocki, G. B., and Dempsey, E. W.: Electron microscopy of the human placenta. Anat. Rec., 123:133, 1955.

Witschi, E.: Embryology of the ovary. In The Ovary, edited by H. G. Grady and D. E. Smith. Baltimore, Williams & Wilkins Co., 1963.

CHAPTER 19

THE MALE REPRODUCTIVE SYSTEM

The male reproductive system comprises the testis, the ducts of the testis, the auxiliary glands associated with them, and the penis.

THE TESTIS

The testis is a double gland since functionally it is both exocrine and endocrine. The exocrine product is chiefly the sex cells, and thus the testis may be referred to as a cytogenic gland. The endocrine product is an internal secretion elaborated by certain specialized cells. The testis is surrounded by a layer of mesothelium (the *tunica vaginalis*), usually destroyed during preparation, beneath which is a thick, white capsule, the *tunica albuginea*. This is composed of dense fibroelastic connective tissue and is thickened along the posterior surface of the testis where it projects into the interior of the gland as the *mediastinum testis*. The innermost zone of the tunica albuginea is looser and more vascular. Thin, fibrous partitions radiate from the mediastinum testis to the capsule and divide the interior of the testis into about 250 pyramidal compartments, the *lobuli testis,* with their apices toward the

444

mediastinum. The septa show numerous deficiencies and the lobules thus intercommunicate quite freely. Each lobule contains one to four highly convoluted *seminiferous tubules,* which are embedded in a loose connective tissue stroma containing vessels, nerves, and several types of cells, principally the specific *interstitial cells* (of Leydig). These are large cells, commonly in groups, and are important because of their endocrine role.

Seminiferous Tubules

Each seminiferous tubule is highly convoluted and is about 0.2 mm. in diameter and 30 to 70 cm. long. At the apex of a lobule, each tubule loses its convolutions and becomes a *straight tubule*. The seminiferous tubule is lined by a complex germinal or seminiferous epithelium, which is a modified stratified cuboidal epithelium. The epithelium rests upon a thin basal lamina and is covered externally by a specialized zone of fibrous tissue, the so-called boundary tissue, which contains numerous connective tissue fibers, flattened fibroblasts, and some smooth muscle cells. It is thought that

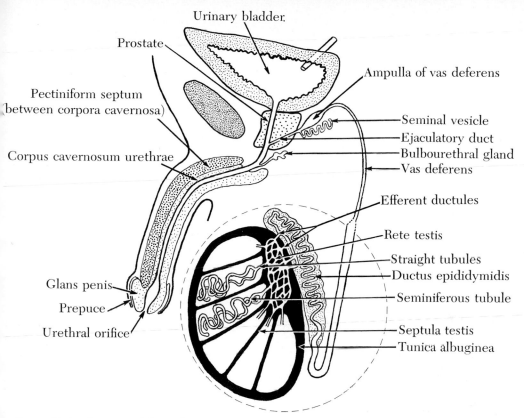

Urinary bladder.

Prostate

Pectiniform septum
(between corpora cavernosa)

Corpus cavernosum urethrae

Glans penis

Prepuce

Urethral orifice

Ampulla of vas deferens

Seminal vesicle
Ejaculatory duct
Bulbourethral gland
Vas deferens

Efferent ductules

Rete testis

Straight tubules
Ductus epididymidis

Seminiferous tubule

Septula testis
Tunica albuginea

Figure 19-1. Diagram of the male reproductive system. The portions of the system within the circle are represented as more highly magnified than the other components of the system.

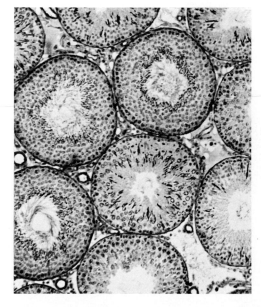

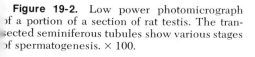

Figure 19-2. Low power photomicrograph of a portion of a section of rat testis. The transected seminiferous tubules show various stages of spermatogenesis. × 100.

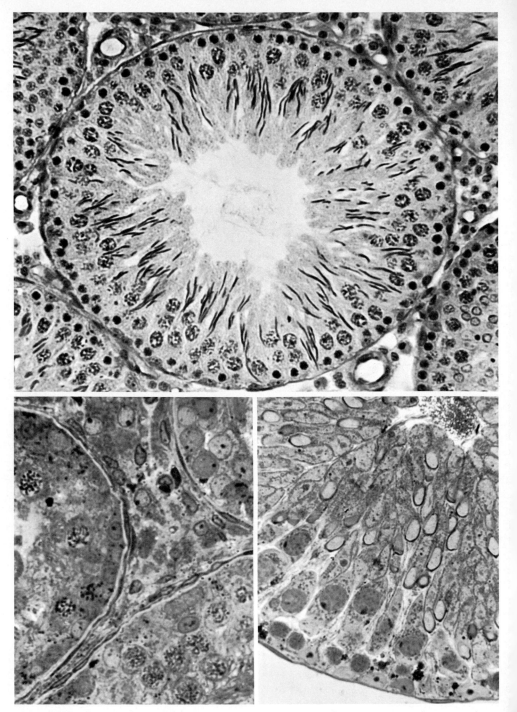

Figure 19-3.   Top: High power photomicrograph of a portion of rat testis. Seminiferous tubules, cut in cross section, are separated by a slight amount of interstitial connective tissue containing groups of Leydig cells. × 300. Bottom left: Portions of three tubules, containing numerous spermatocytes. Note the interstitial cells between tubules. Epon section. × 750. Bottom right: Portion of a tubule with numerous spermatids. Note the supporting cells of Sertoli in relation to the boundary tissue. Epon section. × 900.   See filmstrip II, frames 86 and 87.

the smooth muscle cells, by their contraction, may alter the diameter of the seminiferous tubule and aid in the movement of spermatozoa along the length of the tubule. The thickness of this zone varies with age and shows a great increase in extent in many clinical conditions, particularly those associated with some chromosomal abnormalities (such as Klinefelter's syndrome).

The seminiferous epithelium contains two distinct categories of cells, the nutrient and supporting elements, and the germ or spermatogenic cells. The latter form the vast bulk of the epithelium and, by proliferation and complex differentiation, give rise to the spermatozoa.

Supporting Elements. The supporting cells, or *sustentacular cells* of Sertoli, are relatively few in number and are spaced along the tubule at fairly regular intervals, crowded between the germ cells. They are tall, pillarlike cells, with their bases resting upon the basal lamina of the tubule. The cell outline is irregular, indistinct, and very complex since the heads of maturing spermatozoa lie in deep recesses of the cytoplasm. The nucleus is located some distance above the base of the cell, and is pale and ovoid with its long axis directed radially. The definite nucleolus of these cells readily distinguishes them from the spermatogenic elements within the tubule; it is prominent and of a compound nature, consisting of a central acidophil portion and smaller peripheral concentrations of basophil material. In fixed preparations, the cytoplasm has a reticular appearance and contains small fibrils, lipid droplets, small discrete granules which stain with iron hematoxylin, and small elongated mitrochondria. Occasionally one can also see a tapering crystalloid body near the nucleus. During their period of differentiation, spermatids (immature germ cells) attach to the sustentacular cells and apparently are nourished by them. Sustentacular cells are resistant

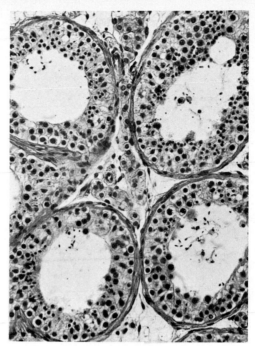

Figure 19-4. Section of the human testis. The wide lumina of the seminiferous tubules contain some spermatozoa. The boundary tissue around the tubules and groups of Leydig cells in the interstitial connective tissue are seen clearly. × 160.

to various noxious influences that destroy the spermatogenic cells.

Spermatogenic Cells. The germ or spermatogenic cells comprise a stratified layer of epithelium, four to eight cells deep, lining the seminiferous tubule. The cells differentiate progressively from the basal region of the tubule to the lumen. Proliferation pushes the cells toward the lumen, and those nearest the lumen transform into spermatozoa and detach from the epithelium, coming to lie free within the lumen. The sequence of events is referred to as *spermatogenesis*, which involves the two processes of cell multiplication, including reduction from the diploid to the haploid number of chromosomes, and cellular differentiation (spermiogenesis). In many lower mammalian orders, spermatogenesis occurs in definite cyclic waves along the length of the seminiferous

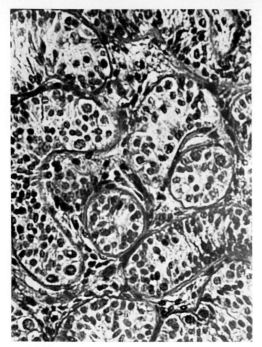

Figure 19-5. Photomicrograph of the human testis from a 21 year old patient suffering from pituitary hypofunction (see page 453). The tubules show no evidence of spermatogenesis, and the appearance is similar to that of a prepubertal gland. × 275.

tubules, but such regular waves of activity do not occur in man. However, not every stage of spermatogenesis will be seen at the same time at a given point along the seminiferous epithelium.

The process of spermatogenesis is thought to occupy about two to three weeks. Spermatogenesis commences with the *spermatogonia*,* which lie immediately adjacent to the basal lamina. These are the only germ cells present until the time of puberty. Each spermatogonium contains a diploid number of chromosomes within its nucleus (44 autosomes and two sex chromosomes, XY). The nucleus has a pale, vesicular appearance and is oval in outline.

Spermatogonia increase in number by a normal mitotic form of cell divi-

---

*G *sperma*, seed; *gonē*, generation.

sion. After several divisions, there is a period of growth during which some spermatogonia move away from the basal lamina, increase in size, and show a change in the character of the nucleus. These gradual changes in the spermatogonia constitute a transformation into *primary spermatocytes*. Some spermatogonia remain close to the basal lamina, undergo none of the changes just mentioned, and form a reservoir of undifferentiated cells.

Primary spermatocytes are the largest germ cells seen within the seminiferous tubule, where they occupy the middle zone of the epithelium. Each cell is spherical or oval in outline, and the nucleus is usually in some stage of karyokinesis. The cell division which occurs within primary spermatocytes is a reduction division, *meiosis*, in which whole chromosomes (synaptic mates, or the halves of the bivalent chromosomes) move to opposite poles of the spindle, unlike a somatic mitosis in which individual chromosomes split and the half chromosomes separate. As a result of the meiotic division, 23 chromosomes (22 autosomes plus one sex chromosome, either X or Y) pass into each daughter cell or *secondary spermatocyte*. The meiotic division also is peculiar in that cytokinesis is incomplete, and the two daughter cells (secondary spermatocytes) resulting from the division of a primary spermatocyte remain connected by a bridge of protoplasm. The two conjoined secondary spermatocytes later divide mitotically, and the resultant four cells (*spermatids*) remain in a syncytial cluster since cytokinesis again is incomplete.

The secondary spermatocytes are about half the size of the primary spermatocytes and lie nearer the lumen. They are seen rarely in sections of seminiferous tubules since they are short-lived and divide quickly to produce spermatids. The division here is a somatic mitosis and a complete set of 23 chromosomes is present in each spermatid (i.e., the haploid number). With the division, there is a further reduction in volume to half that of the secondary spermatocyte. The spermatids lie close to the lumen. No further division occurs and each spermatid is transformed by an extensive differentiation (*spermiogenesis*) into a spermatozoon. The cytoplasmic continuity between clusters of spermatids may constitute a basis for the synchrony of their later differentiation. Soon after their appearance, spermatids become closely applied to the surface of sustentacular cells, where commonly they lie in deep recesses formed by the irregular surface of sustentacular cells. In this environment they undergo metamorphosis into spermatozoa.

SPERMIOGENESIS.   The newly formed spermatid contains a centrally located spherical nucleus with a well delineated Golgi zone nearby, nu-

merous mitochondria, and a pair of centrioles. Spermiogenesis involves marked differentiation of all these cellular structures. Initially, several small granules appear within the numerous small vesicles of the Golgi zone. They coalesce to form a single large granule, the *acrosome*, which lies within an *acrosomal vesicle* (see Figure 19-6). This complex lies between the main components of the Golgi zone and the nucleus. The membrane bounding the acrosomal vesicle, derived from the Golgi zone, then adheres to the outer layer of the nuclear membrane. The acrosomal vesicle grows over the surface of the nuclear membrane and eventually covers about half of the nuclear surface. Part of the enlargement of the acrosomal vesicle and of the acrosome is contributed to by the Golgi zone, which later migrates from the region of the acrosomal

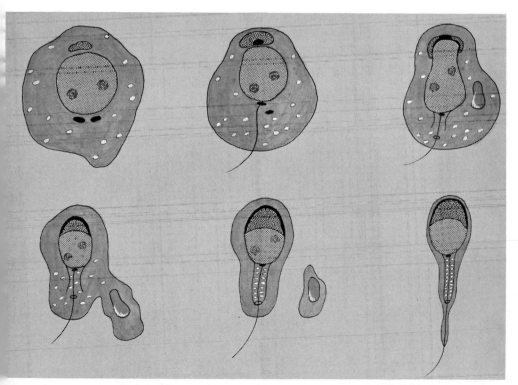

Figure 19-6.   Six successive stages in the transformation of the spermatid into the spermatozoon (spermiogenesis). The nucleus (light mottling) condenses to form the sperm head; the acrosome, which appears within the Golgi zone (heavy mottling), gives rise to the head cap. The flagellum arises in relation to one of the centrioles, and mitochondria migrate around the flagellum to form the sheath of the middle piece.

vesicle and comes to lie at the opposite pole of the nucleus. With the migration of the Golgi zone, there appears to be resorption of the fluid content of the acrosomal vesicle, which collapses onto the acrosome and forms a close-fitting *head cap* over the nucleus, containing the acrosome between its layers.

As acrosome formation is in progress at one pole of the nucleus, the centrioles become associated with the nuclear membrane at the opposite pole and a slender flagellum grows out from one of them. As the flagellum grows, a thin, filamentous sheath, the *caudal tube,* is laid down around the axial filaments of the flagellum, and the other centriole migrates toward the cell surface and encircles the longitudinal axial filaments as a ring or *annulus.* The nucleus becomes condensed, slightly flattened, and elon-

gated, and is displaced toward the cell membrane where it now forms the definitive sperm head. Meanwhile, there is a shift of the bulk of the cytoplasm toward the tail end of the cell. Mitochondria, until now randomly distributed in the cytoplasm, migrate to the region between the basal centriole and the annulus; there they become aligned in a spiral array or helix around the proximal portion of the flagellum as the *mitochondrial sheath,* thus delineating the *middle piece* of the future spermatozoon.

As differentiation proceeds, most of the surplus cytoplasm is cast off as the *residual body,* and only a thin layer of cytoplasm remains as a cover over the nucleus, middle piece, and tail piece of the spermatozoon. The residual bodies are thought to be phagocytosed by sustentacular cells. Their lipid content remains within the cytoplasm of

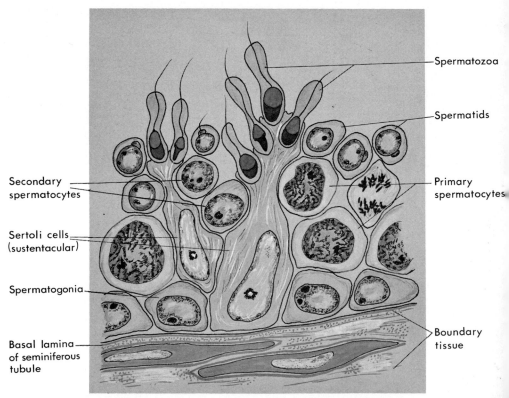

Figure 19-7.   Diagrammatic representation of a segment of a human seminiferous tubule to illustrate the process of spermatogenesis.

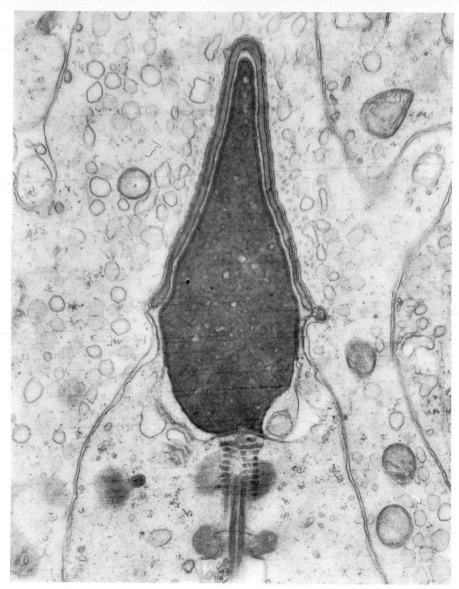

Figure 19-8. Electron micrograph of a section of a human spermatid at an advanced stage of development. The head cap is complete, and the acrosome can no longer be identified as a separate entity. A well-developed flagellum extends from the lower pole of the nucleus. × 27,500.

sustentacular cells and probably constitutes the bulk of lipid seen in these cells to which differentiating spermatids are attached. There is some evidence to suggest that this lipid is utilized by sustentacular cells in the production of a hormone which might play an important role in regulating spermatogenesis locally. The tail piece is similar in structure to a cilium,

containing the same number and arrangement of longitudinal filaments. Upon completion of differentiation, spermatozoa are released from their intimate contact with sustentacular cells and enter the lumen of the seminiferous tubule. At this time they are mature morphologically but are immature functionally in that they are nonmotile and are limited in their

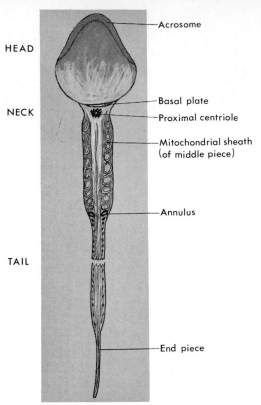

HEAD

NECK

TAIL

— Acrosome

— Basal plate

— Proximal centriole

— Mitochondrial sheath
(of middle piece)

— Annulus

— End piece

Figure 19-9. Diagrammatic representation of a mature spermatozoon.

ability to effect fertilization of the ovum.

Mature Sperm

The mature human spermatozoon consists of a head, middle piece, and tail. The head comprises the condensed nucleus and a head cap, including the dense acrosome at its anterior margin. The head contains the DNA, or genetic material. The function of the acrosome in the human sperm is obscure, but in the rodent sperm there is evidence to suggest that it contains hyaluronidase, an enzyme which facilitates the passage of spermatozoa between the cells that surround unfertilized eggs, thereby aiding fertilization. The

middle piece, which is separated from the head piece by a narrow neck, contains a core of longitudinal filaments surrounded by a mitochondrial sheath, and it is thought that it is responsible for control of movements of the tail. The tail has two central and nine peripheral double filaments (an arrangement essentially identical to that in a cilium), ensheathed by a thin layer of cytoplasm, except for the very tip which is naked.

The Interstitium

The interstitial tissue, within the lobuli testis, lies between the seminiferous tubules. It contains some collagenous fibers, blood and lymph vessels, nerves, and several cell types including fibroblasts, macrophages, mast cells, and some undifferentiated mesenchymal cells. Blood vessels and nerves enter and leave at the mediastinum and form networks around the tubules. The specific interstitial cells of Leydig are a marked feature of this tissue. They lie in compact groups, usually in the angular areas created by the packing of seminiferous tubules. They are large cells in which the cytoplasm often appears vacuolated in light microscopy preparations. The nucleus contains coarse chromatin granules and a distinct nucleolus. Binucleate cells are common. The cytoplasm is rich in inclusions such as lipid droplets and, in the human, it may contain peculiar rod-shaped crystalloids. In electron microscopy the most striking feature of these cells is the extensive development of agranular (smooth-surfaced) endoplasmic reticulum. This appears as a fine meshwork of anastomosing tubules to the surface of which no ribosomes are attached. Unlike the endoplasmic reticulum associated with ribosomes which is concerned with protein synthesis, the agranular reticulum is thought by some to be the site of synthesis of steroid hormones.

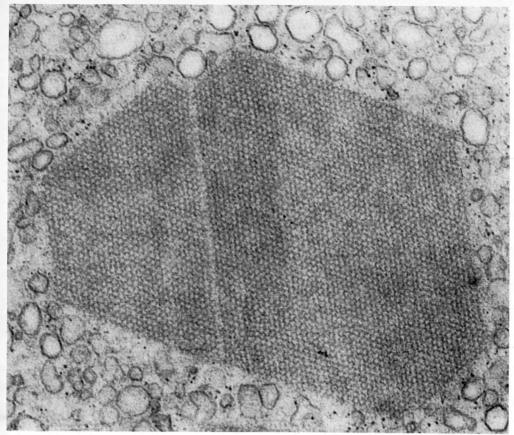

Figure 19-10. Electron micrograph of a portion of a human Leydig cell containing a crystalloid of Reinke. × 40,000.

Functional Considerations of the Testis

The principal exocrine function of the testis, the production of male sex cells, is dependent upon numerous factors. Follicle-stimulating hormone (FSH) of the anterior lobe of the hypophysis stimulates spermatogenesis in mammals, although the effect is not so marked in man as it is in lower forms. A suitable temperature is critical for the process. This is furnished by the position of the testis in the scrotum. In cases of cryptorchism (maldescent of the testis), spermatogenesis does not proceed to completion. In man, spermatogenesis is a continuous process throughout sexual maturity. The sex determining role of

spermatozoa is correlated with the production of two types of spermatozoa. Half of the secondary spermatocytes contain a female determining chromosome (X) and the other half, a male determining chromosome (Y), this distinction continuing into daughter spermatids and into spermatozoa. The principal endocrine secretion of the testis is testosterone, produced by the interstitial cells, which constitute a peculiar type of endocrine gland in that they do not develop from an epithelial surface, as do most glands, but from the mesenchymal stroma of the testis. In the stroma, abundantly supplied with capillaries, they have easy access for their secretory product into the vascular system. The production of testosterone by the testis depends upon stimulation by luteinizing hormone (LH) of the anterior lobe of the hypophysis. Since the target organ here is represented by the interstitial cells, luteinizing hormone often is referred to as interstitial cell-stimulating hormone (ICSH) in this context. Testosterone controls the appearance of secondary sex characters, the sex impulse, and the proper development and maintenance of the genital ducts and accessory glands.

THE MALE GENITAL DUCTS

Tubuli Recti. At the apex of each lobule, the component seminiferous tubules join to form a straight tubule. Each straight tubule is short and devoid of convolutions, and has a diameter of about 25 microns. At the point of continuity with the seminiferous tubules, the spermatogenic cells disappear, and only Sertoli cells remain, forming a simple columnar epithelium. Component cells contain numerous fat droplets.

Rete Testis. The straight tubules course to the dense connective tissue of the mediastinum testis where they enter a network of anastomosing channels, the rete testis. The lining of these irregular spaces is simple cuboidal or squamous epithelium, some component cells of which bear a single cilium. The epithelium rests upon a delicate basal lamina. Passage of spermatozoa through the tubuli recti and the rete testis is thought to occur rapidly, since in sections one rarely sees spermatozoa within the lumina.

Ductuli Efferentes. In the superior portion of the posterior border of the testis, some 10 to 15 spirally wound, efferent ductules emerge from the rete. Each ductule is about 6 to 8 cm. long and about 0.05 mm. in diameter. The ductules are bound by connective tissue, and each is surrounded by a thin layer of circularly arranged smooth muscle fibers; together they constitute the major portion of the

head of the epididymis. The ductuli efferentes are lined by a typical epithelium, mostly simple columnar, which rests upon a thin basal lamina. Externally each tubule has a regular outline, but internally the lumen is irregular in outline owing to the varying height of the epithelium. Groups of tall columnar cells alternate with groups of much shorter cells, the latter forming intraepithelial glands. Cells of these glands appear clear and contain pale secretory material and scattered pigment granules. Some cells bear cilia. The tall cells have a dense acidophil cytoplasm containing fat droplets and pigment granules, and many are ciliated. The cilia of both cell types beat toward the epididymis and thus help in transporting spermatozoa to the epididymis. The efferent ductules possess the only motile cilia in the entire duct system.

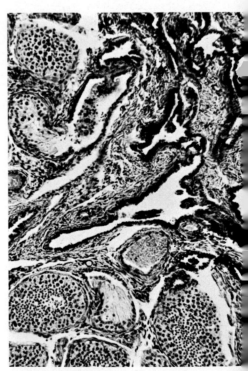

Figure 19-11. Low power photomicrograph of a portion of the human testis and mediastinum. Straight tubules (tubuli recti) pass from the seminiferous tubules into the network of the rete testis (upper right). × 100.

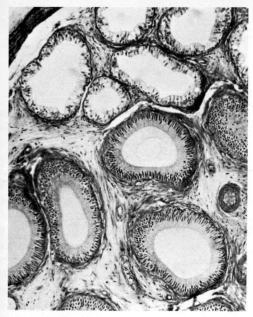

Figure 19-12. Low power photomicrograph of a section of the head of the epididymis. At the top of the picture are cross sections of efferent ductules and below are sections of the ductus epididymidis. Note the tall epithelial cells of the latter and the irregular height of the epithelium of the efferent ductules. × 90.

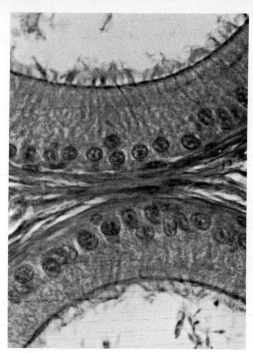

Figure 19-13. High power photomicrograph of a section of the ductus epididymidis. Notice the regular height of the epithelium and the stereocilia projecting into the lumen. × 450.

See filmstrip II, frame 88.

Ductus Epididymidis. The efferent ductules run into a single ductus epididymidis. This duct, which is surrounded by connective tissue, is highly tortuous and forms the body and the tail of the epididymis. It is a long storage duct (5 to 7 meters long) through which spermatozoa pass slowly. In their passage, they acquire motility and optimal fertilizability. The duct has a cylindrical outline both inside and outside, since the epithelium, unlike that of the efferent ductules, is uniform in height. The epithelium is pseudostratified, composed of basal cells and tall columnar cells. Lipid droplets are found in the cytoplasm of both cell types, and the tall columnar cells also contain pigment granules and secretion droplets and bear a tuft of nonmotile stereocilia (long, slender cellular processes, which differ from microvilli in the repeated branching near their bases) on their free surface. The secretory product of the epithelium passes into the lumen through this irregular surface. The duct is surrounded by a definite basal lamina, external to which there is a thin layer of circularly arranged smooth muscle fibers. The muscle is thought to aid by its contraction in transporting spermatozoa down the duct.

Ductus Deferens. The ductus epididymidis straightens out at its termination and becomes continuous with the ductus deferens, which ascends from the scrotum to the inguinal region, traverses the inguinal canal, and courses down the side wall of the pelvis retroperitoneally toward the urethra. Relatively, its wall is thick and the lumen narrow. In the scrotum and inguinal canal, the ductus deferens lies within the spermatic cord, where it is easily palpable because of its thick wall. The spermatic cord contains, in addition to the ductus, arteries, veins of the pampini-

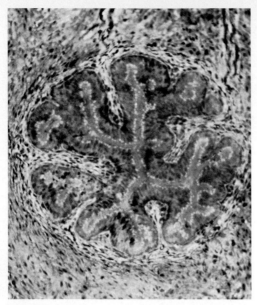

Figure 19-14. Cross section of ductus deferens. Epon section. × 100.

See filmstrip II, frame 89.

form plexus, lymph vessels and nerves of the testis and epididymis, and longitudinal strands of smooth muscle. Prior to its termination, the duct dilates into a spindle-shaped enlargement, the *ampulla*.

The epithelium of the ductus deferens is pseudostratified and many of the tall cells bear stereocilia. A delicate basal lamina intervenes between the epithelium and a thin lamina propria, which is characterized by the presence of numerous elastic fibers. The mucosa rises into longitudinal folds, which are responsible for the stellate outline of the lumen one sees in cross sections. Beneath the lamina propria there is an ill-defined submucosa, containing numerous blood vessels, which separates the mucosa from the muscular coat. This coat is thick and is composed of three distinct layers of smooth muscle. The inner layer is a relatively thin one of longitudinally oriented muscle. The middle or circular layer is markedly robust, and beyond this there is another well-developed layer in which the muscle fibers are arranged longitudinally. A fibrous adventitia surrounds the muscular coat

and blends with that of adjoining tissues.

Ampulla of Ductus Deferens. In the terminal dilatation of the ductus deferens, the lumen is wider and the mucosa much more folded than in the main portion of the ductus. Many of the epithelial folds branch and fuse with each other, producing a number of pocket-like recesses. The simple epithelium may show evidence of secretion. The musculature is much less regularly arranged than in the rest of the ductus deferens. Usually only the external longitudinal layer retains its identity.

Ejaculatory Duct. This is the short, terminal segment of each genital duct system. It is formed by the junction of the ampulla and seminal vesicle. It pierces the prostate gland to open into the urethra just to the side of the prostatic utricle. The ejaculatory duct is lined by a simple columnar or pseudostratified epithelium, probably capable of secretion, which shows some mucosal outpocketings similar to those of the ampulla but less extensive. The supporting wall is fibrous connective tissue only.

THE AUXILIARY GENITAL GLANDS

The glands associated with the duct systems of the testes are the seminal vesicles, the prostate, and the bulbourethral glands.

Seminal Vesicles. Each vesicle is a tortuous, elongated diverticulum of the ductus deferens at the termination of the ampullary portion, situated posterior to the prostate gland. The wall consists of an external connective tissue adventitia containing numerous elastic fibers, a smooth muscle coat thinner than that of the ductus deferens, and a mucosa which is markedly folded. The high primary folds of the mucosa themselves branch into secondary and tertiary folds which project far into the lumen and merge

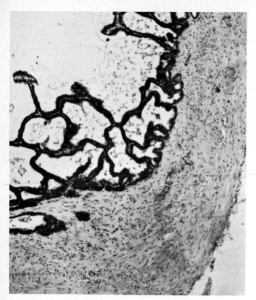

Figure 19-15. Low power photomicrograph of a portion of a cross section of a seminal vesicle. Note the intricate folding of the mucosa. × 70.

Prostate. The prostate surrounds the urethra at its origin from the bladder. It is an aggregate of 30 to 50 small compound tubuloalveolar glands which drain into the prostatic urethra by 15 to 30 small excretory ducts. The glandular elements are distributed in three different areas, more or less concentrically arranged around the urethra. Small glands lie in the mucosa and these are surrounded by submucosal glands. The main, or principal, glandular elements lie peripherally and constitute the bulk of the gland. The whole gland is surrounded by a fibroelastic capsule containing an extensive plexus of veins, and the glandular components are embedded in an abundant, dense stroma which is continuous at the periphery with the capsule. This stroma is again fibroelastic and in addition contains numerous

with one another frequently. As a result, numerous compartments of different sizes are formed. All communicate with the lumen, although in sections many appear to be isolated. The epithelium typically shows many variations. It is usually pseudostratified but may be simple columnar. The height varies with the phase of secretion, age, and other influences. Component cells contain secretory granules and a yellow pigment. The secretion is a yellowish, viscid liquid which in sections appears as a deeply acidophil coagulum within the lumen. The epithelium depends upon hormonal support, testosterone, for its maintenance. Castration is followed by involution and loss of secretory function of the gland, which is promptly restored by the administration of testis extract. The seminal vesicle functions as a gland, secreting and storing the viscid component of the seminal fluid. It is not a site of storage of spermatozoa, although some spermatozoa may be seen within the lumen after death, presumably as the result of backflow.

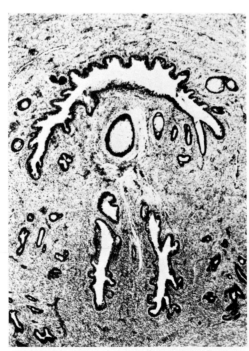

Figure 19-16. Low power photomicrograph of the prostatic urethra and surrounding tissue. Immediately below the urethra, which is crescentic in outline, is the utriculum prostaticus and, below it, portions of both ejaculatory ducts. The surrounding stroma contains portions of some ducts of the prostate gland. × 55.

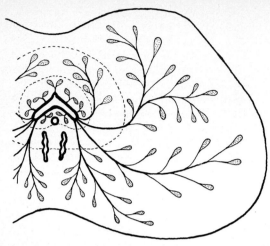

Figure 19-17. Diagram of a cross section of the human prostate. Note the distribution of the mucous, submucous, and main components of the gland.

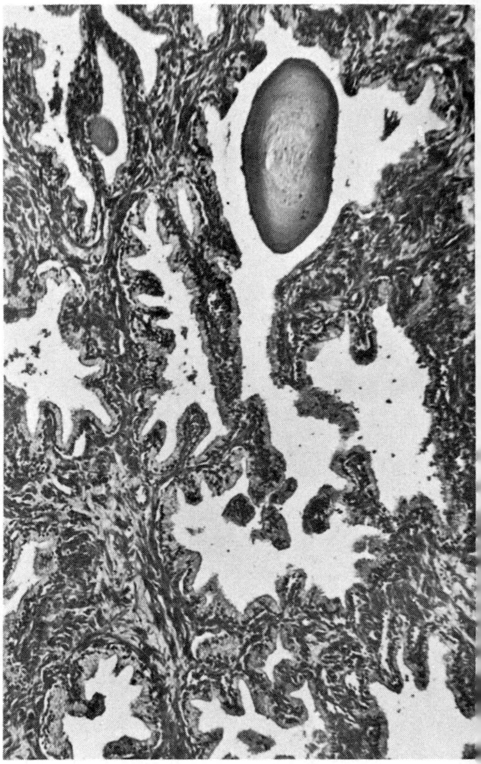

Figure 19-18. Medium power photomicrograph of a portion of the prostate gland. Note the large concretion in the lumen of one alveolus. × 90.

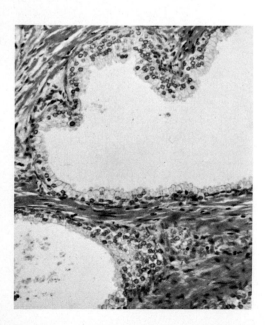

Figure 19-19. High power photomicrograph of a small portion of the prostate gland. Note the character of the epithelium and the presence of numerous smooth muscle fibers in the stroma of the gland. × 160.   See filmstrip II, frame 90.

strands of smooth muscle fibers. The secretory alveoli and tubules are very irregular and vary greatly in size and form. They branch frequently and both alveoli and tubules have wide lumina. There is no distinct basal lamina and the epithelium is very folded and cuboidal to columnar in type. The cytoplasm contains numerous secretory granules and lipid droplets. The ducts, too, have irregular lumina and resemble smaller secretory tubules.

The secretion of the prostate is a thin, milky liquid which is slightly alkaline. In sections, the secretion appears as an acidophil granular mass. It frequently contains spherical or oval bodies, the prostatic concretions (*corpora amylacea*) which are condensations of the secretions and which may become calcified.

Bulbourethral Glands. The bulbourethral glands (of Cowper) are paired bodies, each the size of a pea, lying in the connective tissue behind the membranous urethra. Each is a compound tubuloalveolar gland whose duct enters the posterior portion of the cavernous segment of the urethra. The bulbourethral gland is surrounded by a thin connective tissue capsule, external to which are skeletal muscle fibers. Septa pass into the gland to divide it into lobules. The connective tissue septa contain numerous elastic and skeletal and smooth muscle fibers. The secretory end pieces are variable, being either alveolar, saccular, or tubular. The epithelium, too, is variable, being either cuboidal or columnar. The cytoplasm contains mucigen droplets and some acidophil, spindle-shaped inclusions. Nuclei are basally located. The secretory ducts are lined by a pseudostratified epithelium resembling that of the urethra, and may contain patches of mucous cells. They are surrounded by an incomplete coat of circularly arranged smooth muscle. The secretion is clear, viscid, and mucous.

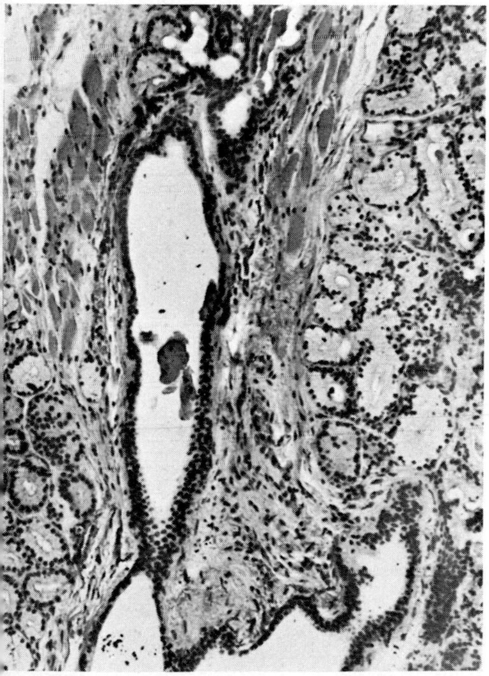

Figure 19-20. Low power photomicrograph of part of a lobule of a human bulbourethral gland. Notice the skeletal muscle fibers present in the stroma around the large duct. × 110.

THE PENIS

The penis serves as the common outlet for urine and for seminal fluid and as the copulatory organ. It is formed by three cylinders of erectile tissue: the paired *corpora cavernosa penis* dorsally and the single *corpus cavernosum urethrae* (corpus spongiosum) ventrally. The latter encloses the cavernous portion of the urethra. The paired corpora cavernosa penis are separated from each other proximally but join beneath the pubic angle and run forward together, united by a common median partition, the *pectiniform septum*, to the region of the *glans penis*. The deep groove beneath the corpora cavernosa is occupied by the corpus spongiosum. This ends in a cupshaped enlargement, the glans penis, which forms a cap over the conical ends of the corpora cavernosa penis. The three cylinders of erectile tissue are surrounded by subcutaneous tissue

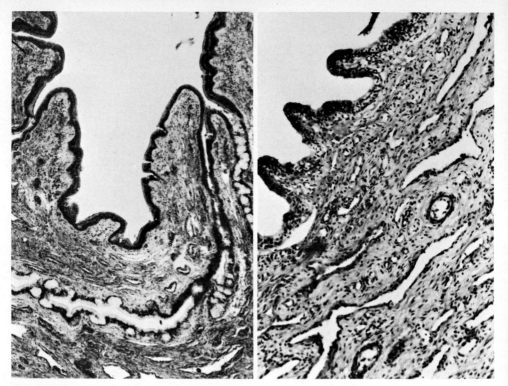

Figure 19-21. Left: Low power photomicrograph of a portion of the cavernous part of the male human urethra together with the glands of Littre. × 90. Right: High power photomicrograph of portion of penile urethra. Note the blood sinuses in the erectile tissue. Epon section. × 150.

which is devoid of fat but contains many smooth muscle fibers. The skin covering the organ is thin and delicate and terminally it reduplicates over the glans as a fold, the *prepuce.* The inner surface of the prepuce, in relation to the glans, is moist and nonkeratinized. The epithelium over the glans itself is firmly adhered to the fibrous tissue beneath. The skin of the penis contains small sweat glands and infrequent sebaceous glands unassociated with hair follicles, there being no hair follicles over the distal part of the penis.

Each cylinder of the corpus cavernosum penis is surrounded by a thick fibrous sheath, the *tunica albuginea.* The collagenous fibers of the sheath are arranged in two layers, outer longitudinal and inner circular. The pectiniform septum, common to both cylinders, is pierced by numerous slit-like openings through which the

cavernous spaces of both sides communicate. Trabeculae, continuous with the fibrous sheath, consist of collagenous, elastic, and smooth muscle fibers and form a dense internal framework. The spaces between the framework are lined by endothelium and constitute the blood sinuses. Owing to the arrangement of the trabeculae, the cavernous spaces are largest in the central zone of each cylinder and gradually diminish in size toward the periphery.

The sheath (tunica albuginea) of the corpus spongiosum is much thinner than that of the corpora cavernosa penis and contains many elastic and smooth muscle fibers. Trabeculae are thinner and more elastic than those present in the paired corpora. The cavernous spaces are small, almost uniform in size, and gradually pass into the small venous spaces around the urethra.

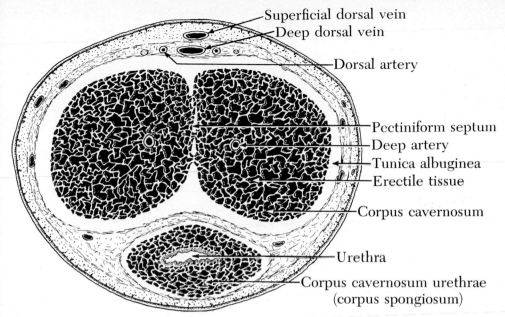

Superficial dorsal vein

Deep dorsal vein

Dorsal artery

Pectiniform septum

Deep artery

Tunica albuginea

Erectile tissue

Corpus cavernosum

Urethra

Corpus cavernosum urethrae
(corpus spongiosum)

Figure 19-22.   Diagram of a cross section of the penis in mid-shaft.

Blood Vessels and the Mechanism of Erection

The principal arterial branches within the penis are the dorsal arteries, which run in the interval between the corpora cavernosa superiorly on either side of the deep dorsal vein, and the deep arteries of the penis traversing each of the corpora. Branches from the dorsal arteries pierce the fibrous capsule along the upper surface to enter the corpora cavernosa, especially near the distal end of the penis. On entering the cavernous spaces, all arteries divide into branches, some of which end in capillary plexuses; others are longitudinal vessels directed distally. In the quiescent state, these vessels, the *helicine arteries,* have a spiral course, their media is thick, and their intima is thrown into longitudinal folds. These vessels open directly into the sinuses of the erectile tissue. Blood from the cavernous spaces and the capillary plexuses is drained by a plexus of venules within the tunica albuginea. Some emerge from the base of the tunica and converge on the dorsum of

the penis to join the deep dorsal vein. Others pass directly out on the upper surface of the corpora cavernosa to enter the same vein. The smooth muscle of the arteries and the trabeculae is supplied both by sympathetic and by parasympathetic fibers.

Under conditions of erotic stimulation, parasympathetic stimulation produces a relaxation of the smooth muscle, and the helicine vessels straighten out and their lumina dilate. Blood flows freely from them into the cavernous spaces, which become engorged with blood. Thus there is a rerouting of blood into a greatly enlarged vascular bed. The venous drainage at the periphery of the corpora is said to be diminished owing to compression of the thin-walled veins under the tunica albuginea by the engorged trabecular spaces. The corpora cavernosa become rigid and enlarged. Since there is less compression of the venous drainage of the corpus spongiosum and a more yielding tunica, there is less rigidity here and the urethra contained within it remains patent to allow for egress of seminal fluid during ejaculation. At the termination of sexual excitement, the penis returns to the flaccid state through a process of *detumescence.* The arteries regain muscular tone owing to sympathetic stimulation, and the amount of blood supplied to the sinuses diminishes. The excess of blood in the corpora cavernosa slowly is pressed out by contraction of the muscle fibers within the trabeculae, and the ordinary route of blood flow through the organ is restored.

Seminal Fluid

Seminal fluid (semen) consists of spermatozoa together with the fluid in which they are suspended. The fluid is a product of all the auxiliary genital glands together with a minor contribution supplied by the system of genital ducts. Semen is a whitish, opaque fluid containing about 100 million spermatozoa in 1 ml., but the number varies greatly. The ejaculate averages about 3 ml., and thus contains about 300 million spermatozoa. The discharge of semen is said to occur in a definite sequence. The bulbourethral glands and the urethral glands of Littre discharge their mucous secretion during erection and lubricate the cavernous urethra. During actual ejaculation, the prostate discharges first. Its alkaline secretion reduces the acidity of the urethra which initially may contain some residual urine. This is followed by the spermatozoa which are forced out of the ductus epididymidis and the ductus deferens by powerful contraction of the muscular walls. Finally, the thick secretion of the seminal vesicles, which contains fructose and is nutrient to the sperm, is added to the mass.

REFERENCES

Albert, A.: The mammalian testis. *In* Sex and Internal Secretion, edited by W. C. Young. Baltimore, Williams & Wilkins Co., 1961, Vol. 1, p. 305.

Brandes, D.: The fine structure and histochemistry of prostatic glands in relation to sex hormones. Int. Rev. Cytol., 20:207, 1966.

Burgos, M. H., and Fawcett, D. W.: Studies on the fine structure of the mammalian testis. J. Biophys. Biochem. Cytol., 1:287, 1955.

Christensen, A. K.: The fine structure of testicular interstitial cells in guinea pig. J. Cell Biol., 26:911, 1965.

Christensen, A. K., and Fawcett, D. W.: The fine structure of interstitial cells of the mouse testis. Amer. J. Anat., 118:551, 1966.

Clermont, Y.: The cycle of the seminiferous epithelium in man. Amer. J. Anat., 112:35, 1963.

Clermont, Y., and Leblond, C. P.: Spermiogenesis of man, monkey, ram and other mammals as shown by the "periodic acid-Schiff" technique. Amer. J. Anat., 96:229, 1955.

Deane, H. W., and Wurzelmann, S.: Electron microscopic observations on the postnatal differentiation of the seminal vesicle epithelium of the laboratory mouse. Amer. J. Anat., 117:91, 1965.

Elftman, H.: Sertoli cells and testis structure. Amer. J. Anat., 113:25, 1963.

Fawcett, D. W., and Burgos, M. H.: Observations on the cytomorphosis of the germinal and interstitial cells of the human testis. *In* Ciba Foundation Colloquia on Ageing. London, J. & A. Churchill Ltd., 1956, Vol. 2, p. 86.

Fawcett, D. W., and Burgos, M. H.: Studies on the fine structure of the mammalian testis. II. The human interstitial tissue. Amer. J. Anat., 107:245, 1960.

Ladman, A. J.: The fine structure of the ductuli efferentes of the opossum. Anat. Rec., 157:559, 1967.

Ladman, A. J., and Young, W. C.: An electron microscopic study of the ductuli efferentes and rete testis of the guinea pig. J. Biophys. Biochem. Cytol., 4:219, 1958.

Leblond, C. P., and Clermont, Y.: Spermiogenesis of rat, mouse, hamster, and guinea pig as revealed by the "periodic acid-fuchsin sulfurous acid" technique. Amer. J. Anat., 90:167, 1952.

Leeson, C. R., and Leeson, T. S.: The postnatal development and differentiation of the boundary tissue of the seminiferous tubule of the rat. Anat. Rec., 147:243, 1963.

Leeson, C. R., and Leeson, T. S.: The postnatal development of the ductus epididymis in the rat. Anat. Anz., 114:159, 1964.

Leeson, T. S., and Leeson, C. R.: The fine structure of cavernous tissue in the adult rat penis. Invest. Urol., 3:144, 1965.

Riva, A.: Fine structure of human seminal vesicle epithelium. J. Anat., 102:71, 1967.

Roosen-Runge, E. C., and Barlow, F. D.: Quantitative studies on human spermatogenesis. Amer. J. Anat., 93:143, 1953.

CHAPTER 20

ORGANS OF
SPECIAL SENSE

Sensory receptor nerve endings functionally are dendrites specialized both morphologically and functionally. They can be classified in several ways. In man, for example, there are several senses. Those for touch, pressure, pain, temperature, and muscle and joint position and movement are distributed widely; those for smell, taste, sight, hearing, and balance are in limited areas. The former group may be referred to as general sensibility; the latter as special or local sensibility. Some have been described where appropriate in previous chapters.

The organs of general sensibility are distributed widely in epithelium, connective tissue, and muscle and tendon. There are none in nervous tissue. Morphologically, they either are *free* or *naked* nerve endings, or are nerve endings which are *encapsulated.*

Touch. The sensation of light touch is received by naked nerve endings associated with hair follicles, and by Merkel's disks in epidermis and Meissner's corpuscles in connective tissue. The naked nerve endings are found as basket-like arrangements, often especially well-developed around hair follicles (the peritrichal endings), the endings being stimulated by movement of the hairs, and as more simple endings between epidermal cells. Some of the latter take the form of a platelike plexus of nerve endings associated with a single epithelial cell. This is the disk of Merkel, found in the deeper layers of the epidermis, in hair follicles, and in the hard palate. Meissner's corpuscles are located in the connective tissues of skin, particularly in the palms and finger tips, soles of the feet, nipples, and external genitalia. They are ellipsoidal in shape and 40 to 150 microns in length, formed by transversely orientated cells embedded in fibrous tissue with a surrounding sheath of fibrous tissue. One or more nerve endings enter at one pole of the corpuscle and spiral between the tactile cells.

Pressure. The sensation of pressure or deep touch is appreciated by large, encapsulated receptors called pacinian or Vater-Pacini corpuscles. They are distributed widely in connective tissues of subcutaneous tissue and near tendons, joints, perimysium, mesentery, and external genitalia. They are large, up to 4 mm. long, and ovoid, with an inner core of protoplasm surrounded by many layers or lamellae of connective tissue arranged

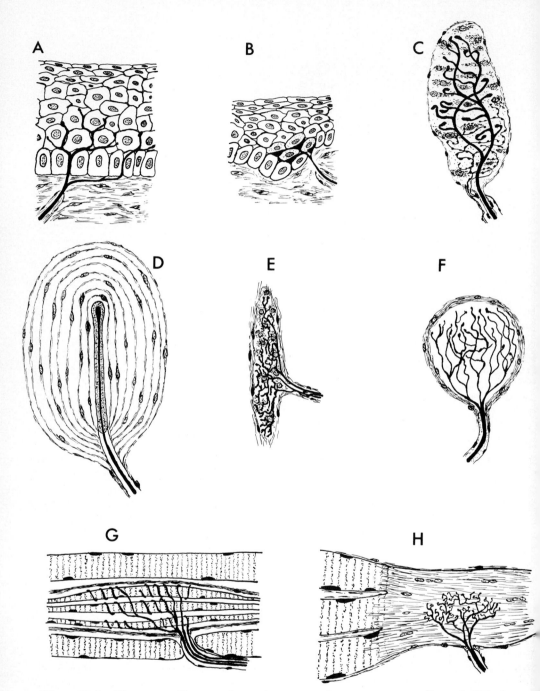

Figure 20-1.   Diagram to illustrate the various types of sensory nerve endings. *A*, Naked nerve endings in cornea (pain). *B*, Merkel's disk in epidermis (touch). *C*, Meissner's corpuscle (tough). *D*, Vater-Pacini corpuscle (pressure). *E*, Ruffini's corpuscle (heat). *F*, Krause's end bulb (cold). *G*, Neuromuscular spindle (proprioception). *H*, Neurotendinous organ (proprioception).

See filmstrip II, frame 91.

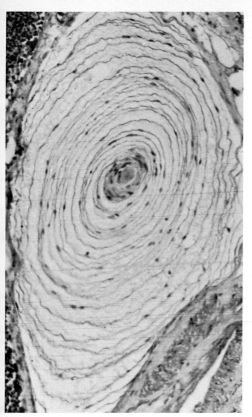

Figure 20-2. Photomicrograph of a cross section through a Vater-Pacini corpuscle. × 100. See filmstrip II, frame 92.

concentrically like the "skins" of an onion. A single nerve fiber enters the corpuscle and runs axially through the central core. It loses its myelin as it enters the corpuscle.

Heat. Heat receptors are the corpuscles of Ruffini, located in dermis and hypodermis. These comprise a loose network of nerve endings with terminal, flattened expansions lying among granular cells, the whole enclosed in connective tissue and of a flattened, disklike shape. These corpuscles also may be involved in proprioception (position sense).

Cold. The sensation of cold is appreciated by the end bulbs of Krause, which are widely distributed in dermis and numerous under the conjunctiva and lingual mucosa and in the external genitalia. They vary in complexity,

the more simple form being a bulblike expansion of the endoneurium containing the terminal nerve fiber which ends blindly in granular material. Particularly in the conjunctiva, the form is more complex with the nerve fiber branching to form a network, each branch terminating in a clublike ending.

Pain. Pain endings take the form of naked terminal endings, there being usually multiple branching of a single nerve fiber. Each terminal twig ends in a small swelling, for example, between cells in the deeper layers of the epidermis, although there are similar endings in many of the connective tissues.

Proprioception. Proprioception, the sense of position of muscles and joints, is subserved by three main types of endings. Neuromuscular spindles lie in muscle, and are fusiform structures consisting of several specialized muscle fibers (usually three to ten) and nerve endings encapsulated in connective tissue. The muscle fibers, termed *intrafusal fibers*, are attached at their ends to tendon or endomysium. They contain numerous nuclei arranged in central axial rows surrounded by peripheral myofibrils. At each end, efferent (motor) nerve fibers terminate at motor end plates; large, myelinated afferent (sensory) nerve fibers terminate as spirals around the central nuclear region. The nerve endings are stimulated by change in length or tension of the muscle fibers. Neurotendinous spindles are similar and are located in tendons and aponeuroses near their junctions with muscle. They are spindle-shaped bundles of tendon fibers with a thin capsule of connective tissue and they contain nerve fibers which branch freely and terminate in club-shaped endings. Ruffini endings are cylindrical in shape and located in ligaments and joint capsules. Although described as nerve endings for heat sensation, in joints they probably also appreciate proprioception.

The specialized endings for taste and olfaction have been described previously in Chapters 14 and 15 respectively.

THE EYE

Structurally the eyeball often has been compared to a camera, but there can be no analogy between the nervous mechanisms involved. The essential component of the eye is the *retina*. This inner, nervous layer serves the function of photoreception and lines the posterior half of the eyeball. Developmentally and functionally it is an isolated part of the central nervous system to which it remains connected by a tract of nerve fibers, the *optic nerve*. As in the central nervous system, the retina is nourished and protected by two sheets, one of vascular and one of fibrous tissue. The outer, fibrous, protective coat, corresponding to dura mater, is white and opaque over the posterior 5/6 of the eye (the *sclera*) and clear and transparent over the anterior 1/6 (the cornea). Between the outer fibrous layer and the retina is a vascular, nutrient layer analogous to pia-arachnoid. This is the *uveal* coat or tunic and it is divided into three zones—posteriorly, the *choroid*; more anteriorly just behind the corneoscleral junction, the *ciliary body*; and anteriorly, reflecting inward to diverge from the cornea, the *iris*. The iris has a central, spherical deficiency of variable diameter termed the *pupil*. The innermost layer (retina) is continued forward, but as a nonnervous layer, to line the inner surfaces of ciliary body and iris. These are the *ciliary* and *iridial portions* of the retina and are not photosensitive.

The fibrous and vascular tunics are attached firmly at the corneoscleral junction anteriorly and at the exit of the optic nerve posteriorly. Between these two regions, they are separated by a potential space, the *perichoroidal* or *subchoroidal space,* across which

pass the nerves entering the eye and the blood vessels which supply and drain the choroid. Anteriorly, where the vascular coat reflects inward as the iris, the space between fibrous and vascular tunics is expanded as the *anterior chamber.* The lens lies immediately posterior to the iris supported by a *suspensory ligament* (the *zonule*) from the ciliary body. The narrow space between iris and lens is termed the *posterior chamber.* Anterior and posterior chambers freely communicate through the pupil and contain a clear fluid, the *aqueous humor,* secreted by the ciliary body. Posterior to the lens, the entire cavity of the eyeball is filled by a transparent gel, the *vitreous humor.* Thus, between the sensory retina and the exterior, there is a series of transparent, refractive media consisting of cornea, aqueous humor, lens, and vitreous body.

The attachment or exit of the optic nerve is not at the posterior pole of the eyeball but is situated about 3 mm. to the nasal side of this, and about 1 mm. below it.

The eyeball is a slightly asymmetrical sphere, somewhat flattened from above down. The central points of corneal and scleral curvatures are termed the *anterior* and *posterior poles,* and the line joining them is the *geometrical axis.* This must not be confused with the *optic* or *visual axis,* which is a line joining the center of the pupil and the *fovea,* the latter being the spot of most distinct vision. The posterior pole of the geometrical axis lies between the fovea and the optic papilla. The *anatomical equator* is a circumferential line joining all points equidistant from the poles, thus dividing the eyeball into anterior and posterior hemispheres. Any circle drawn through the poles and crossing the equator at a right angle is a *meridian.* Two meridionals are important: the *vertical* passing through the fovea and dividing the eye into nasal and temporal halves, and the *horizontal* o

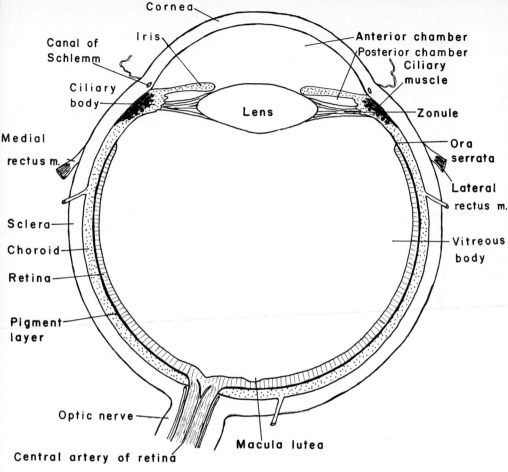

Figure 20-3.   Diagram of a horizontal meridional section of the eye.

transverse dividing the eye into upper and lower halves. These two meridians divide the eye into four quadrants.

The surface of the eye shows two curvatures. The cornea (the anterior 1/6) is curved more acutely, having a radius of about 8 mm., whereas the curvature of the sclera has a radius of 12 mm. At the corneoscleral junction there is a shallow circular sulcus, the *external scleral sulcus*, partially filled by the attachments of the conjunctiva and the bulbar fascia. Around the exit of the optic nerve, the sclera is pierced by the ciliary nerves (about 10 in number) and the short posterior ciliary arteries (about 20), arranged as a ring around the optic nerve. Further forward, two long posterior ciliary arteries pierce the sclera, one on each side of the horizontal meridian. Four veins (the *vortex veins*) draining the choroid emerge a little behind the equator, one for each quadrant, and anterior ciliary arteries and veins pierce the eye just posterior to the corneoscleral junction.

The anteroposterior diameter of the eye is about 24 mm., being slightly greater in the male than in the female. It is about 16 to 17 mm. at birth, increases in size rapidly to a diameter of 22.5 to 23 mm. at age three and virtually is of adult size by age 13.

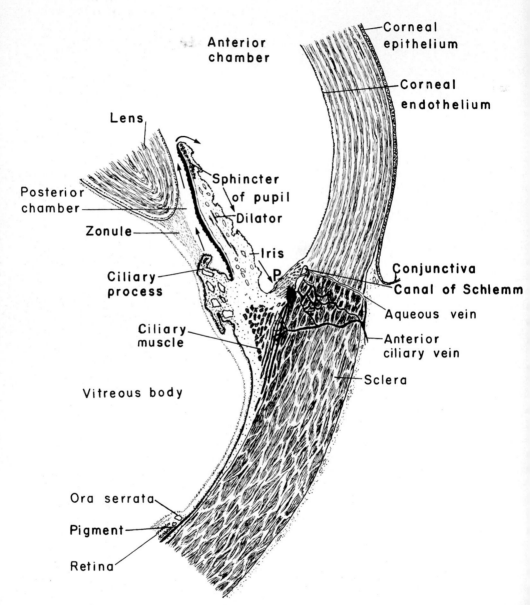

Figure 20-4.   Diagram of a portion of a meridional section to show the angle of the eye. The letter "P" indicates the pectinate ligament or trabecular meshwork. Compare with Figure 20-7. The arrows indicate the course of circulation of aqueous humor.

Fibrous Coat

Sclera. The sclera is composed of dense, white, connective tissue consisting of bundles of collagenous fibers between which are flattened fibroblasts and fine networks of elastic fibers. It is thickest at the posterior pole (about 1.0 to 1.3 mm.), thinnest at the equator (0.3 to 0.4 mm.), and 0.6 to 0.8 mm. at the corneoscleral junction. Although its structure is quite uniform, it can be subdivided into three layers. The outermost layer, the *episcleral* tissue, consists of loose, fibroelastic tissue continuous externally with the dense connective tissue of *Tenon's capsule.* Its deeper surface blends with the middle layer, the *sclera proper.* Here the bundles of collagenous fibers are 10 to 15 microns thick and 100 to 150 microns long, orientated mainly parallel to the surface but with some branching and interweaving. The connective tissue of the tendons of the extraocular muscles is of similar composition and blends with the sclera at their insertion. The innermost layer, termed the *lamina fusca* or dark layer, is composed of much smaller bundles of collagenous fibers than the sclera proper and possesses many more elastic fibers. Between the fibers are branching chromatophores containing melanin, which give the inner aspect of the sclera a brown color. There are very few blood vessels in the sclera, no lymphatics, and a few nerve fibers from the ciliary nerves.

Cornea. The cornea is clear and transparent and has a smooth surface. It is not uniformly curved, the central or optical zone having a smaller radius of curvature than the peripheral parts, and the posterior surface is more strongly curved than the anterior. Thus the cornea is thinner (0.7 to 0.8 mm.) at its center than near its margin (1.1 mm.). The refractive power of the cornea, a function of its refractive index and its radius of curvature, is greater than that of the lens. Anatomically, it is divided into two zones, the *cornea proper* and the *limbus,* the latter being a transitional zone about 1 mm. wide between cornea and sclera, at the periphery of the cornea. This zone differs from the cornea proper in that it contains blood vessels and lymphatics.

Histologically, the cornea is composed of five layers: epithelium, Bowman's membrane, substantia propria (stroma), Descemet's membrane, and endothelium (mesenchymal epithelium).

EPITHELIUM. This is a stratified squamous nonkeratinizing epithelium of a uniform thickness of 50 to 70 microns, consisting usually of five or six layers of cells. There is a single layer of basal, columnar cells, usually

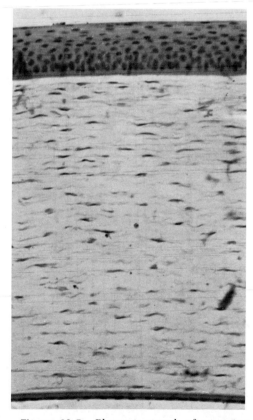

Figure 20-5. Photomicrograph of a section through the cornea, showing, from above down, the epithelium resting upon Bowman's membrane, substantia propria (corneal stroma), Descemet's membrane, and endothelium. × 150.　　　See filmstrip II, frame 93.

three layers of polyhedral or "wing" cells, and one or two layers of squamous surface cells. The epithelium rests upon a fine basal lamina, indistinguishable from Bowman's membrane but visible by electron microscopy. This epithelium contains numerous free nerve endings and is highly sensitive. Mitoses occur only in the basal layer but powers of regeneration after damage are excellent.

BOWMAN'S MEMBRANE. This is a clear uniform membrane about 7 to 12 microns thick lying beneath the epithelium. It is entirely structureless by light microscopy and is regarded as a specially modified layer of the substantia propria. It is perforated for the passage of epithelial branches of the corneal nerves and ends abruptly at the limbus. As shown by electron microscopy, it is composed of a felt-work of fine fibrils of collagen 100 to 150 Å in diameter.

SUBSTANTIA PROPRIA. This comprises some 90 per cent of the total thickness of the cornea, is transparent and is formed by lamellae and cells. The lamellae are broad, tapelike strips of collagenous fibers, the bundles in each lamellae being parallel, with adjacent lamellae at different angles. There is an interchange of fibrils between adjacent lamellae so that all lamellae are held firmly together. Between fibrils in a bundle, bundles in lamellae, and lamellae there is mucoid intercellular material. Individual fibrils of collagen are of a surprisingly uniform diameter, 250 to 300 Å, and show characteristic periodicity. Cells in the substantia propria fall into two groups. Fibroblasts are greatly elongated and flattened cells

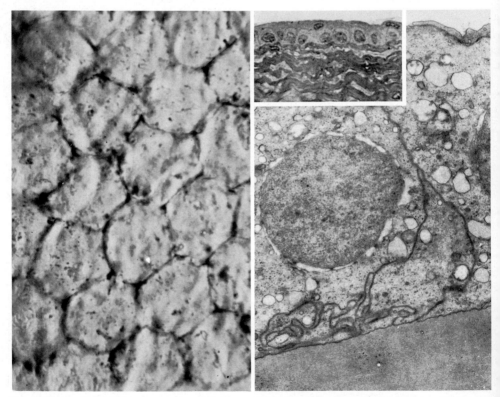

Figure 20-6.   Left: Flat preparation of the corneal endothelium, showing the hexagonal cell pattern and penetration of the stain into the interdigitations between cells. × 950. (Courtesy of J. Speakman.) Insert: Epon section of corneal endothelium. × 550. Right: Electron micrograph of the corneal endothelium with Descemet's membrane beneath. × 7500.

lying parallel to the surface, and have broad protoplasmic extensions which form a pseudosyncytium; i.e., cell processes come into contact but are not in continuity. Also present are "wandering cells," mainly white blood cells, so flattened and deformed as to be difficult to recognize.

DESCEMET'S MEMBRANE. This is an apparently homogeneous layer, 5 to 7 microns thick centrally and 8 to 10 microns thick peripherally, separating substantia propria and endothelium. At the circumference of the cornea, this layer is continuous with material of the pectinate ligament or trabecular meshwork of the iridial angle at the *ring of Schwalbe*. Although apparently a structureless, elastic basal lamina by light microscopy, as shown by electron microscopy, it contains small masses of material composed of granules in a three-dimensional network spaced at 1070 Å and connected by fine fibrils to form a hexagonal pattern of great regularity. Chemically it is considered to be an atypical form of collagen.

ENDOTHELIUM. This is composed of squamous or cuboidal cells arranged in a single layer lining the inner surface of the cornea. It obviously acts as a barrier to aqueous humor contained in the anterior chamber. Usual fixation methods result in vacuolization of the cells, which show by electron microscopy prominent terminal bars and micropinocytotic vesicles. Silver staining appears to demonstrate fine cement substance between cells, but no intercellular cementing material has been demonstrated by electron microscopy.

Limbus Corneae. This is the transition zone, approximately 1 mm. in width, between cornea anteriorly and conjunctiva, episcleral tissue and sclera posteriorly. In relation to the periphery of the cornea, it has a "watch-glass" configuration and is important surgically because it is through this area that surgery for cataract and various filtering procedures is performed. Histologically, it differs from the cornea. Bowman's membrane ends abruptly at the limbus, and Descemet's membrane tapers off and breaks up to become continuous with the trabeculae of the pectinate ligament. Thus, the limbus consists essentially only of epithelium and substantia propria. The epithelium here is thickened to ten or more layers; its basal lamina is thickened as it loses the support of Bowman's membrane, and it becomes continuous with the basal lamina of the bulbar conjunctiva. The stroma at the limbus becomes less regular and gradually changes from the characteristic lamellar arrangement of the cornea to the irregularity of the scleral fibers.

The cornea itself is avascular al-

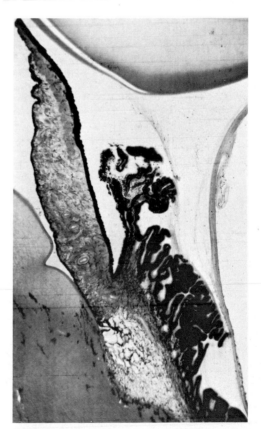

Figure 20-7. Photomicrograph of a portion of a meridional section of the eye, showing corneoscleral junction, iris, ciliary processes, zonule, and part of the lens. Compare with Figure 20-4. × 25.   **See filmstrip II, frame 94.**

though there is a rich circumferential plexus in the limbus. The cornea receives nutrients and maintains its normal condition of hydration by transportation of large amounts of solute and solvent from the aqueous humor which fills the anterior chamber. Nutrient material passes through the corneal endothelium by pinocytosis, and free diffusion occurs through Descemet's membrane and the corneal stroma.

Vascular Coat (the Uvea)

As explained earlier, the vascular coat is divided into three regions from posterior to anterior, the choroid, the ciliary body, and the iris. Uvea means "grapelike," an appropriate term in that this vascular coat has the appearance of the inside of a purple grape skin.

Choroid. The choroid is a spongy, brown membrane characterized by the presence of pigment and extreme vascularity, the venous plexuses being so extensive as to resemble erectile tissue. Thus, its thickness is difficult to determine owing to the collapse of the vessels after death but in general it is about 0.1 to 0.3 mm. thick. Externally the choroid is separated from sclera by the potential *perichoroidal* (suprachoroidal) *space*, the anterior extension of this between ciliary body and sclera being termed the *supraciliary space.* The choroid is divided into four layers from without in: the epichoroid or suprachoroid, vascular layer, choriocapillaris, and lamina elastica (Bruch's membrane).

EPICHOROID. This is only 10 to 35 microns thick and consists of fine lamellae of connective tissue traversing the potential suprachoroid space to attach obliquely to the sclera. The lamellae are separated by flattened fibroblasts, some of which are pigmented, and a rich network of elastic fibers. Melanoblasts are numerous, with scattered macrophages and some smooth muscle cells. Blood vessels traverse this layer to reach the deeper layers. There is no distinct boundary between the epichoroid and the vascular layer.

VESSEL LAYER. This comprises a mass of arteries and veins lying in loose connective tissue containing many melanocytes. In general, the vessels diminish in size from the outer to inner surfaces of this layer. Vessels deep to the fovea are small. The venous plexuses are drained by four large whorls of veins, one in each quadrant, the efferent vein of each being a *vortex vein.* This vessel layer continues anteriorly into the ciliary body.

CHORIOCAPILLARIS. This is a layer of capillaries in which the choroidal arteries terminate. It is described as a plexus but is unique in that it is orientated only in one plane, each capillary being relatively of large diameter. It is particularly rich at the macula posteriorly, and the plexus extends anteriorly only as far as the ora serrata. Between the capillaries is a fine network of elastic and collagenous fibers with some flattened fibroblasts.

LAMINA ELASTICA (BRUCH'S MEMBRANE). The lamina elastica or glass membrane is a shiny, homogeneous layer between the choroid and the pigment layer of the retina, about 1 to 4 microns thick. It comprises two laminae, the outer one (the elastic lamina) being a dense network of fine elastic fibers continuous with those of the choriocapillaris, and the inner (the cuticular lamina) being the homogeneous basal lamina of the pigment epithelium of the retina. This cuticular layer is mucopolysaccharide in nature. Anteriorly, both layers extend forward into the ciliary body; posteriorly the cuticular lamina ends abruptly at the optic disk. The elastic lamina extends posteriorly to contact neuroglia of the optic nerve fibers.

There are nerves in the choroid derived from ciliary (sympathetic) nerves. They terminate on the musculature of the blood vessels, and are associated with a few sympathetic ganglion cells.

Ciliary Body. The ciliary body girdles the eye anterior to the ora serrata. In section it is triangular in shape, the apex lying posteriorly and being continuous with the choroid, its base facing the anterior chamber and tilted toward the center of the cornea. The outer angle is attached to the scleral spur (the inner, anterior extremity of the sclera which projects inward toward the anterior chamber); the inner angle is free and juts internally just anterior to the equator of the lens. The outer surface abuts against sclera, the inner surface against the vitreous, and it is covered by the ciliary (nonnervous) portion of the retina. This surface is irregular posteriorly with shallow grooves (the ciliary striae)

running forward from the ora serrata. Anteriorly, there are radially orientated ridges, the *ciliary processes.*

In its general structure, the ciliary body is an anterior extension of *both* choroid and retina.

CILIARY MUSCLE. This layer, forming the bulk of the ciliary body, replaces the epichoroid. It comprises three layers of smooth muscle fibers with a common origin from the ring-like ciliary tendon attached to the scleral spur and the pectinate ligament. The smooth muscle fibers are meridional, radial, and equatorial in their orientation. Between the bundles of smooth muscle there is a meshwork rich in elastic fibers and containing melanocytes. The role of the ciliary

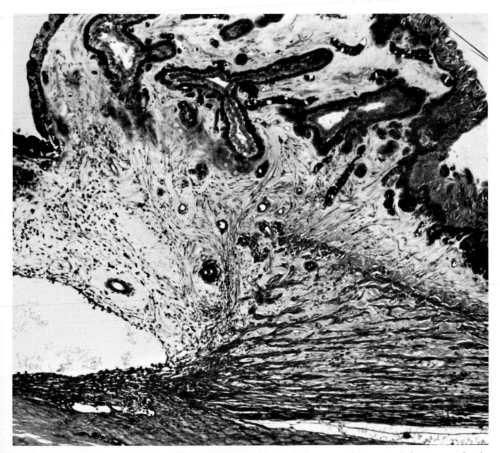

Figure 20-8. Photomicrograph of the angle of the eye, showing the root of the iris and ciliary processes above and the trabecular meshwork, canal of Schlemm, and ciliary muscle arising from scleral spur below. × 125.

muscle in accommodation is discussed later. It probably also aids the drainage of aqueous humor through the trabecular meshwork and possibly affects vascular circulation.

VASCULAR LAYER. This layer consists mainly of capillaries and veins lying in, and constituting the bulk of, the ciliary processes. Arteries enter the processes anteriorly and break up directly into capillaries. The lining endothelium of these is very thin and on electron microscopy it shows perforations. Between the vessels is loose connective tissue in which elastic fibers are prominent.

ELASTIC LAMINA. The internal surface of the vascular layer is lined by a condensation of elastic fibers directly continuous posteriorly with the outer elastic lamina of Bruch's membrane. This becomes thin and inconspicuous near the root of the iris.

INTERMEDIATE LAYER. Between the elastic lamina and the cuticular lamina is developed a narrow zone of collagenous fibers with fibroblasts.

CUTICULAR LAMINA. This is continuous with the cuticular lamina of Bruch's membrane of the choroid and extends anteriorly to the root of the iris. It has here a corrugated surface and is the basal lamina of the pigment epithelium which covers it.

PIGMENT EPITHELIUM. The pigment epithelium is continuous with the corresponding layer of the retina and consists of a single layer of columnar cells so heavily pigmented as to make visualization of individual cells practically impossible. This layer continues forward on the posterior surface of the iris.

CILIARY EPITHELIUM. The ciliary epithelium, which represents the forward prolongation of the entire thickness of the sensory part of the retina, is a single layer of columnar cells, nonpigmented. The cells continue forward on the posterior surface of the iris and here become heavily pigmented.

INTERNAL LIMITING MEMBRANE. This is a fibrillar sheet overlying the epithelium, closely following the irregularities of the surface of the ciliary body. Anteriorly, it blends with the condensation of fibrillar material forming the zonule of the lens, and posteriorly it thins down and is continuous with the internal limiting membrane of the optical portion of the retina.

CILIARY PROCESS. Ciliary processes extend internally from the anterior portion of the ciliary body. In the stroma or core of each are numerous thin-walled capillaries, these probably being the site of formation of aqueous humor. The covering pigment epithelium is not present at the tip of a ciliary process, but the entire process is covered by ciliary epithelium.

Iris. This, the anterior portion of the uvea, literally means a "rainbow"; its central aperture, the pupil, means "little girl" and probably is so termed from the diminutive image reflected in the cornea against the black background of the pupil.

The iris varies in color, appearance, and structure between individuals and in the same individual with age. It is attached to the anterior part of the ciliary body by a root, its thinnest portion. It is thicker centrally, and at its pupillary margin it is thin and rests against the anterior surface of the lens. It has the form of a flat, truncated cone. The anterior surface is irregular, with fissures and clefts, and usually is divided into a peripheral ciliary zone and a central pupillary zone. The posterior surface is more regular, is uniformly black, and shows only shallow furrows.

Histologically, the iris shows several layers, the anterior layers being part of the uvea and mesodermal in origin, the posterior being derived from ectoderm, the pars iridica. The most anterior layer is of endothelium continuous with that of the cornea, underlying which is a delicate connective tissue stroma with relatively few fibers and many fibroblasts and chromatophores. The quantity of pigment in these chromatophores largely

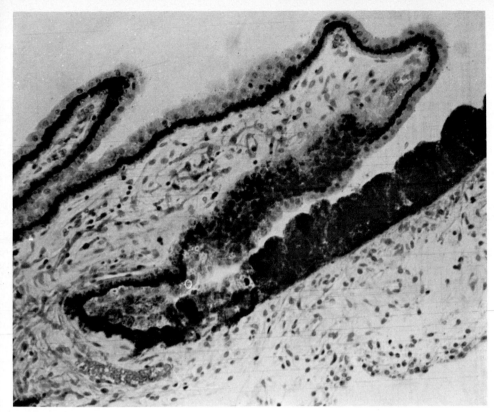

Figure 20-9. Photomicrograph of the root of the iris (right) and ciliary processes. The cells on the posterior surface of the iris are so heavily pigmented as to obscure all cellular detail. × 215.

determines the color of the iris. If little or none is present, the pigment epithelium on the posterior surface imparts a blue color; with increasing pigment, the color becomes gray, green, or varying shades of brown.

Beneath this stroma there is a layer of blood vessels, running mainly in a radial fashion to accommodate easily to changes in length with the changes in pupil diameter. These vessels have unusually thick walls. The vessels are contained in a delicate stroma of connective tissue containing chroma-ophores and primitive mesenchymal fibroblasts. Underlying this layer is connective tissue in which are smooth muscle fibers, arranged as sphincter and dilator pupillae. The sphincter muscle lies around the pupillary mar-gin, closely associated with the pig-ment epithelium on the posterior

surface of the iris. It is supplied by parasympathetic fibers of the third nerve (Edinger-Westphal nucleus) which have synapsed in the ciliary gan-glion. The dilator fibers appear to be more primitive in structure and con-tain some pigment, but both groups of fibers are ectodermal in origin, being derived from pigment epithelium. The dilator muscle is situated posteriorly and blends with the sphincter fibers near the pupillary margin, radiating peripherally from it like the spokes of a wheel. The muscle is thicker peripherally at the ciliary margin of the iris. The dilator is supplied by the sympathetic nervous system through the superior cervical ganglion.

The posterior surface of the iris is covered by a layer of cells continuous with the ciliary epithelium posteriorly. At the pupillary margin, the epithelium is continuous with the anterior endothelial layer. Component cells are so heavily pigmented as to obscure all cellular detail.

The Chambers of the Eye

Anterior Chamber. The anterior chamber is that space bounded anteriorly by the posterior surface of the cornea and posteriorly by the central area of the lens, the iris, and the anterior surface of the ciliary body. At the angle or limbus is the trabecular tissue (pectinate ligament). This angle is the region through which aqueous humor is drained into the canal of Schlemm and is termed also the *"filtration angle."* It should be emphasized that no true filtration occurs; viz., there is no change in constitution of the aqueous with the exception of the removal of some extravasated pigment and red blood cells.

Posterior Chamber. This region is bounded anteriorly by the iris, posteriorly by the anterior surface of the lens and the anterior surface of the zonule, and peripherally by the ciliary processes.

Both chambers contain *aqueous humor,* a thin watery fluid similar to serum in that it contains diffusible materials of blood plasma but with a very low protein content of about 0.02 per cent compared to 7 per cent in serum. It is produced partially by diffusion from capillaries in ciliary processes and partly by an active secretion by the ciliary epithelium and thus enters the posterior chamber. Posterior and anterior chambers communicate freely through the pupil, and aqueous humor is drained through the trabecular tissue into the canal of Schlemm. If the rate of formation of aqueous humor is equal to the rate of drainage, intraocular pressure will remain constant at about 23 mm. of mercury. If, however, there is obstruction to drainage and formation continues, then intraocular pressure will increase. Such a condition is called

glaucoma, which, if untreated, may result in damage to the retina and blindness. The drainage of aqueous thus is important, and the tissues of the filtration angle now require further description.

Canal of Schlemm. This annular vessel encircles the eye just anterior and external to the scleral spur. Usually it has a single lumen but it may be double or even plexiform. Externally and posteriorly the canal is bounded by scleral tissue, medially by the deeper layer of the trabecular tissue. Its wall is only 1 micron thick, consisting of a single layer of endothelium, and it has afferent communications through the trabecular spaces for drainage of aqueous humor from the anterior chamber. Its efferent drainage consists of 20 to 30 endothelial-lined tubes leaving the canal around its circumference to pass into the sclera, in which they anastomose freely to form the deep scleral venous plexus. A few direct channels, together with efferent vessels from the deep scleral plexus, pass to the episcleral venous plexus, lying at the limbus external to sclera and cornea. The anterior channels to the episcleral plexus are clear because they contain aqueous and not blood, and thus they are called the "aqueous veins."

Trabecular Meshwork (Pectinate Ligament). This is a mass of sponge-like tissue interposed between the anterior chamber and the canal of Schlemm. It comprises a meshwork of trabeculae or beams with spaces between the trabeculae in which aqueous humor drains. It is divided, usually, into three zones. All the trabeculae arise from the ring of Schwalbe, which marks the posterior extremity of Descemet's membrane of the cornea, and from subjacent corneal lamellae.

Uveal Meshwork. This is the most internal portion and consists of delicate trabeculae in the form of a fish net arising from Descemet's membrane and Schwalbe's line and passing posteriorly to insert into the root of the

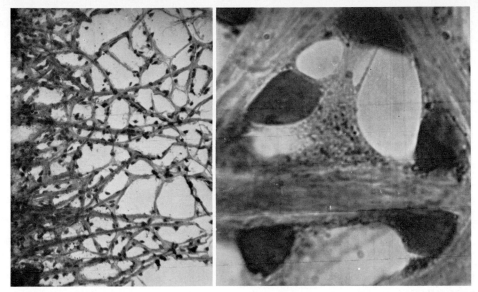

Figure 20-10.   Photomicrographs of flat preparations of the uveal meshwork, showing trabeculae covered by endothelium and trabecular spaces. Left, × 225. Right, × 1500. (Courtesy of J. Speakman.)

iris and its stroma. The trabeculae or beams are only 4 microns or less in diameter with large (inter-) trabecular spaces. Each trabecula has a core of connective tissue fibers and is covered by endothelium.

SCLERAL MESHWORK. This, the bulk of the trabecular tissue, consists of circumferentially orientated, flattened, and perforated bands of tissue attached from Schwalbe's line and corneal lamellae anteriorly to scleral

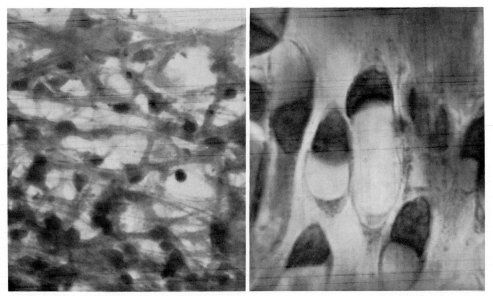

Figure 20-11.   Photomicrographs of flat preparations of, left, the scleral meshwork (× 350) and, right, the endothelial meshwork (× 1500). (Courtesy of J. Speakman.)

spur and ciliary body posteriorly. Each band is a latticework of trabeculae with oval deficiencies between them. Each trabecula is composed of: an innermost core of collagenous fibers, which by electron microscopy have the usual periodicity of 640 to 700 Å, orientated longitudinally in the trabecula; a surrounding sheath of collagenous fibers of a periodicity of 450 to 1000 Å, which is variable in thickness and which may not be present; a "clear zone," continuous with Descemet's membrane, containing collagenous fibers, bundles of "long-spacing collagen" of 1050 to 1250 Å in periodicity, and some elastin; attenuated endothelium lying upon a thin, extracellular basal lamina.

ENDOTHELIAL MESHWORK. This, the outermost portion of the trabecular meshwork, forms the inner wall of the canal of Schlemm and consists of perforated sheets of overlapping endothelium with little or no supporting connective tissue. The pores in it connect on the one side with the trabecular spaces and on the other with the lumen of the canal of Schlemm.

There are numerous fine nerve endings in trabecular tissue, derived mainly from the supraciliary plexus.

The Refractive Media

The refractive media include all transparent structures through which light rays must pass to reach the retina. The cornea and anterior and posterior chambers already have been described, and the remaining components are the lens and the vitreous body.

Lens. The crystalline lens is biconvex, the posterior surface being more highly curved than the anterior. Each surface has a pole. The line joining anterior and posterior poles is the axis, and the peripheral circumferential border is termed the equator. The lens is elastic in the young but becomes harder and sclerosed with age. It is surrounded by a strong, highly elastic capsule which is attached to the ciliary body by the zonule or suspensory ligament. The axis (thickness) is about 3.6 mm., increasing to 4.5 mm. in accommodation; the equatorial diameter in the adult is about 9 mm.

Structurally, there are three components:

LENS CAPSULE. This is clear, of varying thickness, being thinnest at the posterior pole. The deeper part or capsule proper is homogeneous and composed of fine lamellae of collagenous fibers bound by cement substance. Although highly elastic, no elastic tissue is present, elasticity being dependent upon the arrangement of the fibers. The superficial layer or zonular lamella differs in staining reactions from the capsule proper. To it are attached the zonular fibers.

SUBCAPSULAR EPITHELIUM. This is a single layer of cells on the anterior surface, thicker at the equator where they are in the process of transformation into lens fibers. There is no epithelium over the posterior pole.

LENS SUBSTANCE. This is composed of lens fibers, each being of the shape of a six-sided prism, 8 to 10 mm. long, 8 to 12 microns broad, and 2 microns thick. The two long sides are parallel to the surface of the lens. The outer, younger fibers show a very regular pattern, but the central, older fibers become more irregular. Between lens fibers is a small amount of cementing substance of the same refractive index as the fibers. This is thought to allow slight movement between lens fibers during accommodation. The younger fibers contain nuclei but these are lost from the central fibers. Fibers from opposite points of the equator meet at the poles in sutures or junctions to form a triradiate star figure, like a Y. This Y figure stands erect on the anterior surface and inverted posteriorly.

Zonule. The zonule or suspensory ligament is a gel-like structure extending from a broad origin at the ciliary body to the equator of the lens, thus completely covering the lens. The fibrillar material is aggregated to form strands arranged in anterior and

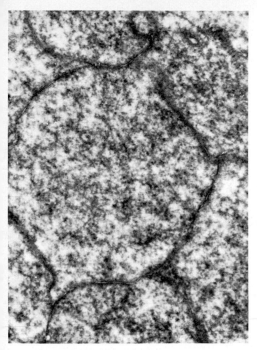

Figure 20-12. Electron micrograph of a cross section through the lens, showing hexagonal lens fibers. × 7500.

posterior sheets to be attached to the superficial layer of the lens capsule on anterior and posterior surfaces. The space between the two main sheets is filled partially by interconnecting strands of similar material but with wide spaces between the fibers for free circulation of aqueous humor. The fibrillar elements appear to arise from the internal limiting membrane which lines the internal surface of the ciliary epithelium. The fibers insert into the zonular lamella of the lens capsule. As seen by electron microscopy, the fibers are composed of microfibrils 80 to 120 Å in diameter.

Vitreous Body. The vitreous body is a clear, transparent gel filling the space posterior to the lens. Its shape is determined by the space in which it lies, being spheroidal with an anterior depression to accommodate the posterior convexity of the lens. It is adherent to the ciliary epithelium, particularly at the ora serrata, and posteriorly around the optic disk.

It is structureless, consisting of a gel containing a fibrillar protein related to collagen and hyaluronic acid. It is not homogeneous, the component fibrils being denser peripherally and around an anteroposterior tubular canal, the "hyaloid canal." This canal, originally around the embryonic hyaloid artery, contains a clear fluid in adult life. There are a few cells in the vitreous, more numerous anteriorly in the region of the zonule. They possibly are macrophages and lymphocytes. Around the surface of the vitreous is the hyaloid membrane, a surface condensation composed of true fibrils, but which appears structureless and homogeneous.

The Retina

The retina is the innermost layer of the eyeball and comprises the anterior, nonsensitive iridial and ciliary portion (already described) and the posterior, functional portion, which is the photoreceptor organ. As stated previously, the retina is developmentally and functionally part of the central nervous system. The retina develops as an evagination of the forebrain, termed the optic vesicle, and remains connected to the brain by the optic stalk, the future optic nerve. The optic vesicle becomes transformed into a double-layered optic cup, the outer layer forming the pigment epithelium and the cuticular layer of Bruch's membrane, the inner layer forming the optical portion of the retina. A potential space remains between the two layers, traversed only by processes of the pigment cells. The outer layer is attached firmly to the choroid, but the inner layer is detached readily during histological preparation and also in life after trauma. Clinical detachment of the retina is actually a separation between inner and outer layers.

The optical portion of the retina lines the choroid from the papilla of the optic nerve posteriorly to the ora serrata anteriorly and shows a shallow depression, the *fovea centralis*, situ-

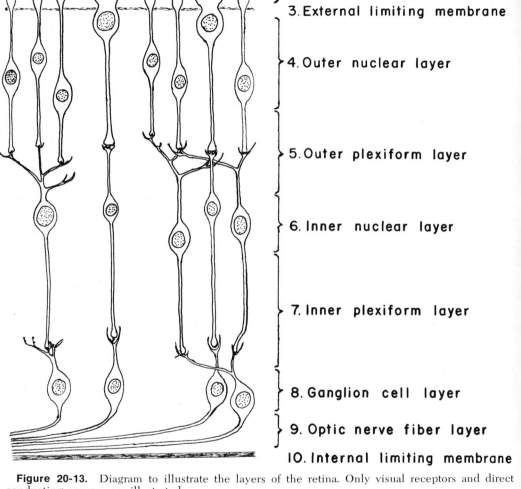

1. Pigment epithelium

2. Layer of rods and cones

3. External limiting membrane

4. Outer nuclear layer

5. Outer plexiform layer

6. Inner nuclear layer

7. Inner plexiform layer

8. Ganglion cell layer

9. Optic nerve fiber layer

10. Internal limiting membrane

Figure 20-13. Diagram to illustrate the layers of the retina. Only visual receptors and direct conducting neurons are illustrated.

ated about 2.5 mm. to the temporal side of the optic papilla. In the region of the fovea and immediately surrounding it, the retina contains a yellow pigment; hence this area is termed the yellow spot or *macula lutea.* The fovea is the area of most clear vision. There are no photoreceptors over the optic papilla and this region is called the *blind spot.*

Layers of the Retina. In cross section, from external to internal, these are:

1. Pigment epithelium
2. Layer of rods and cones
3. External limiting membrane } 1st neuron
4. Outer nuclear layer

5. Outer plexiform layer ⎫
6. Inner nuclear layer   ⎬ 2nd neuron
7. Inner plexiform layer ⎭
8. Ganglion cell layer
9. Optic nerve fiber layer ⎫ 3rd neuron
10. Internal limiting membrane ⎭

The retina is a complex structure, but the complexity becomes simplified with appreciation of the fact that it is only three neurons deep. Each rod or cone (the first neuron) has a sensory end organ lying outermost against the pigment epithelium, a nucleus, and an inner terminal fiber, and these parts of the cells account for the outer layers. The nuclei of the rods are placed more centrally than those of the cones. At the fovea, there are many layers of cone nuclei, but over the remainder of the retina, layer four comprises a single outer row of cone nuclei with four rows of rod nuclei lying more centrally. The outer plexiform layer marks the junction between first and second (intermediate) neurons. The inner nuclear layer appears as a closely

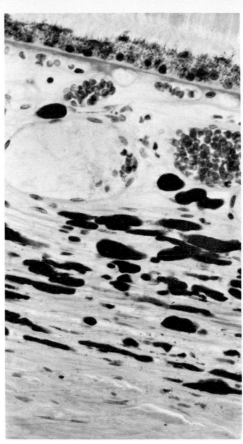

Figure 20-15. Photomicrograph of pigment epithelium (above) resting upon the lamina elastica (Bruch's membrane) with choriocapillaris, vessel layer, and epichoroid. A small portion of the sclera lies below. Note the pigment cells in the choroid. × 500.

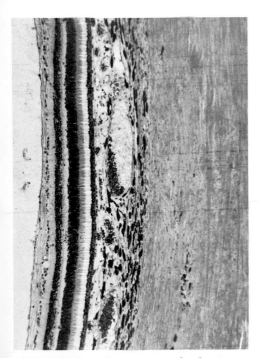

Figure 20-14. Photomicrograph of a section through the thickness of the eye, showing from left to right, retina, choroid, and sclera. × 70.

packed mass of nuclei of bipolar (second neuron) cells, association cells, and supporting elements. The inner plexiform layer is the site of junction between second and third neurons, the ganglion cell layer containing ganglion (third neuron) cells and neuroglia. The central processes of the ganglion cells form the optic nerve fibers, all of which pass to the optic papilla and thus to the optic nerve. These fibers are unmyelinated but obtain a myelin sheath as they pass through the cribriform plate at the optic papilla. Thus, it should be recognized that the retina is gray matter of the central nervous system

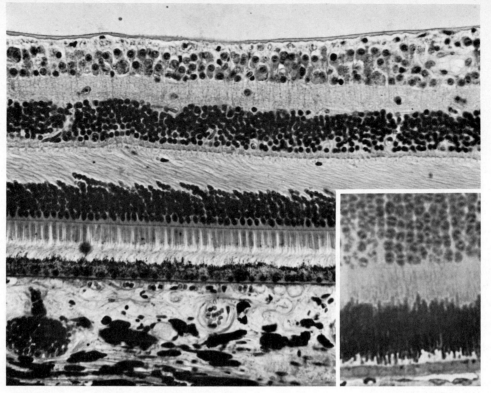

Figure 20-16. Photomicrograph to show all layers of the retina. Compare with Figure 20-13. Part of the choroid appears below. × 350. Insert: Epon section to show pigment epithelium (below), outer and inner segments of rods, and rod nuclei. × 1050.   See filmstrip II, frames 95 and 96.

and the optic nerve is white matter. The internal limiting membrane separates the retina from the vitreous body.

Pigment Epithelium. This is a single layer of polygonal cells, regular in height (8 microns) except at the macula where they are taller (11 to 14 microns) and at the ora serrata where they are large, irregular, and often multinucleate (60 microns in diameter). The spherical nucleus lies peripherally against the basal lamina (of Bruch), and each cell has a cytoplasmic process containing a large content of pigment (melanin) extending centrally between the rods and cones. With changes in illumination, pigment moves into the cell processes to prevent diffusion of light between the photoreceptors. In the dark, most of the pigment lies in the cell body adjacent to the nucleus.

Elements of the Retina. There are four groups: visual receptors (rods and cones); direct conducting neurons (bipolar and ganglion cells); association and other neurons (horizontal, "amacrine," and centrifugal bipolar cells); and supporting elements (Müller's fibers and neuroglia).

VISUAL RECEPTORS. Both rods and cones are divided into inner and outer segments situated outside the external limiting membrane, and a conducting nucleated portion lying inside the external limiting membrane. Each conducting portion includes an outer conducting fiber (physiologically a dendrite), a cell body in the outer nuclear layer, and an inner conducting fiber (physiologically an axon) extending into the outer plexiform layer. It is important to appreciate that light must pass through the thickness of the retina to reach the photoreceptors in the outer layer.

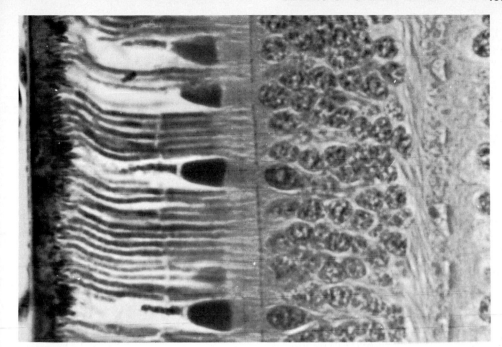

Figure 20-17. Photomicrograph of rods and four cones — Bruch's membrane at the left, outer plexiform layer at the right. × 1500.

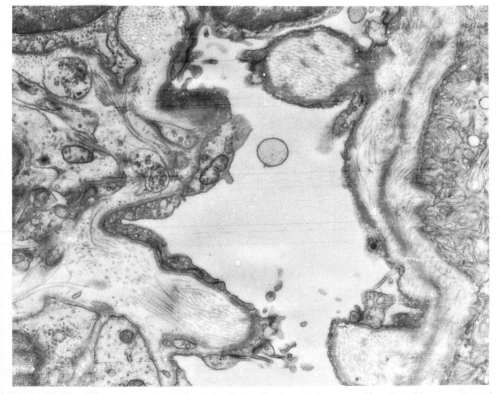

Figure 20-18. Electron micrograph of choriocapillaris with large capillary lined by type II endothelium. Bruch's membrane and bases of pigment epithelial cells, showing infoldings of basal plasma membrane, appear at the right. × 8500.

The Rod. The rod is a modified neuron. Each rod has a cylindrical outer segment about 28 microns long containing the photopigment rhodopsin (visual purple), and a slightly thicker inner segment about 32 microns long. Both parts are 1.5 to 2 microns thick. The tip of the outer segment is surrounded by pigment of the pigment epithelium. The outer segment shows transverse striations, and the two segments are connected by a narrow "neck" region containing a cilium.

As shown by electron microscopy, the outer segment is composed of double membrane lamellae 140 Å thick, separated by intervals of 100 Å, but connected in series by short processes. There are about 700 of these lamellae. The inner segment comprises an outer "ellipsoid" composed of longitudinally oriented mitochondria and an inner "myoid" containing

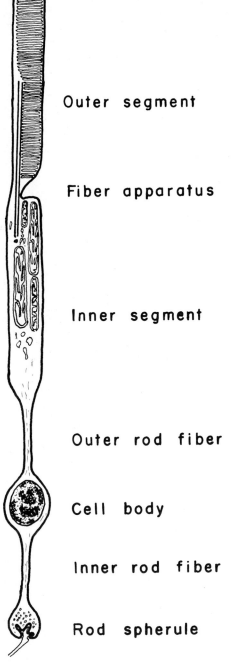

Outer segment

Fiber apparatus

Inner segment

Outer rod fiber

Cell body

Inner rod fiber

Rod spherule

Figure 20-19. Diagram of a single rod as seen with the electron microscope.

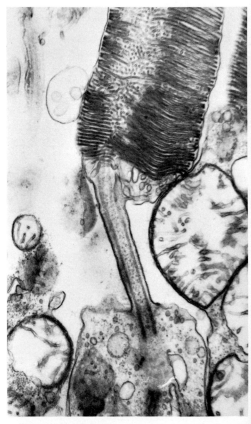

Figure 20-20. Electron micrograph of parts of the outer (above) and inner (below) segments of a retinal rod with connecting cilium. × 12,000.

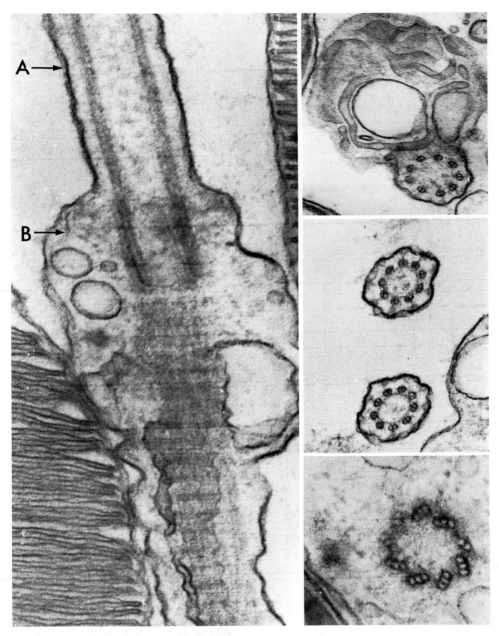

Figure 20-21. Electron micrographs of parts of a retinal rod. Left: Longitudinal section through fibrillar apparatus and outer part of the inner segment. Note the basal body, showing periodicity, and a portion of an outer segment with membrane lamellae (left). × 90,000. Top right: Cross section through the inner portion of an outer segment, showing membrane lamellae and nine pairs of peripheral filaments or microtubules in the fibrillar apparatus. × 85,000. Center right: Cross section through two fibrillar apparatuses. × 85,000. Bottom right: Cross section through the fibrillar apparatus in an inner segment. × 120,000. Arrows A and B indicate approximate levels of sections at right center and right bottom respectively.

large quantities of particulate glycogen. Outer and inner segments are joined by an eccentrically situated fibrillar structure similar to a cilium with longitudinally orientated fibrils.

The rod proper is connected to its cell body by a delicate outer rod fiber which traverses the external limiting membrane. The cell body is composed of a nucleus with a thin rim of cytoplasm, and from it the inner rod fiber extends into the outer plexiform layer to terminate as a small end knob, the rod spherule. This is similar to boutons terminaux and is in contact with dendrites of bipolar cells of the inner nuclear layer and with axons of horizontal cells.

The Cone. The cone, like the rod,

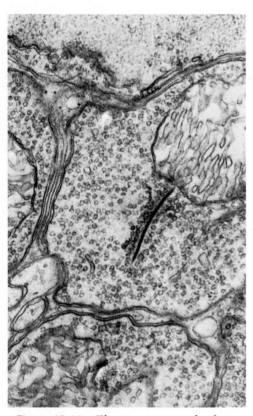

Figure 20-22. Electron micrograph of a section from the outer plexiform layer. Above is a portion of the nucleus of a receptor cell, and the remainder of the field is occupied by rod cell axon terminals. Note the numerous "synaptic" vesicles and the peculiar rodlet structure. × 35,000.

is a modified neuron and has a somewhat similar appearance. It has a long, slightly tapered outer segment swelling to a conical inner segment, the two together resembling a flask, this being external to the outer limiting membrane. In the outer segment are lamellae similar to those of rods, but in some of them the membranes are continuous with the covering plasma membrane, thus forming narrow clefts open at the surface to the extracellular space. The inner segment contains numerous, elongated mitochondria and, as in the rod, the two segments are connected by a cilium. The cones contain no visual purple.

Cones vary in different parts of the retina. Those at the fovea are long and slender with inner and outer segments of the same diameter; i.e., they are not truly cone-shaped. At the periphery of the retina, they are shorter and thicker.

The cone nucleus is larger and shows less densely packed chromatin than the rod nucleus and usually lies just inside the external limiting membrane. Thus, the outer cone fiber is short. The inner cone fiber is much thicker than that of the rod, runs through the outer plexiform layer, and widens at its termination in the center of this layer to form the cone pedicle. From it emerges one or more basal filaments. In the fovea, each cone pedicle is connected to a single bipolar cell.

There are estimated to be 130 million rods and six to seven million cones in the human retina.

DIRECT CONDUCTING NEURONS. These comprise the bipolar and ganglion cells.

Bipolar Cells. The cell bodies of these cells lie mostly in the central zone of the inner nuclear area. They can be divided into two main groups: the diffuse bipolars contacting several photoreceptors and the midget or monosynaptic bipolars connecting with a single cell. The dendrites of the diffuse bipolars contact rod spherules or groups of about six cone pedicles in the outer plexiform layer. The dendrites may be long ("mop" bipolars) or short ("brush" bipolars). As just stated, the dendritic expansions penetrate the rod spherules. Axons are straight and pass vertically into the inner plexiform layer where they contact dendrites of ganglion cells. The midget bipolars synapse with only a single cone pedicle. The axon passes into the inner plexiform layer and divides into several small telodendrons which synapse with the dendrites of a single midget ganglion cell, thus providing a one-to-one pathway from cone to optic nerve fiber.

Ganglion Cells. These are situated in the inner nuclear layer (ganglion cell layer) with their dendrites in the inner plexiform layer and their axons constituting the optic nerve fibers. The axons never branch. They are large cells, closely resembling cerebral neurons with a mass of chromophil material (Nissl body) in the cell body. They are of two main types, the diffuse type with dendrites contacting several bipolar cells, and the small or monosynaptic type with dendrites synapsing with a single, midget, cone, bipolar cell.

ASSOCIATION AND CENTRIFUGAL NEURONS

Horizontal Cells. The bodies of these cells lie in the outer part of the inner nuclear layer with dendrites and axons in the inner part of the outer plexiform layer. The cell bodies are larger than most bipolar cells in the same layer. The dendrites terminate in cuplike "baskets" around numerous cone pedicles, and the single axon branches at its termination into an elaborate telodendron to synapse with both rod spherules and cone pedicles. The horizontal cells thus connect a group of cone cells in one area with a group of rods and cones in another area and perhaps function to raise or lower the functional threshold between rods and cones and the bipolar cells.

Amacrine Cells. These cells lie in the inner two or three rows of the inner nuclear layer. They are pear-shaped with a single process passing inward to terminate in the inner plexiform layer. Probably they are association cells.

SUPPORTING ELEMENTS. In the retina, as in the brain, an elaborate framework of neuroglia serves functions of support, insulation, and nutrition. This framework comprises a main network of Müller's fibers with astroglia and perivascular glia, and microglia, the last being mesodermal in origin, the others ectodermal.

Fibers of Müller. They traverse the retina in a radial fashion, except at the fovea where they are oblique. The cell nuclei are large and situated mainly in the inner nuclear layer with a few in the ganglion cell layer and even in the optic nerve fiber layer. Cytoplasmic processes of the cells (Müller's fibers) pass between nerve cells into the plexiform layers, extending internally to the internal limiting membrane.

Other Glial Elements. These form the finer neuroglial network and include "interstitial spongioblasts" in the inner nuclear layer and astrocytes, which are more numerous in the optic nerve and the region of the disk than in the retina itself. In the retina, the astrocytes are star-shaped cells in the ganglion cell layer and the inner and outer plexiform layers, and small cells usually only with two processes (the lemmocytes) situated in the nerve fiber layer. Microglia are found in all layers and are phagocytic.

The Limiting Membranes. The external limiting membrane between the rods and cones and their nuclei is not a complete layer but is fenestrated to permit the visual cells to perforate it. It is composed of glia which at the optic disk is continuous with the limiting membrane on the internal surface of the pigment epithelium. The internal limiting membrane lines the vitreal surface of the retina. Its inner surface is smooth, but the external surface is connected to the innermost terminal expansions of Müller's fibers.

Central Area of Retina. The human retina can be divided into a central area 5 to 6 mm. in diameter and a peripheral area comprising the remainder of the retina. This distinction is both morphological and functional, the central area with a high concentration of photoreceptors being specialized for accurate diurnal vision, and the peripheral area being of coarser structure and more suitable for reception of weak stimuli in dim illumination.

Morphologically, in the central area there is an accumulation of ganglion cells in more than one row and a density of cones and bipolar cells. The *macula lutea* is a more vague area characterized by the presence of a yellow pigment in the inner layers of the retina. This is an area about 3 mm. in diameter surrounding the *fovea,*

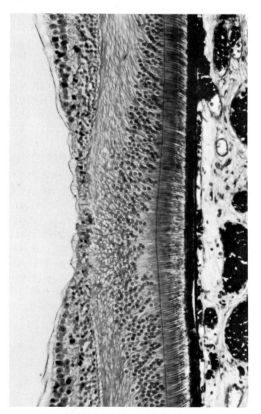

Figure 20-23. Section through the fovea centralis. Notice the disappearance of the inner layers of the retina and the closely packed, elongated cones in the floor of the depression. × 275.   See filmstrip II, frame 97.

which itself contains very little pigment and thus appears pale.

The fovea centralis is a shallow, rounded pit lying 4 mm. to the temporal side of the optic disk and about 0.8 mm. below the horizontal meridian. The depression is caused by the virtually complete absence of the inner layers of the retina in this region, the visual cells in the floor of the fovea all being cones, closely packed and longer than those in the peripheral retina. These cones synapse with bipolar cells obliquely placed around the margins of the fovea. There are no capillaries in the central area of the fovea.

Optic Papilla and Nerve. The retinal aspect of the optic nerve is termed the *optic disk.* This includes the slight prominence, the optic papilla, formed by the heaping up of nerve fibers as they leave the retina to enter the optic nerve, and a small central depression (the "physiological cup") through which the central artery and vein of the retina emerge. The central artery in the great majority of cases is the sole arterial supply to the retina, and its occlusion results in permanent blindness. In some people, the retina also is supplied partially by a cilioretinal artery to the macula. Occlusion of the central artery in these people causes only a loss of peripheral vision, the macula being spared. The optic disk usually is slightly oval, about 1.5 mm. in diameter, situated to the nasal side of the posterior pole. At the margin of the disk all the retinal tissues except the optic nerve fibers cease abruptly. The opening in the sclera is filled by the lamina cribrosa, a dense fibrous plate perforated by bundles of optic nerve fibers, and continuous with the tissue of the sclera at its periphery.

The optic nerve itself is not a peripheral nerve but is a tract of the central nervous system between the retinal ganglion cells and the midbrain. It extends posteriorly to the optic chiasma and contains over 1000 bundles of myelinated nerve fibers supported by neuroglia and not endoneurium. The

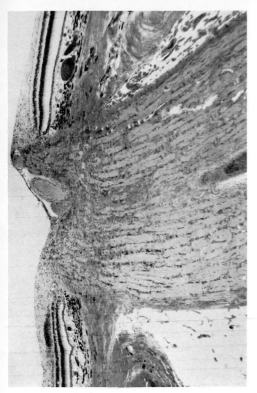

Figure 20-24. Section through the optic disk and optic papilla. Note the central artery to the retina within the optic nerve (right center, dark). × 25.

meninges and subarachnoid space continue from the brain as sheaths of the optic nerve. In addition to afferent fibers from the retinal photoreceptors, the optic nerve also contains fibers running to the tectum of the brain for the pupillary reflex, fibers to the superior colliculus, some autonomic nerve fibers, and a few efferent fibers passing to the retina, of unknown function. The central artery and vein reach the retina by entering the optic nerve some distance posterior to the eyeball.

Accessory Organs of the Eye

The eyeball is situated in the bony orbit which, of course, is open anteriorly. This opening is closed by the upper and lower eyelids which, when they are opposed, meet at the trans-verse *palpebral* tissue. Conjunctiva covers the anterior surface of the cornea and is reflected from its perimeter to line the deep surface of the eyelids, the reflections being termed superior and inferior *fornices*. With the eyelids closed, the conjunctival sac is a closed space anterior to the eyeball filled with a small amount of fluid.

Eyelids. Essentially, each eyelid consists of a central supporting plate of connective tissue and skeletal muscle covered by skin externally and a mucous membrane internally. The skin anteriorly is thin with small hairs, sweat and sebaceous glands, and a dermis of delicate connective tissue rich in elastic fibers. The dermis is more dense at the lid margin and here contains three or four rows of long, stiff hairs, the *eyelashes,* which penetrate deeply into the dermis. Between and posterior to the eyelashes are large, modified sweat glands characterized by straight and not coiled terminal ducts (the glands of Moll).

Beneath the skin is a layer of striated muscle fibers, this being the palpebral part of the orbicularis oculi muscle which is the bulk of the core of the eyelid, and the fibers of insertion of levator palpebrae superioris. Slender slips of smooth muscle, the palpebral muscles (of Müller), also are present.

Posterior to the muscle layer is a fibrous layer consisting of a thin sheet of fibrous tissue peripherally (the septum orbitale) and the tarsal plate. The tarsal plates are sheets of dense connective tissue curved to the shape of the eyeball, the upper being D-shaped with its lower horizontal border coextensive with the lid margin. The upper plate is 10 to 12 mm. broad, but the lower plate is a narrow (5 mm.) band lying in the central region of the lower lid. Present in both tarsal plates is a single row of very large sebaceous glands, the tarsal (meibomian) glands, the ducts of which open at the lid margin. From the main ducts, numerous lateral branches pass out to drain single or multiple secretory alveoli. The deep, posterior surface of each tarsal plate blends with conjunctiva which is continuous with epidermis at the inner edge of the lid margin.

Conjunctiva. The conjunctiva is the mucous membrane lining the inner surface of the eyelids from which it is reflected onto the anterior surface of the eyeball. It is continuous with corneal epithelium at the corneal margin and with skin at the lid margins.

The conjunctival epithelium varies with location but consists of a basal layer of cuboidal cells, a surface layer of cone or cylindrical shaped cells, and, particularly over the lower lid,

one to three intermediate layers of polygonal cells. Scattered among the epithelial cells are some mucus-secreting goblet cells.

At the edge of the cornea, the conjunctival epithelium becomes stratified squamous identical to the corneal epithelium. Underlying the epithelium is a lamina propria, superficially composed of fine fibroelastic connective tissue with numerous lymphocytes (the "adenoid" layer) and deeply composed of dense fibroconnective tissue.

The Lacrimal Apparatus. The lac-

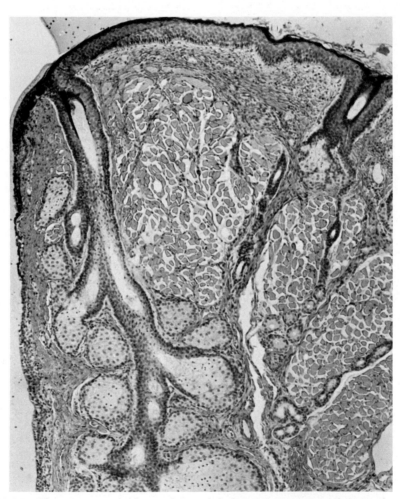

Figure 20-25. Photomicrograph of part of an eyelid, showing conjunctiva (left), epidermis (above), and the large modified sebaceous glands (tarsal or meibomian glands). The striated muscle fibers (right) are part of the palpebral portion of orbicularis oculi muscle. Between the muscle fibers are portions of three glands of Moll (apocrine type sweat glands). × 25.

rimal apparatus comprises the lacrimal glands and their ducts draining into the conjunctival sac, and the lacrimal passages which drain excess tears from the conjunctival sac into the nasal cavity.

The main lacrimal gland lies in the superolateral corner of the orbit, just within the orbital margin, in relation to the tendon of levator palpebrae superioris and just beneath the conjunctiva of the superior fornix. It is the size of an almond, tubuloacinar, and serous, with prominent myoepithelial cells. The separate lobes of the gland drain via 10 to 15 excretory ducts into the lateral part of the superior conjunctival fornix. There also are numerous accessory lacrimal glands situated in the lamina propria of upper and lower eyelids.

After entering the conjunctival sac, the tears (the sterile secretion of the lacrimal glands) partially evaporate. They serve to keep the conjunctival epithelium moist, the blinking eyelids spreading the tears over the cornea like windshield-wipers, and to wash out foreign matter, e.g., dust particles. Excessive evaporation is prevented by a film of mucus (from the tarsal conjunctival goblet cells) on the film of water and a film of oil (from the meibomian glands). Excess tears pass medially to a slight expansion of the conjunctival sac (the lacus lacrimalis) and then into the lacrimal canaliculi, one in each eyelid, which open on the surface at a minute orifice termed the lacrimal puncta. These ducts pass to the lacrimal sac situated in the medial corner of the eye from which tears pass down the nasolacrimal duct to enter the inferior meatus of the nose.

Function of the Eye

The eye functions as the receptive organ of the visual system. Light rays entering the eye are focused by cornea and lens to form an inverted, real, reduced image of the object on the photosensitive layer of rods and cones of the retina. Focusing is accomplished by alteration of the convexity of the lens. In the position of rest with the ciliary muscle relaxed, the lens is flattened by elastic tension of the zonule. Contraction of the ciliary muscle, particularly of the outer, meridional fibers, pulls the choroid and ciliary body anteriorly. This relaxes the tension of the zonule and permits the lens, which is elastic, to become more convex, thus increasing the refractive power.

In the outer segments of rods and cones are two visual pigments: *rhodopsin* in the rods, which is sensitive to scotopic (dark-adapted) vision and *iodopsin* in the cones. These pigments consist of a specific protein bound to vitamin A aldehyde. Visible light falling on these pigments by a series of chemical changes results in depolarization of the receptor cell membrane and the formation of an action poten-

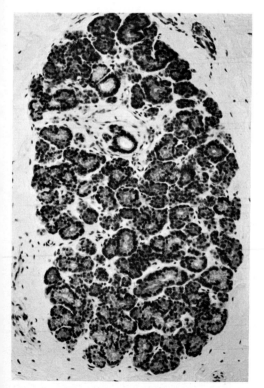

Figure 20-26. Photomicrograph of a lobe of the lacrimal gland, showing secretory serous acini and an intralobular duct (center). × 100.
See filmstrip II, frame 98.

tial, which is then conducted by a series of neurons (including bipolar and ganglion cells) to the brain.

THE EAR

The ear is divided into three portions: the *external ear,* the *middle ear,* and the *inner ear,* the latter containing the organs both of hearing and of balance.

The external ear comprises the auricle (the visible appendage), the external auditory meatus extending deeply in the temporal bone, and the tympanic membrane or eardrum, which closes the deep extremity of the external auditory meatus. The middle ear is a cavity shaped like a biconcave lens, the lateral wall of which is the tympanic membrane and the medial wall of which is the external surface of the inner ear. Its cavity is traversed from tympanic membrane to inner ear by a chain of three small bones or ossicles (the malleus or hammer, the incus or anvil, and the stapes or stirrup). The inner ear consists of an irregular system of canals (the membranous labyrinth) walled in by bone (the bony labyrinth).

The External Ear

Auricle. The characteristic and complicated shape of the auricle is

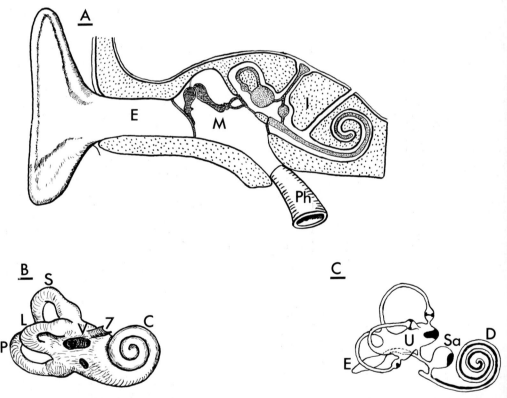

Figure 20-27. Diagrams to illustrate the parts of the ear. *A,* External ear consisting of pinna and external auditory meatus (E); middle ear (M), separated from the external ear by the tympanic membrane and traversed by the three ossicles (malleus, incus, and stapes); and internal ear (I). The pharyngotympanic (eustachian) tube (Ph) extends inferiorly from the middle ear. *B,* Right osseous or bony labyrinth viewed from the lateral side. Superior (S), posterior (P), and lateral (L) semicircular canals, vestibule (V), and cochlea (C) are shown. The oval and round windows and the canal for the facial nerve (7) also can be seen. *C,* Membranous labyrinth with semicircular canals, utricle (U), saccule (Sa), cochlear duct (D), and endolymphatic sac (E). Neuroepithelial areas are indicated in black.

due to a plate of yellow elastic cartilage of 0.5 to 1 mm. thickness, covered by a perichondrium with a high content of elastic fibers. On all surfaces, it is covered by thin skin with a very thin subcutaneous layer (hypodermis) on the anterolateral surface. Hairs and sebaceous and sweat glands are present but in general are poorly developed. Contained in the subcutaneous layer and attached to perichondrium are a few small slips of striated muscle. These are vestigial in man, but in lower animals that are capable of ear movements they are more prominent.

External Auditory Meatus. The external auditory meatus extends from the auricle to the tympanic membrane. It is oval in section and held patent by the rigidity of its wall. The external third has a wall of elastic cartilage continuous with that forming the support of the auricle, and the inner two-thirds is of bone. The canal is lined by thin skin with no subcutaneous tissue, the deeper layers of the dermis blending with perichondrium or periosteum. Numerous hairs associated with sebaceous glands are present in the outer portion, and some small hairs and sebaceous glands are present in the roof only of the inner portion. Contained in the external meatus is *cerumen*, a brown, waxy material bitter to the taste and protective in function. It is the combined secretion of the sebaceous and ceruminous glands, which are large, modified, coiled, tubular sweat glands, the ducts of which open either directly onto the skin surface or with sebaceous glands into the necks of hair follicles.

Tympanic Membrane. This is oval and placed obliquely to close the innermost extremity of the external meatus. It has a core of connective tissue in two layers, the fibers of the outer layer being radial, those of the inner layer being circular. Externally it is covered by very thin skin and internally by the mucosa of the middle meatus, here only 20 to 30 microns

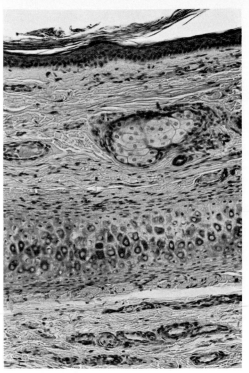

Figure 20-28. Photomicrograph of a section of the external auditory meatus. Note the thin epidermis, the sebaceous gland, and the elastic cartilage. × 100.

thick and with a cuboidal epithelium. Attached to the tympanic membrane is the malleus, one of the middle ear ossicles, the handle of which extends to the center of the membrane and causes it to bulge into the middle ear cavity. The upper portion of the tympanic membrane lacks collagenous fibers and is termed the flaccid part (Shrapnell's membrane).

The Middle Ear

The middle ear comprises a cleftlike cavity in the temporal bone, the *tympanic cavity*, and a canal or duct which connects it with the nasopharynx, the *auditory (eustachian) tube*.

The tympanic cavity is a flat, boxlike air space about 1.3 cm. high and the same in length, but measuring only 2 to 3 mm. transversely. The lateral wall is formed largely by the tympanic membrane, the medial wall by the inner ear. The bony roof separates it from the middle cranial fossa and temporal lobe of the brain, the floor from the retropharyngeal area and contents of the carotid sheath. Its posterior wall opens into another, smaller chamber, the tympanic antrum, into which open the numerous mastoid air cells. The anterior wall is partially deficient as the opening of the pharyngotympanic or auditory tube.

The epithelium lining the cavity and every structure it contains is squamous or low cuboidal over most of the area, but is columnar and ciliated anteriorly at the opening of the auditory tube. The lamina propria is thin and blends with periosteum.

The three ossicles, composed of compact bone without a marrow cavity, pass across the cavity of the middle ear, the malleus being attached to the tympanic membrane. Both the malleus and the incus are suspended by tiny ligaments from the roof. The base plate of the stapes is attached by a fibrous joint to an oval window or opening (the fenestra ovalis) in the medial wall. Between the three ossicles are two synovial joints. The thin periosteum of the ossicles blends with a thin lamina propria underlying the squamous epithelium lining the entire tympanic cavity. Associated with the chain of ossicles are two small muscles. The tensor tympani muscle lies in a canal above the auditory tube, its tendon passing at first posteriorly and then hooking around a small bony projection to cross the tympanic cavity from medial to lateral walls to insert into the handle of the malleus. The tendon of the stapedius muscle issues from a pyramidal bony projection in the posterior wall and passes anteriorly to insert into the neck of the stapes. These muscles are protective in that they "damp down" high frequency vibrations.

The oval window in the medial wall, occluded by the base plate of the stapes, separates the tympanic cavity from the perilymph in the scala vestibuli of the cochlea. Thus vibrations of the tympanic membrane are transmitted by the chain of ossicles to the perilymph of the inner ear. The perilymph spaces, however, are closed spaces and, because fluid is incompressible, a "safety valve" is necessary. This is the round window or fenestra rotunda, situated in the medial wall of the tympanic cavity below and behind the oval window and closed by an elastic membrane (the secondary tympanic membrane), separating the tympanic cavity from the perilymph of the scala tympani of the cochlea.

The auditory tube, connecting the tympanic cavity and the nasopharynx, is about 3.5 cm. in length, the posterior third having a bony wall, the anterior two-thirds a cartilaginous wall. The lumen is flattened, and medial and lateral walls of the cartilaginous part usually are opposed to occlude the lumen. The epithelial lining varies from ciliated columnar near the tympanic cavity to pseudostratified, ciliated columnar with goblet cells near the pharynx. The lamina propria near the pharynx contains seromucous glands. By the act of swallowing, the walls of the tube are separated, thus opening the lumen and allowing air to enter the middle ear cavity to equalize pressure on both sides of the tympanic membrane.

The Inner Ear

The inner ear is a system of canals and cavities in the petrous part of the temporal bone, the osseous labyrinth, within which is a further series of canals and cavities, the membranous labyrinth. The membranous labyrinth is filled with fluid, the *endolymph,* the walls of the membranous labyrinth separating endolymph from *perilymph,* which fills the remainder of the osseous labyrinth.

Osseous Labyrinth. Centrally situated is the *vestibule* lying medial to the tympanic cavity, with the wall between the two containing the fenestra ovalis. Posterior to the vestibule and opening into it are three *semicircular canals*. By their position, they are named superior, posterior, and lateral, each being at right angles to the others. The two lateral canals of right and left ears are in the same plane approximately, and the superior of one side is parallel to the posterior canal of the other side. Each canal has a dilatation or *ampulla* at one end. Those of the superior and lateral canals lie close together above the fenestra ovalis; that of the posterior canal opens into the posterior part of the vestibule. Although there are three canals, there are only five and not six openings into the vestibule, the non-ampullated posterior end of the posterior canal fusing with the nonampullated medial end of the superior canal to open into the medial part of the vestibule by the *crus commune*. The nonampullated end of the lateral canal opens separately into the upper part of the vestibule. From the medial wall of the vestibule, a narrow canal extends inferoposteriorly to reach the posterior surface of the petrous temporal bone in the posterior cranial fossa.

Anteriorly, the cavity of the vestibule is continuous with the bony *cochlea*, a spirally coiled tube like a snail shell. Its total shape is conical with a base about 9 mm. in diameter and a height from base to apex of 5 mm. with two and three-quarter turns. The axial bony stem of the cochlea, the *modiolus*, is orientated across the long axis of the petrous temporal bone with the base toward the posterior cranial fossa and the apex pointing forward and laterally. A shelf of bone which projects from the modiolus forms a spiral ridge, the *spiral lamina*, like the thread of a screw around its stem.

It should be emphasized that the term "osseous labyrinth" may be confusing. It is *not* a separate bone, but simply a system of canals and cavities in the petrous part of the temporal bone, which, like the ossicles, is composed of compact bone.

Membranous Labyrinth. Within the osseous labyrinth is the membranous labyrinth, a system of interconnected parts lined by epithelium and containing endolymph. In a few regions, the wall of the membranous labyrinth is adherent to periosteum lining the osseous labyrinth, but in general it lies free and separated from the wall of the osseous labyrinth by perilymph. However, thin strands of connective tissue containing blood vessels pass across the perilymph space to suspend the membranous labyrinth within the osseous labyrinth.

The form of the membranous labyrinth is similar to that of the osseous labyrinth with the exception that the vestibule is occupied not by one but by two chambers and connecting channels. Posteriorly the *utricle* communicates via five orifices with the three membranous semicircular canals, which, like the osseous semicircular canals, have a crus commune between superior and posterior canals. The ampullae of the membranous semicircular canals are large. Anteriorly the *saccule* is nearly spherical in shape and is joined to the utricle by a slim Y-shaped tube, the short stems being the utricular and saccular ducts. These ducts join to form the *endolymphatic duct*, which passes posteroinferiorly to the posterior surface of the petrous temporal bone where it terminates as a blind sac, the *endolymphatic sac*. Anteriorly from its lower part, the saccule communicates with the *cochlear duct* by the short, narrow *ductus reuniens*.

There are sensory nerve endings in the ampullae of the semicircular canals (*cristae ampullares*) and in the utricle and saccule (*maculae utriculi and sacculi*) which subserve static and kinetic senses. The organ of hearing is the *organ of Corti* located along the length of the cochlear duct.

Utricle and Saccule. The connective tissue layer of the wall of the utricle and saccule is delicate and contains some fibroblasts and melanocytes. Fine trabeculae extend from its outer surface across the perilymphatic space to the inner surface of the periosteum lining the vestibule. They consist of a core of connective tissue covered by mesothelium. Interposed between the connective tissue layer of the wall of the utricle and saccule and the lining squamous epithelium is a fine basal lamina.

The macula utriculi lies in the lateral wall and is ovoid, 2 by 3 mm., and the macula sacculi is in the medial wall of the saccule and of similar size and shape. The two are orientated perpendicular to each other and have a similar structure. Two cell types are present: *supporting* or *sustentacular cells* and *hair cells.* The supporting cells are columnar and slender with a single small cilium. The hair cells are flask-shaped and do not reach the basal lamina, and their nuclei are located nearer the lumen than those of the supporting cells. Apically, they have a tuft of long, nonmobile cilia which do not float free in endolymph but are embedded in a surface, gelatinous layer about 22 microns thick. This is the *otolithic membrane,* and it contains numerous, small crystalline bodies, the *otoconia* or *otoliths,* composed of calcium carbonate and a protein. Changes in position of the head result in changes in pressure or tension in the otolithic membrane and consequent stimulation of the hair cells. The stimulus is detected by nerve endings lying between the hair cells.

Semicircular Canals. All are oval in cross section, the greatest convexity being closely apposed to periosteum, but each is smaller than the osseous

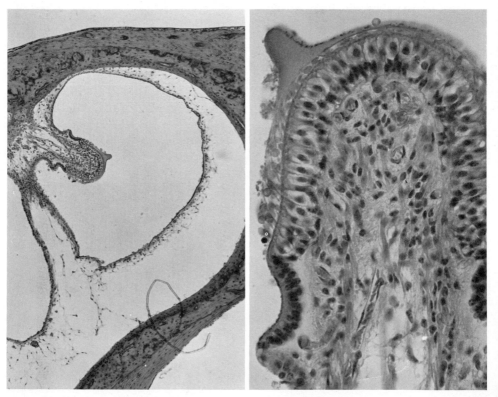

Figure 20-29. Left: Photomicrograph of the crista ampullaris of the lateral semicircular canal. × 40. Right: A higher magnification of the crista ampullaris. × 250.   See filmstrip II, frame 99.

semicircular canal and, on the opposite surface, there is a wide perilymph space traversed by trabeculae.

A crista is present in each ampulla. Each crista is orientated across the long axis of the duct and is formed by sustentacular and hair cells with tufts of hairs embedded in a gelatinous mass termed a *cupula,* similar to the otolithic membrane but lacking otoconia.

Cochlea. The osseous cochlea, as explained previously, spirals for two and three-quarter turns around the modiolus, from which projects the spiral lamina. Extending from the spiral lamina to the outer wall of the cochlea is the *basilar membrane,* the cochlear periosteum being thickened at its outer attachment as the *spiral ligament.* A second membrane, the vestibular membrane (of Reissner) extends across the cochlea from the spiral lamina to the outer wall. These two membranes thus divide the osseous canal into three cavities: an upper cavity, the *scala vestibuli,* a lower cavity, the *scala tympani,* and an intermediate cavity, the *cochlear duct.* The scala vestibuli and the scala tympani contain perilymph, and their walls, like those of other perilymph spaces, consist of connective tissue covered by a squamous layer of mesenchymal cells. The connective tissue blends externally with periosteum. The scala vestibuli is continuous with the perilymphatic space of the vestibule and thus reaches the inner surface of the fenestra ovalis. The scala tympani extends laterally to the fenestra rotunda and the secondary tympanic mem-

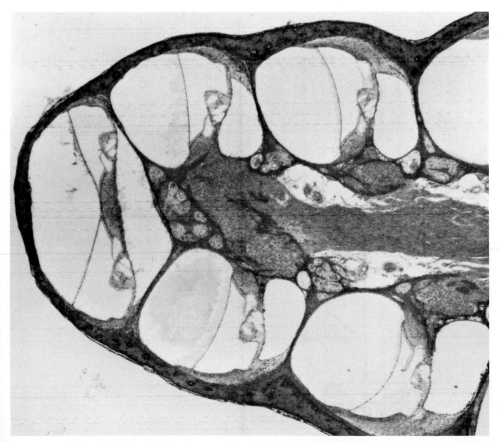

Figure 20-30.   Photomicrograph of the cochlea of a guinea pig. × 25.

brane which separates it from the tympanic cavity. At the apex of the cochlea, the scala vestibuli and scala tympani are in communication through a narrow canal termed the *helicotrema*. .

The cochlear duct, via the ductus reuniens, connects with the saccule but terminates blindly near the helicotrema at the *cecum cupulare*.

At the junction of osseous spiral lamina and modiolus lies the *spiral ganglion,* incompletely surrounded by bone. From the entire length of the ganglion, bundles of nerve fibers perforate the bone of the spiral lamina to reach the organ of Corti. The periosteum above the spiral lamina is thickened and bulges into the cochlear duct as the *limbus spiralis*. Its lower part is continuous with the basilar membrane, which extends outward across the cochlear duct to attach to the spiral ligament. Contained in the basilar membrane are the *basilar fibers (auditory strings),* these differing in composition from both collagen and elastin. They are embedded in some amorphous ground substance. Their length increases from the base to the apex of the cochlea (from about 100 to 425 microns), and they number about 24,000. The cochlear duct surface of the basilar fibers is covered by a thin, homogeneous basal laminar material, whereas its lower, tympanic surface is covered by delicate fibroconnective tissue in which there are a few blood capillaries.

The vestibular membrane is a thin sheet of connective tissue covered on its upper, vestibular surface by the mesenchymal, squamous lining of perilymph spaces. The lower, cochlear duct surface is covered by flat epithelium.

Cochlear Duct. The epithelium lining the cochlear duct varies with location. That over the vestibular membrane is squamous and may contain pigment. Over the limbus it is higher and irregular. Laterally, the epithelium is low columnar and is underlain by connective tissue containing many capillaries. This region

is termed the *stria vascularis,* which is considered to be the site of secretion of endolymph. The epithelium over the basilar membrane is highly specialized as the organ of Corti.

Organ of Corti. As in other sensory areas in the inner ear, the organ of Corti comprises supporting and hair cells.

The *supporting cells* all are tall, columnar cells, but various groups are described. Within the organ of Corti is a tunnel extending the length of the cochlea, triangular in cross section and bounded basally by the basilar membrane and medially and laterally by the inner and outer pillar cells. The *inner pillar* cell is of a narrow cone shape with a broad base containing the nucleus lying against the basilar membrane and a narrow column expanding slightly at the apex. The apex overlies the outer pillar cell. The outer pillar cell is longer than the inner but of similar shape, with an expanded apex fitting into a depression of the undersurface of the head of an inner pillar cell. The inner pillar cells are more numerous than the outer, roughly in the proportion of three to two.

The inner phalangeal cells and the outer phalangeal cells (of Deiters) lie on the basilar membrane adjacent to the pillar cells. The phalangeal cells are smaller; together with the pillar cells they surround the hair cells. However, there are spaces between the processes of phalangeal cells, although their bases fit tightly together along the basilar membrane. The innermost part of the basilar membrane near the limbus gives attachment to a slender row of border cells, whereas toward the spiral ligament there are elongated, polygonal cells arranged in more than one row and decreasing in height. These are the cells of Hensen and of Claudius respectively.

The *hair cells* of the organ of Corti lie as a single row between the inner pillars on one side and the inner phalangeal and border cells on the other (the inner hair cells) and as three rows

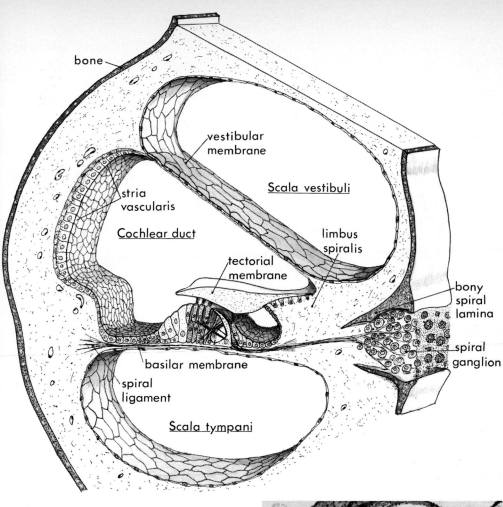

bone

vestibular
membrane

Scala vestibuli

stria
vascularis

Cochlear duct

limbus
spiralis

tectorial
membrane

bony
spiral
lamina

basilar membrane

spiral
ganglion

spiral
ligament

Scala tympani

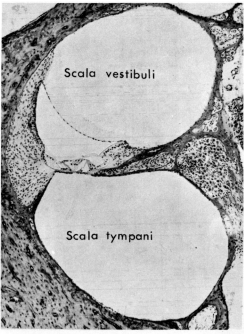

Scala vestibuli

Scala tympani

Figure 20-31. Top; Three-dimensional diagram of the organ of Corti. Lower left: Photomicrograph of the organ of Corti. × 40.

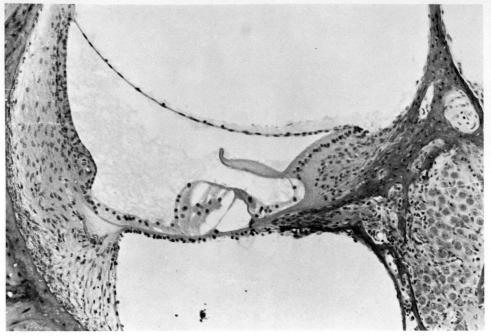

Figure 20-32.   Photomicrograph of the organ of Corti. Compare with Figure 20-33. × 125.

See filmstrip II, frame 100.

between the outer pillars and the outer phalangeal cells (the outer hair cells). They are cylindrical cells with basal nuclei and apical hairlike processes.

The surface of the organ of Corti is covered by a ribbon of gelatinous material termed the *tectorial membrane.* This membrane, composed of homogeneous ground substance containing fibrillar material, in the living

or fresh specimen rests upon the hairs of the hair cells.

Spiral Ganglion.   This is composed of bipolar neurons, the central processes (axons) being myelinated and running together to form the acoustic nerve. The peripheral myelinated processes (dendrites) run through canals in the bone surrounding the ganglion, lose their myelin sheaths, and terminate by entering the organ of

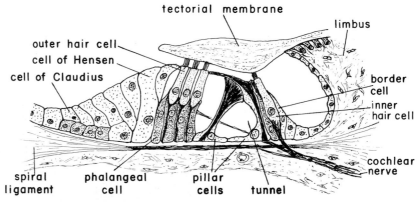

Figure 20-33.   Diagram of the cellular types in the organ of Corti.

Corti to lie between hair cells. The mode of stimulation remains uncertain. Sound waves are conducted from the perilymph of the scala vestibuli to the endolymph of the cochlear duct and in some manner affect the hair cells.

The eighth (acoustic) cranial nerve in addition to its cochlear division has a vestibular division for the sensory supply of the remainder of the labyrinth. Its ganglion is located in the internal auditory meatus of the temporal bone, and its axons run with those of the spiral ganglion. The peripheral dendrites pass to the three ampullae of the semicircular canals and to the maculae of the utricle and saccule. Additionally, some fibers join with those of the cochlear nerve. The function of these fibers is not understood.

REFERENCES

Bast, T. H., and Anson, B. J.: The Temporal Bone and the Ear. Springfield, Ill., Charles C Thomas, 1949.

Cohen, Adolph I.: New evidence supporting the linkage to extracellular space of outer segment saccules of frog cones but not rods. J. Cell Biol., 37:424, 1968.

Duke-Elder, S., and Wybar, K. C.: System of Ophthalmology. The Anatomy of the Visual System, Vol. 2. London, Henry Kempton, 1961.

Duvall, A. J., 3rd, Flock, A., and Wersall, J.: The ultrastructure of the sensory hairs and associated organelles of the cochlear inner hair cell, with reference to directional sensitivity. J. Cell Biol., 29:497, 1966.

Fine, B. S., and Zimmerman, L. E.: Observations on the rod and cone layer of the human retina. Invest. Ophthal. 2:446, 1963.

Garron, L. K., and Feeney, M. L.: Electron microscopic studies of the human eye. Arch. Ophthal., 62:966, 1959.

Granit, R.: Receptors and Sensory Perception: A Discussion of Aims, Means, and Results of Electrophysiological Research into the Process of Reception. New Haven, Yale University Press, 1955.

Iurato, S.: Submicroscopic Structure of the Inner Ear. Oxford, Pergamon Press Ltd., 1967.

Jakus, M. A.: Studies on the cornea. II. The fine structure of Descemet's membrane. J. Biophys. Biochem. Cytol., 2:243, 1956.

Jakus, M. A.: Ocular Fine Structure. London, J. & A. Churchill Ltd., 1964.

Last, R. J.: Wolff's Anatomy of the Eye and Orbit, 6th edition. Philadelphia, W. B. Saunders Co., 1968.

Leeson, T. S.: Tarsal (meibomian) glands of the rat. Brit. J. Ophthal., 47:222, 1963.

Leeson, T. S.: The outer layer of the optic cup and associated tissue. Canad. J. Ophthal. 3:77, 1968.

Leeson, T. S., and Leeson, C. R.: Choriocapillaris and lamina elastica (vitrea) of the rat eye. Brit. J. Ophthal., 51:599, 1967.

Leeson, T. S., and Speakman, J. S.: The fine structure of extracellular material in the pectinate ligament (trabecular meshwork) of the human iris. Acta. Anat., 46:363, 1961.

Raviola, G., and Raviola, E.: Light and electron microscopic observations on the inner plexiform layer of the rabbit retina. Amer. J. Anat., 120:403, 1967.

Robertson, J. D.: The existence of continuity between the membranes of rod outer segment lamellae. Anat. Rec., 151:405, 1965.

Rohen, J. W. (editor): The Structure of the Eye. II. Symposium. Stuttgart, F. K. Schattaner-Verlag, 1965.

Sjöstrand, F. S.: The ultrastructure of the outer segments of rods and cones of the eye as revealed by the electron microscope. J. Cell Comp. Physiol., 42:15, 1953.

Sjöstrand, F. S.: The ultrastructure of the inner segments of the retinal rods of the guinea pig eye as revealed by electron microscopy. J. Cell Comp. Physiol., 42:45, 1953.

Smelzer, G. K. (editor): The Structure of the Eye (A Symposium). New York, Academic Press, 1961.

Vosteen, K. H.: Neue Aspekte zur Biologie und Pathologie des Innenohres. Arch. Ohr. Nas. Kehlkopfheilk., 178:1, 1961.

Wislocki, G. B., and Ladman, A. J.: Selective and histochemical staining of the otolithic membranes, cupulae and tectorial membrane of the inner ear. J. Anat., 89:3, 1955.

INDEX

Page numbers in *italics* refer to illustrations;
numbers in **boldface** refer to supplementary filmstrip frame
numbers.

Chapter 11

CIRCULATORY SYSTEM

Frame 42. Arteriole, venule, and lymphatic capillary in loose areolar tissue, Epon section. Toluidine blue, safranin. *Fig. 11-7*

Frame 43. Medium-sized artery. Resorcin fuchsin. *Fig. 11-11*

Frame 44. Medium-sized artery, Epon section. PAS, toluidine blue. *Fig. 11-11*

Frame 45. Aorta (elastic artery). Resorcin fuchsin. *Fig. 11-12*

Frame 46. Medium-sized vein. Weigert's stain. *Fig. 11-13*

Chapter 12

LYMPHOID ORGANS

Frame 47. Lymph node. H and E. *Fig. 12-3*

Frame 48. Lymph node. Silver stain. *Fig. 12-3*

Frame 49. Lymph node, medulla. H and E. *Fig. 12-5*

Frame 50. Thymus. H and E. *Fig. 12-11*

FILMSTRIP II

Chapter 13

THE SKIN AND ITS APPENDAGES

Frame 51. Thick skin. H and E. *Fig. 13-2*

Frame 52. Thin skin, Epon section. Toluidine blue, safranin. *Fig. 13-3*

Frame 53. Thick skin, intercellular bridges. Masson trichrome. *Fig. 13-4*

Frame 54. Hair, longitudinal section. Iron hematoxylin, aniline blue. *Fig. 13-7*

Frame 55. Hair, cross section. H and E. *Fig. 1*

Frame 56. Sweat gland. Iron hematoxylin, anil blue. *Fig. 13-11*

Chapter 14

THE DIGESTIVE TRACT

Frame 57. Circumvallate papilla. H and *Fig. 14-4*

Frame 58. Tongue, taste buds. H and E. *Fig. 1*

Frame 59. Submandibular salivary gland. Mas trichrome. *Fig. 14-19*

Frame 60. Esophagogastric junction. H and *Fig. 14-23*

Frame 61. Stomach, base of fundic glands. L aldehyde fuchsin; right, Epon section, toluid blue and safranin. *Fig. 14-26*

Frame 62. Stomach, fundic glands, Epon secti Toluidine blue, safranin. *Fig. 14-26*

Frame 63. Duodenum. PAS. *Fig. 14-28*

Frame 64. Jejunum. Iron hematoxylin. *Fig. 14*

Frame 65. Ileum, Epon section. Toluidine bl safranin. *Fig. 14-35*

Frame 66. Pancreas, Epon section. Toluid blue. *Fig. 14-39*

Frame 67. Liver, Epon section. PAS, toluid blue. *Fig. 14-51*

Chapter 15

RESPIRATORY SYSTEM

Frame 68. Nasal concha: olfactory and respirat epithelia. H and E. *Fig. 15-3*

Frame 69. Olfactory epithelium. H and *Fig. 15-6*

Frame 70. Trachea, respiratory epithelium, E<sub>section. Toluidine blue, safranin. *Fig. 15-10*